Textbook of
Human Reproductive Genetics

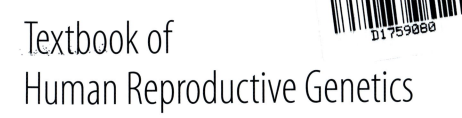

Textbook of Human Reproductive Genetics

Edited by

Karen Sermon

Professor, Research Group Reproduction and Genetics, Vrije Universiteit Brussel, Brussels, Belgium

Stéphane Viville

Professor, Institut de Génétique et de Biologie Moléculaire et Cellulaire (IGBMC), Institut National de Santé et de Recherche Médicale (INSERM)
U964/Centre National de Recherche Scientifique (CNRS) UMR 1704/Université de Strasbourg, Illkirch, and Centre Hospitalier Universitaire; Strasbourg, France

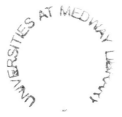

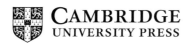

CAMBRIDGE
UNIVERSITY PRESS

CAMBRIDGE
UNIVERSITY PRESS

University Printing House, Cambridge CB2 8BS, United Kingdom

Published in the United States of America by Cambridge University Press, New York

Cambridge University Press is part of the University of Cambridge.

It furthers the University's mission by disseminating knowledge in the pursuit of education, learning and research at the highest international levels of excellence.

www.cambridge.org
Information on this title: www.cambridge.org/9781107683587

© Cambridge University Press 2014

First published 2014

Printed in the United Kingdom by TJ International Ltd. Padstow Cornwall

A catalogue record for this publication is available from the British Library

Library of Congress Cataloguing in Publication data
Textbook of human reproductive genetics / edited by Karen Sermon, Stéphane Viville.
   p.   ;   cm.
Includes bibliographical references and index.
ISBN 978-1-107-68358-7 (pbk.)
I. Sermon, Karen, 1964–, editor of compilation.
II. Viville, Stéphane, editor of compilation.
[DNLM: 1. Reproduction – genetics.   2. Embryonic Development.
3. Genetic Services.   WQ 205]
QM28
573.6 – dc23   2013048908

ISBN 978-1-107-68358-7 Paperback

Contents

Contributors

Esther B. Baart
Division of Reproductive Medicine, Department of Obstetrics and Gynecology, Erasmus MC, University Medical Center, Rotterdam, the Netherlands

Alison Bagshawe
Altrui Ltd, North Yorkshire, UK

Ashwini Balakrishnan
Magee-Womens Research Institute, Department of Microbiology and Molecular Genetics, University of Pittsburgh School of Medicine, Pittsburgh, PA, USA

Déborah Bourc'his
Institut Curie, Centre National de Recherche Scientifique (CNRS) UMR 3215/Institut National de Santé et de Recherche Médicale (INSERM) U934, Paris, France

J. Richard Chaillet
Magee-Womens Research Institute, Department of Microbiology and Molecular Genetics, University of Pittsburgh School of Medicine, Pittsburgh, PA, USA

Wybo Dondorp
Department of Health, Ethics, and Society, Research School GROW, Maastricht University, Maastricht, the Netherlands

Ursula Eichenlaub-Ritter
University of Bielefeld, Faculty of Biology, Institute of Gene Technology/Microbiology, Bielefeld, Germany

Elias El Inati
Institut de Génétique et de Biologie Moléculaire et Cellulaire (IGBMC), Institut National de Santé et de Recherche Médicale (INSERM) U964/Centre National de Recherche Scientifique (CNRS) UMR 1704/Université de Strasbourg, Illkirch, France

Masoud Zamani Esteki
Laboratory of Reproductive Genomics, Department of Human Genetics, KU Leuven, Leuven, Belgium

Patricia Fauque
Hôpital de Dijon, Université de Bourgogne, Laboratoire de Biologie de la Reproduction, Dijon, France

Parveen Kumar
Laboratory of Reproductive Genomics, Department of Human Genetics, KU Leuven, Leuven, Belgium

Alison Lashwood
Clinical Genetics, Guy's Hospital, London, UK

Inge Liebaers
Center for Medical Genetics, UZ Brussel, Brussels, Belgium

Willy Lissens
Center for Medical Genetics, UZ Brussel, Brussels, Belgium

Aafke P. A. van Montfoort
Department of Reproductive Medicine, Maastricht University Medical Center, Maastricht, the Netherlands

Aleksandar Rajkovic
Department of Obstetrics, Gynecology, and Reproductive Science, University of Pittsburgh, Pittsburgh, PA, USA

Karen Sermon
Research Group Reproduction and Genetics, Vrije Universiteit Brussel, Brussels, Belgium

Catherine Staessen
Center for Medical Genetics, UZ Brussel, Brussels, Belgium

Jan Traeger-Synodinos
Laboratory of Medical Genetics, National, and Kapodistrian University of Athens, Athens, Greece

Niels Van der Aa
Laboratory of Reproductive Genomics, Department of Human Genetics, KU Leuven, Leuven, Belgium

Diane Van Opstal
Department of Clinical Genetics, Erasmus MC, University Medical Center, Rotterdam, the Netherlands

Willem Verpoest
Center for Reproductive Medicine, UZ Brussel, Brussels, Belgium

Stéphane Viville
Institut de Génétique et de Biologie Moléculaire et Cellulaire (IGBMC), Institut National de Santé et de Recherche Médicale (INSERM) U964/Centre National de Recherche Scientifique (CNRS) UMR 1704/Université de Strasbourg, Illkirch, and Centre Hospitalier Universitaire; Strasbourg, France

Thierry Voet
Laboratory of Reproductive Genomics, Department of Human Genetics, KU Leuven, Leuven, Belgium

Guido de Wert
Department of Health, Ethics, and Society, Research School GROW, Maastricht University, Maastricht, the Netherlands

Svetlana A. Yatsenko
Department of Obstetrics, Gynecology, and Reproductive Science, University of Pittsburgh, Pittsburgh, PA, USA

Preface

Genetic advances in the reproductive sciences are arguably occurring with greater rapidity than those in any other organ system. Not only have the dazzling technological advances of molecular genetics become applicable in reproduction, but meteoric advances are occurring in diagnosis and treatment. Assisted reproductive technology (ART) has rendered infertility far less daunting. Yet treating those couples, that once would not have conceived, may generate offspring who differ from the general population.

Textbook of Human Reproductive Genetics addresses pivotal topics of clinical and scientific interest. There is much for the student, practicing physician, and laboratory scientist alike. Crisply edited by renowned geneticists of international repute – Stéphane Viville and Karen Sermon – the book begins with a précis of genetic principles – molecular, single gene, and cytogenetic. The novice quickly gets up to speed.

The basic science landscape targets fields of most immediate relevance to reproduction. Techniques suitable for analyzing a single cell are explained, one cell's (6 picograms) DNA obviously necessitates different approaches than if larger amounts of DNA were available. Thus, Kumar *et al.* explain where we are now and where we will soon be (microarrays and next generation sequencing). Cell division and the consequences of its perturbation are framed, respectively, by Eichenlaub-Ritter in her chapter on meiosis and by Baart and Van Opstal in their chapter on the role of aneuploidy in human embryonic development. Yatsenko and Rajkovic extend the dialogue to cytogenetic disorders affecting infertility. Monogenic causes are not neglected, Liebaers and colleagues covering infertility in pleiotropic presentation. This is especially relevant because it has become clear that common conditions like premature ovarian failure or polycystic ovarian syndrome are heterogeneous. Thus, looking at rare genes whose perturbations cause syndromes could be a fruitful strategy in identifying more common disorders like premature ovarian failure.

Van Monfoort covers epigenetic phenomena as related specifically to ART. The basic science component of this text also lets us know that genes must be *expressed*, without which it matters little whether they are present or absent. To this end, Balakrishnan and Chaillet discuss transgenerational effects mediated by epigenetic alteration. Fauque and Bourc'his shed light on transposons as newly appreciated determinants of male reproductive fitness.

The scientific framework having been established, specific clinical aspects of human reproduction are then systematically addressed. Traeger-Synodinos and Staessen cover clinical preimplantation genetic diagnosis. Individualized ART tests are discussed by Verpoest. Lashwood and Bagshawe review genetic counseling, providing not only traditional "how to" checklists but also discussing the emotional impact experienced by client families. Defense mechanisms like denial and anger impede patients from gaining requisite knowledge, and must be overcome. Dondorp and de Wert extend this theme by their treatise on ethical considerations.

Our authors have thus provided us with a text broad in coverage. Contributions by an international spectrum of authors – European and American – assure us provincial views are eschewed. Here we have a text that students, practitioners, and scientists involved in reproduction genetics should have on their shelves, or readily accessible in their computer.

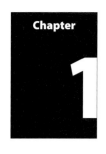

Chapter

1

Basic genetics and cytogenetics: a brief reminder

Karen Sermon

Introduction

This brief reminder chapter aims to freshen up what professionals in reproduction may have learned a while ago at university, and will also serve the reader as a source of information to comprehend the following, more complex chapters. At the end of this chapter, basic study books recommended for further reading are given to help the reader in the further understanding of this textbook [1, 2].

Human reproduction and genetics are intimately intertwined and indeed often confused and rolled into one. Understanding reproduction is impossible without a firm basis in genetics, and the readiness to acquire more knowledge when needed. However, human genetics is much broader than just reproduction – think of for instance oncogenetics – so in this chapter I will summarize what basic genetics is indispensable for the specialists in reproduction.

In this chapter, I will introduce the general organization of our genome, how this genome behaves when it goes through a reproductive cycle (meiosis), how our genome is used as a template for making proteins, and how this is broadly regulated, major genetic and hereditary abnormalities both at the chromosome and at the monogenic level, and a brief overview of current genetic diagnostic techniques.

The organization of the human genome

The basic building material: DNA

Deoxyribonucleic acid (DNA) consists of four different nucleotides [1, 2]. Each nucleotide consists of sugar, which is deoxyribose in DNA, a phosphate group, and a base. Four different bases are present in

the nucleotides of DNA: adenine (A), cytosine (C), guanine (G), and thymine (T) (Fig. 1.1A [3]). These four nucleotides are strung together in long strands of DNA, alternating a sugar (with a base attached) and a phosphate group, and where the order of the different bases defines the genetic code (Fig. 1.1B). The phosphate group can be either bound to the 5′ carbon of the sugar, or to the 3′ carbon of the sugar, while the base is bound to the 1′ carbon. When strung together, the first sugar in the DNA strand has a free 5′ carbon, while its 3′ carbon is covalently bound to a phosphate group. This phosphate group is bound further down the strand to the 5′ of the next sugar. This is why in a DNA strand the 5′ carbon of the first sugar is free and at the end of the strand the 3′ carbon of the last sugar is free. This is why DNA base pairs are always read from 5′ to 3′.

Moreover, cellular DNA is usually found in a double helix form. The bases A and T on one hand and C and G on the other hand are complementary to each other and will pair up by forming hydrogen bonds, thus stabilizing the double helix (Fig. 1.1C). According to the Ensembl database [4], our nuclear DNA contains 3 287 209 763 base pairs (bp). An estimated half of the human genome consists of transposons, also known as mobile DNA elements or "jumping genes," and will be extensively discussed in Chapter 6.

DNA is organized in chromosomes

The DNA of our whole genome is not ordered in one long strand, nor does it lie naked and unprotected in the nuclei of our cells. Nuclear DNA is organized in 46 separate strands, so each chromosome contains one long DNA strand. Twenty-two of these chromosomes are paired, one inherited from the mother and one from the father. These are called the autosomes.

Textbook of Human Reproductive Genetics, eds Karen Sermon and Stéphane Viville. Published by Cambridge University Press. © Cambridge University Press 2014.

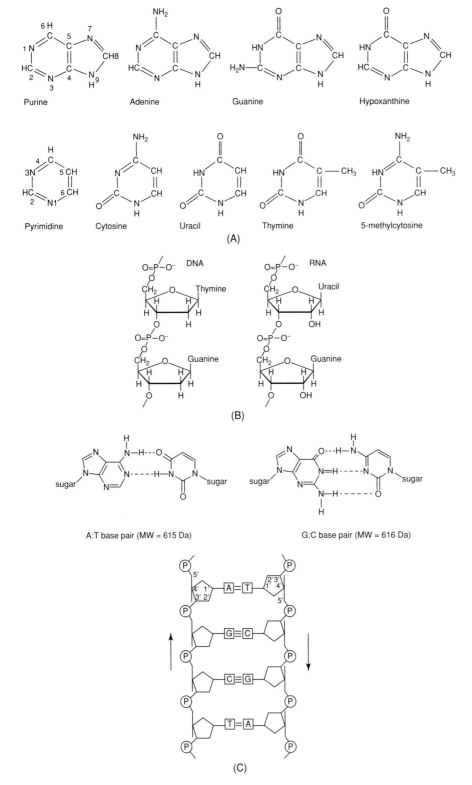

Figure 1.1 (**A**) The four bases in DNA and RNA. (**B**) Sugar–phosphate backbone of nucleotides. DNA has 2′-deoxyribose as sugar, RNA has ribose as sugar. (**C**) A and T form two hydrogen bonds while G and C form three hydrogen bonds. Together with the sugar–phosphate backbone this forms the double helix of DNA. Source: Figs 2.4 and 2.7– 2.9 from Ringo [3].

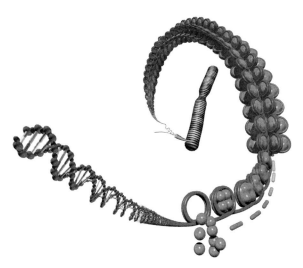

Figure 1.2 DNA is organized in chromatin. See plate section for color version. © Science Photo Library.

The two remaining chromosomes are the sex chromosomes: females have two X chromosomes, while males have one X and one smaller Y chromosome.

When the cell is not dividing, the DNA is organized in chromatin. The double helix is wound around protein structures called histone octamers, which in their turn are further coiled into structures called solenoids. These solenoids are attached to a protein scaffold within the nucleus to form loops (Fig. 1.2). The way the chromatin is organized in a specific cell, and the way for instance some histones are chemically modified, defines which genes can or cannot be transcribed and expressed. For instance, some genes will be so tightly packed in the chromatin that the transcription machinery cannot reach them and thus these genes are silenced in this particular cell. The chromatin structure is thus one of the determinants of the cell's expression pattern and therefore its function.

A particular type of DNA can be found in mitochondria. Mitochondria are cell organelles that are essential for the respiration and energy production of the cell. They carry their own circular DNA of about 16 000 bp which replicates independently of the DNA in the nucleus. The genes on the mitochondrial DNA encode for their own ribosomal RNA (rRNA), transfer RNA (tRNA), and ribosomal proteins, as well as a handful of aerobic metabolism enzymes. Many mitochondrial proteins are however encoded by the nuclear DNA and are later imported into the mitochondrion to contribute to the mitochondrial function.

The functional genetic entity: the gene

A gene can be defined as "a sequence of DNA in the genome that is required for the production of a functional product which can be a polypeptide or a functional RNA molecule" [2]. The number of genes in our genome is estimated to be around 25 000 ([4]). These are not equally scattered along the chromosomes: some parts of chromosomes are very gene-rich while other stretches of more than a million base pairs contain no genes at all and are called gene deserts. Some genes are quite small and count only a few kilobase pairs, while others span a million or more base pairs. One such large gene is the dystrophin gene spanning more than two million base pairs. The two gene copies on the autosomes are usually both transcribed (or both silenced), except for a number of developmentally important genes where only one copy is transcribed. In these so-called imprinted genes, either the paternal or the maternal copy is exclusively expressed. Some of these genes have been implicated in congenital defects occurring more frequently after assisted reproductive technology (ART): this topic is discussed in Chapter 13.

Genes that typically code for a polypeptide have recurring structural features (Fig. 1.3 [3]). Not all base pairs in a gene will be translated into a protein: genes typically contain exons that are the translated

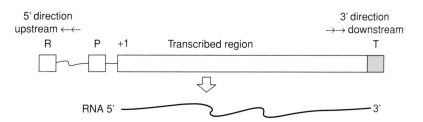

Figure 1.3 Anatomy of a gene: R is a regulatory sequence, P is the promoter sequence, and T is the terminator sequence. Source: Fig. 7.4 from Ringo [3].

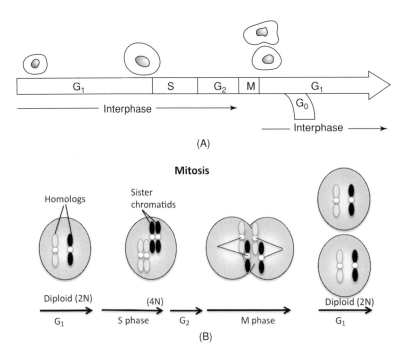

Figure 1.4 (**A**) The cell cycle of a somatic cell and (**B**) the different steps in mitosis. Source: Figure 19.1 from Ringo [3] and Chapter 3.

parts interspersed with introns that are not translated. In many genes, the introns represent a significantly larger proportion of the gene than the exons. Other recurring structural features are sequences conserved among many different genes that give the transcription machinery of the cell appropriate signals of when and where to transcribe specific genes. Every gene has a start and a stop signal, as well as a promoter sequence in the 5′ end. This promoter specifies the pattern as well as the level of expression of a gene. Other regulatory elements include enhancers, silencers, and locus control regions and can be either in the 5′ or 3′ untranslated region, or in intronic sequences of the gene. Some can even lie far away from the coding sequence of a gene.

Alleles are alternative forms of the same gene: changes in the DNA sequence will lead to a different protein with different function. A well-known example of multiple alleles is the ABO blood group system.

Making more copies: the cell cycle

Different parts of the cell cycle

In order to get from the fertilized zygote to the estimated 100 trillion cells in the human body, cells need to undergo continuous divisions. Cell division and mitosis are also crucial for differentiation.

When a cell is not in mitosis, it is said to be in interphase (Fig. 1.4A,B [3]). The first part of the interphase, immediately after mitosis, is called the G_1 phase. In this phase, the chromosomes each contain only one copy of the DNA strand. This G_1 phase typically lasts for several hours until the S phase is reached, although some terminally differentiated cells (neurons or white blood cells) may withdraw from the cell cycle altogether and are said to be in G_0.

When the cell starts to replicate its DNA, it is said to enter the S phase. The two DNA strands are separated, and a complementary strand is made of each strand. The chromosomes at the end of the S phase consist of two sister chromatids, each containing an identical DNA strand. The chromatids are held together at the centromere that, associated with specialized proteins, forms the kinetochore by which the chromatids will be attached to the mitotic spindle. Before the cell enters mitosis, it goes through a brief control G_2 phase in which the cell visibly grows after the accumulation of synthesized proteins during the whole cell cycle. The whole interphase of a typical cell lasts between 16 and 24 hours but may extend to months, whereas mitosis is completed in a couple of hours.

Passing on the information: mitosis

At the end of G_2, every chromosome consists of two chromatids and one of each of these chromatids needs to end up in one of the daughter cells in orderly chromosome segregation. The first step in mitosis is the prophase, in which chromosomes start to condense and a mitotic spindle starts to form (see Figs 1.4B, and 3.1A in Chapter 3). The formation of the mitotic spindle is organized through two centrosomes from which microtubules will radiate to form the spindle. During prometaphase, the nuclear membrane breaks up and the chromosomes are attached to the mitotic spindle by their kinetochore. Led by the microtubules of the spindle, the chromosomes move to the metaphase plate in a process called congression. During the metaphase, the chromosomes have reached their maximal condensation at the equatorial plane and are easiest to visualize. The anaphase starts when the chromosomes separate into two chromatids and each chromosome moves to the different poles. The mitosis is ended by the telophase during which the chromosomes decondense and the nuclear membrane is built up again, this process is called karyokinesis. Concomitantly to telophase, the cytoplasm is divided over the two daughter cells and karyokinesis is completed.

Making more humans: meiosis

During the process of mitosis, two daughter cells are produced that carry exactly the same genetic information both in content as in volume. Mitosis could thus not be used to form gametes, since with every generation the amount of DNA would double. Meiosis as a specialized form of cell division solves this problem by resulting in cells (gametes) with only half of the DNA content, i.e. one of each chromosome, of the somatic cells. An added bonus is that during meiosis, the DNA from the two parental chromosomes is exchanged to form new chromosomes built with genetic material from the two parents. This process of recombination is important to generate genetic diversity in a species and thus to secure its evolution. Meiosis is the most important step for the survival and evolution of sexually reproducing species.

The different steps in male and female meiosis are discussed in depth in Chapter 3.

From DNA to protein: the transcription and translation machinery

RNA comes in many forms and functions

If DNA is important as the keeper of genetic information, the role of RNA is at least as important – some say more important – because of the versatility in form and function of RNA. In three aspects RNA differs from DNA: (1) the sugar moiety is different and is ribose instead of deoxyribose; (2) the thymine base is replaced by a uracil base; and (3) RNA can be found in many different three-dimensional structures, usually as a single strand [1, 2].

RNA is transcribed from the DNA template by RNA polymerases that first unwind the DNA and then synthesize an RNA strand that forms a temporary double helix with the DNA. The RNA is synthesized on the $3'$–$5'$ DNA strand in the $5'$-$3'$ direction. This $3'$–$5'$ template DNA strand is often called the antisense strand because it is in the opposite sense from the RNA, while the $5'$-$3'$ DNA strand, which does not serve as a template, has the same nucleotide sequence as the synthesized RNA strand (except that thymine is replaced by uracil) and is often called the sense strand.

Different examples of RNA forms and functions are messenger RNA (mRNA) that is transcribed from polypeptide-encoding genes, ribosomal RNA (rRNA) that will make up the ribosomes and transfer RNA (tRNA) that will ultimately translate the information in the mRNA sequence to an amino-acid sequence. When RNA is transcribed from the DNA strand, it will need to undergo a lot of processing before it can fulfill its function. Introns will have to be spliced out of the mRNA so that only the exons are translated into protein and a polyA tail will be added to the mRNA to ensure its stability. The rRNA and tRNA also undergo extensive changes before they are functional.

A more recently discovered type of RNA is transcribed from non-coding RNA genes. These RNAs have an important function in the regulation of other genes. Well-known examples of this are the microRNAs that can regulate the amount of mRNA available for translation. Other examples are other small noncoding RNAs such as piwi-protein interacting RNA (piRNA) and short interfering RNA (siRNA) as well as long non-coding RNAs. After the chromatin structure, this is the second example of how gene expression is regulated and explains the increasing importance that scientists are giving to RNA.

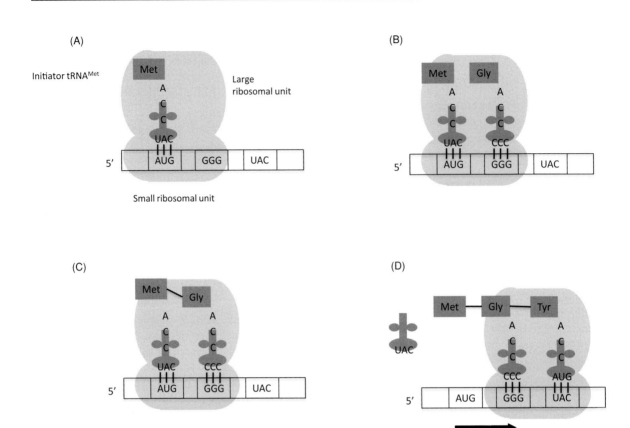

Figure 1.5 Translation of mRNA into protein (A–D). For explanation, see text.

Different RNAs work together to translate DNA into protein

Genetic code

In the DNA sequence of a polypeptide gene, a set of three base pairs constitutes a codon. One codon codes for one amino acid. Looking at all the possible codons using combinations of three of the four base pairs, we get to 4^3 or 64 possibilities. These 64 codons are the genetic code. Because there are only 20 amino acids, one amino acid can be represented by more than one codon. There is only one codon for the amino acid methionine, and this codon also represents the start of the polypeptide. Finally, three codons represent a stop signal that tells the translation machinery that the end of the polypeptide is reached [1, 2].

Translation machinery

Once the mRNA, rRNA, and tRNA have been transformed into their mature and functional forms, they are transported to the cytoplasm of the cell where the translation into proteins takes place. The large ribosomes, built of several rRNA molecules, will start to read the mRNA at the start codon, which is always AUG coding for methionine (Fig. 1.5A–D). Within the ribosome, a tRNA that carries an anticodon that is complementary to the methionine codon on the mRNA will then bind to the methionine codon. The other end of the tRNA carries a methionine amino acid. The ribosome then moves one codon along the mRNA to the next codon. In Figure 1.5, this codon is GGG coding for glycine. A tRNA that has CCC as anticodon binds to the mRNA codon and carries a glycine amino acid. This glycine amino acid is then bound to the first methionine amino acid, and the two first amino acids of the polypeptide are formed. The whole mRNA is read in this fashion until the ribosome reaches one of the three stop codons. The synthesis of the polypeptide is then terminated, and the polypeptide is released from the ribosome to be further processed into a functional protein by other cytoplasmic organelles such as the endoplasmic reticulum before reaching its cellular localization.

Behold the genome: tools in human genetics

We will discuss here only a handful of tools as they appear in the next chapters. This should help the reader to understand the contents, but is by no means a complete story. We refer the interested reader to the study books in the reference list for additional information [1, 2].

The big view: cytogenetics

Know your classics: G-banding and karyotypes

Cytogenetics is the study of chromosomes, their structure, and their inheritance. At the end of the 1950s, the exact number of chromosomes was known and, at the first Conference on Standardization in Human Cytogenetics in Denver, the chromosomes were classified according to their size: the largest chromosome is chromosome 1, the smallest is chromosome 22, and, in addition, chromosome X and chromosome Y were also included. Later on, banding techniques became available and the current classification was established in Paris in 1971 (Fig. 1.6) [5]. The complete picture with every chromosome of an individual arranged from the largest to the smallest is called a karyotype.

Most commonly, chromosomes are visualized from lymphocytes from peripheral blood. These are put in culture and forced to divide and then arrested when they go into metaphase. Once in metaphase, the microtubules in the spindle are stopped, the cells lysed and spread on a glass slide. The spread metaphases can be dyed with Giemsa staining, which is the classical G-banding found on most karyotype protocols. According to the position of the centromere, three types of chromosomes can be distinguished: metacentric chromosomes, with a centromere approximately in the middle, submetacentric chromosomes with two arms of clearly unequal length, and acrocentric chromosomes with centromeres at or near an end. Each chromosome has a long arm, called the q-arm and a short arm called the p-arm. The banding patterns visible after G-banding characterize each individual chromosome, and allow cytogeneticists to classify and number the chromosomes and to identify possible rearrangements (Fig. 1.6).

Fluorescence *in situ* hybridization: count the dots

Although fluorescence in situ hybridization (FISH) was the first step from classic cytogenetics to molecular cytogenetics, the method gives only limited information in contrast to currently developed molecular cytogenetics methods. Fluorescence *in situ* hybridization is a relatively quick and easy method that allows fast screening of, for example, prenatal samples for the most common aneuploidies such as trisomy 13, 18, and 21. The sampled cells are spread on a glass slide, fixed, and the DNA is denatured so that the single-stranded DNA is accessible for fluorescently labeled DNA probes. These probes are chosen so that they are complementary to the DNA region of interest, are allowed to form double-stranded DNA with the DNA in the sample ("to hybridize"), after which the place in the nucleus where the probe has bound can be seen as a fluorescent spot. The FISH probes are carefully chosen to serve a particular purpose. For a quick chromosome count such as for aneuploidy detection in prenatal samples, centromere probes are usually chosen, because they give large, easy-to-read signals. For the detection of more specific chromosome regions, such as in translocations involving small fragments or microdeletion syndromes such as DiGeorge syndrome, more care has to be taken in the design of the FISH probes. If the probes are mixtures covering a whole chromosome, they are called chromosome paints and are very useful for visualizing a chromosomal translocation.

More on FISH and its application in preimplantation genetic diagnosis and screening can be found in Chapters 4 and 11.

The detailed view: DNA and RNA analysis

Polymerase chain reaction

Before the advent of polymerase chain reaction (PCR), the only way to amplify a DNA fragment of interest was to clone it into a vector (say a plasmid), introduce the vector in a host (say an *Escherichia coli* bacteria), culture the bacteria, and then isolate the expanded plasmid with the DNA of interest. This was very time consuming, necessitating a large amount of DNA starting material and special equipment for bacteria culture. Polymerase chain reaction very quickly took its place in many applications in molecular biology: PCR products are used as templates for restriction enzymes or sequencing reactions; probes used

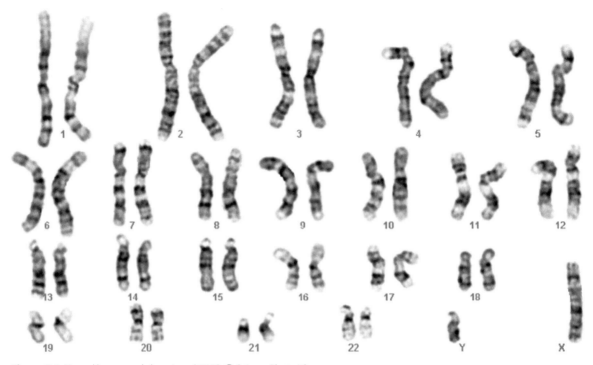

Figure 1.6 Normal human male karyotype (46,XY). © Science Photo Library.

in other applications (FISH, hybridizations of all kinds) are synthesized using PCR; even making transgenic animals has become much simpler thanks to PCR.

Polymerase chain reaction is in essence a DNA copier machine (Fig 1.7 [3]). In a first step, the native DNA strands are denatured, i.e. the two strands are separated by heating them up, typically to 95°C. In the second step, at a lower temperature, two single-strand short DNA fragments bind to the complementary DNA. These short DNA fragments are called the primers, and are chosen so that they delineate a fragment of the genomic DNA that has to be amplified; for instance, because a disease-causing mutation resides in that fragment. The primers then serve as an anchor for the polymerase, which synthesizes the complementary DNA strand resulting in double-stranded DNA at a higher temperature, typically 72°C, during the third part of the reaction. Ordinary DNA polymerases are not heat resistant and will thus be destroyed at each PCR cycle. Therefore, the discovery of thermophilic DNA polymerases was a major breakthrough in PCR technology. Taq DNA polymerase was the first and most widely used thermophilic DNA polymerase and was first described in *Thermus aquaticus*, a

thermophilic bacterium isolated from the hot springs of Yellowstone National Park in the USA.

Like any ordinary chemical reaction, PCR reactions have typical kinetics. First, during the exponential phase, the number of PCR fragments generated increases in an exponential fashion. At a certain point, the reaction components are depleted and PCR reaches a plateau phase, meaning that the number of PCR molecules does not increase anymore. When PCR fragments are analyzed on agarose gels, or other means of fragment analyses, the reaction usually had reached this plateau phase.

Sequencing

The still most widely used chemistry for DNA sequencing is called Sanger sequencing. The chemical principle has remained the same, whether using radioactively labeled nucleotides for detection or the currently widely used fluorescence sequencing. The starting material is nowadays usually a PCR product, but before the advent of PCR, DNA fragments cloned into vectors and flanked by known primers were used. The principle is shown in Fig. 1.8: the DNA of interest is denatured and primers are allowed to bind to the complementary sequences. Then, a polymerase

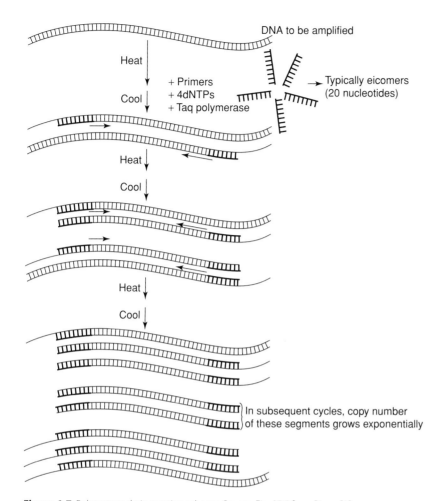

DNA to be amplified

Heat

Cool + Primers
+ 4dNTPs
+ Taq polymerase

Typically eicomers
(20 nucleotides)

Heat

Cool

Heat

Cool

In subsequent cycles, copy number
of these segments grows exponentially

Figure 1.7 Polymerase chain reaction scheme. Source: Fig. 27.7 from Ringo [3].

reaction is initiated. In the reaction mix, four nucleotides with a different chemistry are added next to the usual deoxynucleotides: the dideoxynucleotides. There are four dideoxynucleotides: dideoxy A, dideoxy C, dideoxy G, and dideoxy T. Each dideoxynucleotide is labeled with a different fluorescent dye, represented as shades of gray in Fig. 1.8. In the example, dideoxy G is labeled black, dideoxy T is labeled white, dideoxy A is light gray and dideoxy C is labeled dark gray.

When the polymerase synthesizes the complementary strand, each time a normal nucleotide is incorporated, the synthesis continues. If a dideoxy is incorporated, the synthesis is stopped. This reaction creates a mixture of fragments of different lengths, each differing only one nucleotide in size. The last nucleotide of the fragment is always a fluorescent dideoxynucleotide, and is complementary to the last nucleotide

in the analyzed fragment. By separating the different fragments according to their length, and analyzing which fluorescence they emit, the sequence can be read.

Quantitative-real time-reverse transcription PCR

To know if a specific gene is transcribed in a particular cell type, and to what level, quantitative-real time PCR is often used. After RNA extraction from the cells, the mRNA is reverse transcribed into complementary DNA (cDNA). This cDNA can then be used as a template for real-time PCR. The difference between regular PCR and real time PCR is that the number of fragments generated is read during the PCR reaction, through the exponential phase and to the plateau phase, and not at the end after the PCR has reached the plateau phase. For this, special PCR machines are

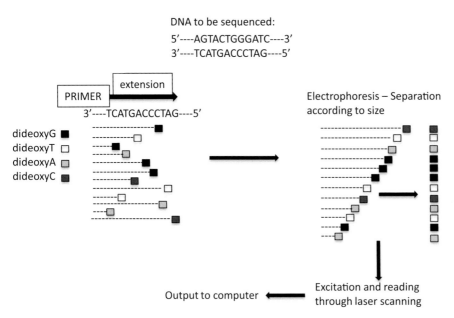

Figure 1.8 Sanger sequencing – dideoxy termination method. For explanation, see the text.

necessary that can read fluorescence incorporated in the PCR fragments after each PCR cycle. The more cDNA of the gene of interest is present in the original sample, the earlier, or the lower number of PCR cycles, the exponential phase of the PCR will start. An often-used measure of the abundance of the cDNA in the original sample is the C_t or threshold cycle. The C_t is defined as the cycle where the number of detected PCR fragments reaches a previously set threshold, usually when the exponential phase has started without doubt. It is a measure of the number of fragments in the original sample. The abundance of the mRNA of interest is usually normalized to the abundance of mRNA from household genes supposed to be expressed in all cells such as HPRT or GAPDH. This allows for the comparison of the expression of a gene of interest between different samples (e.g. *OCT4* in human embryonic stem cells) or for changes that can be measured in time.

The holistic view: modern tools in genetic analysis

Microarrays

Microarrays were developed in the 1990s when the need was first felt to analyze the whole genome or transcriptome of cells. They are always built following the same principles: DNA fragments are spotted upon a suitable support, mostly glass, according to a very precise location, hence the name array. The sample to be analyzed can be DNA or cDNA in solution and fluorescently labeled. After hybridization to the support, the amount of fluorescence for every spot in the array can be read in a high-resolution laser scanner. The abundance of a given DNA fragment or cDNA in a sample will determine the amount of fluorescence. Hence, the amount of fluorescence is a measure for the abundance of the DNA fragment or cDNA.

Originally, DNA fragments from large Bacterial Artificial Chromosome (BAC) libraries were spotted onto the glass slides. The more versatile and amenable oligonucleotide arrays (i.e. very short DNA fragments of only about 20 bp) have now largely taken over, except for very specific applications such as array comparative genomic hybridization (aCGH). Single nucleotide polymorphism (SNP) arrays interrogate SNPs dispersed over the human genome and can be used for haplotyping (i.e. identification of the maternal or paternal origin of the chromosome) and copy number analysis.

Despite the development of higher resolution technologies, aCGH is still a method of choice in prenatal diagnosis because of its robustness and low cost. In reproductive medicine, it is now of course widely used in chromosome analysis in embryos. Chapters 2, 4, and 11 will go more deeply into this topic.

Whole genome sequencing

Sanger sequencing allows for the determination of the sequence of only a short stretch of DNA. In the wake of the Human Genome Project, the need was felt to develop methods to sequence the whole genome of one individual in one go. Several large biotech companies took up the challenge and developed methods based on different chemistries and using different platforms [6]. This new technology was termed "next generation sequencing", a term which a couple of years after its introduction is already obsolete and replaced by "third generation sequencing". As the fourth and fifth generation are certainly already in the pipeline, we will refer to this type of technologies as "whole genome sequencing," or "high throughput sequencing."

Whole genome sequencing includes a number of methods that are grouped broadly as template preparation, sequencing and imaging, and data analysis. According to what methodology each provider applies in each step, different types of data are produced from each platform. Factors to take into consideration when choosing a platform are the depth of the sequencing (i.e. the efficiency with which rare sequences are detected such as is required for RNA sequencing); the length of the sequences (which vary from 26 bp to more than 1000 bp); whether the platform amplifies the DNA fragments first before sequencing; or whether the sequencing is done on single molecules; and, of course, the cost of the platform and of running the samples. For more detail on the chemistry and the possibilities of the different platforms, I refer the reader to Metzker [6] and Schadt et al. [7]. These authors also point out the difficulties in whole genome sequencing, which are mainly a result of the large amount of data produced and the complex bio-informatics necessary to isolate relevant information from these data.

The applications of whole genome sequencing are innumerable. The most prominent application has been in human genetics of rare monogenic diseases. Because these diseases are so rare that only a handful of individuals worldwide are affected – sometimes only one family – these diseases were not amenable to gene identification using classical genetics. Sequencing the whole genome in family trios (parents and one affected child) and comparing the whole sequence obtained using high-brow bio-informatics means that genes have been identified for several rare diseases. As most mutations in human genetic diseases can be found in the exons, targeted sequencing of exons alone, called exome sequencing, has now become the method of choice as it is much more cost-effective than to sequence the whole genome [8]. If exome sequencing does not yield results, whole genome sequencing can be considered.

Whole genome sequencing is currently also becoming the method of choice for transcriptome analyses, very swiftly overtaking microarray analysis. Methylome analysis is another important emerging application.

Causes and effects in human genetic disease

Chromosomal abnormalities

Chromosome abnormalities have traditionally been defined as a change that produces a visible change in the chromosomes. However, as we have seen previously, this greatly depends on the technique used. If classic G-banding is considered, the minimal visible change is about 4 Mb. A more functional definition is any abnormality that arises from specific chromosomal mechanisms, such as incorrect segregation of chromosomes during mitosis or meiosis, or misrepair of broken chromosomes, or improper recombination events. Chromosomal abnormalities can be constitutional, i.e. they are present in every cell of the individual, or the individual can be mosaic, meaning that two or more cell lines are present originating from the same zygote. In postnatal cytogenetics, usually only two cell lines will be analyzed but, as we will see in Chapter 4, preimplantation embryos can carry many different cell lines and are then called chaotic mosaics.

Two categories of abnormalities are distinguished: chromosomal abnormalities with altered copy number, i.e. the numerical abnormalities, or structural abnormalities, where chromosomes show abnormal structure.

Numerical abnormalities

Triploidy and tetraploidy are forms of polyploidy, i.e. all cells in the individual carry respectively three or four haploid genomes. Triploidy is usually caused by the fertilization of the oocyte with two sperms, while tetraploidy is due to an incomplete first division: the DNA is replicated to 4N but the cell does not divide. Both triploidy and tetraploidy are lethal.

11

Aneuploidy means that one or more individual chromosomes are either missing or present with an extra copy. The best known trisomy is Down syndrome, where one extra chromosome 21 is present (47,XY,+21). Monosomies are lethal in the embryonic period except for monosomy of the X chromosome, such as in Turner syndrome (45,X). One mechanism through which aneuploid cells arise is nondisjunction, which can arise during meiosis leading to abnormal gametes, or during mitosis, leading to mosaicism. During meiosis, paired chromosomes fail to separate or sister chromatids fail to disjoin during mitosis. Another mechanism is anaphase lag, in which a chromosome or a chromatid lags behind the other chromosomes during movement in anaphase, and is lost.

The consequences of numerical abnormalities are dire: nullisomies and monosomies (except Turner syndrome) are never viable, while only individuals with trisomies of 13, 18, and 21 may survive to term. Of these, only those with trisomy 21 can reach adult life. Sex chromosomes again form an exception: 47,XXX, 47,XXY, and 47,XYY are all known to cause very few clinical problems and these individuals have normal lifespans.

Chromosomal rearrangements

Chromosome breaks can be caused by DNA damage or faulty recombination during meiosis. Cellular mechanisms will try to repair these breaks by rejoining the ends, or by adding telomeres to the ends. If such repair mechanisms lead to a chromosome with no centromere, i.e. an acentric chromosome, or a dicentric chromosome, these chromosomes will be lost during segregation in the next mitosis.

When two breaks occur in the same chromosome, a fragment can be lost (deletion), or inserted after turning the fragment around (inversion), or included in a circular chromosome (a ring chromosome).

When two chromosomes each suffer one break, the resulting fragments can be exchanged. This is called a translocation. If acentric fragments are exchanged, this leads to a stable centric chromosome that can be passed on in mitosis, and this is termed a reciprocal translocation (see Fig. 7.5 in Chapter 7). Any acentric or dicentric product arising from exchange of a centric and an acentric fragment are lost during mitosis.

Robertsonian translocations are a peculiar type of translocation involving two of either chromosomes 13, 14, 15, 21, or 22. These chromosomes have very small short arms that are very similar in DNA sequence. When the short arms of two of these chromosomes break, acentric and centric fragments are exchanged resulting in acentric and dicentric fragments. The acentric fragment is lost, while in the dicentric fragment the centromeres are so close to each other that they fuse and form one large centromere (centric fusion). This chromosome is stable during mitosis.

Individuals that carry a balanced rearrangement have a normal phenotype, although the term balanced has come under pressure since the advent of higher resolution chromosomal analysis. However, carriers' gametes run into problems when entering meiosis. As explained previously, in order to go through meiosis the chromosomes have to pair in order to allow recombination. The cell that carries two abnormal chromosomes has to form special structures to allow for the pairing of the abnormal chromosome with the normal chromosomes. In a carrier of a Robertsonian translocation, no less than six different haploid cells can be formed. Only one of these gametes will lead to a normal individual, while a second one will lead to a balanced (and thus normal) individual; the other four will either lead to monosomy or trisomy.

Monogenic diseases

Modes of transmission

How a monogenic disease is transmitted mainly depends on two factors: firstly, is the disease dominant or recessive, and secondly is the gene located on an autosome or on a sex chromosome (mostly the X chromosome) [9]. In autosomal recessive disorders, the carriers have a normal phenotype while only homozygous carriers of the disease are affected. This can mostly be explained by the fact that recessive mutations are usually loss-of-function mutations. If one gene copy coding for an enzyme is therefore eliminated, the second copy will see to it that enough enzyme activity remains. If, however, the two copies are disabled, then the individual that carries this disease is affected. This explains why in recessive diseases both parents of an affected child are phenotypically normal carriers. A few of the most frequent autosomal recessive diseases are hemochromatosis and cystic fibrosis in Caucasian populations, sickle cell anemia in African populations, and beta-globinopathies in Mediterranean countries.

In autosomal dominant inheritance, individuals that carry only one copy of the defective gene are affected. The genes responsible for the diseases then often carry a gain-of-function mutation. The protein that is synthesized from the gene causes problems, e.g. in Huntington's disease because the abnormal protein forms toxic aggregates. Loss of function can also lead to dominant transmission, if there is so-called haploinsufficiency, i.e. one copy of the gene does not produce sufficient protein for normal functioning. Other well-known examples of autosomal dominant diseases are neurofibromatosis (Von Recklinghausen's disease of Elephant Man fame) and myotonic dystrophy or Steinert's disease.

Monogenic diseases that lie on the X chromosome have a particular mode of transmission, because women carry two X chromosomes, and men only one. Thus, in male patients, mutation on their one X chromosome is not balanced by the second X chromosome as it is in women. Here too, both recessive and dominant modes of inheritance exist. Examples of well-known recessive X-linked disorders are color blindness (very common but quite harmless) and the hemophilias. Dominant X-linked disorders are quite rare: Online Mendelian Inheritance in Man (OMIM)'s catalog [9] lists 821 of them. One striking example is incontinentia pigmenti: in affected males the disease is usually lethal in the prenatal period, while affected females show abnormalities in skin, hair, and central neural system, and a high rate of X-chromosome skewing. This is because the cells with an active mutation-carrying chromosome are lost around birth. Fragile X syndrome is also classified as dominant, but we will see below that this is related to the particular type of mutation.

Mutation types

Changes in one or a few base pairs are the most common mutations. A missense mutation means that one base pair in a sequence is changed, and causes one amino acid in the protein to be changed. This can lead to both loss-of-function mutations, such as when an active site of an enzyme is changed, or gain-of-function, because the three-dimensional structure of the protein is changed. Nonsense mutations change one codon to a stop codon, leading to a shortened mRNA, which is usually degraded and not translated into protein. This type of mutation thus mostly leads to loss-of-function. However, if the stop codon is at the end of the mRNA, protein can still be translated.

This truncated protein can cause many problems. In frameshift mutations, deletions or insertions of a few base pairs cause a frameshift in the downstream translational reading frame. A well-known example is the most common mutation in Tay–Sachs disease: a four-base pair insertion in the α-chain of hexosaminidase A. Other examples are splice-site mutations, causing whole exons to be missing or introns to be included in the mature mRNA, and mutations in the promoter regions, causing too little or too much of the mRNA to be transcribed.

Dynamic mutations are a special class of mutation, and mentioned here separately because a significant number of preimplantation genetic diagnosis (PGD) patients (see Chapter 11) undergo treatment for this type of disease [10]. Small repeats, usually of three nucleotides, are present in many genes. They are usually transmitted in a stable, Mendelian way [10]. However, if their size increases over a certain threshold, they become unstable and tend to enlarge during replication and/or meiosis. In some of these diseases, the triplet repeat codes for a stretch of amino acids: in Huntington's disease, this is a stretch of glycines. If the stretch of glycines becomes too large, this will cause the protein to misfold and form toxic aggregates. In other diseases, the repeats are located outside the coding sequence in the 5′ or 3′ untranslated region, or in an intron. This very long repeat then usually prevents expression of the gene, such as is the case in fragile X syndrome. Myotonic dystrophy type 1 (DM1) however has a different molecular pathology: the mRNA transcribed from the DMPK gene that carries an expanded repeat in the 3′ region, forms aggregates and sequesters mRNAs of other genes, thus causing dysfunctions in these genes. Moreover, the enlarged repeat has an effect on the transcription of genes nearby to the DMPK gene. This explains – in part – the pleiomorphic character of DM1.

References

1. Strachan T, Read A. *Human Molecular Genetics*, 4th edn. New York, NY: Garland Science, 2010.

2. Nussbaum R, McInnes R, Willard HF. *Thompson and Thompson Genetics in Medicine*, 7th edn. Philadelphia, PA: Saunders Elsevier, 2007, p. 28.

3. Ringo J. *Fundamental Genetics*. Cambridge, UK: Cambridge University Press, 2004.

4. Ensembl project: www.ensembl.org

5. Shaffer LG, McGowan-Jordan J, Schmid M, eds. *ISCN 2013: An International System for Human Cytogenetic Nomenclature*. Basel, Switzerland: Karger, 2012.

6. Metzker, ML. Sequencing technologies – the next generation. *Nat Rev Genet* 2010; 11: 31–46.

7. Schadt EE, Turner S, Kasarskis A. A window into third-generation sequencing. *Hum Mol Genet* 2010; 19: R227–40.

8. Gilissen C, Hoischen A, Brunner HG, Veltman JA. Disease gene identification strategies for exome sequencing. *Eur J Hum Genet* 2012; 20: 490–7.

9. Online Mendelian Inheritance in Man (OMIM): www.omim.org

10. Brouwer JR, Willemsen R, Oostra B. Microsatellite repeat instability and neurological disease. *Bioessays* 2009; 31: 71–83.

How to analyze a single blastomere?

Application of whole genome technologies: microarrays and next generation sequencing

Parveen Kumar, Masoud Zamani Esteki, Niels Van der Aa, and Thierry Voet

Introduction

Although a cell in general produces an arsenal of products that protect, inspect, and if necessary heal its valuable genetic content, DNA mutations can accumulate during a cell's cycle and division. This is exemplified by the creation of somatic genetic lesions underpinning the development of cancer, but also by the birth of handicapped children burdened with a genomic aberration arisen during gametogenesis or early embryogenesis. In fact, chances are high that we all are genetic mosaics early-on or later in our life, when part of our cells contain a genetic repertoire that deviates from the original zygotic genome. As a consequence, the ability to characterize the entire genome of a single human cell for all classes of genetic variants – including DNA copy number variants, structural DNA variants, small insertions, or deletions (indels), single nucleotide substitutions, and many other deviations – will be of paramount importance to understand genome evolution and to unravel genomic instability during a variety of processes such as tumorigenesis [1], gametogenesis [2], and embryogenesis [3]. In particular, cleavage-stage embryogenesis in humans appears to have an extraordinary rate of chromosome malsegregation and breakage [3]. Not the least, such single-cell genomics will be a stepping-stone towards the development of novel clinical methods for genetic diagnosis of cells derived from preimplantation human embryos or tumors.

This chapter provides an overview of modern high-throughput technologies, as well as their basic concepts, that allow capturing one or more classes of genetic variants in a single human cell (Fig. 2.1). As will

become clear in the chapter, a large variety of single-cell genome analysis methods is available. However, importantly, all current methods not only have limitations in the spectrum of DNA mutations and genetic variants that can be detected in the cell, but also have limitations in terms of resolution, accuracy, and reliability for detecting genetic variants.

Whole genome amplification

While a single human diploid cell contains only ~7 picograms of DNA, state-of-the-art genomic technologies require hundreds of nanograms to micrograms of input DNA to perform only one genomic scan of a DNA sample. Hence, a critical step for single-cell genomics is whole genome amplification (WGA) during which the cell's DNA is amplified thousands of times to yield sufficient input DNA. Since these single-cell WGA products will ultimately produce the signals for interpretation on the genome-wide platform, it is of paramount importance to understand the *modus operandi* as well as the various imperfections of the different WGA methods.

All current WGA approaches are underpinned by either multiple displacement amplification (MDA) or a polymerase chain reaction (PCR) on a cell lysis product in microliter volumes [1–24].

Multiple displacement amplification starts with the annealing of random primers onto the cell's denatured DNA template and subsequently copies the genome many times by a mechanism of strand displacement amplification in an isothermal reaction at 30°C. During MDA, DNA chain elongation proceeds

Textbook of Human Reproductive Genetics, eds Karen Sermon and Stéphane Viville. Published by Cambridge University Press.
© Cambridge University Press 2014.

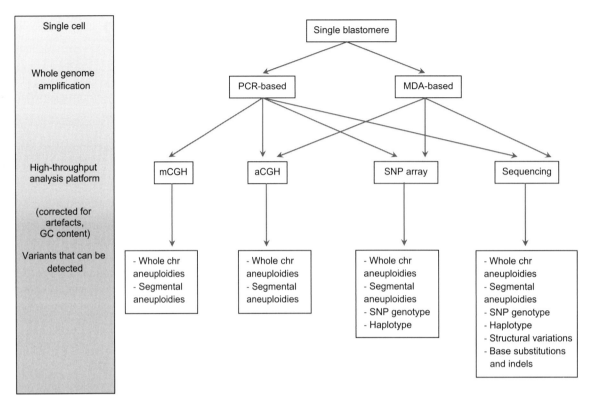

Figure 2.1 Single-cell genomics. Flowchart summarizing the different approaches for single-cell genomics, comprising the single-cell whole genome amplication (WGA) method, the high-throughput genome-wide analysis platform, and the genetic aberrations that can be detected in the cell by following a specific approach. aCGH, array comparative genomic hybridization; GC, guanine-cytosine; mCGH, metaphase comparative genomic hybridization; MDA, multiple displacement amplification; PCR, polymerase chain reaction; SNP, single nucleotide polymorphism; Whole chr, whole chromosome.

from annealed primers in the 5' to 3' direction. As soon as a 3' extending end of one nucleotide chain reaches the 5' end of the neighboring primed chain, it displaces the latter, and hence new random primers can anneal to the liberated single-stranded DNA chain and be extended again (Fig. 2.2). The end result is branches of DNA rather than the conventional DNA molecules. All DNA is synthesized by a Bacillus BstI or bacteriophage ϕ29 DNA polymerase, which can generate nucleotide chains of 10 kilobases (kb) or more. In addition, ϕ29 has proficient proofreading capacity using 3'->5' exonuclease activity. These properties make MDA the WGA method of choice for a number of specific single-cell analyses, in particular base mutation detection and single nucleotide polymorphism (SNP) genotyping [16, 19, 23] (see below).

In contrast, WGA methods based on PCR make use of thermostable DNA polymerases and recursive cycling between temperatures for denaturation and synthesis of the DNA. Commercial products

that convert the cell's DNA into a library of amplifiable semi-random DNA fragments are available – e.g. PicoPLEX (Rubicon Genomics), SurePlex (Blue-Gnome), and GenomePlex (Sigma-Aldrich). In contrast, Ampli1 (Silicon Biosystems) also applies PCR, but involves restriction digestion of the cell's DNA, followed by adapter ligation and amplification with universal primers, and thus relies on absolutely efficient restriction digestion, ligation, and unbiased amplification between the identical primed regions. All PCR-based methods typically produce DNA fragments of 200–1500 base pairs (bp) in length [1, 19]. Older versions of PCR-based single-cell WGA based on degenerate-oligonucleotide primed PCR (DOP-PCR) or primer extension preamplification PCR (PEP-PCR) suffered from vast incomplete genome coverage and limited amplification efficiencies.

Although WGA methods have obvious advantages for single-cell analysis, all have various imperfections that make the downstream analysis of the single-cell

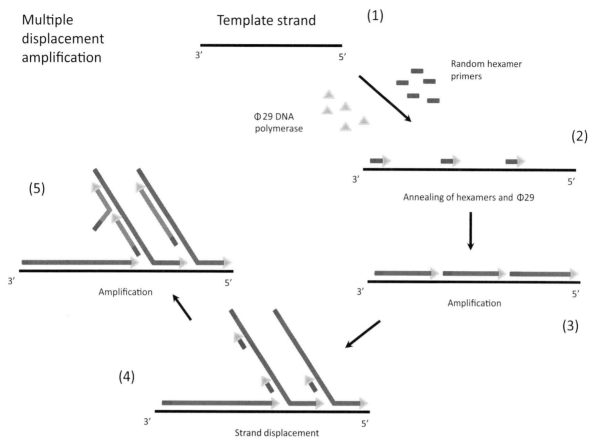

Figure 2.2 Multiple displacement amplification (MDA). The MDA method is an isothermal whole genome amplification method involving: (**1**) the annealing of random primers onto the denatured DNA template; (**2–3**) amplification of the DNA strands at constant temperature using, for example, the φ29 DNA polymerase; (**4**) strand displacement that (**5**) exposes the newly synthesized DNA strands for further amplification. See plate section for color version.

WGA product conceptually challenging. No WGA method produces a linear amplification product of the original cell's DNA template. Random loss of one allele (called allele drop-out or ADO), preferential amplification (PA) of an allele, or over-amplification or under-amplification of both alleles of a certain locus of the genome occurs during every single-cell WGA, and even varies significantly between different WGA methods [16] (see later). Also other less-known and less-characterized artefacts, including the production of chimeric DNA molecules [25] and the incorporation of wrong nucleotides [2] during WGA, can distort the DNA picture of the original cell. Chimeric DNA molecules have first been identified by single-end sequencing of MDA products of single bacterium cells [25] and later also by paired-end sequencing of human genetic material amplified by MDA.

Single-end sequencing methods sequence linear DNA fragments from only one end up to a specific length. In comparison, paired-end sequencing methods sequence both ends of the linear DNA molecules up to a specified length, but in the opposite direction, allowing a more in-depth analysis of the structure of the sequenced DNA (see later). The majority of the chimeric DNA molecules following MDA have architectures of DNA inversions, but also artefacts typical for deletions and other structural DNA anomalies are created. Mechanistic models that can explain the generation of such chimeric DNA artefacts during MDA have been described [25]. Whether similar artefacts are created by the other single-cell WGA methods is still unknown. Evidently, such artefacts tremendously complicate downstream analyses and the interpretation of the signals obtained with the WGA product on the genome-wide analysis platform. A systematic screen of the advantages and disadvantages of the various commercial and in-house WGA protocols, preferably with next generation sequencing, is thus required to enable decisions on which WGA method to best use for which single-cell genetic test.

Furthermore, a number of microfluidics devices have become available that allow us to perform WGA reactions in volumes that are several orders of magnitude below a microliter. Applying the same WGA method in a different reaction volume may have drastic effects on the number of artefacts introduced in the single-cell WGA product. For instance, decreasing the reaction volume will increase the concentration of DNA molecules in the reaction, and hence artefacts between the different DNA molecules may be primed more efficiently when compared to larger reaction volumes. However, the exact effects of reaction volumes on single-cell WGA artefacts remain to be investigated thoroughly.

Detection of genetic variants in single-cell WGA products

Incontrovertibly, the major difficulty in the analyses downstream of single-cell WGA is to discriminate the WGA artefacts from the cell's true genetic variants. Uneven allelic amplification artefacts (e.g. under- or over-amplification of both alleles of a locus, ADO, and PA) have to be discriminated from true copy number variants; also chimeric DNA molecules fabricated by WGA have to be distinguished from genuine structural variants in the cell; and nucleotide WGA copying errors may be misinterpreted as true nucleotide changes in the single-cell genome. Hence, standard algorithmic approaches that extract genetic variants from the signals obtained with non-preamplified DNA (extracted from many cells) on the platform become inadequate, and novel parameters and algorithms have to be defined for the analysis of one cell. Evidently, such novel approaches must first be tested thoroughly on individual cells that contain known genetic variants in order to establish resolution, false-negative and false-positive discovery rates of the new method. Furthermore, depending on (1) the purpose of the genetic screen (e.g. which genetic variants have to be captured? is the variant known or expected?), (2) the desired resolution (e.g. complete chromosome aneuploidies versus submicroscopic copy number variants), and (3) the time frame available (e.g. for preimplantation genetic

diagnosis only < 48 hours may be available), one combination of single-cell WGA, genome-wide screening platform, and mathematical–statistical algorithm may be more favorable than another (Fig. 2.1; Table 2.1). For instance, detecting the DNA copy number changes resulting from an unbalanced translocation with known DNA breakpoints in a single blastomere allows the application of specific platforms and computational approaches not suited for blind *de novo* discovery of segmental DNA copy number aberrations present in the cell genome-wide. Finally, particular single-cell genetic screens require not only expertise in genetics and molecular biology, but importantly also in bioinformatics and statistics. Current genome-wide screening platforms – including metaphase and microarray comparative genomic hybridization platforms, SNP array platforms, and next generation sequencing platforms – can involve complex analyses, in particular for the analysis of single-cell WGA products.

Table 2.1 provides a comprehensive overview of the variety of combinations of WGA, platform, and algorithms that have been reported thus far to detect specific genetic variants in a cell [1–20, 23].

Single-cell metaphase comparative genomic hybridization

Metaphase comparative genomic hybridization (mCGH) allows discovering DNA imbalances in a cell. The method is based on the hybridization of a fluorescently labeled WGA product of a single cell (= test sample) against a normal DNA sample (= reference sample) that is labeled with a different fluorophore onto karyotypically normal male metaphase chromosomes. The fluorescence intensity ratios across the chromosomes are subsequently analyzed for DNA copy number imbalances in the test versus the reference sample using quantitative fluorescent image analysis. Fluorescent signals of the single-cell WGA product that are more intense when compared to the reference sample for a particular locus of a chromosome indicate putative DNA gains, while less intense signals for the test sample point to DNA losses. In spite of low cost, the method is time consuming, labor intensive, and the resolution of mCGH is limited and not clear cut. Voullaire *et al.* reported that single-cell mCGH enables the detection of DNA copy number aberrations that encompass 40 megabases (Mb) or

Table 2.1 Milestone single-cell mCGH, aCGH, SNP array, and sequencing studies

Author [Ref no.]	Variants detected	Applied to single blastomere (Yes/No)	Approach	WGA method	Platform	Analysis software	Best resolution for copy number detection
Voullaire et al. [4]	Whole-chr, segm-chr	Yes	mCGH	DOP-PCR	Male-metaphase	Commercial	40 Mb
Rius et al. [15]	Whole-chr, segm-chr	Yes	mCGH	DOP-PCR	Male-metaphase	Commercial	NM
Le Caignec et al. [5]	Whole-chr, segm-chr	Yes	aCGH	MDA-GenomiPhi	3K BAC array	Custom	34 Mb
Fiegler et al. [6]	Whole-chr, segm-chr	No	aCGH	PCR-GenomePlex	32K BAC array	Custom	8.3 Mb
Geigl et al. [8]	Whole-chr, segm-chr	No	aCGH	PCR-GenomePlex	385K chr 22 and 2.1M whole-genome Nimblegen oligoarrays, 240K custom Agilent oligoarray		3 Mb
Alfarawati et al. [12]	Whole-cnr, segm-chr	Yes	mCGH/aCGH	DOP-PCR (mCGH)/ PCR-SurePlex (aCGH)	Male-metaphase (mCGH)/ BlueGnome (24Sure-V2/CytoChip V3)	Commercial	10 Mb mCGH, 2.8 Mb aCGH
Fiorentino et al. [13]	Whole-chr, segm-chr	Yes	aCGH	PCR-SurePlex	BlueGnome (24Sure+)	Commercial	2.5 Mb
Gutierrez-Mateo et al. [14]	Whole-chr	Yes	aCGH	PCR-GenomePlex, SurePlex	BlueGnome (CytoChip)	Commercial	NM
Bi et al. [18]	Whole-chr, segm-chr	No	aCGH	PCR-PicoPlex	44K, 180K, and 400K Agilent oligoarrays	Commercial	1.2 Mb
Iwamoto et al. [7]	Whole-chr, segm-chr, SNP genotyping	No	SNP array	MDA-GenomiPhi V2	50K Affymetrix SNP array	Commercial	NM
Vanneste et al. [3] and Konings et al. [20]	Whole-chr, segm-chr, SNP genotyping	Yes	aCGH/SNP array	MDA-GenomiPhi V2	3K BAC array, 250K Affymetrix SNP array	Custom (package downloadable)/ commercial	10 Mb
Handyside et al. [9]	Whole-chr, SNP genotyping	Yes	SNP array	MDA-REPLI-g	HumanCNV370 (Illumina)	Custom	NM
Treff et al. [11]	Whole-chr, SNP genotyping	Yes	SNP array	PCR-GenomePlex	250K Affymetrix SNP array	Commercial	NM
Johnson et al. [10]	Whole-ch , segm-chr, SNP genotyping	Yes	SNP array	PCR-Rubicon and MDA	HumanCNV370 and CytoSNP-12 (Illumina)	Custom	NM
Treff et al. [16]	Whole-chr, SNP genotypirg	No	SNP array	PCR-GenomePlex, MDA-(GenomiPhi,REPLI-g)	250K Affymetrix SNP array	Commercial	NM
Voet et al. [17]	Whole-chr, segm-chr, SNP genotyping	Yes	SNP array	MDA-GenomiPhi V2	250K Affymetrix SNP array	Custom/ commercial	10 Mb
Navin et al. [1]	Whole-chr. segm-chr	No	Single-end sequencing	PCR-GenomePlex	Illumina-seq	Custom (package downloadable)	NM
Xu et al. [23]	SNP genotyping	No	Exome sequencing	MDA-REPLI-g	Illumina-seq	Custom	NA
Hou et al. [19]	SNP genotyping	No	Exome sequencing	MDA-REPLI-g	Illumina-seq	Custom	NA
Wang et al. [2]	Whole-chr, segm-chr, SNP genotyping	No	Sequencing	MDA-REPLI-g	Illumina-seq	Custom	NM

aCGH, array comparative genomic hybridization; DOP-PCR, degenerate-oligonucleotide primed PCR; mCGH, metaphase comparative genomic hybridization; MDA, multiple displacement amplification; NA, not applicable; NM, not mentioned; PCR, polymerase chain reaction; segm-chr, segmental chromosomal aneuploidy; SNP, single nucleotide polymorphism; Whole-chr, whole-chromosome aneuploidy.

more [4], while Alfarawati *et al.* reported a resolution of approximately 10 Mb [12].

Nevertheless, many studies using mCGH of DOP-PCR-based WGA products have successfully pinpointed nullisomies, monosomies, and trisomies, as well as large-scale structural DNA imbalances in the genome of a cell, including blastomeres [4]. The technology enabled for the first time the *de novo* discovery of such DNA imbalances genome-wide in individual cells of human embryos [4].

Single-cell aCGH

Like mCGH, comparative genomic hybridization of a test single-cell WGA product versus a reference sample onto DNA microarrays also allows the detection of numerical DNA aberrations, including chromosome aneuploidies and segmental DNA imbalances, but at much higher resolution and robustness. In addition, microarrays allow interrogating parts of a cell's genome of particular interest to the investigator at ultra-high resolution, while less interesting parts of the genome can be neglected or examined at lower resolution by the production of custom microarrays [8, 18].

In general, microarrays are composed of thousands to millions of DNA spots attached to a solid surface, usually a glass slide. Each spot or probe contains the DNA of a very small locus in the genome (Fig. 2.3A–C). Subsequently, as for mCGH, a fluorescently labeled and denatured WGA product of a single cell is hybridized simultaneously with a denatured reference DNA sample that is labeled with a different fluorophore onto the DNA microarray containing single-stranded DNA probes. By interpreting the fluorescence intensity ratios obtained on each spot, DNA copy number aberrations can be identified. When multiple probes, which interrogate consecutive loci in the genome, demonstrate fluorescence intensity ratios that approximate the value of -1 following $\log_2$ transformation (i.e. a $1 : 2$ test : reference ratio) or a value of 0.58 (i.e. a $3 : 2$ test : reference ratio), then this segment can represent a putative deletion or duplication, respectively. $\log_2$-transformed fluorescence intensity ratios rippling around 0 (i.e. $2 : 2$ test : reference ratio) indicate normal diploid loci (Fig. 2.3A–C).

Although this simple principle is very efficient with test DNA extracted from many cells that have not undergone preamplification, the artifacts associated with WGA remain the biggest challenge in copy number profiling of a single cell. Not only ADO and PA, but also the chimeric DNA molecules and nucleotide copy errors resulting from WGA, can tilt the fluorescent signal obtained at a particular spot in favor of one or the other allele. For instance, nucleotide WGA copy errors may interfere with the hybridization efficiency of the amplified DNA molecule to the complementary probe's DNA sequence and, depending on the amount of nucleotide copy errors as well as the time of occurrence of the error in the WGA reaction, this effect may be more pronounced for a particular allele of the cell. As a consequence of this cocktail of WGA artefacts, the standard deviation of fluorescence intensity ratio signals on probes representing consecutive domains in the genome will be significantly higher when compared to an identical analysis of a non-preamplified DNA test sample on the same platform. Importantly, high standard deviations across the signals for consecutive probes reduce the sensitivity and specificity for detecting DNA copy number changes in the single-cell WGA product, because the more noise that is present in the data the harder it becomes to detect statistically reliable genetic variations. In addition, WGA biases over longer distances in the genome can even easily be misinterpreted for genuine copy number changes in the cell. For instance, parts of the genome rich in guanine and cytosine bases may amplify less efficiently and yield less product in the single-cell WGA test sample when compared to neighboring loci in the cell's genome. After conventional microarray analysis, such parts of the single-cell genome where both alleles are under amplified may be detected and falsely interpreted as genuine deletions in the cell. Furthermore, such WGA artefacts and effects on data analyses can differ tremendously between WGA methods. Various studies indicate that most MDA-based WGA protocols lead to higher standard deviations of the $\log_2$ intensity ratios than PCR-based WGA protocols making MDA currently less favorable for high resolution DNA copy number screening, but instead more favorable for detecting other genetic variants in a cell [6, 16] (see previous and following paragraphs). Hence, standard array CGH (aCGH) methods do not suffice to analyze aCGH signals downstream of the single-cell WGA product, but specific approaches are required.

Furthermore, different types of DNA microarrays exist depending on the DNA content of each spot. Bacterial artificial chromosome (BAC) arrays

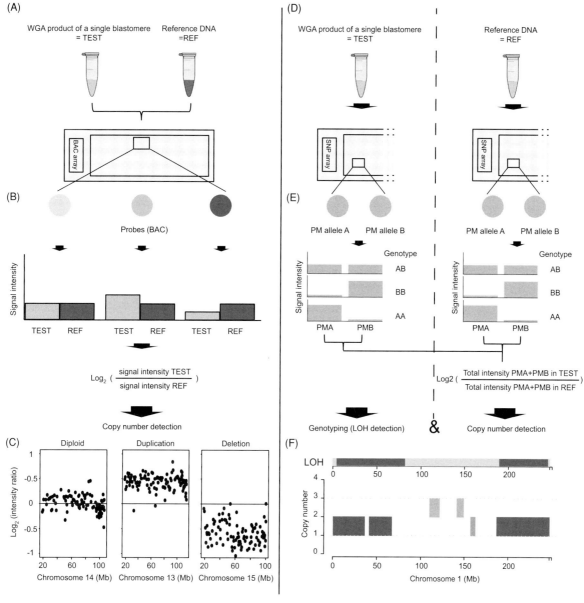

Figure 2.3 Single-cell aCGH and SNP array analysis. Analyzing the genome of a single blastomere using bacterial artificial chromosome (BAC) arrays (**A–C**) or SNP arrays (D–F). (**A**) The whole genome amplification (WGA) product of a single blastomere "TEST" sample is fluorescently labeled (green) and a reference DNA "REF" sample is marked with a different fluorophore (red). The labeled TEST and REF samples are hybridized simultaneously on a BAC array, and (**B**) the intensities of the fluorescent signals resulting from hybridized TEST and REF DNA are measured for each spot containing DNA of a specific BAC probe. The ratio of both signals is representative of the relative copy number in the TEST sample compared to the REF sample. Equal signal intensities for TEST and REF indicate a diploid region in the TEST sample (left bars) if the REF sample is diploid for the locus interrogated by the BAC probe. In this scenario, a higher or lower TEST signal versus the REF signal indicates a DNA gain (middle bars) or DNA loss (right bars) in the TEST respectively. Log$_2$ intensity ratios across all BAC probes are normalized, segmented, and used for copy number detection. (**C**) Log$_2$ intensity ratios (Y-axis) for each probe according to their genomic location (X-axis). The left panel shows a diploid chromosome 14 in a single blastomere demonstrating log$_2$ intensity ratios rippling around 0. The middle and right panel show, respectively, a duplication of chromosome 13 and a deletion of chromosome 15 in the same single blastomere. (**D,E**) The WGA product of a single blastomere is labeled and hybridized to a SNP array (left of panel **D,E**). Reference DNA sample(s) are hybridized each to a separate SNP array (right of panel **D,E**). (**E**) The labeled DNA will bind a set of single-stranded probes interrogating, respectively, the A and B allele for each SNP on the array. These are depicted as perfect-match probes (PM) for the A and B allele of a SNP (gray dots). Gray bar-plots represent different examples of signal intensities for PM-A and PM-B allele probes that can be obtained in scenarios of AB, BB, or AA genotypes for this SNP, respectively. The genotypes inferred from PM-probe signals can be used to detect stretches of loss of heterozygosity (LOH) in the genome. Log$_2$ intensity ratios per SNP can be calculated *in silico* from the PM-A and PM-B probe signals obtained for both the TEST sample and REF sample(s). The log$_2$ intensity ratios are used to detect copy number aberrations in the TEST sample as compared to the REF sample(s). (**F**) The bottom panel shows the calculated copy number (Y-axis) for chromosome 1 (X-axis) in a single blastomere as deduced from SNP array analysis. Red signifies deletions, green duplications. The top panel of (**F**) shows the detection of regions of LOH (red) using the same SNP array data. The LOH is detected in the deleted 1p- and 1q-terminal regions, confirming that these deletions are real. See plate section for color version.

apply the DNA inserts of BACs that can accommodate from 150 to 350 kb of DNA. Bacterial artificial chromosome arrays were one of the first platforms for comparative genomic hybridization, and are still very popular for analyses of single-cell WGA products (see below). Oligonucleotide arrays, in contrast, contain synthesized oligonucleotide probe sequences that are usually 25–80 nucleotides in length. Since many thousands-to-millions of spots, each with specific short oligonucleotide sequences, can be deposited on a solid surface, oligonucleotide arrays offer theoretically a better coverage and higher resolution for aCGH analysis of a genome. Although this is certainly the case for analyses of non-preamplified DNA samples that have been extracted from many cells, single-cell aCGH is burdened with the variety of WGA biases that are introduced in the single-cell WGA product influencing the hybridization signal from probe to probe. In this respect, single-cell fluorescent signals on BAC probes may be more robust and lead to less standard deviation across the probes because larger regions of the genome are interrogated in the single-cell WGA product, thus ironing out the effects of small WGA artefacts. Data of single-bacterium genome sequencing indicate that the majority of DNA artefacts due to MDA encompass less than 10 kb [25].

The following paragraphs will give a brief overview of milestone studies on single-cell aCGH analysis. Each applies a unique pipeline combining a specific single-cell WGA protocol with a microarray platform and custom algorithmic analyses still applied today.

Le Caignec et al. developed customized BAC arrays and applied single-cell DNA amplified with MDA in combination with non-amplified genomic DNA as a reference for comparative hybridization onto the array [5]. For each of the ∼3000 BAC probes on the array, a normalized log$_2$ intensity ratio was determined. Subsequently, to detect whole-chromosome aneuploidies they calculated for each chromosome a single average log$_2$ value and evaluated these against thresholds that were determined for each chromosome discretely using data of multiple single cells that were karyotypically normal for the chromosome and analyzed on the same platform. Chromosome-specific average log$_2$ values that surpassed the threshold in the positive direction indicated a DNA gain for that chromosome in the cell, while in the negative direction it

Table 2.2 Chromosomal aberrations used to validate single-cell array comparative genomic hybridization (aCGH)

Author [Ref.]	Best resolution	Abberation validated
Le Caignec et al. [5]	34 Mb	Trisomy (13, 18, 21), Monosomy X and del4q (34 Mb) in fibroblasts delXq (58 Mb) and dup14q (47 Mb) in Epstein–Barr virus (EBV) cells
Fiegler et al. [6]	8.3 Mb	Trisomy 21 and del15q (10.8 Mb)* del1p (30 Mb) and dup1q (90 Mb) in the renal cell carcinoma cell line (769P)
Geigl et al. [8]	3 Mb	del22 (1.2, 2.8, and 3 Mb)* del9p (6.3 Mb), del1p (30 Mb) and dup1q (90 Mb) in the renal cell carcinoma cell line (769P) del16p (1.29 Mb) and del20p (1.81 Mb) in the colorectal cancer cell line (HT29)
Bi et al. [18]	1.2 Mb	Trisomy 21, del7q (1.2 Mb), del22q (2.5 Mb), del17p (3.8 Mb) and del15q (6.6 Mb), dupXq (0.6 Mb), dup17p (1.3 and 3.8 Mb) in lymphoblastoid cell lines

* Human cell type not mentioned

indicated a DNA loss. In contrast to characterizing partial aneuploidies with known chromosomal breakpoints and uncovering unknown whole-chromosome imbalances, de novo discovery of segmental DNA imbalances in single cells with this method remains difficult (Table 2.2 [5, 6, 8, 18]).

Fiegler et al. reported the first high resolution aCGH analysis of individual cells using a customized 32K BAC array in combination with PCR-based single-cell WGA (GenomePlex) test samples and non-amplified male reference DNA [6]. They were able to detect whole-chromosome aneuploidies as well as previously unknown segmental DNA imbalances down to approximately 10 Mb. To enable interpretation of the data, they normalized all the raw ratios by dividing with the median ratio across all autosomal BAC probes. The variability of the single-cell genome-amplification process necessitated smoothing of the data by averaging the signals across 10 BAC probes. Subsequently, to detect the chromosomal DNA imbalances, at least 3 consecutive data points had to be above or below 1.5 times the experimental variability (Table 2.2).

Later, Geigl *et al.* analyzed PCR-amplified (GenomePlex) single-cell genomes versus amplified reference DNA samples on high density oligonucleotide tiling arrays [8]. Aneuploidy detection was based on an algorithm that includes running means of intensity ratios in different window sizes and analyses at progressively greater levels of smoothing. The data of these recursive analyses was integrated for the detection of DNA imbalances. They showed that imbalances as small as 2.8 Mb could be detected using high-resolution oligonucleotide arrays (Table 2.2).

Bi *et al.* used customized 44K, 180K, and 400K oligonucleotide arrays and PCR-based PicoPLEX WGA to detect *a priori* known or expected chromosomal changes as small as 1.2 Mb in a cell [18]. In their approach, they designed custom arrays on which the genomic regions of interest were densely coated with oligonucleotide probes. For instance, on the 400K array approximately 1 probe every 425 base pairs interrogated the region of interest and only 1 probe every 500 kb interrogated the remainder of the genome. This increment of the probe density in specific regions in combination with specific algorithms and filters allowed the authors to push the resolution of single-cell aCGH to ~1.2 Mb for the targeted region (Table 2.2).

While all of the above studies required multiple days for single-cell DNA copy number analysis, Gutiérrez-Mateo *et al.* [14], Alfarawati *et al.* [12], and Fiorentino *et al.* [13] used a recent commercially available BAC microarray approach that allows the detection of single-cell DNA imbalances down to ~2.5 Mb within 24 hours.

Single-cell SNP array analysis

Single nucleotide polymorphisms or SNPs are places in the genome characterized by the substitution of one nucleotide (e.g. A) for another (C, G, or T). Once this variant allele reaches a frequency of 1% in the population, it is regarded as a SNP. Single nucleotide variants with an allele frequency lower than 1% in the population are rather referred to as rare variants. In a diploid situation, a cell is either homozygous (AA or BB) or heterozygous (AB) for a particular SNP, where A and B refer to the two possible variant alleles at that base position. Currently, more than 15 million SNPs are known in the human genome.

While SNP array technology is a fast and easy way to characterize or genotype a DNA sample simultaneously for thousands to millions of SNPs that are known in the population, it does not allow discovering SNPs *de novo*. In addition, the technology enables detecting copy number variants (Fig. 2.3D–F). This gives SNP array technology a distinct advantage over conventional aCGH-analysis for single-cell DNA copy number analysis, as DNA copy number calls can now be integrated with single-cell SNP genotypes and can thus be discriminated from WGA artefacts. This results in increased reliability of the detected single-cell DNA copy number landscape. For example, a hemizygous deletion detected by SNP-array DNA-copy number analysis can be affirmed by the concurrent detection of lacking heterozygous SNP calls in the deleted locus, termed as loss of heterozygosity (LOH). Although LOH at a particular SNP can result from WGA ADO (or PA producing an overwhelming signal of one allele over the other), ADO and/or PA are unlikely to occur at each heterozygous SNP over vast consecutive distances in the genome. Hence, LOH detection is very powerful to confirm large-scale deletions in single cells and thus to discriminate false from true deletions. This strength is best illustrated for GC-rich loci of the genome. These regions are known to amplify less efficiently and variably using particular WGA methods (e.g. MDA) resulting in lower fluorescence intensity signals for those regions when compared to non-preamplified reference signals and neighboring loci of the cell's genome [3]. As a consequence, copy number calling algorithms may interpret and report such regions as putative deletions. However, an algorithm scanning the same single-cell data for LOH-regions will not detect loss of heterozygosity in these regions because both alleles have been amplified, be it less well, and thus heterozygosity of the SNPs has been preserved in the WGA product. Not only deletions but also duplications can be confirmed by SNP genotype analysis based on the distorted frequency of one allele versus the other, e.g. if the B allele of a heterozygous SNP is duplicated, one expects to find ABB instead of AB SNP calls (see below). Furthermore, SNP arrays enable the detection of copy neutral loss of heterozygosity, indicating uniparental isodisomy in single cells [3, 17].

Currently, there are two main manufacturers of SNP array platforms (underpinned by different chemistries and analyses) that are applied for single-cell genome analysis: Affymetrix and Illumina SNP arrays.

Single-cell SNP and copy number variation typing using Affymetrix chemistry

The Affymetrix platform typically utilized for single-cell analysis is the GeneChip Human Mapping 250K NspI Array [3, 11, 16, 17, 22]. In the analysis, single-cell WGA DNA is first subjected to restriction digestion using the NspI enzyme, DNA adapters are then ligated and a PCR amplification using universal primers follows. Hence, DNA fragments following single-cell WGA must be long enough to allow restriction digestion at both ends, subsequent adaptor ligation, and Affymetrix's PCR. Both MDA-based (yielding fragments encompassing multiple kilobases) and PCR-based (yielding smaller fragments) single-cell WGA products have been successfully analyzed with Affymetrix SNP arrays, but important differences were detected [16] (see below). The resulting Affymetrix amplicons of 200–1100 bp in size are further fragmented, labeled, and hybridized without a reference DNA sample to the Affymetrix SNP array (Fig. 2.3D–F). After hybridization, the arrays are washed and stained to detect the hybridization signals on the probes following scanning.

On the GeneChip Human Mapping 250K arrays, two sets of 25-mer oligonucleotide probes that hybridize specifically to the A or B allele of a particular SNP respectively are used for single-cell genotyping and copy number typing. Besides these perfect match (PM) probes, other probe sets, including mismatch (MM) probes, are synthesized on the array that are applied to interpret background noise and hybridization efficiencies. The labeled single-cell WGA DNA binds to PM (and MM) probes, but depending on the degree of sequence match, PM and MM probes will reveal different fluorescent intensities. Subsequently, computational algorithms interpret the observed intensities at each SNP probeset and infer SNP genotype calls. For instance, for a homozygous AA SNP call, one expects a strong signal on the PM probes for the A allele, but background signals on the PM probes for the SNP's alternative B allele (Fig. 2.3E). For subsequent SNP copy number analysis, signal intensities obtained with a test cell are compared *in silico* against signal intensities obtained for a reference set of DNA samples that have been hybridized individually to the same platform (Fig. 2.3E–F). For instance, the publicly available SNP probe intensity data from 41 HapMap female DNA samples can be applied as a reference [20]. Subsequently, $\log_2$ intensity ratios including PM probe fluorescent intensities summarized over both alleles per SNP of test versus reference sample are computed, normalized, segmented, and converted to integer DNA copy number profiles using a Hidden Markov Model (HMM) embedded in the "Copy Number Analysis Tool (CNAT – Affymetrix)" or other software.

Iwamoto *et al.* [7] and Treff *et al.* [16] both applied Affymetrix SNP arrays to detect DNA copy number aberrations in single cells using CNAT approaches. The concept of integrating SNP copy number with SNP LOH profiles was first presented by Iwamoto *et al.*, who in addition took WGA bias into account by using both non-WGA and single-cell WGA signals as the *in silico* reference for SNP copy number profiling of a test cell [7]. In this way, they successfully corrected single-cell test WGA samples for insufficiently amplified DNA regions following MDA, like chromosomes 19 and 22 that are GC-rich. However, this method uses older low-resolution 50K SNP arrays, and the false-positive and false-negative rates for detecting segmental DNA imbalances are unclear. Treff *et al.*, in contrast, called whole-chromosome aneuploidies in single cells according to the copy number state of the majority of the chromosome-specific SNPs and thus failed to detect segmental DNA aberrations using GeneChip Human Mapping 250K NspI arrays in combination with GenomePlex single-cell WGA test samples [11]. However, they used LOH probabilities to integrate with whole-chromosome copy number profiles, and thus obtained more confidence in detected aneuploidies.

In contrast, Vanneste *et al.* attained a resolution of ≥9.3 Mb to detect DNA copy number aberrations in a cell by hybridizing single-cell WGA products to both a 3K BAC array as well as an Affymetrix 250K NspI SNP array [3]. Subsequent copy number profiling of the cell was based on the integration of: (1) BAC probe specific copy number probabilities; (2) SNP copy number states; and (3) SNP LOH states. Specifically, single-cell MDA DNA was first hybridized against differentially labeled non-preamplified genomic DNA (47,XXY) on a 3K BAC array. An algorithm, based on a statistical mixture model, then corrected probe-specific intensity ratios for recurrent WGA bias, which was assessed using cells with normal chromosomes. For each locus that was interrogated by the BAC array, the algorithm estimated three probabilities that reflected whether in the test cell the interrogated locus was likely to be normal diploid, deleted, or duplicated. Advantageously, this algorithm also provided a quality control measurement. Detection of equal probabilities for the three copy number states across a single-cell genome indicated that an imbalance could not be statistically discriminated from the other copy number states. Hence, such single-cell WGA products could be excluded from further analysis. Subsequently, single-cell MDA DNA samples interpretable for DNA copy number were hybridized to Affymetrix 250K NspI SNP arrays for independent SNP copy number and genotype confirmation. The SNP copy number and LOH states were estimated by HMMs using optimized parameters. The data resulting from the BAC- and SNP-array single-cell analyses were integrated and conservative genetic-variant calling rules for single cells were applied. Furthermore, the recurrence and reciprocity of DNA aberrations detected amongst blastomeres of the same embryo were exploited. Besides a resolution of ~10 Mb, the method was demonstrated to be proficient in reliable detection of copy neutral uniparental isodisomies in single human blastomeres as well. The method was validated on individual cells of Epstein–Barr virus (EBV) -transformed cell lines containing either a trisomy 21 plus monosomy X, a 9.3 Mb 18pter duplication plus a 1.7 Mb 20pter deletion, a 47.5 Mb 14qter duplication plus a 58 Mb Xqter deletion, or a 14 Mb 18pter deletion. The 1.7 Mb deletion could not be reliably detected with this approach.

Voet *et al.* subsequently used additional parental genotype information and developed a novel parent-of-origin algorithm that interprets Affymetrix 250K SNP calls of a single blastomere amplified by MDA for Mendelian errors to detect DNA anomalies [17]. Whole chromosome as well as segmental DNA gains and losses, and even copy neutral uniparental disomies, could not only be captured in a cell but also the rearranged parental allele could be pinpointed using the following principle genome-wide: if for a particular SNP the maternal and paternal genotypes are "AA" and "BB" respectively, the blastomere's genotype for the same SNP is expected to be "AB." But, if the blastomere's genotype for that specific locus is typed as e.g. "AA," this could be due to ADO of the paternal B allele, a PA of the maternal A allele, a true deletion of that locus on the paternally inherited chromosome, or a true amplification of the locus on the maternally inherited chromosome. Although it is impossible to distinguish between these possibilities on the basis of this one SNP, by including neighboring SNPs, DNA copy number aberrations can be confirmed in the cell because WGA artefacts like ADO and PA occur randomly and are highly unlikely to indicate systematically the same parental allele. The method was validated using blastomeres with known DNA imbalances.

Recently, van Uum *et al.* used similar principles for copy number typing, genotyping, and parent-of-origin analysis of DNA imbalances resulting from unbalanced translocations in blastomeres [22]. They attained a resolution of 5 Mb using REPLI-g MDA products of single cells and Affymetrix 250K NspI arrays.

Importantly, the amount of SNPs that are called, as well as the resulting SNP genotype and copy number call accuracy, can differ significantly when individual cells of the same cell line are amplified with different WGA methods and hybridized to the same 250K NspI SNP array platform. Treff *et al.* evaluated two MDA-based WGA methods, QIAgen's "REPLI-g" and GE healthcare's "GenomiPhi," as well as one PCR-based WGA method (GenomePlex) [16]. Approximately 74, 78, and 88% of the $\sim 2.5 \times 10^5$ SNPs could be genotyped following GenomiPhi WGA, GenomePlex, and REPLI-g respectively, suggesting significant differences in attained genome coverage following different single-cell WGA methods. Furthermore, the accuracy of the single-cell SNP genotypes when compared to the corresponding genotypes of non-preamplified multicell DNA samples were 86, 89, and 96% following GenomiPhi, GenomePlex, and REPLI-g WGA, respectively. Falsely called SNPs for each WGA technology were also interrogated by the computation of ADO. The ADO rates for GenomiPhi, GenomePlex, and REPLI-g were 14, 11, and 4%, respectively. In addition, single-cell SNP copy numbers were 62, 95, and 99% accurate following GenomiPhi, REPLI-g, and GenomePlex WGA, respectively [16].

Single-cell SNP and copy number variant typing using Illumina chemistry

Infinium HD assays, like the HapMap CNV370Quad or CytoSNP-12 arrays, based on the different SNP typing chemistry provided by Illumina, have also been used for single-cell SNP copy number profiling and genotyping. In this assay, single-cell preamplified DNA is subjected to an additional isothermal amplification. The final amplification product is fragmented and hybridized to oligonucleotide probes that have a sequence complementary to the bases immediately flanking a particular SNP in the reference genome. A single-base extension using labeled nucleotides subsequently produces the quantitative signal. These fluorescent signals are interpreted algorithmically for the SNP genotype, copy number, and LOH.

Johnson *et al.* reported, however, that commercial software packages underperform for copy number profiling single cells analyzed by Illumina technology and developed a novel algorithm called Parental Support [10]. The Parental Support methodology uses the genotype of the parents to detect copy number aberrations in the embryo, as well as the parental and meiotic or mitotic origin of the DNA anomaly. While the method analyzes PCR-based and MDA-based single-cell WGA products within 24 hours (standard SNP array protocols require ~3 days) and does take single-cell WGA bias into account for variant calling, its ability to detect segmental copy number aberrations remains limited. This is because for *de novo* segmental DNA imbalance discovery each chromosome is subdivided in five different segments to which the algorithm is applied thereby reducing the resolution and the sensitivity. The method has a false-negative proportion of 2.1% and a false-positive proportion of 3.9% following the analysis of 330 cells that carry trisomy 21 and 129 single euploid cells. Unfortunately, a similar validation experiment was not performed for individual cells with various segmental DNA anomalies. Johnson *et al.* [10] and Rabinowitz *et al.* [21] subsequently applied the Parental Support algorithm to profile hundreds of blastomeres biopsied from cleavage-stage embryos. Various nullisomies, monosomies, trisomies, UPDs, and segmental DNA aberrations, including the parental and meiotic or mitotic origin, could be deduced from the data.

Single-cell genome sequencing

Next generation sequencing (NGS) technologies allow enormous amounts of sequencing reactions in parallel in a time- and cost-effective manner. Genome sequencing projects that previously required decades of "first-generation" or Sanger "chain-termination" sequencing can now be accomplished in a matter of days at 10^4 to 10^5 times the cost reduction. Various second-generation systems, each based on a different sequencing chemistry or technology, have been developed and are able to sequence a genome for the full spectrum of DNA mutations – ranging from base substitutions and indels, over balanced and imbalanced structural DNA variants, to full chromosome and genome ploidy changes – using hundreds of nanograms of non-amplified DNA extracted from many cells. Current prominent commercially available NGS platforms include the Roche 454 system, the Illumina HiSeq2000 system, and the Life Technologies SOLiD platform. The most popular system for sequencing a single-cell WGA product is the Illumina HiSeq2000 sequencer.

In order to grasp fully the advantages of sequencing over other technologies to analyze a single-cell WGA product, it is important to understand the basic workflow. First, the test DNA sample – e.g. a DNA product from a single cell that underwent MDA- or PCR-based WGA – is shattered into smaller pieces from which a library of DNA templates is created ready for massively parallel sequencing (Fig. 2.4). Even PCR-based single-cell WGA methods that immediately generate a library of DNA molecules ready for Illumina sequencing during the WGA reaction are becoming available. Either way, before sequencing, the templates have to be immobilized on a solid surface to allow the thousands to millions of simultaneous sequencing reactions, each at a separate site on the surface. Since the imaging systems used in second-generation sequencers cannot detect a fluorescent event resulting from a sequencing reaction of a single DNA molecule, the DNA template molecules adhered to the solid surface must first be PCR amplified clonally into a cluster of molecules on the surface prior to sequencing. Subsequently, many clusters of individually amplified DNA templates are sequenced in parallel. Roche 454 applies a DNA polymerase-based pyrosequencing method, while Illumina sequences by cycles of single-base extensions using a modified DNA polymerase and a mixture of four differentially labeled nucleotides with reversible terminators. SOLiD does not use a DNA polymerase but a DNA ligase and differentially labeled probes for sequencing in a cyclic fashion. The obtained short sequence reads, typically ≤100 bases after Illumina sequencing, obtained from only one end or both ends of each clonally amplified-test DNA molecule are mapped back to the established GRCh37 human reference genome. This is also known as single-end and paired-end sequencing respectively. Following mapping of the short sequence reads to the reference genome, the mapped reads can be used for copy number profiling [1] or genetic variant detection

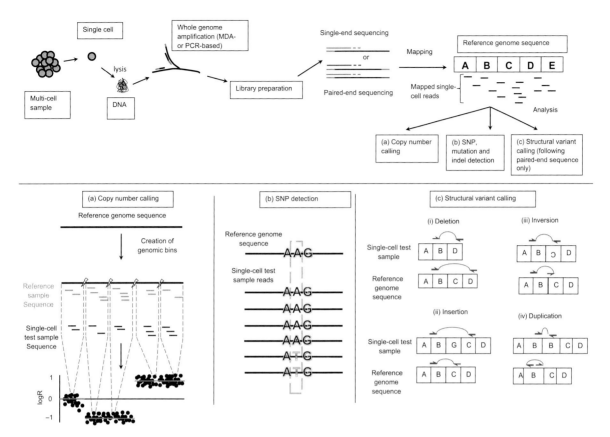

Figure 2.4 Single-cell genome sequencing and variant detection. Top panel shows the pipeline to sequence a single cell. The cell is lysed, subjected to whole genome amplification (WGA) and followed by either single-end or paired-end sequencing, meaning that only one end or both ends of each DNA fragment is sequenced respectively. Following sequencing the reads are mapped to the reference genome sequence allowing various analyses including copy number calling, SNP detection, structural variant calling (only following paired-end sequencing), as well as base mutation and indel detection. The bottom left panel depicts the basics of copy number detection from mapped single-cell reads. Sequences of a single-cell test sample (and optionally of a sequenced reference DNA sample as depicted in this figure) are mapped to the sequence of the human reference genome. Subsequently, the human reference genome is portioned into genomic bins and the amount of reads from the test and reference sample mapping to each bin are counted. By computing $\log_2$ ratios (logR) of test versus reference sample focal read-depth counts per bin, the DNA copy number can be deduced. The bottom middle panel shows a SNP detection pipeline. Any nucleotide mismatch of mapped single-cell sequence reads with the sequence in the human reference genome indicates a putative SNP or base mutation in the cell. However, putative genetic changes have to be discriminated from WGA artefacts (see main text). The bottom right panel depicts how structural variants can be detected following paired-end sequencing and mapping of the obtained read-pairs. After mapping, any violation to the expected insert size and/or mapping orientation of the paired reads indicates a putative structural variant in the cell. Scenarios for (i) a deletion, (ii) an insertion, (iii) an inversion, or (iv) a tandem duplication are depicted.

using computational methods. The DNA copy number analysis can be done using focal read-depth analysis, in which the genome is divided into bins and the number of mapped reads per bin is compared to the number of reads in this bin in a sequenced reference sample of known ploidy (Fig. 2.4). In turn, structural variants can be detected by identifying groups of aberrantly mapping paired-end reads demonstrating a violation against the expected insert size or orientation when a read-pair is mapped back to the reference genome sequence (Fig. 2.4, right panel, see also below).

In contrast, nucleotide mismatches of mapped single-cell sequence reads with the sequence in the human reference genome indicate putative SNPs or base mutations in the cell (Fig. 2.4, middle panel). Depending on the amount of bases that are sequenced in total (e.g. 12×10^9), the GRCh37 reference genome becomes covered ($4\times$ in the example; $= 12 \times 10^9$ divided by 3×10^9, i.e. the size of the haploid human genome) with mapped short sequence reads accordingly. Subsequently, depending on which type of genetic variants one wants to extract from the mapped reads of a sequenced DNA sample, a deep coverage is necessary – e.g. for SNP or indel detection, 30× coverage is common – or a more shallow coverage suffices – e.g. for copy number or structural variant discovery (Fig. 2.4).

Next generation sequencing thus has a number of important advantages when compared to DNA microarrays that can increase the resolution, accuracy, reliability, and scope of single-cell genomics tremendously. Firstly, massively parallel sequencing of single-cell WGA products can interrogate virtually every base amplified by the WGA method, while microarrays only interrogate specific loci of the single-cell WGA product defined by the location of the DNA probes. Hence, single-cell WGA products can be characterized with digital precision (digital unit = mapped read) in terms of genomic breadth and depth following sequencing, which is unattainable with microarray analysis. Secondly, in contrast to SNP arrays, sequencing allows not only the characterization of SNPs known in the population but, in fact, *de novo* discovery of the full spectrum of DNA mutations and genetic variants genome-wide with digital information on allelic frequency. Thirdly, principles applied for SNP array analysis of single-cell WGA products can be applied on sequences of single cells as well, at much higher resolution and for the full spectrum of genetic variants. Last, but not least, DNA fragments in the library may not only be sequenced from one end but also from both ends of each DNA molecule in opposite directions with an intervening non-sequenced portion. The latter is called the insert of paired-end sequencing libraries and typically encompasses 200–700 bp. Hence, not only can the basic insertions and deletions be detected by simply comparing the distance between mapped read pairs to the average insert size between the paired-ends in the sequencing library (Fig. 2.4), but also inversions and translocations can be disclosed by altered orientation and chromosomal identity of the mapped read pairs respectively. Thus, paired-end sequencing allows discovery of types of structural variants that cannot be unveiled by microarray analysis (e.g. translocations), revealing the architecture of DNA imbalances and confirming DNA copy number changes detected in a single-cell WGA product by finding matching aberrantly mapping read-pair(s).

Although NGS presents a number of advantages, the interpretation of single-cell sequencing data is complex. Since NGS portrays a single-cell WGA product in more detail than microarrays, more WGA artefacts in number and type are also detected. Small uneven allelic amplification artefacts have to be discriminated from true submicroscopic copy number variants, chimeric DNA molecules created by WGA have to be distinguished from genuine structural variants in the cell following paired-end sequence analysis, and nucleotide WGA copying errors may be misinterpreted as true nucleotide changes in the single-cell genome. Hence, dedicated approaches to sift these amplification artefacts from true genetic changes are required but still remain to be largely established for single-cell genome sequence analyses. Although none of the methods reported and described below have been used to analyze single blastomeres, there is conceptually no restriction.

Navin *et al.* recently demonstrated that low coverage (<1× haploid genome coverage) single-end sequencing of sorted nuclei could increase the resolution of single-cell copy number analyses beyond the level possible with microarray approaches [1]. To study genetic heterogeneity in breast cancers, the methodology was applied to 100 cells of a polygenomic breast tumor, as well as 100 cells of a monogenomic breast tumor and liver metastasis. Following sequencing of the single-nuclei GenomePlex-amplification products, the obtained single-end reads were mapped to the reference genome. Subsequently, the genome was distributed in several bins (average bin size ~54 kb) and the amount of sequence reads mapping uniquely to each bin was calculated. These digital signals of each bin are then used to estimate the DNA copy number state of the bin using, actually, principles very similar to aCGH analysis where, instead of a probe's signal, the read depth across a genomic bin is applied (e.g. Fig. 2.4). Before copy number prediction, Navin *et al.* first corrected these focal read-depth signals for GC content-dependent WGA bias [1]. Unfortunately, however, a comprehensive representation of the sensitivity and specificity of the method for the detection of copy number variants in single cells is lacking, as well as a robust method to discriminate true copy number changes from WGA artefacts. Furthermore, the detection of structural variants like inversions and translocations is still not efficiently feasible using their method.

Besides full-genome sequencing, parts of the genome can be selected for targeted sequencing by using, for example, DNA pull-down approaches. Even all exons can be cherry-picked from a DNA library for sequencing, which is also known as exome sequencing. Since the exons only represent ~1% of a genome, multiple exomes can be sequenced in a multiplexed reaction at the same cost and time-span as required for one full genome sequence. Xu *et al.* [23] and Hou *et al.* [19] recently investigated subclonal single nucleotide mutations in a renal carcinoma and a myeloproliferative neoplasm respectively by single-cell exome sequencing. Following sequence library preparation of single-cell MDA products, the DNA molecules representing the exons were captured and sequenced. However, despite the proofreading of the φ29 polymerase, WGA nucleotide copy-errors, allelic WGA amplification bias as well as sequencing errors prohibited the detection of mutations present in only one diploid or polyploid cell. Only mutations detected recursively in at least 3–5 single-cell exomes could be called. Detecting the same variant across multiple cells increases the reliability of the variant and allows discriminating it from a WGA artefact.

In contrast to diploid or polyploid cells, WGA products of single haploid cells can be used for *de novo* mutation detection [2]. In these cases WGA nucleotide copy errors can be discriminated from true base variants in the cell, because no heterozygous base variants are to be expected for unique loci in a haploid cell. Wang *et al.* [2] also profiled DNA copy number landscapes of single-spermatozoa sequences, but these were very low resolution and at best comparable to the resolution of aCGH.

Haplotype reconstruction from genotyped single-cell WGA products

The ability to characterize a single-cell genome for its copy number and SNP profile offers a stepping-stone towards the development of a generic method for preimplantation genetic diagnosis (PGD). This diagnosis is offered to couples that wish to circumvent the transmission of heritable genetic defects to their offspring [26]. However, not all couples can be helped via the current PGD strategies – e.g. couples burdened with a complex chromosomal rearrangement (CCR) – and current routine methods for chromosome analysis still result in carrier offspring – e.g. distinguishing between an embryo that carries an inherited balanced translocation or has a normal karyotype is not normally available off the shelf.

While DNA imbalances resulting from unbalanced translocations or CCRs can be detected in a single blastomere using the technologies described above, the ability to SNP genotype a single blastomere also enables reconstruction of the haplotype of the cell's entire genome, provided that genotype information from close relatives is available. As a consequence, this allows following the segregation of any disease allele in a pedigree using genetic linkage principles, and thus the development of a generic approach for PGD (Fig. 2.5). Indeed, a haplotype represents the genetic variants that are present on the same stretch of DNA and can be determined *in silico* from observed genotype data. Such a method would not only replace labor-intensive locus and family-specific PCR or fluorescence *in situ* hybridization (FISH) designs required in current PGD practice in IVF centers worldwide, but also opens the daunting capability to select embryos for many Mendelian traits at once as well as for risk factor, polygenic, or complex disease variants, which are increasingly being uncovered in recent genome-wide association studies. A genome-wide single-cell haplotyping approach not only can determine the parental origin of DNA copy number alterations, like that offered by the Parental Support algorithm, but it can also distinguish in copy-neutral scenarios the presence of a genetic risk allele on the homologous chromosomes of the potential offspring. The latter is possible, by observing the SNPs linked with the genetic risk allele in the embryo or putative offspring and, as such, the parental haplotype block demarcated by two homologous recombination sites, or a homologous recombination site and a chromosomal end, in which the risk allele is embedded (see below).

One step in this direction has been made with the development of karyomapping [9]. This method allows following the inheritance of alleles from the parents to the zygote as well as the segregation of the inherited alleles in the embryo. To this end, single-blastomere SNP genotypes are phased according to parental and sibling genotype information determined by SNP array analysis. For SNP genotyping of the individual cells (amplified by MDA) as well as the parental and sibling non-WGA DNA, the authors applied Illumina HumanCNV370 arrays of which the hybridization signals were converted to genotypes using Illumina's BeadStudio software. To avoid errors caused by ADO, karyomap analysis was restricted to those informative SNP loci which were heterozygous in the cell being analyzed. Although this decreased the resolution of the obtained karyomap, recombination sites

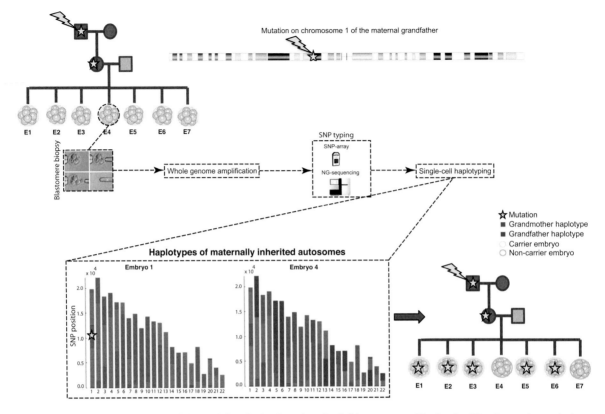

Figure 2.5 A schematic overview of the workflow for haplotyping single blastomeres of *in vitro* fertilization embryos. In the depicted pedigree, a blue color represents the grandfather's homologous chromosomes and a red color represents the grandmother's homologous chromosomes in the maternal lineage of an embryo. After a single blastomere biopsy of the Day 3 cleavage-stage embryos and genotyping of the whole genome amplification (WGA) products, single-cell haplotypes can be deduced. Following haplotyping of the single blastomere genotypes, the homologous recombinations that occurred between the homologous chromosomes in maternal meiosis I are revealed by the transitions of red and blue haplotype blocks on the maternally inherited chromosomes. The X-axis represents the 22 autosomes and the Y-axis represents the relative SNP position along the chromosome. The transmission of the genetic risk allele (depicted as a star) can now be tracked through the pedigree, and carrier embryos (embryos 1, 2, 3, 5, and 6) as well as non-carrier embryos (embryos 4 and 7) can be identified. See plate section for color version.

between parental homologous chromosomes could still be accurately identified genome wide. The method was validated using DNA samples of two families segregating mutations in the *CFTR* gene. In the first family, two children were affected by cystic fibrosis and were compound heterozygous carriers of the parental mutations, while three other siblings were unaffected. Using non-preamplified DNA of the children and parents, the sibling's haplotypes were determined using SNP genotyping and karyomapping. Subsequently, the haplotypes of five individual EBV-transformed lymphoblastoid cells of a child not affected by cystic fibrosis were aligned with the haplotype determined from the respective non-WGA DNA sample to demonstrate the accuracy of karyomapping. Similarly, in the second family, both parents were carriers of a p.F508del

mutation and, following PGD, five preimplantation embryos, which were not selected for transfer, were applied to evaluate the technology. The PGD result could be confirmed by karyomapping DNA from embryo biopsies. In addition, karyomapping allowed detecting chromosome aneuploidies and their parental origin.

Conclusion

A variety of WGA methods, genome-wide analysis platforms, and algorithms have been developed allowing the detection of primarily megabase-sized copy number aberrations and/or genotyping SNPs in a single cell. However, robust methods for *de novo* discovery of submicroscopic copy number variants, structural variants, and base mutations still need to be established. Besides WGA artefacts burdening downstream analyses of the cell, biological characteristics of the cell itself may affect its analysis. For instance, since a genetic snapshot of a diploid cell in S phase will demonstrate alternating loci of copy number state 2, 3, or 4, it is imperative to investigate to what extent cell-cycle status may introduce aberrations in DNA copy number profiles of individual cells. Furthermore, since WGA is performed on a lysed cell rather than purified DNA, WGA of the same genome in cells of a different type may be slightly altered and even render single-cell WGA products biased according to cell type. Hence, we have an exciting number of years ahead to tackle these challenges.

References

1. Navin N, Kendall J, Troge J *et al*. Tumour evolution inferred by single-cell sequencing. *Nature* 2011; 472: 90–4.

2. Wang J, Fan HC, Behr B *et al*. Genome-wide single-cell analysis of recombination activity and *de novo* mutation rates in human sperm. *Cell* 2012; 150: 402–12.

3. Vanneste E, Voet T, Le Caignec C *et al*. Chromosome instability is common in human cleavage-stage embryos. *Nat Med* 2009; 15: 577–83.

4. Voullaire L, Wilton L, McBain J *et al*. Chromosome abnormalities identified by comparative genomic hybridization in embryos from women with repeated implantation failure. *Mol Hum Reprod* 2002; 8: 1035–41.

5. Le Caignec C, Spits C, Sermon K *et al*. Single-cell chromosomal imbalances detection by array CGH. *Nucleic Acids Res* 2006; 34: e68.

6. Fiegler H, Geigl JB, Langer S *et al*. High resolution array-CGH analysis of single cells. *Nucleic Acids Res* 2007; 35: e15.

7. Iwamoto K, Bundo M, Ueda J *et al*. Detection of chromosomal structural alterations in single cells by SNP arrays: a systematic survey of amplification bias and optimized workflow. *PLoS One* 2007; 2: e1306.

8. Geigl JB, Obenauf AC, Waldispuehl-Geigl J *et al*. Identification of small gains and losses in single cells after whole genome amplification on tiling oligo arrays. *Nucleic Acids Res* 2009; 37: e105.

9. Handyside AH, Harton GL, Mariani B *et al*. Karyomapping: a universal method for genome-wide analysis of genetic disease based on mapping crossovers between parental haplotypes. *J Med Genet* 2010; 47: 651–8.

10. Johnson DS, Gemelos G, Baner J *et al*. Preclinical validation of a microarray method for full molecular karyotyping of blastomeres in a 24-h protocol. *Hum Reprod* 2010; 25: 1066–75.

11. Treff NR, Su J, Tao X *et al*. Accurate single cell 24 chromosome aneuploidy screening using whole genome amplification and single nucleotide polymorphism microarrays. *Fertil Steril* 2010; 94: 2017–21.

12. Alfarawati S, Fragouli E, Colls P *et al*. First births after preimplantation genetic diagnosis of structural chromosome abnormalities using comparative genomic hybridization and microarray analysis. *Hum Reprod* 2011; 26: 1560–74.

13. Fiorentino F, Spizzichino L, Bono S *et al*. PGD for reciprocal and Robertsonian translocations using array comparative genomic hybridization. *Hum Reprod* 2011; 26: 1925–35.

14. Gutiérrez-Mateo C, Colls P, Sanchez-Garcia J *et al*. Validation of microarray comparative genomic hybridization for comprehensive chromosome analysis of embryos. *Fertil Steril* 2011; 95: 953–8.

15. Rius M, Daina G, Obradors A *et al*. Comprehensive embryo analysis of advanced maternal age-related aneuploidies and mosaicism by short comparative genomic hybridization. *Fertil Steril* 2011; 95: 413–16.

16. Treff NR, Su J, Tao X *et al*. Single-cell whole-genome amplification technique impacts the accuracy of SNP microarray-based genotyping and copy number analyses. *Mol Hum Reprod* 2011; 17: 335–43.

17. Voet T, Vanneste E, Van der Aa N *et al*. Breakage-fusion-bridge cycles leading to inv dup del occur in human cleavage stage embryos. *Hum Mutat* 2011; 32: 783–93.

18. Bi WM, Breman A, Shaw CA *et al*. Detection of ≥ 1 Mb microdeletions and microduplications in a single cell using custom oligonucleotide arrays. *Prenat Diagn* 2012; 32: 10–20.

19. Hou Y, Song L, Zhu P *et al*. Single-cell exome sequencing and monoclonal evolution of a JAK2-negative myeloproliferative neoplasm. *Cell* 2012; 148: 873–85.

20. Konings P, Vanneste E, Jackmaert S *et al*. Microarray analysis of copy number variation in single cells. *Nat Protoc* 2012; 7: 281–310.

21. Rabinowitz M, Ryan A, Gemelos G *et al*. Origins and rates of aneuploidy in human blastomeres. *Fertil Steril* 2012; 97: 395–401.

22. van Uum CM, Stevens SJ, Dreesen JC *et al*. SNP array-based copy number and genotype analyses for preimplantation genetic diagnosis of human unbalanced translocations. *Eur J Hum Genet* 2012; 20: 938–44.

23. Xu X, Hou Y, Yin X *et al.* Single-cell exome sequencing reveals single-nucleotide mutation characteristics of a kidney tumor. *Cell* 2012; 148: 886–95.

24. Spits C, Le Caignec C, De Rycke M *et al.* Optimization and evaluation of single-cell whole-genome multiple displacement amplification. *Hum Mutat* 2006; 27: 496–503.

25. Lasken RS, Stockwell TB. Mechanism of chimera formation during the Multiple Displacement Amplification reaction. *BMC Biotechnol* 2007; 7: 19.

26. Sermon K, Van Steirteghem A, Liebaers I. Preimplantation genetic diagnosis. *Lancet* 2004; 363: 1633–41.

Meiosis
How to get a good start in life

Ursula Eichenlaub-Ritter

Introduction

Meiosis comprises fundamental processes that permit sexual reproduction and species evolution. Indeed, in addition to producing haploid gametes, it provides a stochastic distribution of maternally and paternally inherited chromosomes, which undergo allelic recombination. Thus it generates diversity within the population, and is essential for the formation of euploid germ cells that will contribute to a euploid, healthy embryo after fertilization. Meiosis is therefore the basis for maintaining genomic integrity, high developmental potential, and health of the embryo and offspring, and normal fertility in males and females [1]. This chapter will introduce the principles underlying the meiotic process including pairing and recombination, chromosome segregation at meiosis I and meiosis II, and formation of oocytes and sperm that will form a euploid embryo after fertilization. Since many of the genes in meiosis are highly conserved between species, the chapter will also give a brief overview on experimental studies. Sexual dimorphism that contributes to gender-specific predisposition to disturbances is briefly discussed. This may increase risks for specific chromosomal aberrations in oogenesis or spermatogenesis (for instance, aneuploidy, predivision, or genomic instability), as well as meiotic delay, arrest, or cell death that cause subfertility or infertility.

Principles of chromosome segregation at meiosis

During mitosis of a diploid cell there is typically one round of replication of all chromosomes during the S phase. The separation of chromatids at mitotic division results therefore in the formation of two diploid daughter cells, each containing a set of originally maternally and paternally derived chromosomes (see Chapter 1 and Fig. 3.1A). In contrast, to obtain haploid gametes for fertilization in meiosis two consecutive meiotic divisions occur after only one S phase resulting in formation of four haploid gametes (Fig. 3.1B) that can form a diploid zygote after fertilization. Meiosis, with these two specialized divisions, takes place during germ-cell formation of most sexually reproducing animals not only in order to obtain haploid gametes but also gametes and zygotes with new combinations of genes from the originally maternally and paternally derived chromosomes (Fig. 3.1B,C). So, in terms of DNA content, meiosis allows the germ cell to go from 2N to 4N and to end with 1N DNA (Fig. 3.1B). At prophase I of meiosis, homologous chromosomes originally obtained from father (gray in Fig. 3.1B) and mother (black in Fig. 3.1B) first pair side-by-side and there is usually at least one genetic exchange (crossover) between chromatids of the two homologs (in non-sister chromatids) that results in recombination. This is visible by the presence of one or several chiasmata at late prophase I to metaphase I of meiosis I on the bivalent chromosomes (Fig. 3.1B). At meiosis I a reductional division of the homologous chromosomes derived originally from father and mother occurs at anaphase I (Fig. 3.1B). Separation at first meiosis occurs by chiasma resolution to release the physical attachment between homologs. Then the homologs with both of their sister chromatids separate from each other. This leads to two cells with only half the number of chromosomes at meiosis II (2N). Unlike in the mitotic G_1 phase, each daughter cell from the first meiotic division contains either only the maternally or the paternally derived chromosome with its two sister chromatids, except for parts that were

---

Textbook of Human Reproductive Genetics, eds Karen Sermon and Stéphane Viville. Published by Cambridge University Press.

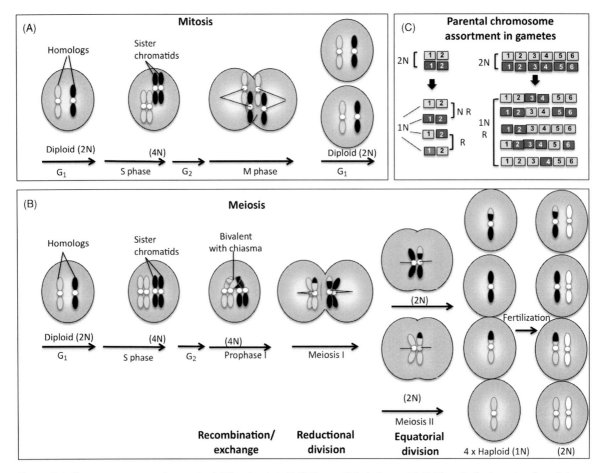

Figure 3.1 Chromosome segregation at mitosis (**A**) and meiosis (**B,C**). Gray and black chromatids (**A,B**) symbolize homologs from father and mother. Note, during mitotic M phase/anaphase sister chromatids disjoin (**A**), while in meiosis I the two homologous maternally and paternally derived chromosomes separate from each other reductionally with both of their sister chromatids (**B**). New assortment of originally paternally and maternally derived chromosomes (2N, diploid status) in gametes (1N, haploid after reductional separation) (**C**), NR: non-recombinant; R: recombinant. For further explanation, see text.

intrachromosomally exchanged. In meiosis II, which commences without an intervening S phase, the two sister chromatids of each homolog separate (termed "equatorial division") to form four haploid gametes (Fig. 3.1B). The latter contain only one chromatid of each chromosome with genes (alleles) derived from either father or mother (Fig. 3.1C), except for parts where an exchange occured between non-sister chromatids [1]. The haploid gametes can subsequently form a chromosomally normal diploid zygote (2N) after fertilization with a single haploid set of chromosomes (white and gray/black in Fig. 3.1B) from gametes of both sexes and are thus forming a euploid (diploid) embryo (2N).

Since different chromosomes randomly segregate to either one or the other daughter cell at anaphase

I, the haploid gametes can contain a new assortment of the different originally maternally and paternally derived chromosomes (Fig. 3.1C). By random separation and assortment of different parental chromosomes (e.g. chromosomes 1 and 2, left side of Fig. 3.1C) at meiosis I, two gametes with only two maternal or two paternal chromatids are formed (non-recombinants, NR in Fig. 3.1C) plus two gametes (50%) which are recombinant (R in Fig. 3.1C). The latter possess one maternal and one paternal chromosome each. According to the number of chromosomes in the haploid complement therefore 2^N (N referring to haploid chromosome number) of recombinant gametes can be formed (another example is shown on the left side of Fig. 3.1C with six chromosomes and various recombinant gametes). In the human the random distribution of homologs from father or mother can result in the formation of 2^{23} combinations of parental chromosomes, so more than eight million different gametes.

Key events in meiosis

Meiotic entry

Determination of the fate to enter female or male meiosis is not triggered by the sex of the primordial germ cell, i.e. the precursor of the gamete. Instead meiosis is regulated by the sex of the somatic cells in the fetal gonads. Without a Y chromosome containing sex-determining genes, an ovary and oocytes are formed [2]. After migration of the primordial germ cells to the fetal gonads, some mitotic divisions occur in both sexes. One of the key factors in gamete formation and initiation of meiosis is Dazl (or human DAZ ortholog), an RNA-binding protein. Another gene involved in meiotic entry and expressed at different times in the female and male gonads is *Stra8* (Stimulated by Retinoic Acid gene 8), a transcription factor and protein required for premeiotic DNA replication. Furthermore, retinoic acid receptors regulate gene expression in the developing gamete, and the CYP26B1 enzyme that oxidizes retinoic acid (RA) to transcriptionally non-active metabolites is also important (reviewed in [2, 3]).

In the mouse, RA concentration is high in the fetal female gonad and induces alterations in gene expression through the *Stra8* transcription factor in the expression of genes important for meiosis. This occurs already in the fetal ovary when mitotically dividing oogonia are first formed which then enter meiosis and form primary oocytes (Fig. 3.2). In the human fetal ovary, meiosis is initiated between 8 and 13 weeks of gestation (left side, Fig. 3.2). Meiosis becomes arrested two times in oogenesis: first after completion of prophase I when primary oocytes enter interphase and become surrounded by granulosa cells in primordial follicles (Fig. 3.2; Table 3.1). Meiosis continues and becomes completed only after oocyte growth in a few or single oocytes at each cycle (in monoovulatory species like human only in one oocyte) from puberty to the end of the reproductive period. The second meiotic arrest is after maturation to metaphase II and ovulation (Fig. 3.2). Meiosis in the female is only completed after fertilization by sperm. It is unknown whether resumption of maturation occurs in the same order as

the oocytes entered meiosis in fetal life, according to a "production line."

Retinoic acid is also produced in the fetal testis. However, due to the presence of a Y chromosome, somatic cells of the testis express CYP26B1, that inactivates RA. Retinoic acid levels remain locally low, and *Stra8* is not induced. Precursor germ cells therefore remain arrested in the mitotic G_0 stage and do not enter meiosis until after birth at puberty when RA concentration rises (Fig. 3.2). In contrast to the female, mitotic divisions of spermatogonia followed by meiosis in the primary and secondary spermatocytes occurs continuously in the male from puberty until old age (right side, Fig. 3.2). During spermiogenesis complex morphogenetic processes and compaction of chromatin occur before sperm become competent to fertilize an oocyte (Fig. 3.2 and Table 3.1).

The relationship between meiosis initiation, RA signaling, and resumption of meiosis in adult life in humans remains to be further elucidated [3]. The differences in meiotic entry have a profound impact on fertility since all oocytes ever to become ovulated initiate meiosis already prior to birth in the female. In human and most mammals the pool becomes reduced and even depleted by oocyte death and follicular atresia prior to and after birth and throughout the reproductive period. This restricts fertile life in the human female to the time when the pool of primordial follicles has reached a critical size. Thus oocytes are amongst the most long-lived cells in the body, entering meiosis in the embryo and completing it decades later.

Chromosome pairing and formation of the synaptonemal complex

Meiosis is characterized by an extended prophase I in preparation for the first reductional chromosome segregation in both sexes. In male and female meiosis, during the meiotic prophase I, homologous chromosomes replicate, pair, synapse, and recombine, which is a prerequisite for faithful chromosome segregation at the first and second meiotic divisions (Fig. 3.3). After the premeiotic S phase, chromosomes start to condense at the leptotene stage and homologs begin to pair (Fig. 3.3). This is facilitated by attachment of the chromosome ends, the telomeres, to the inner nuclear membrane, which then glide to achieve a gradual assembly at one side of the nuclear envelope during the following meiotic stages. This eventually results in

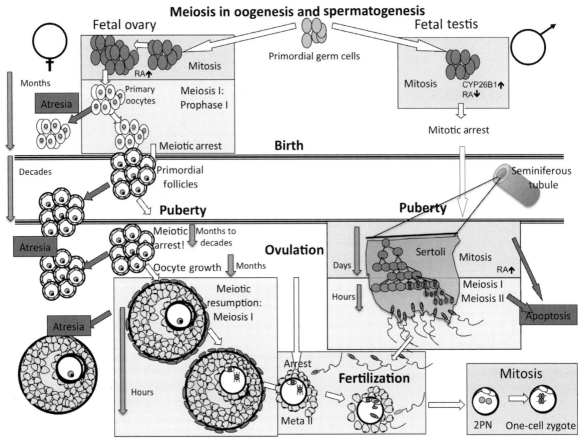

Figure 3.2 Germ-cell formation and timing of meiosis in oogenesis (left side) and spermatogenesis (right side). For further explanation, see text. See plate section for color version.

clustering in a "bouquet"-like arrangement with chromosome ends all close to each other (Fig. 3.3). During zygotene, the process of chromosome condensation and pairing continues until homologs with their two sister chromatids are fully paired (synapsis) at the pachytene stage. In male meiosis, telomeres of all homologs are attached to the nuclear membrane next to a morphologically distinct site in the nucleus, the sex body. The sex body contains the transcriptionally inactive X and Y chromosomes that are only partially paired. Pairing occurs in a region of the sex chromosomes which contains homologous genes, termed the "pseudoautosomal region" (PAR) [3]. In the diplotene stage, the homologs lose contacts all along chromosome arms while the two sister chromatids remain glued to each other. Therefore, homologs separate from each other except at the sites where recombination (crossover) and exchanges occurred.

These sites of exchange are cytologically recognized as chiasmata that physically attach homologous chromosomes (Figs 3.1 and 3.3). Further meiotic progression is at diakinesis when the nuclear membrane breaks down, chromosomes continue to condense, and the centromeres of the homologs become attached to spindle fibers. In female meiosis, oocytes become arrested after the diplotene stage, when chromosomes decondense and primary oocytes remain blocked in the dictyate stage within primordial follicles (Fig. 3.2). Meiosis remains arrested until oocytes have fully grown in the adult, sexually mature female.

The synaptonemal complex (SC) is a meiosis-specific large proteinaceous structure that plays an important role in the organization of chromatin, and the deposition and activity of a structural framework for pairing and recombination in meiotic prophase I

Table 3.1 Differences between mitosis and meiosis and male and female meiosis

	Mitosis	Male meiosis	Female meiosis
Location	All tissues	Testis	Ovary
Product	Diploid somatic cell	4 haploid sperm from each spermatocyte	One metaphase II arrested oocyte and one PB at ovulation/ haploid oocyte that also contains sperm chromatin and second PB after fertilization
DNA replication	One S phase between each division	One S phase before two subsequent meiotic divisions	One S phase before two subsequent meiotic divisions
Cell cycle	Usually continuous from S phase to G_1 phase in absence of disturbances	Uninterrupted progression from prophase I to completion of meiosis, and from round spermatid to mature sperm	Interrupted at two stages: first arrest after completion of prophase I up to diplotene (in dictyate stage); resumption of meiosis after growth and acquisition of maturational competence up to metaphase II; second arrest at metaphase II; completion of meiosis II only after fertilization
Duration	Usually short prophase and M phase of about 30 min to 1 hour	Days in male meiosis	Days to months in prophase I in fetal ovary; meiotic arrrest up to several decades in dictyate stage; about 36 hours for resumption of maturation to ovulation *in vivo*
Time in life	Throughout embryonic, fetal, and adult life	From puberty throughout reproductive period up to death	Begins in fetal ovary, followed by arrest until puberty and sequential resumption from puberty to menopause/depletion of primordial follicle pool
Pairing	Usually no pairing	Pairing between all homologs; X/Y pairing in pseudoautosomal region of the heterologous gonosomes. Unpaired regions inactivated	Pairing of all autosomal chromosomes; reactivation of the second X chromosome and full pairing and recombination between both X chromosomes
Recombination	Some sister chromatid exchange; usually no recombination; aberrant recombination may be induced by adverse conditions	Usually at least one exchange between all autosomal homologs and an obligatory exchange between the gonosomes in the pseudoautosomal region	Usually at least one crossover and exchange between all autosomal homologs and between the two X chromosomes; overall more interstitial and higher recombination rates in female meiosis compared to male meiosis
Daughter cells	Two genetically identical cells	Four haploid sperm containing different combinations of chromosomes from each parent and recombinant chromatids with some maternally and paternally derived alleles	One diploid and one haploid first and second PB, and a haploid set of chromatids in the egg after fertilization comprising different combinations of chromatids from each parent as well as recombinant chromatids with some maternally and paternally derived alleles
Size	Similar or different size, depending on type of division (equal or unequal/ symmetric or asymmetric) and tissue	Four sperm of same size containing highly condensed chromatin in nucleus and little cytoplasm with some specific organelles for fertilization (e.g. acrosome, sperm tail, Nebenkern with mitochondria)	Asymmetric divisions at meiosis I; formation of one small PB and one large oocyte arrested at metaphase II that contains an eccentrically localized spindle with well-aligned chromosomes and cytoplasm with maternal products for early development as well as numerous organelles (e.g. cortical granules, large numbers of mitochondria). Oocyte surrounded by a thick extracellular coat (the Zona pellucida). Fertilization triggers second asymmetric divsion and second PB formation
Chromosome errors	Nondisjunction is very rare	Aneuploidy from meiotic errors is usually low (1–4%) and especially involves gonosomes and short chromosomes. No or minor increase with paternal age	Aneuploidy from meiotic errors is common in oocytes (average 20%), and risks for errors increase exponentially with advanced maternal age, then involving frequently more than one chromosome

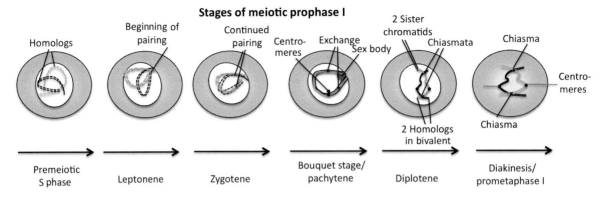

Figure 3.3 Chromosome pairing and chiasma formation during prophase I of meiosis. For further explanation, see text.

of both sexes (for references, see [4]). Structurally, the synaptonemal complex (SC) is highly conserved between plant and animal cells. It consists of three main morphologically recognizable components first identified by electron microscopy: outer electron-dense lateral or axial elements (LE) and an inner central element (CE) (Fig. 3.4A). In the space between the lateral and central element, transversal fibers are usually recognizable (Fig. 3.4A). The SC formation proceeds in distinct steps: the lateral protein axes (LE) are formed during leptotene on which loops of chromatin of each paternal and maternal homolog each with two chromatids (light and dark blue and green, chr 1 and chr 2 in Fig. 3.4A, respectively) become organized. The two sister chromatids (chr 1 and chr 2) are physically connected to each other and to the lateral elements by cohesion complexes (red rings in Fig. 3.4A). From leptotene to zygotene the transversal fibers interact with each other and the central element of the synaptonemal complex is formed. In the center of the SC, protein complexes assemble (gray ovals in Fig. 3.4A). Pairing often proceeds in a zipper-like fashion, starting from chromosome ends at the site of attachment at the inner membrane of the nuclear envelope (NE; Fig. 3.4B). In pachytene homologs are fully paired (synapsed) (Fig. 3.4A). The SC with the LE and the inner CE and some ladder-like transversal fibers extends at this stage from one end to the other of each pair of homologous chromosomes. Many components of the SC, like the synaptonemal proteins SYCP1 to SYCP3, SYCE1 to SYCE3, and TEX12 (depicted in Fig. 3.4A), have now been identified [4].

Ultrastructural analysis by electron microscopy revealed also the presence of electron-dense, knobby structures on top of the SC termed "recombination nodules" (RN green ovals in Fig. 3.4A). The latter contain recombination enzymes. At late prophase I, the RNs appear spaced at a distance from each other along the chromosome axis consistent with sites where exchanges occur and chiasmata are present. The relative length of the SC in the fully synapsed state corresponds to the relative length of the different chromosomes. The RN numbers are related to SC length and chromatin conformation status, species, and sex, as are the chiasmata [5, 6].

Meiotic recombination

Studies in model organisms have provided information on highly conserved mechanisms and molecules in intrachromosomal meiotic recombination, and a road map of events that mediate genetic exchange, homologous recombination, and formation of chromosomally balanced but genetically different germ cells (Fig. 3.4B). In short, meiotic recombination is initiated by homology search and homologous pairing of DNA molecules from the originally maternally and paternally derived homologous chromosomes. An essential next step is the introduction of DNA double-strand breaks (DSBs) into one of the chromatids of a homolog containing just one DNA double helix (step 1 in Fig. 3.4B) [7]. This involves activity of meiosis-specific recombination enzymes (e.g. SPO11) [7]. Specific sites on DNA with open chromatin (hot spots) and enzymes for histone methylation appear essential for male and female meiosis (for references, see [7, 8]). Other complexes of conserved proteins are involved in the next steps in recombination: strand invasion in which one single strand of nucleotides invades the double strand of a chromatid of the other homolog

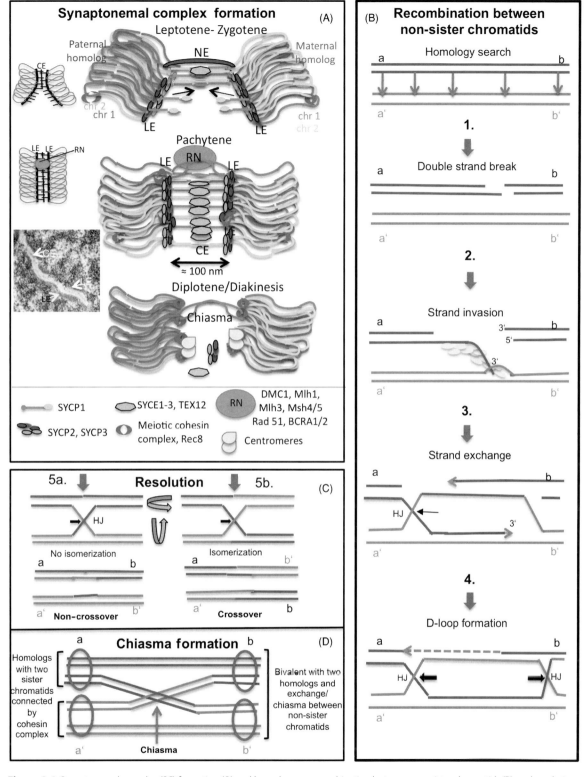

Figure 3.4 Synaptonemal complex (SC) formation (**A**) and homologous recombination between non-sister chromatids (**B**), and resolution of recombination after non-crossover or crossover (**C**), and chiasama formation (**D**). DNA strands from parental homologs are symbolized by different colors (blue and green, respectively). Proteins involved in the SC (**A**) in lateral elements (LE) with SYCP2 and 3 proteins, central element (CE) containing SYCE1–3 and TEX12 proteins, cohesion (red clips) with meiotic Rec8 cohesin that physically attach the sister chromatids to each other or to the LE, transversal fibers (orange) containing SYCP1 protein, and recombination nodules (RN) containing recombination enzymes (DMC1, Mlh1, Mlh3, Msh4/5, Rad 51, BCRA1/2) are presented. Chr 1 and Chr 2: sister chromatids in paternal and maternal homolog. Left: top view, right tangential section of SC and homologs are depicted at successive stage of prophase I (**A**). Events in recombination between non-sister chromatids (steps 1.–4. and 5a. and 5b., in **B** and **C**, respectively) leading to chiasma formation (**D**) are shown. See plate section for color version.

(depicted in step 2 in gray in Fig. 3.4B). Recombinase enzymes can polymerize to form a "presynaptic filament" (shown in yellow in step 2 of Fig. 3.4B) that catalyses binding of the single-stranded DNA, opening of the double strand of the homolog for strand invasion, and exchange (step 3) [7]. Eventually, a D-loop is formed, in which there are two crosses by single-stranded DNA molecules (termed "Holliday Junctions"; HJ in Fig. 3.4B) [7]. The different alleles of homologous genes on two chromatids are depicted in black and gray (a,b and a',b', respectively) in Fig. 3.4B–D. If the crossing is resolved (i.e. cut by nucleases, black arrows in 3.4C) without further change in the conformation of the DNA (panel A in 3.4C; no isomerization) there is only a very small stretch of DNA that contains DNA strands from both partners. However, if the DNA undergoes a conformational change (termed isomerization; indicated by two arrows representing twists around the intercrossed DNA strands) followed by resolution by nucleases (panel B in Fig. 3.4C, black arrow), the two double-stranded DNA molecules in the chromatids have exchanged DNA fragments between the original maternal and paternal chromosomes left and right of the crossover (panel B in Fig. 3.4C).

If the recombinant chromatids are not further physically connected after resolution of the crossover, they would fall apart and might randomly segregate at first meiosis. However, within a bivalent, the two sister chromatids in each homolog are connected by complexes of cohesion proteins (red circles in Fig. 3.4D). Thus, arms and centromeres of sister chromatids are tied together by cohesion proteins (like a glue or rubber band, red ovals in Fig. 3.4D). Physical attachment of homologs in a bivalent is achieved by the cohesion proteins together with the chiasmata located at the sites where crossover occurred. They also help the homologs to attach and orient to opposite spindle poles at first metaphase I and anaphase I of meiosis [9–12].

In conclusion, crossover serves two purposes:

1. Providing for intrachromosomal recombination of originally paternally and maternally derived alleles on non-sister chromatids to form recombinant chromosomes.
2. Physically attaching the two homologs such that they can stably align on the spindle, with centromeres of each homolog's sister chromatid attaching to only one spindle pole.

Number and localization of crossovers

There is evidence that the number of DNA double-strand breaks that are initially introduced far exceeds the rate of crossover and exchanges in a meiocyte. Sites of true crossovers can be identified by staining with antibody to DNA repair proteins like MLH1, components of the recombination nodules in pachytene and diplotene stage (Fig. 3.4C), or by examining the numbers and localization of chiasmata at diakinesis and prometaphase I. In combination with fluorescence *in situ* hybrization (FISH) to identify individual chromosomes, this has been used to characterize the events at meiotic prophase I in human oocytes and spermatocytes [5, 6]. This showed that on average about 50 crossovers are characteristic for human spermatocytes and about 50–70 for human oocytes. Recombination "hot spots," where double-strand breaks occur frequently, appear conserved between species and have been recently mapped in the mouse; however, the distribution of double-strand breaks maturing to a chiasma differs between sexes and their distribution can also differ greatly between individual meiocytes. Analysis of fetal oocytes revealed an unexpected high number of oocytes with pairing failures at early meiotic stages [5]. When oocytes containing such chromosomes that are not stabilized by chiasmata, survive to metaphase I, the single, physically non-connected homologs (termed "univalents," Fig. 3.5C) have a high risk of undergoing meiotic errors at meiosis I.

Although the number of intrachromosomal exchanges by crossover may differ greatly between individuals and individual meiocytes, the numbers of exchanges appears overall similar and characteristic for each species and gender. Chiasmata are usually spaced and not formed in the immediate vicinity of each other. This has been termed "chiasma interference." Generally it is known that the longer the chromosome, the more likely it will have several chiasmata. The likelihood of inheriting a chromatid with a new combination of originally paternally or maternally derived alleles is thus dependent on the relative distance of the genes/alleles on the chromosome. The analysis of the frequency of recombination between two genes on one chromosome by markers and phenotype of the offspring can therefore be used to construct a recombination map following traits in subsequent generations [1]. While the recombination rate between genes on different chromosomes is 50%, because segregation is random it becomes lower

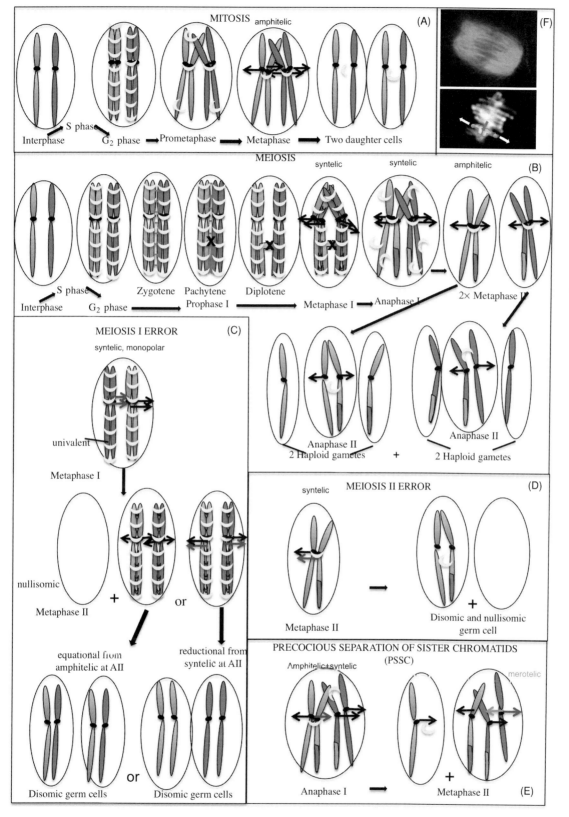

Figure 3.5 Loss of cohesion along sister chromatid arms and centromeres and attachment to spindles (arrows) in mitosis (**A**) and meiosis (**B–F**). Homologs with their two sister chromatids are colored in blue and red, respectively (**A–E**), cohesion complexes between sister chromatids in yellow and exchanges by crossover/chiasmata by black X (**B**). Aberrant chromosome attachment/orientation is indicated by

when genes are located close to each other on one chromosome. Certain areas of the chromosomes are particularly accessible for recombination enzymes and form recombination hot spots. One such recombination hot spot is on the pseudoautosomal region of the X and Y chromosomes where they share homology. In male meiosis, an obligatory exchange provides for the presence of a chiasma physically linking the sex chromosomes. This is important for the separation of the X from the Y chromosome at first meiosis of spermatogenesis [3]. In oogenesis, the two X chromosomes pair all along their length and may possess chiasmata on long and short chromosome arms.

Role of chromosome cohesion in meiosis

At prophase of mitosis and meiosis I (Fig. 3.5C), sister chromatid arms become attached to each other by complexes of cohesin proteins (yellow clamps in Fig. 3.5). This occurs usually already at or prior to S phase [11] (Fig. 3.4C). While in mitosis arm cohesion is lost already at late prometaphase, the chromatids in homologous chromosomes in meiosis remain physically attached to each other by chiasmata until anaphase I. Thus, cohesion complexes between sister chromatids' arms and centromeres of homologs are present throughout meiotic prometaphase I (e.g. zygotene, pachytene, diplotene) and metaphase I (Fig. 3.5B). At first anaphase the cohesin complexes at the arms but not at the centromeres of chromatids in the homologs are released by proteolytic cleavage of meiotic cohesion proteins (Fig. 3.5B) [11–13]. This results in resolution of chiasmata and provides for homolog separation at anaphase I. However, it is essential that the two sister chromatids within each homolog remain attached to each other at their centromeres by cohesion complexes throughout first and second meiosis until anaphase II (Fig. 3.5B), unlike in mitosis where they separate at each division (Fig. 3.5A).

In first meiosis, the centromeres of both sister chromatids attach to only one spindle pole (termed syntelic, Fig. 3.5B). In contrast, the centromeres of the two sister chromatids attach to opposite spindle poles at metaphase II (amphitelic, right side of Fig. 3.5B).

The loss of cohesion between sister centromeres at anaphase II allows sister chromatids to disjoin and segregate from each other to form four haploid germ cells (lower part of Fig. 3.5B) [1, 11–13].

If there is no recombination or when the cohesion between arms of sister chromatids in homologous chromosomes is lost and chiasmata precociously become resolved, pairs of homologs termed "univalent chromosomes" are present at metaphase I (Fig. 3.5C). Such physically unattached univalents have a high risk of attaching to the same spindle poles instead of migrating to opposite poles (as indicated in top of Fig. 3.5C). If both univalents migrate to the same pole at anaphase I, one of the products will be nullisomic for the respective chromosome (middle of Fig. 3.5C) at metaphase II. The other will contain both homologs. Attachment of sister chromatids to opposite spindle poles (indicated by arrows in metaphase II), will give rise to disomic germ cells that will possess sister chromatids from each of their parent (red and blue; Fig. 3.5C, left side). When the univalents separate by chance because both sister chromatids become attached to only one spindle pole (right side of Fig. 3.5C) the disomic germ cell products will contain two chromatids of only the maternally or paternally derived chromosome (indicated by red and blue color).

If chromatid cohesion is lost precociously at meiosis I on chromosome arms (precocious separation of sister chromatids, PSSC, also termed "predivision") (Fig. 3.5D), two sister chromatids of one or both univalent chromosomes may attach to opposite spindle poles (amphitelic) at metaphase I instead of at metaphase II [9, 13]. Upon progression to metaphase II this produces a gonocyte with pairs of chromatids or single chromatids (right side of Fig. 3.5D). The single, unattached chromatid or the two chromatids derived from PCCS at meiosis I have a high risk of randomly migrating to one or other spindle pole at anaphase II, and therefore pose a high risk for meiotic errors and formation of aneuploid gametes. If single centromeres attach to both spindle poles (merotelic, blue arrows in Fig. 3.5D), or fail to acquire attachment, normal chromosome migration can be hindered and result

Figure 3.5 (cont.) blue arrows in typical meiotic errors at first meiosis (**C**), second meiosis (**D**), and precocious separation of sister chromatids (PSSC) (**E**), or by green arrow in case of merotelic attachment of one centromere to both spindle poles (**E**). Alignment of bivalents (blue and white) in the spindle (green fluorescence) in mouse meiosis I oocyte (**F**): one condensed bivalent is outlined in blue in which the centromeres of the homologs are attached to opposite spindle poles (white arrows) while the chiasma physically connecting the parental homologs lies at the spindle equator (red arrow). For further explanation, see text. See plate section for color version.

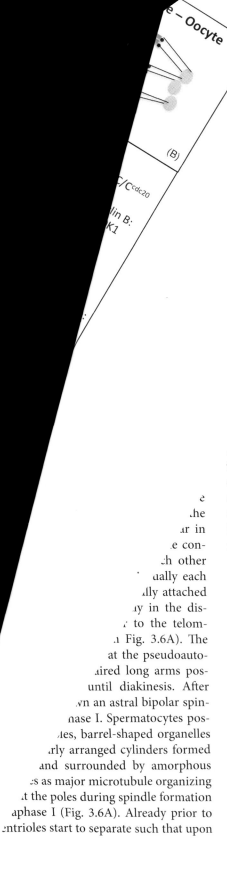

– Oocyte

(B)

C/Ccdc20

lin B:
K1

ne

f the nuclear membrane a short bipolar
⁴v present (for review see [9]). The
⁺es possesses characteristically
ntubules anchor the spin-
tral spindle). During
of each homolog
ers, and the biva-
stable attachment is
A,C) [11, 12]. Attach-
poles leads to alignment
omosome congression").
gs by their centromeres to
auses the first chiasma next
keep the homologs together so
ated at the equator until separa-
J, 12, 13]. Centromeres are located
y from the central spindle, depend-
some length and where the first chi-
ed (Fig. 3.5F). The centromeres of sper-
recruit proteins of the spindle assembly
t (SAC) prior to and at prometaphase I. The
nses unattached chromosomes [14], renders
aphase factor (APC/C) inactive, and will cause
lay or arrest in meiotic progression until proper
achment is achieved (Fig. 3.6C). Spermatocytes are
therefore sensitive to the presence of univalents or disturbances in spindle formation resulting from insufficient chromosome attachment. This safeguards against
errors in chromosome segregation. Prometaphase I is
a fairly long stage in meiosis. Homologs in a bivalent repeatedly reorient until a stable bipolar attachment is achieved. Improper attachments of chromosomes to the spindle are resolved by specific enzymes
(for discussion, see [12, 13]). Sister chromatids remain
attached to each other by cohesion complexes on arms
and centromeres containing meiotic cohesion proteins
like REC8 (indicated in red clamps in Fig. 3.4B and D,
and open or gray circles in Fig. 3.6C) (for references,
see [11–14]). At anaphase of meiosis I, homologs
migrate to two daughter cells. Transiently a nucleus is
formed in spermatogenesis (Fig. 3.2 and the gray in
Fig. 3.6D) before chromosomes recondense, and spermatocytes progress to prometaphase II. Prometaphase
II is usually a short stage in which centromeres of sister
chromatids attach to spindle fibers from opposite poles
(amphitelic attachment) (Figs 3.5B and 3.6D). Once
they congress to the equator and all centromeres are
bipolarly attached to spindle fibers the SAC is released
and anaphase II takes place (Fig. 3.6D). From each
spermatocyte, four haploid gene products are formed

e
he
ar in
e con-
ch other
ually each
lly attached
y in the dis-
to the telom-
Fig. 3.6A). The
at the pseudoauto-
ired long arms pos-
until diakinesis. After
vn an astral bipolar spin-
nase I. Spermatocytes pos-
les, barrel-shaped organelles
rly arranged cylinders formed
and surrounded by amorphous
s as major microtubule organizing
t the poles during spindle formation
aphase I (Fig. 3.6A). Already prior to
entrioles start to separate such that upon

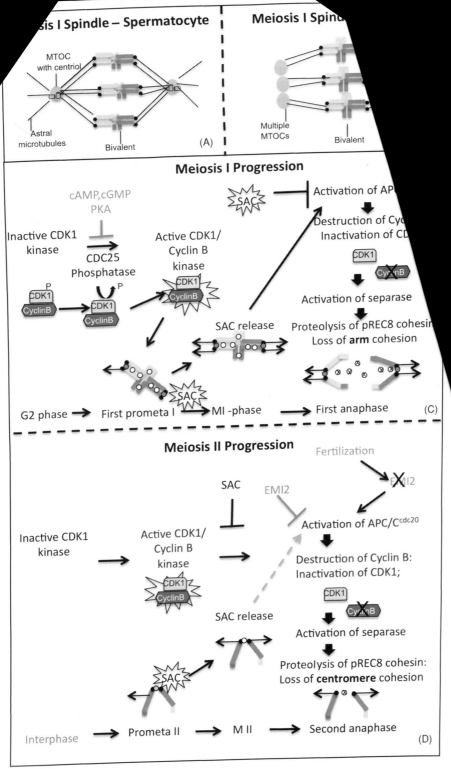

Figure 3.6 Spindles in spermatocytes (astral, **A**), oocytes (unastral, **B**) and major factors driving the cell cycle and sensing chromosom[e] attachment (spindle attachment control, SAC) in meiosis I (**C**) and meiosis II (**D**). Inhibitory pathways/inhibitors that are involved in oogenesis or spermatogenesis are marked in black; pathways that are only active in either spermatogenesis or oogenesis are in gray. CDK1, cyclin-dependent kinase 1; P, phosphorylation; white and gray circles, cohesin complex with phosphorylated REC8 (white) or dephosphorylated REC8 (gray); X indicates proteolytic cleavage/destruction of protein; EMI2, early mitotic inhibitor in meiosis II arrest at oogenesis. For further explanation, see text.

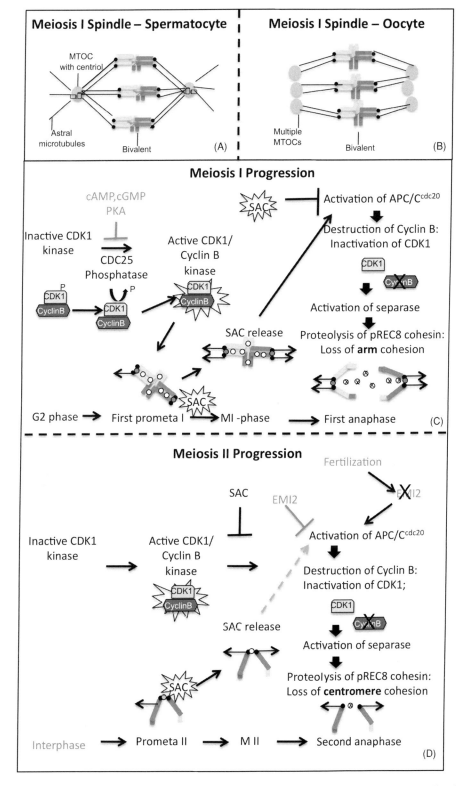

Figure 3.6 Spindles in spermatocytes (astral, **A**), oocytes (unastral, **B**) and major factors driving the cell cycle and sensing chromosome attachment (spindle attachment control, SAC) in meiosis I (**C**) and meiosis II (**D**). Inhibitory pathways/inhibitors that are involved in oogenesis or spermatogenesis are marked in black; pathways that are only active in either spermatogenesis or oogenesis are in gray. CDK1, cyclin-dependent kinase 1; P, phosphorylation; white and gray circles, cohesin complex with phosphorylated REC8 (white) or dephosphorylated REC8 (gray); X indicates proteolytic cleavage/destruction of protein; EMI2, early mitotic inhibitor in meiosis II arrest at oogenesis. For further explanation, see text.

in lagging behind of a chromosome at anaphase I or anaphase II. Thereby it induces chromosome loss or random inclusion in one of the daughter cells.

A meiotic error at anaphase II (Fig. 3.5E) may occur due to a syntelic attachment of sister chromatids, when cohesion fails to be lost in time, or when single chromatids attach randomly to only one spindle pole and segregate together (Fig. 3.5E). The disomic daughter cell from such a typical meiosis II error will usually possess centromeres, chromatids, and alleles of only one of the parental homologs (blue in Fig. 3.5D) except for sites on chromatids that underwent an exchange.

In any case, after fertilization the zygote from a disomic germ cell will contain three chromatids; two chromatids from the aneuploid and one from the euploid germ cell. A nullisomic daughter cell from a first meiotic nondisjunction event or a meiosis II error will form a monosomic embryo after fertilization. Monosomy or trisomy can cause altered gene expression that in most cases results in implantation failures, congenital abnormalities, and spontaneous abortion.

Spindle formation and chromosome segregation at meiosis

Spermatocytes that complete prophase I of meiosis up to the pachytene stage progress without delay to diplotene stage, diakinesis, and first meiotic metaphase (Fig. 3.2; Table 3.1). In normal male meiosis the central and lateral elements of the SC disappear in diplotene/diakinesis, the chromosomes become condensed, and the homologs detach from each other except for the chiasma sites (Fig. 3.3). Usually each pair of homologs in a bivalent is physically attached by at least one chiasma, predominantly in the distal part of the chromosomes (closer to the telomeres) in male meiosis (indicated in Fig. 3.6A). The X and Y chromosome are paired at the pseudoautosomal region whereas the unpaired long arms possess only a lateral element until diakinesis. After nuclear membrane breakdown an astral bipolar spindle is formed at prometaphase I. Spermatocytes possess two pairs of centrioles, barrel-shaped organelles with two perpendicularly arranged cylinders formed from microtubules and surrounded by amorphous material. This serves as major microtubule organizing center (MTOC) at the poles during spindle formation at meiotic metaphase I (Fig. 3.6A). Already prior to metaphase, centrioles start to separate such that upon

breakdown of the nuclear membrane a short bipolar structure is already present (for review see [9]). The spindle in spermatocytes possesses characteristically fusiform poles. Astral microtubules anchor the spindle centrally in the cytoplasm (astral spindle). During prometaphase I, the sister chromatids of each homolog within bivalents attach to spindle fibers, and the bivalents migrate on the spindle until a stable attachment is achieved (Figs 3.1B, 3.5B, and 3.6A,C) [11, 12]. Attachment of the bivalents to both poles leads to alignment at the equator (termed "chromosome congression"). The attachment of homologs by their centromeres to opposite spindle poles causes the first chiasma next to the centromere to keep the homologs together so that they remain located at the equator until separation (Fig. 3.6A) [10, 12, 13]. Centromeres are located more or less away from the central spindle, depending on chromosome length and where the first chiasma is located (Fig. 3.5F). The centromeres of spermatocytes recruit proteins of the spindle assembly checkpoint (SAC) prior to and at prometaphase I. The SAC senses unattached chromosomes [14], renders an anaphase factor (APC/C) inactive, and will cause a delay or arrest in meiotic progression until proper attachment is achieved (Fig. 3.6C). Spermatocytes are therefore sensitive to the presence of univalents or disturbances in spindle formation resulting from insufficient chromosome attachment. This safeguards against errors in chromosome segregation. Prometaphase I is a fairly long stage in meiosis. Homologs in a bivalent repeatedly reorient until a stable bipolar attachment is achieved. Improper attachments of chromosomes to the spindle are resolved by specific enzymes (for discussion, see [12, 13]). Sister chromatids remain attached to each other by cohesion complexes on arms and centromeres containing meiotic cohesion proteins like REC8 (indicated in red clamps in Fig. 3.4B and D, and open or gray circles in Fig. 3.6C) (for references, see [11–14]). At anaphase of meiosis I, homologs migrate to two daughter cells. Transiently a nucleus is formed in spermatogenesis (Fig. 3.2 and the gray in Fig. 3.6D) before chromosomes recondense, and spermatocytes progress to prometaphase II. Prometaphase II is usually a short stage in which centromeres of sister chromatids attach to spindle fibers from opposite poles (amphitelic attachment) (Figs 3.5B and 3.6D). Once they congress to the equator and all centromeres are bipolarly attached to spindle fibers the SAC is released and anaphase II takes place (Fig. 3.6D). From each spermatocyte, four haploid gene products are formed

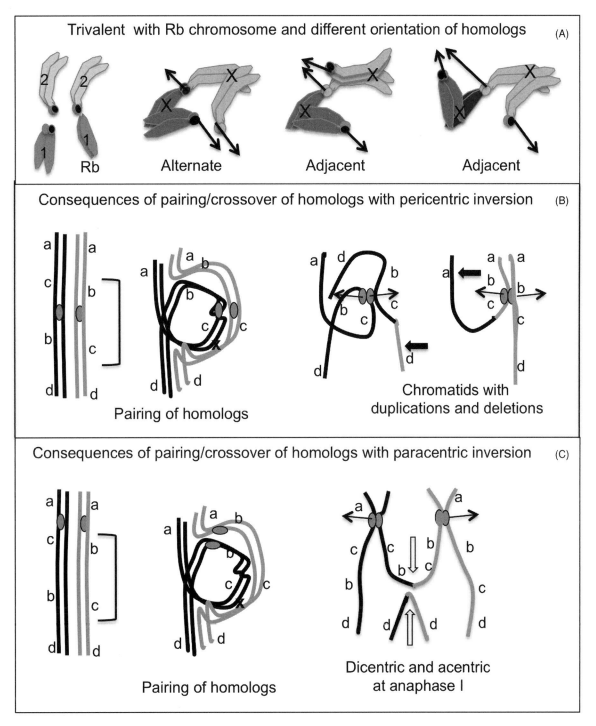

Figure 3.7 Pairing, recombination, and separation of chromosomes in meiocytes that are heterozygous for a Robertsonian translocation chromosome (Rb) (**A**), a balanced pericentric inversion (**B**), or a paracentric inversion (**C**). For further explanation, see text. See plate section for color version.

Spermatocytes differentiate to spermatids and sperm, and finally become released into the lumen of the tubules (Table 3.1). Extensive nuclear and cytoplasmic remodeling (known as spermiogenesis) takes place upon completion of meiosis before haploid, mature sperm are released into the tubules together with residual bodies from shed cytoplasm (Fig. 3.2).

Sexual dimorphism plays an important role in the behavior of chromatin in the germ cells and in meiotic progression, meiotic arrest, or apoptosis [18–20]. For example, epigenetic changes by genomic imprinting are completed in spermatogenesis prior to the pachytene stage while they take place after pachytene, during oocyte growth in the female (see Chapter 12). The inactivated second X chromosome of the female becomes reactivated prior to meiosis and can fully synapse with the active X chromosome, comparable to pairing between the homologs of autosomes (Table 3.1). By contrast, in male meiosis, only the homologous part of the X and Y chromosomes, the PAR, fully synapses while unsynapsed non-homologous parts of the X and Y chromosome form the sex chromatin that is transcriptionally inactivated and retained in a cytologically visible structure (sex body) until cells enter first meiotic metaphase [2, 18]. Failure to transcriptionally inactivate the unpaired chromatin of the X and Y chromosomes induces meiosis arrest in spermatocytes at the pachytene stage [2].

The meiotic process is controlled by feedback mechanisms that cause meiotic arrest in cases of failures of chromosomes pairing, of DNA repair, or of chromosomes failing to properly attach to the spindle. Primary chromosomal imbalance (e.g. in constitutional or mosaic Turner syndrome, XXX, or presence of duplication, deletions, etc.) predispose to pairing failures or non-homologous pairing events in prophase I of meiosis. In male meiosis, specific sensitive checkpoints exist that become activated by failures in synapsis in early prophase that cause death of germ cells and can contribute to oligospermia or azoospermia [2, 18]. A pachytene checkpoint also exists in oocytes, which contributes to loss of germ cells, and possibly a low primordial follicle pool and premature ovarian insufficiency in cases with meiotic failures. However, oocytes may escape the earlier meiotic arrest as a folding back of single unpaired chromosomes or other non-homologous pairing more frequently occurs. However, later they become prone to random segregation of univalent chromosomes and aneuploidy at resumption of maturation [13, 19].

Errors in meiosis that affect germ-cell formation or genomic integrity of the embryo and predisposition to genetic disease

Failures in recombination and checkpoints, mutations, and deletions

Models from mouse to yeast have revealed that the recombination proteins are highly conserved. Altered expression of the genes of components of the synaptonemal complex or the DNA recombination and repair proteins can cause sex-specific infertility or subfertility in animal models and in the human (see [2, 18, 19] and Chapter 8). Non-homologous recombination, or excess or low recombination as well as recombination at unusual sites, can contribute to disturbances in chromosome segregation or formation of aneuploid or chromosomally unbalanced gametes. The influence of constitutional chromosomal aberrations (e.g. deletions, duplications, or gonosomal abnormalities and microdeletions) on meiotic arrest, meiotic failures, and infertility are discussed in Chapters 7, 10, and 11.

Translocations

In cases where recombination occurs between more than two chromosomes, trivalents of 3 or quadrivalents and multivalents of 4 or more homologous chromosomes may be formed. For instance, presence of a single Robertsonian translocation (Rb) chromosome in a heterozygote can give rise to meiotic errors, depending on how chromosomes orient on the meiosis I spindle (Fig. 3.7A). When the Rb chromosome segregates to one pole and the two non-Rb chromosomes to the other (alternate), gametes will have a balanced constitution. If one of the non-Rb chromosomes attaches to the same spindle pole as the Rb chromosome (adjacent) the gametes will be unbalanced (see Fig. 3.7A and Chapter 7).

Presence of a balanced inversion also poses a risk for meiotic errors. Pairing and exchanges between homologous parts of the inversion chromosomes at meiosis can lead to the formation of a loop for pairing between homologous parts of the normal and the inverted segment on homologous chromosomes (Fig. 3.7B,C). When there is an exchange in this part in a heterozygous carrier of a pericentric inversion

chromosomes are not properly attached to the spindle. Once all chromosomes are attached, the anaphase-promoting complex (APC/C^{cdc20}) is activated in meiocytes of both sexes [14]. This initiates the degradation of cyclin B and the inactivation of the CDK1 kinase (Fig. 3.6C). It also initiates the activation of a proteolytic enzyme separase, that recognizes a phosphorylated meiotic cohesin protein (REC8) at the arms of the sister chromatids (open circles in Fig. 3.6C). Upon cleavage of phosphorylated REC8 (pREC8 in Fig. 3.6C), cohesion on arms of sister chromatids is lost, chiasmata resolve and homologs can separate at anaphase I.

Spermatocytes transiently enter interphase without undergoing replication (Fig. 3.6D) while oocytes immediately progress to prometaphase II. Activation of CDK1 causes entry into second meiotic division while APC/C^{cdc20} causes exit from it. After inactivation of CDK1 by proteolysis of cyclin B the phosphorylated cohesin REC8 at centromeres of sister chromatids becomes cleaved in second meiosis and thus allows for separation of the sister chromatids at anaphase II (Fig. 3.6D) [13]. Alignment of metaphase II chromosomes at the spindle equator in oocytes does not induce the immediate activation of the APC/C^{cdc20}. The EMI2 inhibits the activation of the APC/C^{cdc20} and thereby prevents meiotic progression until fertilization. Ovulated metaphase II oocytes resume maturation after sperm entry has induced cytoplasmic calcium release and activation of a cascade of events leading to destruction of EMI2, activation of the APC/C^{cdc20} and separase, and proteolysis of pREC8 and anaphase II progression (Fig. 3.6D).

Deregulation of the synchrony and timing of anaphase I and anaphase II or of the loss of chromosome cohesion, attachment, and separation in a sequential, timely fashion predisposes to meiotic errors [13].

Differences in male and female meiosis during the formation of germ cells

Sexual dimorphism not only exists with respect to the obvious differences in size of the germ cells in male and female meiosis [1]. Thus the large oocyte contains the most products needed for early development until zygotic gene activation is completed. The comparatively small sperm contributes mainly the nucleus and enzymes causing calcium release (Table 3.1). Furthermore, four mature gametes are present at the end of meiosis in the male and only one mature egg plus the two polar bodies (PBs) at the end of female meiosis [1].

All primary oocytes ever to become ovulated form prior to birth and constitute the pool of primordial follicles in the human. Therefore, they can be exposed to adverse conditions over long periods and are subject to aging. Oocytes acquire the competence to resume meiosis only after a long meiotic arrest and growth in interphase. During this period chromatin typically remains decondensed and transcriptionally active. Many follicles become recruited and start to grow but most become atretic and only one (in monoovulatory species such as the human) will resume meiosis. For high developmental competence it appears important that the fully grown, competent germinal vesicle (GV) oocyte becomes transcriptionally repressed and its chromatin condensed. The surge in LH initiates a cascade of signaling events in dominant large antral follicle(s) that result in the release of one or few fully grown oocytes from the meiotic block. Both cGMP and cAMP concentrations drop and PKA is inactivated (Fig. 3.6D) [13, 15]. This ultimately results in activation of CDK1, chromosome condensation, nuclear membrane breakdown, spindle formation, progression through meiotic metaphase I to metaphase II, and ovulation (Fig. 3.2). Only one or few oocytes become ovulated and can be fertilized to complete meiosis in each cycle [11, 14].

Spermatogenic stem cells can continuously replenish the pool of spermatogonia and undergo many more mitoses compared to oogonia before entering meiosis throughout the reproductive period. With increased numbers of mitotic divisions, mutations may increase [16]. Furthermore, stem cells with some specific rare mutations leading to different signaling and cell selection can clonally expand and increase mosaicism of mutant gonocytes in testes [17]. This increases the risk for "paternal age-effect mutations" causing disorders like Apert syndrome, achondroplasia, and missense mutations in the FGFR2, FGFR3, and RET protein, and a relative enrichment of mutant sperm with increasing paternal age [16, 17]. Primary spermatogonia undergo several mitotic divisions before premeiotic S phase and meiosis is initiated. Meiosis from S phase to completion of meiosis II occurs continuously in spermatocytes embedded in the Sertoli cells and is much shorter in spermatocytes compared to oocytes.

in male meiosis (Table 3.1). These remain connected by intercellular bridges until mature sperm are formed such that gene products may be shared between spermatocytes and spermatids. After completion of meiosis spermatids undergo an extensive remodeling, chromatin becomes compacted, a sperm tail grows out, mitochondria fuse, and an acrosome is formed before the mature sperm is released into the seminiferous tubules (Fig. 3.2).

Progression from diakinesis to prometaphase I is fundamentally different between oogenesis and spermatogenesis. Oocytes remain meiotically arrested in dictyate stage after progressing through diplotene, and therefore meiosis I is much longer in the female compared to the male (Fig. 3.2; Table 3.1). Only the fully grown oocyte in antral follicles can resume meiosis. During the resting and growth phase, chromatin decondenses and oocytes are transcriptionally active and acquire maternal products and organelles before they become transcriptionally quiescent, prior to resumption of meiosis [13]. This is fundamental not only for the survival of the oocytes but also for the accumulation of maternally inherited mRNAs, proteins, and organelles needed for the first days of embryonic development and zygotic gene activation. Oocytes are unusual cells since they do not possess pairs of centrioles, but instead MTOCs assemble at the flat spindle poles of a barrel-shaped spindle upon prometaphase I of meiosis (Figs 3.5F and 3.6B) [12, 13]. Attachment to spindle fibers is mostly at chromosome arms in early stages of prometaphase I. Only at a later stage centromeric bipolar attachment occurs and SAC proteins are recruited. This may be an inefficient step since initially many centromeres of homologs appear connected to one instead of both spindle poles (monopolar, example shown in Fig. 3.5C). Frequently centromeres of sister chromatids or a single chromatid are attached to both poles (amphitelic or merotelic, Fig. 3.5E). Such improper attachments need to be resolved before progression to anaphase I [13, 14]. Prometaphase I in female meiosis appears to be characterized by frequent reorientation and reattachments of homologs in each bivalent [13]. However, similar to spermatocytes, at metaphase I the centromeres of both sister chromatids are under tension from spindle fibers pulling at the first chiasma. This holds homologs together (indicated by red arrow in Fig. 3.5F). The signaling by the SAC to block oocytes from progressing to anaphase I may not be so efficient compared to spermatocytes and will allow metaphase I to proceed although some chromosomes failed to properly align (for references, see [13]). This can contribute to susceptibility to female meiotic errors. Oocytes immediately progress to metaphase II without forming a transient interphase nucleus. Unlike in male meiosis, congression of the metaphase II chromosomes at the spindle equator does not induce immediate progression to anaphase II even if the SAC is satisfied. A meiotic inhibitor maintains oocytes in metaphase II arrest. The inhibitor (early mitotic inhibitor 2; EMI2; Fig. 3.6D) is only destroyed after sperm has fertilized the oocyte. In oogenesis, first and second meiosis are asymmetrical [1, 12, 13]. A small first polar body is formed after the first meiosis that contains one set of homologs (also termed "dyads"), each with two chromatids (2N). After fertilization, a second polar body is emitted which contains a haploid set of chromatids (also termed "monads"). The haploid set of chromatids in the oocyte decondenses and becomes surrounded by a nuclear membrane within the maternal pronucleus (PN), while the haploid sperm chromatin decondenses and forms the male pronucleus in the 2PN one cell embryo (Fig. 3.2). After replication, all paternal and maternal chromosomes align on a common spindle in the zygote before it undergoes the first mitotic division.

Cell cycle regulation at meiosis

The major enzymes driving the cell cycle in mitosis and meiosis are the cyclin-dependent kinases (CDKs). In male and female meiosis, CDK1 becomes activated after it has formed a complex with a cyclin B. Activation is regulated by dephosphorylation of residues on the CDK1 by phosphatase (CDC25) at progression from interphase to metaphase (Fig. 3.6C). Oocytes remain arrested in G_2 phase for long periods and are prevented from entering first metaphase by high cyclic adenosine monophosphate (cAMP), cyclic guanosine monophosphate (cGMP), and active protein kinase A (PKA) (Fig. 3.6C). Upon the surge in lutenizing hormone (LH) prior to ovulation the levels of cGMP and cAMP in ooplasm drop, the PKA becomes inactive, and the CDC25 phosphatase activated [15]. CDK1 inhibitory phosphorylation is removed and oocytes progress to first meiotic metaphase.

Oocytes and spermatocytes will usually only progress to anaphase I when they are released from the SAC [14]. The SAC prevents activation of the anaphase-promoting complex (APC/C^{cdc20}) when

(inversion includes the centromere), this may lead to the formation of gametes with a normal number of alleles (only gray- or black-colored chromatids in Fig. 3.7B). However, gametes that are chromosomally unbalanced can also be formed (closed large arrows in Fig. 3.7B). When recombinant chromatids separate at meiosis II they may contain duplications or deletions. Paracentric inversions in which crossover occurs in the inverted segment outside of the centromere can also result in the formation of acentric fragments or chromatids with more than one centromere at anaphase I (open arrows in Fig. 3.7C). This condition may cause lagging of the dicentric chromosome (indicated by open arrow) when the centromeres become attached to opposite spindle poles (Fig. 3.7C). Acentric fragments (open arrow) cannot attach to spindle fibers and may be lost or randomly segregate to one of the daughter cells. Consequences of meiotic disturbances due to inversions and translocations are discussed in Chapters 7, 10, and 11.

Aneuploidy

Most of the clinically recognized aneuploidies from errors in chromosomal distribution at meiosis result in implantation failures of the embryos, spontaneous abortions, or stillbirths. Thus it is estimated that a large majority of embryos from recurrent implantation failure are aneuploid (see Chapter 4). More than 35% of spontaneous abortions carry numerical chromosomal aberrations. In stillbirths the chromosomal aberration rate is still about 4% and in newborns about 0.3% [20]. Trisomies of all chromosomes have been recognized in spontaneous abortions. Most autosomal monosomies appear incompatible with survival in the uterus, and only monosomy for the X chromosome has a higher probability to develop to term. Unfortunately, although most aneuploidies are meiosis-derived, aneuploidy cannot be recognized by altered morphology of oocytes or sperm *per se* or in preimplantation embryos obtained through assisted reproduction (see Chapter 4).

Overall, chromosomal analysis suggests that on average only 1–4% of sperm of karyotypically normal males are aneuploid with a large interindividual variation [21, 22]. Rates of aneuploidy tend to be increased in patients with male idiopathic infertility and in azo- oligo-, asteno-, and teratozoospermia

(see Chapter 7). Disomy of the sex chromosomes and of the small acrocentric chromosomes are the major contributing factors to sperm aneuploidies, while autosomal disomies of the longer chromosomes contribute to only a low percentage of aneuploidy in sperm [21, 22] (see Chapter 7). Fathers of Down syndrome, Turner syndrome, and Klinefelder syndrome children of paternal meiotic origin tend to have a significantly increased disomy rate for XY sperm compared to controls (see Chapter 7). The contribution of paternal age to increases in sperm aneuploidy appears minimal and paternal age mostly affects the sex chromosomes [21].

From analysis of spare or donated oocytes, polar bodies, and preimplantation embryos, it appears that between 10 and 70% of human oocytes from stimulated cycles are aneuploid; rates depending mainly on maternal age (see [10, 22] and Chapter 4). Thus it has been known for a long time that the risk to conceive a trisomic child becomes dramatically increased with advanced maternal but not with advanced paternal age [10, 21, 22]. Incidence of trisomies exponentially increase from about 35 years of maternal age to the end of the female reproductive period. Concomitantly, the pool of non-growing primordial follicles becomes depleted and success rates in natural or assisted reproduction decrease [23]. Polar body analysis points to premature separation of sister cromatids (PSSC) as main mechanism of meiotic error [24] (see Chapter 11).

Chromosome-specific differences in the recombination history and exchange patterns on extra chromosomes in trisomies appear to influence susceptibility to a first or second meiotic error and to age-related aneuploidy. As may be expected, achiasmatic, univalent chromosomes lacking an exchange/chiasma (e.g. in chromosome 21) present a risk for meiotic nondisjunction over all maternal ages. However, for trisomy 21 it was shown that chromosome 21, with a single exchange in the distal part of the chromosome, appears highly susceptible to meiotic errors in first meiosis independent of maternal age. In contrast, a single proximal exchange close to the centromere appears related to a high risk for an error involving sister chromatid segregation at anaphase II especially in an aged oocyte (for references, see [13, 24]). In conclusion, there is now increasing evidence that the presence and localization of exchanges influence the risks for meiotic errors of specific chromosomal configurations differentially in young and in aged oocytes. This may be influenced by presence/absence of chromosome cohesion and other factors.

Thus, there is evidence that the cohesion proteins holding arms and centromeres of sister chromatids together are not renewed during the long meiotic arrest in oogenesis (for references, see [13]). Particularly, aged oocytes that rested for decades in the dictyate stage in primordial follicles may therefore lose chromatid cohesion resulting in PSSC at first or second meiosis and presence of chromatids in polar bodies [24]. Univalents and chromatids have a high risk to randomly segregate leading to aneuploidy (Fig. 3.5D). Aging at metaphase II (post-ovulatory aging) contributes to loss of cohesion between sister chromatid centromeres. This is relevant in assisted reproduction when fertilization is delayed.

Aged human oocytes frequently possess aberrant spindles and there is some tentative evidence for epigenetic changes in the post-translational modification of histones in aged oocytes (for references, see [13]). Furthermore, from transcriptome analysis of young and aged oocytes it appears that an abundance of gene products controlling meiotic progression, metabolism, spindle formation and the SAC may be altered in aged oocytes (for references, see [13]). It was suggested that this contributes to relaxed cell cycle control and increases the risks that oocytes enter anaphase I or anaphase II in presence of unattached chromosomes, defective spindles, and/or with chromosomes that precociously lost cohesion or fail to resolve chiasmata in time.

Studies in human and animal models have shown that exposures to therapeutic drugs, namely those affecting spindle formation, occupational agents like pesticides, and lifestyle factors may lead to increases of aneuploidy frequency in sperm [25, 26]. Analysis of chromosomal constitution, spindles, and chromosome congression in human oocytes and embryos, as well as in animal models, have also suggested that certain stimulation protocols, exposures to environmental chemicals, and chemotherapeutic agents, as well as lifestyle and diet, may contribute to meiotic errors in males and females, independent of age (for references, see [13, 26].) Furthermore, there is emerging evidence that exposures of adult males or females *in utero* to endocrine-disrupting chemicals that might alter pairing and recombination of chromosomes can contribute to susceptibility to meiotic errors in sons and daughters, but much more research is needed to confirm this [27].

Conclusions and future perspectives

Formation of euploid functional germ cells is essential to maintain fertility and genetic stability from one generation to the next. Recent years have provided a wealth of information on conserved genes and processes in germ-cell formation and meiosis. These have confirmed that there are gender-specific processses and sensitivities, and that our species is exceptionally prone to nondisjunction and germ cell aneuploidy in the female. Although we now have more information on what causes increased risks for nondisjunction in oogenesis with advanced maternal age, there is currently no way of prevention. More research is required to understand what may go wrong in meiosis to induce germ cell death and abnormalities that lead to subfertility or infertility. Meiotic errors that occur at first division can occasionally be compensated at second meiosis or mitosis so that a balanced constitution arises in all or some of the blastomeres of the embryo (see Chapter 4). However, if both chromosomes are exclusively derived from the mother or the father this results in uniparental disomy. When genes on such chromosomes are only expressed from the paternal or maternal allele, i.e. they are imprinted (see Chapter 5), this may result in a gene-dosage effect and aberrant expression that causes genetic disease (see Chapter 12). The advent of novel sensitive and reliable methods for analysis of the chromosomal constitution of parents, single cells like PBs, and gametes and embryos (see Chapters 2 and 11) is promising to detect even such disturbances and to provide information on genetic and etiological factors that affect genomic stability. This can be used to inform patients and hopefully develop strategies for prevention and treatment, or selection of germ cells or euploid embryos with high developmental potential for assisted reproduction. Currently, it is of prime importance to inform men and women about their prospects and chances to have a healthy child in order to make appropriate decisions on family planning and preserving fertility and to raise interest in processes in normal meiosis and germ-cell formation in either gender. For the clinician, embryologist, and geneticist it is of prime importance to develop best strategies that are least invasive, cost- and time-efficient, and of greatest reliability to test and determine risks for abnormal meiosis and improve benefits of treatments for patients to conceive a healthy child.

References

1. Alberts B, Johnson A, Lewis J *et al.* Meiosis. In *Molecular Biology of the Cell*, 4th edn. New York, NY: Garland Science, 2002: http://www.ncbi.nim.gov/books/NBK26840/

2. Bowles J, Koopman P. Sex determination in mammalian germ cells: extrinsic versus intrinsic factors. *Reproduction* 2010; 139: 943–58.

3. Bolcun-Filas E, Schimenti JC. Genetics of meiosis and recombination in mice. In *International Review of Cell and Molecular Biology*, Vol. 298, Ed. K W Yeon; Burlington, MA: Academic Press, 2012.

4. Davies OR, Maman JD, Pellegrini L. Structural analysis of the human SYCE2–TEX12 complex provides molecular insights into synaptonemal complex assembly. *Open Biol* 2012; 2: 120099.

5. Hassold T, Sherman S, Hunt P. Counting cross-overs: characterizing meiotic recombination in mammals. *Hum Mol Genet* 2000; 9: 2409–19.

6. Tease C, Hultén MA. Inter-sex variation in synaptonemal complex lengths largely determine the different recombination rates in male and female germ cells. *Cytogenet Genome Res* 2004; 107: 208–15.

7. San Filippo J, Sung P, Klein H. Mechanism of eukaryotic homologous recombination. *Annu Rev Biochem* 2008; 77: 229–57.

8. Lichten M, De Massy B. The impressionistic landscape of meiotic recombination. *Cell* 2011; 147: 267–70.

9. Eichenlaub-Ritter U, Vogt E, Yin H, Gosden R. Spindles, mitochondria and redox potential in ageing oocytes. *Reprod Biomed Online* 2004; 8: 45–58.

10. Nagaoka SI, Hassold TJ, Hunt PA. Human aneuploidy: mechanisms and new insights into an age-old problem. *Nat Rev Genet* 2012; 13: 493–504.

11. Nasmyth K. Cohesin: a catenase with separate entry and exit gates? *Nat Cell Biol* 2011; 13: 1170–7.

12. Watanabe Y. Geometry and force behind kinetochore orientation: lessons from meiosis. *Nat Rev Mol Cell Biol* 2012; 13: 370–82.

13. Eichenlaub-Ritter U, Gosden R. Cellular origin of age-related aneuploidy in mammalian oocytes. In *Biology and Pathology of the Oocyte, Role in Fertility and Reproductive Medicine*, Eds. A Trounson, R Gosden, U Eichenlaub-Ritter; Cambridge, UK: Cambridge University Press, 2013.

14. Musacchio A. Spindle assembly checkpoint: the third decade. *Philos Trans R Soc Lond B Biol Sci* 2011; 366: 3595–604.

15. Conti M. Hormones and growth factors in the regulation of oocyte maturation. In *Biology and Pathology of the Oocyte, Role in Fertility and Reproductive Medicine*, Eds. A Trounson, R Gosden, U Eichenlaub-Ritter; Cambridge, UK: Cambridge University Press, 2013.

16. Kong A, Frigge ML, Masson G *et al.* Rate of *de novo* mutations and the importance of father's age to disease risk. *Nature* 2012; 488: 471–5.

17. Goriely A, Wilkie AO. Paternal age effect mutations and selfish spermatogonial selection: causes and consequences for human disease. *Am J Hum Genet* 2012; 90: 175–200.

18. Burgoyne PS, Mahadevaiah SK, Turner JM. The consequences of asynapsis for mammalian meiosis. *Nat Rev Genet* 2009; 10: 207–16.

19. Hunt PA, Hassold TJ. Sex matters in meiosis. *Science* 2002; 296: 2181–3.

20. Hassold T, Hunt P. To err (meiotically) is human: the genesis of human aneuploidy. *Nat Rev Genet* 2001; 2: 280–91.

21. Hann MC, Lau PE, Tempest HG. Meiotic recombination and male infertility: from basic science to clinical reality? *Asian J Androl* 2011; 13: 212–18.

22. Hassold T, Hall H, Hunt P. The origin of human aneuploidy: where we have been, where we are going. *Hum Mol Genet* 2007; 16: R203–8.

23. Alviggi C, Humaidan P, Howles CM, Tredway D, Hillier SG. Biological versus chronological ovarian age: implications for assisted reproductive technology. *Reprod Biol Endocrinol* 2009; 7: 101.

24. Handyside AH, Montag M, Magli MC *et al.* Multiple meiotic errors caused by predivision of chromatids in women of advanced maternal age undergoing *in vitro* fertilisation. *Eur J Hum Genet* 2012; 20: 742–7.

25. Pacchierotti F, Eichenlaub-Ritter U *et al.* Environmental hazard in the aetiology of somatic and germ cell aneuploidy. *Cytogenet Genome Res* 2011; 133: 254–68.

26. Martin RH. Cytogenetic determinants of male fertility. *Hum Reprod Update* 2008; 14: 379–90.

27. Hunt PA, Lawson C, Gieske M *et al.* Bisphenol A alters early oogenesis and follicle formation in the fetal ovary of the rhesus monkey. *Proc Natl Acad Sci USA* 2012; 109: 17 525–30.

Chromosomes in early human embryo development

Incidence of chromosomal abnormalities, underlying mechanisms and consequences for development

Esther B. Baart and Diane Van Opstal

Introduction

Reproduction in humans is considered to be a relatively inefficient process, as the chance of achieving a spontaneous pregnancy after timed intercourse is only approximately 30%. This is much lower than the 70–90% estimated for other species such as the rhesus monkey, the captive baboon, or rodents and rabbits. The inefficiency of human reproduction is mainly explained by the high incidence of preclinical losses, an estimated 60% of all conceptions. Early pregnancy loss is mainly explained due to the occurrence of chromosome abnormalities, which have been identified in the majority of spontaneous abortion samples investigated.

The introduction of assisted reproductive technology (ART) and specifically *in vitro* fertilization (IVF) has allowed better insight into human early embryo development and it has become clear that chromosomal abnormalities identified in abortion material from *in vivo* conceptions are also frequently identified in preimplantation embryos generated by IVF. This indicates that chromosome instability is an inherent feature of human conceptions. So far, advanced maternal age remains the only etiological risk factor identified for chromosomal aneuploidy [1]. However, increasing evidence has made it clear that most preimplantation embryos do not have a uniform chromosomal constitution in all cells and are said to be mosaic as a result of post-meiotic errors in chromosome segregation. The mechanisms underlying this phenomenon and its consequences for developmental potential of the preimplantation embryo are still poorly understood.

This chapter aims to provide insight into the type and frequency of chromosomal abnormalities commonly found in human early embryos. It will explore molecular mechanisms that may contribute to the observed high error rate, and to what extent it could be induced by IVF procedures. The developmental capacity of mosaic embryos will be investigated by analyzing *in vitro* data on blastocyst development. Furthermore, by giving an overview of the type and frequency of chromosome abnormalities observed after implantation, we aim to investigate the implications of chromosomal mosaicism for implantation and further embryonic development.

Chromosome abnormalities in human preimplantation embryos

Contribution of meiotic errors to embryo aneuploidy and consequences for embryo development

Despite the high frequency and clinical importance of human aneuploidy, the underlying mechanisms leading to an abnormal chromosome constitution remain poorly understood. As detailed in Chapter 3, the incidence of aneuploidy is strongly related to maternal age and is also dependent on the stage of development: only 0.3% of newborns are aneuploid, which increases to 4% in stillbirths, and 35% when spontaneous abortions are investigated. Interestingly, the type of abnormalities that are observed also differ. Among newborns and stillbirths, the most

Textbook of Human Reproductive Genetics, eds Karen Sermon and Stéphane Viville. Published by Cambridge University Press.
© Cambridge University Press 2014.

common abnormalities are trisomy of chromosome 13, 18, or 21, or sex-chromosomal aneuploidies (i.e. 45,X, 47,XXX, 47,XXY, and 47,XYY). In contrast, trisomies of all chromosomes have been described in spontaneous abortions with the most common ones being trisomy 15, 16, 21, and 22. With the exception of trisomy 21, these aberrations are lethal early in pregnancy, and only allow fetal survival beyond the first trimester of pregnancy if present in mosaic form. In contrast, trisomy 13, 18, and 21 and sex chromosomal aneuploidy can be tolerated and may lead to the birth of an affected child. The only significant monosomy observed at the different stages of development is 45,X, and this condition accounts for at least 10% of all spontaneous abortions [1].

By using analysis of DNA polymorphisms in trisomic cases, the origin of the extra chromosome can be examined. Results from such studies reveal that, depending on the chromosome investigated, there is variation in the parental origin (maternal or paternal) and also in the meiotic division where the segregation error occurred. For example, paternal errors are observed to account for 30–50% of cases of 47,XXY and trisomy 2, but they are rarely observed in other trisomies. Trisomy 16 is almost exclusively from maternal origin and seems to be solely derived from errors during meiosis I, whereas trisomy 18 also frequently arises due to an error during meiosis II. However, despite the variation, errors during maternal meiosis I overall explain most of the abnormalities observed [1].

These observations in clinically recognized pregnancies were confirmed by analyses of oocytes and sperm cells. Whereas only 1–4% of sperm carry aneuploidy, this was found to vary between 10 and 70% in human oocytes, depending on maternal age and method of investigation. Interestingly, although abnormalities involving all chromosomes have been observed in oocytes, the most common aneuploidies were those involving chromosomes 15, 16, 18, 21, and 22 [1]. Thus, findings in oocytes correlate well with findings in liveborns and pregnancy losses. From this it can be concluded that meiotic aneuploidy originates mostly during maternal meiosis I, it arises in an age-dependent manner, and certain chromosomes are more frequently involved. However, as the application of IVF made human preimplantation embryos available for chromosome analysis, it soon became clear that the contribution of meiotic errors to preimplantation embryo aneuploidy is rather small.

Incidence of aneuploidy and mosaicism in cleavage-stage embryos

Most of our current knowledge concerning the chromosomal constitution of human preimplantation embryos comes from the analysis of cleavage-stage embryos by preimplantation genetic screening (PGS) performed 3 days after fertilization, when embryos are usually composed of 6–10 blastomeres (see Chapter 11). Molecular cytogenetic analysis of interphase nuclei by fluorescence *in situ* hybridization (FISH) has been the most frequently used technique for the analysis of chromosomal abnormalities in human embryos. Data obtained by such studies have indicated that on average 60% of human cleavage-stage embryos generated by *in vitro* fertilization (IVF) contain chromosomally abnormal cells [2]. These abnormalities may arise from an error during meiosis, resulting in a uniform abnormality present in all cells, or from segregation errors occurring during the first mitotic divisions. The latter event results in chromosomal mosaicism, defined as the coexistence of karyotypically distinct cell lineages derived from a single zygote. Mosaic embryos can be composed of a mixture of chromosomally normal and abnormal cells (diploid–aneuploid mosaic) or of abnormal cells with different abnormalities (aneuploid mosaic) [2]. The rate of mosaic embryos described in the literature is highly variable (15–90%). This depends on the method of chromosome analysis, the number of chromosomes analyzed, the developmental stage of the embryo, and the definition of mosaicism. A systematic review and meta-analysis of studies analyzing the chromosomal constitution of all cells of 815 human embryos showed 22% to be uniformly diploid, and only 5% were either uniformly abnormal (i.e. aneuploid, haploid, polyploid) or complex abnormal [3]. Chromosomal mosaicism was found in 73% of the embryos. Within the group of mosaic embryos, 80% was found to be diploid–aneuploid mosaic, with the remainder showing aneuploid mosaicism.

The first reports on chromosomal mosaicism in human embryos were much debated. It was hypothesized that the observed high error rate was due to technical artifacts of the FISH procedure, potentially leading to overlapping or non-specific signals and hybridization failure, as proper control material was lacking. However, several studies using novel comprehensive molecular cytogenetic methods based on comparative genomic hybridization (CGH) or microarray technologies, such as array CGH that allow the screening of all chromosomes, have confirmed that three-quarters of normally developing human embryos display chromosomal mosaicism at this early stage of development and only one quarter are uniformly diploid [2]. Although these novel techniques also have issues of validation and lack of proper controls (see Chapter 2), they support findings by FISH [2]. It is now increasingly accepted that chromosomal mosaicism is a common phenomenon in human cleavage-stage embryos.

Although errors during female meiosis are thought to explain most of the aneuploidy observed in stillbirths and liveborns, this is not the case for preimplantation embryos. Detailed analysis of preimplantation embryos from young women undergoing IVF indicated that only 10–20% of the abnormalities observed can be explained by a chromosome segregation error during meiosis [4, 5]. This proportion corresponds to aneuploidy rates reported in a large set of IVF oocytes from young women [1]. The remaining proportion of abnormalities observed in embryos can only be explained by errors occurring during the first cleavage divisions, indicating that these divisions are especially error prone.

Mitotic mechanisms leading to chromosomal abnormalities

As stated above, most of the abnormalities observed in human cleavage-stage embryos were the result of post-meiotic events. As illustrated in Fig. 4.1, losses and gains of whole chromosomes during mitosis can be explained in several ways [6]. Mitotic nondisjunction occurs when during mitosis the sister chromatids do not separate properly, or have separated prematurely. Both defects can result in aberrant segregation, where one daughter cell ends up with both chromatids and the other with the reciprocal loss. Alternatively, nondisjunction can also be the result of defective attachment of the chromosome to the spindle in combination with a weakened mitotic checkpoint that fails to prevent anaphase before all chromosomes are properly attached to the spindle in a bipolar fashion (Fig. 4.1). Anaphase lagging occurs when improper attachments of the chromosome to the spindle have formed, in which one sister chromatid is simultaneously attached to microtubules emanating from both poles. This will result in one chromatid being pulled

correctly to one spindle pole, whereas the other chromatid is pulled from both directions and remains at the spindle midzone. With ingression of the cleavage furrow it can be lost, so one daughter cell will have the normal chromosome complement, whereas the other daughter cell has a chromosome loss. Aberrant cytokinesis can also cause chromosome malsegregation. Cells can skip cytokinesis or undergo cell fusion, resulting in polyploidization. This can lead to the formation of a multipolar spindle in a subsequent division, giving rise to complex abnormalities in the daughter cells.

Analysis of the abnormalities observed within mosaic embryos show that they are most often consistent with anaphase lagging, followed by nondisjunction. Both mechanisms can also occur within the same embryo, and are also frequently found in combination with meiotic errors [7].

Next to numerical chromosome abnormalities, studies using CGH and array CGH in human preimplantation embryos have also demonstrated the presence of structural abnormalities ([8] and references therein). When investigating good quality embryos from young and fertile women undergoing IVF, 70% of the embryos were shown to be mosaic for segmental deletions, duplications, and amplifications. These partial aneuploidies are thought to be the result of DNA double-strand breaks followed by fusion in the zygote or the two-cell embryo, but the significance of these findings is still poorly understood.

Molecular mechanisms regulating chromosome segregation during preimplantation embryo development

Research into the origin of embryo aneuploidy has so far focused on the contribution of the oocyte, and a link between maternal age and an increased risk for meiotic errors has been well established. Meiotic errors in oogenesis are currently explained by a "two-hit" hypothesis: homologous chromosomes can form more susceptible crossover configurations during the meiotic pairing process, resulting in segregation errors as the result of multifactorial perturbations in the oocyte's spindle and checkpoint function [1]. However, this model does not explain the high rate of chromosomal mosaicism in human embryos, which can occur independently of meiotic

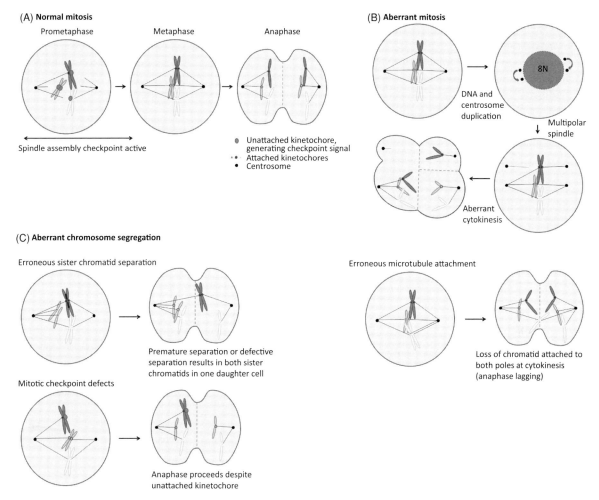

Figure 4.1 (**A**) Schematic representation of normal chromosome alignment and segregation. At prometaphase, the spindle assembly checkpoint is activated at each unattached kinetochore. Microtubule capture of both kinetochores of a chromosome results in silencing of the checkpoint and chromosome alignment at the metaphase plate. Anaphase is not initiated until all chromosomes have achieved bipolar attachment to the spindle and congression to the spindle midzone. During anaphase, the sister chromatids are pulled apart. After invagination of the cell membrane and completion of cytokinesis, the sister chromatids are equally separated to the two daughter cells. (**B**) Losses and gains of whole chromosomes during mitosis can be explained in several ways. Aberrant mitosis can cause chromosome loss. Too many centrosomes can result from errors in centrosome duplication or skipping cytokinesis, producing polyploidization (8N). Multiple centrosomes induce multipolar spindles and chromosome malsegregation. (**C**) Mitotic nondisjunction results in reciprocal loss and gain of a chromosome in the two daughter cells. This can be caused by erroneous sister chromatid separation (chromatids separate prematurely or not at all) or mitotic checkpoint defects that fail to prevent anaphase before all chromosomes are properly attached. Anaphase lagging results in loss of a sister chromatid from one daughter cell and can be the result of erroneous microtubule attachment (merotelic attachment). See plate section for color version.

segregation errors and does not appear to correlate with maternal age [7]. In order to better understand this high chromosome segregation error rate, this section will explore contributing factors by analyzing differences in mechanisms regulating chromosome segregation in adult somatic cells and the early embryo.

The first embryonic cleavage division differs from normal mitotic divisions

The formation of the bipolar spindle is a crucial event for cell division, which ensures correct chromosome segregation to daughter cells. The centrosome, which comprises a pair of centrioles surrounded by the pericentriolar material, is the organizing center of the mitotic spindle in somatic cells. At prophase, the duplicated centrosomes separate to form two spindle poles. Chromosome condensation initiates and two functional kinetochores are formed on the sister chromatids at the primary constriction. After nuclear envelope breakdown and entry to prometaphase, each chromosome is captured at both kinetochores by microtubules emanating from the spindle poles (Fig.4.1A). After capture, chromosomes congress and align at the spindle midzone (metaphase). Cells can then enter anaphase where sister chromatids are separated and equally pulled to the daughter cells. The chromatin decondenses (telophase) and the nuclear envelope reforms while cytokinesis is completed.

According to the classic definition, the first embryonic cleavage division is a mitotic division, as opposed to preceding meiotic divisions. However, intriguing differences exist between a zygote and a somatic mitotic cell. Mature human oocytes are arrested at metaphase of the second meiotic division (MII). Upon fertilization by a sperm cell, the oocyte completes the second meiotic division and the highly condensed chromatin of the sperm nucleus decondenses, resulting in the formation of the haploid paternal pronucleus. The parental pronuclei are maintained physically separate in the ooplasm during the subsequent G_1, S, and G_2 phase of the first embryonic cell cycle. Upon entry into mitosis, maternal and paternal chromatin is condensed into chromosomes that align for the first time at a common metaphase plate.

Fertilization and the transition from maternal to embryonic control

Oocytes and early embryos are transcriptionally inactive. During oogenesis, mammalian oocytes store an abundance of mRNAs, proteins, and macromolecular structures in the ooplasm to sustain the first cell cycles following fertilization and to facilitate the transition from maternal to embryonic control, a process called embryonic genome activation (EGA). In humans, EGA was believed to occur at the four- to eight-cell stage, but recent reports suggest that it starts as early as the two-cell stage for a select number of genes followed by a major wave of transcription between the six- and eight-cell stage [9]. In somatic cells, transcription of most of the genes that regulate mitosis and faithful chromosome segregation is tightly cell cycle regulated and disturbances in expression levels and timing cause chromosome instability [6]. The quality and quantity of this maternal store of transcripts and proteins in the oocyte is therefore likely to be crucial for chromosome segregation regulation during the first embryonic divisions.

The human sperm cell contributes the centrosome to embryonic spindle formation

Compromised spermatogenesis is associated with increased chromosome segregation errors, as evidenced by an increased incidence of mosaicism in embryos derived from non-obstructive azoospermia patients, compared with those from ejaculated sperm [2]. This raises the question whether the sperm contributes to chromosome malsegregation in the early embryo. Interestingly, mammalian oocytes, with the exception of mouse oocytes, lack the centrosome needed to form a bipolar spindle. During fertilization in humans, the centrosome is contributed by the sperm cell and responsible for spindle assembly in the zygote. The sperm centrosome contribution is essential for spindle formation in human zygotes and therefore directly related to faithful chromosome segregation.

An increased incidence of mosaicism is observed in dispermic human zygotes compared to monospermic or digynic embryos and can be considered evidence of a sperm contribution to abnormal spindle organization [7]. This may result from the presence of an extra centrosome delivered by the second sperm cell, as extra centrosomes have been shown to induce transient multipolar spindles. Although these poles can fuse to reform a bipolar spindle, this can result in chromosomes where one sister kinetochore attaches to both spindle poles resulting in anaphase lagging [2]. The transfer of a defective centrosome from the sperm to the oocyte has also been proposed to contribute to chromosome segregation errors in the embryo. Attempts have been made to assess functionality of the sperm centrosome by insemination of rabbit or bovine oocytes with human sperm and evaluation of its ability to organize microtubules. However, so far no clear relationship between sperm quality, centrosomal dysfunction, and spindle formation in the zygote has been established in human IVF [10]. However, multipolar spindles are frequently observed at all stages of human preimplantation development and the presence of multiple or defective centrosomes may thus

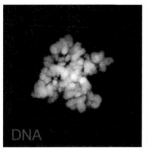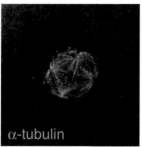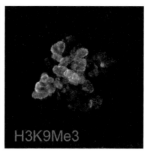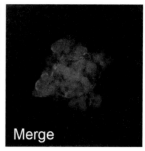

Figure 4.2 Confocal image of a human tripronuclear zygote at prometaphase, showing chromosomes (DNA) together with immunolocalization of tubulin protein in the spindle (α-tubulin) and trimethylation of histone 3 on lysine 9 (H3K9Me3). Z-stack images were merged into a single image. Maternal and paternal chromosomes are in the process of congression in a spindle that displays multiple poles. Staining for H3K9Me3 reveals a parental epigenetic asymmetry: maternal chromosomes can be observed to be enriched for H3K9me3, whereas paternal chromosomes have very low levels. See plate section for color version.

contribute to the incidence of complex aneuploidies (Fig. 4.2).

Compromised functionality of the spindle assembly checkpoint?

The spindle assembly checkpoint (SAC) is a complex surveillance mechanism that delays anaphase until biorientation of all chromosomes at the metaphase plate. The SAC is composed of Mad1, Mad2, and Bub3 proteins and BubR1, Bub1, and Mps1 kinases. When activated, it generates an inhibitory signal that stops cells from entering anaphase [6]. Once all pairs of sister kinetochores are properly captured by the spindle microtubules and are under tension, the SAC is silenced, resulting in sister-chromatid separation and cells being able to enter anaphase (Fig.4.1A).

The SAC improves chances of a successful mitosis by delaying anaphase to provide the cell with an opportunity to correct attachment errors (Fig. 4.3). However, it is not necessary for the completion of mitosis [6]. The high incidence of chromosome aneuploidies and mosaicism during the first cleavage divisions in human embryos has been proposed to result from a dysfunctional SAC, allowing embryonic cells to divide while not all chromosomes have achieved proper attachment. However, human embryos readily arrest at prometaphase of the cell cycle when microtubule–kinetochore interactions are disturbed by treatment with spindle poisons [11]. Although this is a strong indication of an active SAC, the checkpoint can in fact be weakened. The biochemical signal produced by each unattached kinetochore can be quantitatively reduced in concentrations of signal-producing components [6]. This creates a situation in which more than one unattached kinetochore is needed to produce enough signal to inhibit anaphase onset, and in which chromosome separation can occur with unaligned chromosomes. Only when all kinetochores are unattached due to the addition of spindle poisons, is the amount of signal generated enough to activate the SAC. It is feasible that the large cytoplasmic volume present in cells of the early embryo may dilute kinetochore signaling to the SAC. Alternatively, a weakened signal may also be caused by reduced expression of SAC proteins. Interestingly, experimental studies in rhesus macaque oocytes have demonstrated oocyte quality related differences in *BUB1* expression [12]. This illustrates that immature oocytes may not have acquired an optimal maternal store of relevant transcripts during oocyte growth and maturation, and this is expected to have an impact on chromosome segregation in the embryo.

We can easily imagine that such a phenomenon may arise during ovarian stimulation, as explained in more detail below, and/or that some subfertile women will be more prone to produce such oocytes with reduced mitotic competency.

Distinct constitution of the chromosomal passenger complex during the cleavage divisions

Kinetochore capture by the mitotic spindle is a trial-and-error process. While unattached chromosomes activate the SAC to delay anaphase until biorientation is achieved, erroneous attachments cannot induce

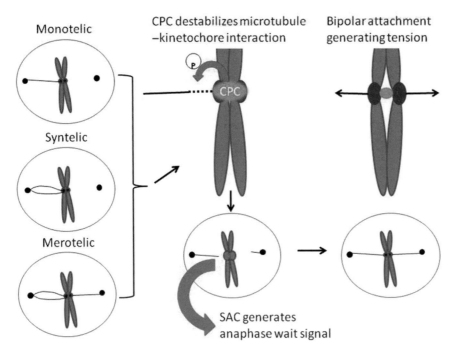

Figure 4.3 Schematic representation of erroneous, non-bipolar, attachments and how they are corrected by joint action of the chromosomal passenger complex (CPC) and the spindle assembly checkpoint (SAC). The CPC localizes to the region between the kinetochores and phosphorylates several proteins present in the kinetochore, resulting in destabilization of microtubule–kinetochore attachments. The CPC thereby generates unattached kinetochores that activate the SAC. The SAC in turn prevents anaphase, providing the chromosome the opportunity to form new attachments. As soon as bipolar attachment is achieved, tension is generated across the kinetochores, pulling them apart. The CPC can no longer reach its targets, enabling microtubule–kinetochore attachments to become stable and resulting in deactivation of the SAC. See plate section for color version.

a SAC response. Therefore, non-bipolar microtubule–kinetochore interactions are corrected by the chromosomal passenger complex (CPC, Fig. 4.3) [13]. This complex consists of Aurora B kinase, survivin, borealin, and INCENP. To be able to function properly, targeting of this complex to the region between the kinetochores is crucial. One of the kinases involved in the SAC, BUB1, is essential for correct localization of the CPC by providing one of the recruiting marks (Fig. 4.4). In turn, the CPC plays an important role in proper activation of the SAC [13].

In human zygotes, Aurora C is the main active subunit in the CPC as opposed to Aurora B in normal mitotic cell division [11]. Aurora C was first identified in the testis and has been coined the meiotic counterpart of Aurora B. It has been shown to compensate for Aurora B to support mitotic progression in somatic cells and mouse embryos. However, structural differences between the proteins exist, with so far unknown implications for CPC localization and/or function. This different composition of the CPC in

human cleavage-stage embryos underscores the need for research to further elucidate differences in mechanisms regulating chromosome segregation in the early embryo (Fig. 4.5).

The role of epigenetics in chromosome segregation in early embryonic mitosis

In somatic cells, DNA is wrapped around nucleosomes, which consist of a histone H3–H4 tetramer and two histone H2A–H2B dimers, together forming chromatin. The N-terminal tails of these core histones can undergo a range of post-translational modifications, including acetylation, methylation, phosphorylation, and ubiquitination. Such post-translational "marks," together with variants of the canonical histones and chromatin-associated proteins, determine chromatin structure and thereby functional chromatin domains. Heterochromatin domains, as opposed to euchromatin, remain condensed and transcriptionally silent throughout the cell cycle.

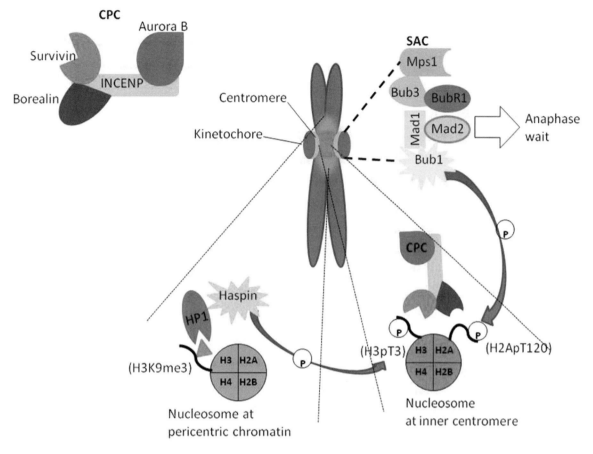

Figure 4.4 Schematic representation of the molecular mechanisms ensuring chromosomal passenger complex (CPC) recruitment to the inner centromere. Phosphorylated H3T3 is generated by haspin kinase, which is recruited to pericentric heterochromatin by HP1 bound to H3K9me3. During prometaphase, phosphorylated H2AT120 is generated by Bub1 kinase, which is recruited to the kinetochore as part of the spindle assembly checkpoint (SAC). This recruitment is promoted by Aurora B. The overlap between H3pT3 and H2ApT120 defines the inner centromere and recruits the CPC: Survivin binds H3pT3, whereas Borealin binds indirectly to H2ApT120. Aurora B is then correctly placed to phosphorylate different protein targets to destabilize chromosome-microtubule attachment errors until bipolar attachment is achieved. The SAC in the mean time generates a signal that prevents anaphase and Aurora B activity is required for maintenance of this signal. See plate section for color version.

In the context of chromosome segregation, the constitutive heterochromatin domains at the centromeric and pericentric regions are of particular importance. In humans these domains consist of DNA sequences of α-satellite repeats for centromeric, and satellite II and III repeats for pericentromeric heterochromatin. However, these regions are not purely specified by DNA sequences, but epigenetic mechanisms play a dominant role. The centromere is determined by incorporation of a variant of histone H3.1, named CENP-A, and forms the basis of the kinetochore and attachment of the chromosome to the spindle. The pericentric region has a distinct epigenetic signature, with enrichment for DNA methyla-

tion, trimethylation of lysine residue 9 on histone H3 (H3K9me3) (Fig. 4.6), as well as certain histone variants, such as H2A.Z and H3.3 [14]. This region is also enriched for a protein called heterochromatin protein 1 (HP1) that binds to H3K9me3. Disturbances in this signature have been shown to cause chromosome segregation errors (see references in [14]).

In the complex regulatory process that ensures correct chromosome segregation, trimethylation of H3K9 seems to be an important upstream component, in association with its recruitment of HP1. HP1 provides a direct link between pericentric heterochromatin and kinetochore formation by recruiting a component of the kinetochore (the Mis12 complex) to the

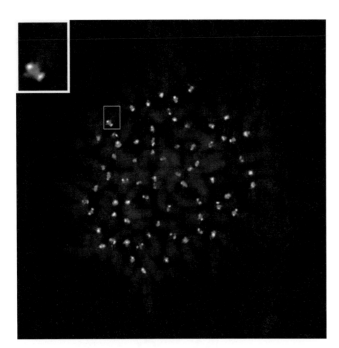

Figure 4.5 Immunolocalization of the CPC subunit INCENP and the centromere on a chromosome spread from a human tripronuclear zygote. Each chromosome (blue) displays two paired signals for the centromeres (white). INCENP (red) is located between the centromeres, on the region referred to as the inner centromere. The insert shows an enlargement of the boxed chromosome. See plate section for color version.

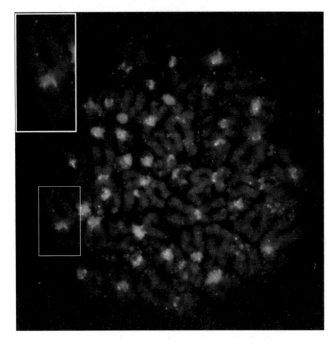

Figure 4.6 Immunolocalization of trimethylation of histone 3 on lysine 9 (H3K9Me3) and the centromere on a chromosome spread from a human fetal fibroblast cell line. Each chromosome (blue) displays two paired signals for the centromeres (red). Enrichment for H3K9Me3 can be observed on the regions surrounding the centromeres, referred to as the pericentric heterochromatin. The insert shows an enlargement of the boxed chromosome. See plate section for color version.

centromeric region during interphase. HP1 also binds to INCENP and may thus be involved in targeting of the CPC (Fig. 4.4) [13].

A role for pericentric heterochromatin in CPC localization is further demonstrated by an experimental model consisting of a human cell line incorporat-ing a mutated copy of chromosome 4 (see references in [13]). This chromosome 4 contains an epigeneti-cally silenced centromere and a neocentromere has formed, meaning that the CENP-A containing nucleo-somes have translocated to a different location, devoid of centromeric and pericentric DNA repeat sequences.

This was found to result in an altered distribution of the CPC and impairment of its error-correction ability. As a result, the chromosome containing the neocentromere was more frequently involved in misattachment and failed alignment at the metaphase plate. Thus, mounting evidence indicates that the epigenetic signature of the pericentric region is intricately linked to mechanisms regulating chromosome segregation, although the underlying molecular mechanisms are still the subject of much research.

A crucial epigenetic process after fertilization is the reestablishment of the paternal chromatin structure in order to form a functional embryonic genome. At the time of fertilization, the maternal genome is marked by histone modifications inherited from the oocyte, and the majority of somatic epigenetic heterochromatin marks are retained on the meiotic chromosomes and transferred to the zygote. In contrast, most heterochromatin marks are lost from the sperm nucleus, as histones are replaced by protamines during spermiogenesis. After fertilization, dramatic changes occur in the paternal chromatin organization, as the protamines are replaced by maternally provided nucleosomes. This process has been extensively studied in mouse zygotes, showing that these newly provided nucleosomes are initially mostly devoid of modifications [14]. To compensate for the lack of typical pericentric heterochromatin modifications found in somatic cells (and maternal chromatin), mouse paternal pericentric heterochromatin regions were shown to be enriched in maternally provided proteins from the Polycomb Repressive Complexes. This alternative repressive pathway thus compensates for the absence of H3K9me3 and the classic pericentric heterochromatin signature, until it is reestablished. The remarkable epigenetic asymmetry in the maternal and paternal pericentric heterochromatin signatures can be observed until the eight-cell stage. In human embryos, it remains to be investigated how paternal pericentric heterochromatin is reestablished, but a similar parental asymmetry for the H3K9me3 mark has been observed (Fig. 4.2).

As explained above, early mouse and human embryos show parental asymmetry at the pericentric regions for an epigenetic mark that has shown to be crucial for faithful chromosome segregation in somatic cells. It is therefore tempting to speculate on the impact of this parental asymmetry on chromosome segregation. It appears that the epigenetic signature of paternal pericentric heterochromatin may be underdeveloped in comparison to maternal chromosomes and somatic cells. It is conceivable that this may affect CPC localization and the capacity of CPC to correct erroneous attachments, predisposing chromosomes for malsegregation. These mechanisms may thus constitute a "first hit." The "second hit" would then be oocyte-quality-related perturbation of the chromosome segregation machinery or defective or additional centrosomes contributed by the sperm cell, resulting in chromosomally mosaic embryos.

Clinical implications of the high rate of chromosomal abnormalities in IVF embryos

Impact of IVF procedures on chromosome abnormalities and mosaicism

Our knowledge on the high rate of chromosomal abnormalities is almost exclusively derived from embryos generated by IVF. It is therefore possible that these abnormalities are induced by ovarian stimulation and/or suboptimal *in vitro* culture conditions. Following recruitment into the growing pool, the oocyte expands from 35 to 120 µm in diameter, which represents a 100-fold increase in volume over a period of several months. Oocyte growth and maturation are linked to follicle development, and bidirectional signaling occurs between oocytes and granulosa cells. Oocytes must achieve both nuclear and cytoplasmic maturity in order to sustain the early stages of embryonic development. Control of the late stages of follicle development lies primarily with follicle-stimulating hormone (FSH) and luteinizing hormone (LH), but granulosa cell-derived growth factors play a major role in modulating the action of these gonadotrophins during follicle development. The orderly expression of these somatic and oocyte-derived factors allows the follicle to acquire a number of properties at a precise time and in a specific sequence. So far, it is largely unknown how ovarian stimulation and the development of multiple preovulatory follicles interfere with these intraovarian factors. Experimental evidence from studies in mice shows that disturbances in the complex interplay of signals that regulate folliculogenesis alter the late stages of oocyte growth, increasing the risk of chromosome malsegregation in subsequent meiotic divisions [1]. Human IVF studies confirm that ovarian stimulation affects chromosomal competence, and a comparison of different stimulation regimens suggests that this mainly affects the incidence of post-zygotic errors [7]. Still, ovarian stimulation may not be the only contributing factor, as a high rate of mosaicism is also observed in embryos obtained from young women undergoing natural cycle IVF [2].

Different levels of mosaicism have been reported by different IVF centers. Next to differences in stimulation approaches, this may also reflect variation in culture conditions such as pH and composition of the culture medium, temperature differences, air quality, and oxygen concentration. Supraphysiological oxygen levels (i.e. atmospheric oxygen levels) have been shown to increase malsegregation in cleavage-stage *in vitro*-cultured embryos from a nondisjunction prone mouse model [7].

Chromosomal mosaicism is not exclusively observed in human embryos. Incidences of 20–40% of chromosomal mosaicism have also been described in bovine, equine, porcine, and non-human primate embryos by FISH analysis for 2–5 chromosomes. Interestingly, although mosaicism was observed both in *in vitro*- and *in vivo*-produced embryos, the proportion of mosaic embryos and the proportion of aberrant cells were significantly lower in *in vivo*-produced embryos (see references in [11]). In contrast, wild-type mouse preimplantation embryos are apparently devoid of chromosomal mosaicism, as they show very low rates of aneuploidy regardless of whether they are produced *in vivo* or *in vitro*. From this we can conclude that, in humans and other non-rodent mammals, chromosome segregation in cells of the preimplantation embryo is predisposed to errors and that this can be exacerbated by (suboptimal) IVF procedures.

Implications of chromosomal mosaicism for preimplantation genetic screening

As an increasing body of evidence suggested that the incidence of chromosomal abnormalities in IVF embryos was extremely high, it also became clear that good embryo morphology did not necessarily exclude an abnormal chromosomal constitution. It was hypothesized that screening of IVF embryos for chromosomal abnormalities before transfer would increase pregnancy rates after IVF. This lead to the introduction of preimplantation genetic diagnosis for aneuploidy screening (PGD-AS) or in short, preimplantation genetic screening (PGS), where FISH analysis was combined with biopsy of Day 3 embryos and the removal of one or two blastomeres for analysis. Although PGS was offered in many IVF centers around the world, its clinical value remained uncertain. Although positive effects on implantation and ongoing pregnancy rates were observed in retrospective studies, prospective randomized trials failed to show a positive effect of PGS on clinical outcomes, or even showed detrimental effects [15].

The observed high rate of diploid–aneuploid mosaicism likely undermines the reliability of the PGS diagnosis, as in this case the blastomere biopsied is not representative for the remaining embryo. If a diploid cell is biopsied from a diploid–aneuploid mosaic embryo, it will be transferred, while the remaining embryo in fact contains aneuploid cells. Moreover, the proportion of diploid cells decreased as a result of the biopsy. If an aneuploid cell is biopsied, the embryo is not transferred, while the proportion of diploid cells has in fact increased [3].

As the proportion of mosaic embryos appears to be highest at the cleavage stages, accuracy can be improved by analyzing the blastocyst stage. This has the additional advantage that several (5–10) trophectoderm cells can be removed, while being less damaging to the embryo than cleavage-stage biopsy [15]. Moreover, most studies of cleavage-stage embryos have been performed using FISH, allowing the screening of only a limited number of chromosomes. It is likely that high-throughput molecular cytogenetic methods and the screening of all chromosomes are necessary to gain the desired diagnostic accuracy. Although preliminary results are promising, several large randomized controlled trials (RCTs) using this approach to PGS are now under way to investigate if this can improve take-home baby rates in IVF.

Impact of chromosomal mosaicism on embryo development and implantation

Development from the cleavage stage to the peri-implantation blastocyst

So far, the majority of the studies investigating the chromosomal constitution of human blastocysts have suggested no definite selection against most of the chromosomal abnormalities observed at the cleavage stage [15]. According to an early model proposed by Evsikov and Verlinsky in 1998, there is self-elimination (arrest) of the whole embryo if the number of aneuploid cells at the morula stage reaches a certain threshold level. Embryos with a number of aneuploid cells below this threshold level develop further and reach the blastocyst stage [7]. So far this hypothesis of a threshold has not been directly investigated, but mouse knockout models have shown that up to 30% of aneuploid cells can be tolerated in apparently healthy animals. However, this model does not take into account the type and number of chromosomes involved in the aberrations that may influence this threshold. Certain chromosome abnormalities, for example trisomy 21, may be tolerated in a higher proportion of cells as an extra chromosome 21 is compatible with (abnormal) development.

Alternatively, it has been shown in human and mouse embryonic stem cells (ESCs) containing chromosomal abnormalities, that these cells do not initiate apoptosis. However, there is apoptosis of chromosomally abnormal cells upon differentiation of ESCs. It has been proposed that similar to this, elimination or non-proliferation of chromosomally abnormal cells may occur at the blastocyst stage, in response to cavitation and initiation of differentiation with the formation of the inner cell mass and trophectoderm compartments (see references in [5]).

Although there are reports of an increase in the proportion of blastocysts showing chromosomal mosaicism, compared to early cleavage-stage embryos, the proportion of aneuploid cells within an embryo seems to decline towards the blastocyst stage [3, 15]. Although not well studied, the proportion of mosaic embryos on Day 4 of embryo development appears to be even higher than at the eight-cell stage [5, 8]. Thus, the process of compaction does not provide a developmental barrier for mosaic embryos. The proportion of mosaic embryos subsequently declines from over 80% in Day 4 embryos to less than 60% in Day 5 developing blastocysts (10 chromosomes investigated with FISH), suggesting that a proportion of mosaic embryos undergo developmental arrest between compaction and cavitation [5].

In an attempt to learn about the fate of mosaic blastocysts around the time of implantation, we subjected embryos to extended culture in an *in vitro*-implantation model up to Day 8 post-fertilization. It was found that, at that time, the incidence of chromosomal mosaicism had further declined to 42%. Furthermore, we found a positive correlation between the total number of cells in the embryo and the number of normal cells in Day 5 and Day 8 developing blastocysts, but not in Day 4 morulas or embryos arrested before cavitation. This finding provided indirect evidence that cavitation, but not compaction, may be critical for elimination of chromosomally abnormal cells or for the establishment of a growth advantage of normal over abnormal cells. On the other hand, we and others have found that new segregation errors can occur after cavitation [4, 5] and that the incidence of mosaicism is still high at Day 8 (42% if only the copy number of 10 chromosomes was investigated). This raises the question about the fate of these mosaic blastocysts after implantation. To explore this question, we will give an overview of what is known about the incidence of chromosomal mosaicism during further embryonic and fetal development.

The incidence of chromosomal mosaicism in chorionic villi and amniotic fluid during prenatal diagnosis

Chromosomal mosaicism is a well-known phenomenon in chorionic villi (CV). Although fetus and placenta originate from the same zygote, their chromosomal constitution can be different which was discovered soon after the introduction of chorionic villus sampling (CVS) for prenatal diagnosis in the first trimester of pregnancy. There are numerous reports of abnormal karyotypes in CV that were later not confirmed in fetal cells. Chorionic villus can be processed for cytogenetic studies in two ways: the direct or semi-direct technique, also called short-term cultured villi (STC-villi) and the long-term preparation method (long-term cultured villi, LTC-villi) [16]. These techniques differ in the origin of the cells that are investigated in the cytogenetic preparations: the cells in STC-villi are derived from the cytotrophoblast of CV and those of LTC-villi are predominantly of mesenchymal origin. Cytotrophoblast and mesenchymal core of CV have a different embryonic origin: the cytotrophoblast is derived from the trophoblast of the blastocyst, whereas the mesenchymal core of the CV is derived from the inner cell mass, and more particularly the hypoblast (see [17] and references herein).

Chromosome analysis of both cell types in fact represents the investigation of two different embryonic compartments that may be chromosomally different as a consequence of post-zygotic mitotic division errors. Due to its embryonic origin, the karyotype of the mesenchymal core better represents the karyotype of the fetus than does that of the cytotrophoblast. Conventional prenatal cytogenetic diagnosis in CV revealed chromosomal mosaicism in 1–2% of the samples. The time and place of a post-zygotic mitotic error during embryonic development, as well as the mitotic or meiotic origin of the chromosome aberration, will determine the pattern of mosaicism. While early division errors of an originally normal zygote may cause generalized mosaicism involving both placental and fetal compartments, later errors, affecting specific cell lineages, will lead to confined placental mosaicism (CPM) and, more rarely, confined fetal mosaicism (CFM). A total of nine different types of mosaicism, five generalized and four confined, can be differentiated [18]. In daily practice of prenatal cytogenetic diagnosis all categories can be found, which implicates a considerable cytogenetic variability along the trophoblast–embryo axis.

If chromosomal mosaicism is encountered in CV, it mostly represents CPM with a fetal confirmation rate of only about 10%, primarily depending on the cell type in which the chromosome abnormality is seen (cytotrophoblast and/or mesenchymal core) and on the type of chromosome abnormality [18]. Confined placental mosaicism involving a trisomy, which accounts for about 50% of all CPM cases, may result from a somatic duplication of a whole chromosome in placental progenitor cells originating from a diploid zygote, or from a trisomic conceptus with loss of the extra chromosome in embryonic but not placental progenitor cells. This phenomenon is called trisomic zygote rescue and is associated with a theoretical 1 in 3 risk of uniparental disomy (UPD) (i.e. both copies of a chromosome pair derived from one parent only) in the normal cell line [19]. The incidence of UPD in a series of 24 unselected cases of CPM involving a trisomy was 4%, confirming the mitotic nature of most CPM cases of trisomy [20]. Although the majority of pregnancies with CPM proceed uneventfully, CPM is associated with an increased risk for intrauterine growth retardation, fetal loss or poor perinatal outcome potentially caused by disturbed placental function, UPD (if an imprinted chromosome is involved or if homozygosity of a recessive allele leads

to a recessive disease), or hidden fetal mosaicism with the abnormal cell line in fact also present in fetal tissues [20].

Chromosomal mosaicism in amniotic fluid (AF) cell cultures, as determined with classical cytogenetic techniques, is even rarer then it is in CV. The frequency ranges from 0.1 to 0.3% with a fetal confirmation rate of about 70% [21].

Do we underestimate chromosomal mosaicism in prenatal diagnosis?

It is important to mention that the incidence of chromosomal mosaicism in CV (1–2%) and AF (0.1–0.3%) may be underestimated because of several reasons. These figures are determined in the course of prenatal cytogenetic diagnosis by using karyotyping of banded chromosomes. This usually involves the analysis of about 10 metaphases excluding a level of mosaicism of 26% with 95% confidence. This means that a low level of mosaicism (<26%) is disregarded during routine chromosome studies, probably leading to an underestimation of the real frequency of mosaicism in CV and AF. Moreover, classical cytogenetic techniques make use of cell cultures, because they depend on metaphases for chromosome analysis. However, in vitro cell cultures may change the in vivo level of mosaicism in favor of normal cells and, therefore, mosaicism can go undetected. Finally, the resolution of karyotyping is limited to 5–10 megabases (Mb) and therefore mosaicism of some structural chromosomal rearrangements that appear to be common in preimplantation embryos [8] can easily be missed during prenatal diagnosis if smaller than 10 Mb. This is illustrated by a case of mosaic 5p submicroscopic/5p microscopic deletion that led to a false negative diagnosis in CV due to presence of only the cell line with the submicroscopic deletion and absence of cells with the microscopically visible deletion in STC- and LTC-villi [16].

Chromosomal mosaicism in CV of spontaneous versus IVF pregnancies

As discussed above, it is important to realize that the high incidence of mosaicism may in part be the result of the IVF procedures, and whether this high frequency is also found in in vivo-generated embryos is not known. Therefore, it could be hypothesized that the incidence of chromosomal mosaicism found during prenatal diagnosis is higher in IVF as compared to non-IVF pregnancies. Two studies investigated the incidence of CPM in IVF/intracytoplasmic sperm injection (ICSI) pregnancies as compared to that in spontaneous conceptions and both found no significant difference [22]. So, it can be concluded that mosaicism associated with ART persists beyond the preimplantation embryo at a rate similar to that associated with pregnancies conceived spontaneously, so that by the end of the first trimester no difference is found in rate of mosaicism between IVF and non-IVF pregnancies. Whether a difference exists before this time remains to be investigated.

Chromosomal mosaicism in spontaneous abortions

About 15% of clinically recognized pregnancies end up in a first trimester spontaneous abortion, mostly due to a chromosome aberration. In a recent review of studies reporting cytogenetic findings with conventional karyotyping, an incidence of chromosome aberrations of 45% was found [23]. Mosaicism accounted for less than 6% of the chromosome abnormalities in this study.

Due to the high incidence of culture failures and maternal cell contamination (MCC), which may account for about 30% of all 46,XX abortion samples [23], researchers have searched for other techniques that are able to determine cytogenetic abnormalities in uncultured abortion tissue. A few studies on tissues of spontaneous abortions used interphase FISH and they concluded that at least 50% of spontaneous abortions with an abnormal karyotype have mosaic forms of chromosome abnormalities [24]. There have also been numerous studies using array CGH. An advantage of using this technique is the high sensitivity for detection of chromosomal mosaicism. A detection level of 10% for whole chromosomes could be achieved [25]. However, none of these studies found a higher incidence of chromosomal mosaicism as compared to karyotyping. An even more sensitive technique for the detection of mosaicism is a genome-wide SNP array, which uses a combination of genomic dosage and genotyping data. The dual property of this tool has proven to be very useful for detection and quantification of chromosomal mosaicism even below 5%, amongst other advantages [26]. Two studies that used SNP arrays for cytogenetic investigation of spontaneous abortions revealed mosaicism in 5.4% and 0%, respectively (see [27] and references therein).

Do we underestimate chromosomal mosaicism in spontaneous abortions?

One of the reasons for this low incidence of mosaicism in spontaneous abortion tissue, despite the use of sensitive cytogenetic techniques such as array CGH or SNP arrays, is probably the use of routine detection criteria. One study was able to detect mosaicism of 10%, but only by lowering the algorithm thresholds [25]. But lowering the algorithm thresholds means the specificity also decreases. Therefore, if mosaicism is not suspected, or is not searched for, a laboratory will not use these specific criteria, potentially leading to underestimation of the true incidence of mosaicism in spontaneous abortions. This is in fact the same as with classical karyotyping that will also miss cases of mosaicism if a routine number of metaphases is investigated, as is discussed above.

Another important biological reason for the underestimation of the frequency of mosaicism is the fact that most studies of spontaneous abortions only investigated one germ layer. For karyotyping, mostly cultured CV (LTC-villi) are used, which involves cytogenetic analysis of predominantly the mesenchymal core of the villi that is derived from the compartment of the extraembryonic mesoderm [17]. By doing so, the karyotype of cytotrophoblast and embryo itself is left undetermined. Sometimes only direct preparations of CV were investigated, determining the karyotype of the cytotrophoblast, while just a few studies investigated both placental cell lineages [28]. Unfortunately, the embryo itself is most of the time not investigated. The existence of discordant cytogenetic results between direct and long-term CV, cultured amniotic membrane, and chorionic plate was detected in 20% of 54 miscarriages [28]. Thus, by analysis of only one compartment in most spontaneous abortion studies, mosaicism can easily go undetected. Dependent on type of chromosomal trisomy, the timing of mitotic segregation error, and the mitotic or meiotic origin of the trisomy, different tissue-specific compartmentalization patterns can be found for the different autosomal trisomies [19]. For instance, trisomy 3 is mostly found in cytotrophobast and will go undetected when the mesenchymal core is investigated. The opposite is true for trisomy 2 [19]. Despite this knowledge, most of the studies using array CGH or SNP array, which are all of rather recent date, isolated DNA out of the whole CV. This potentially dilutes the percentage of abnormal cells to fall beneath the detection level of both techniques, which may contribute to an underestimation of the real incidence of mosaicism.

More cytogenetic studies investigating all placental and embryonic compartments with techniques able to detect (low-level) mosaicism will be necessary to determine the actual incidence of chromosomal mosaicism. Since FISH cannot differentiate between numerical and structural chromosome aberrations, SNP array seems to be the preferred method at this moment.

Summary and conclusions

Screening of human IVF-derived embryos for chromosomal aneuploidies before transfer revealed that the majority of embryos are chromosomally abnormal, with the bulk of abnormalities originating from errors during the first mitotic divisions of early preimplantation development, resulting in chromosomally mosaic embryos. This phenomenon undermines the reliability of PGS at the cleavage stage. We hypothesize that zygotic chromosomes may be predisposed to incorrect attachments to the spindle, due to the remarkable parental epigenetic asymmetry at the pericentric region. This can in turn be exacerbated by oocyte-quality-related perturbation of the chromosome segregation machinery, or by spindle abnormalities induced by a defective or additional sperm centrosome, leading to chromosome malsegregation.

The extent of chromosomal mosaicism observed in preimplantation embryos has so far not been reported in clinically recognized pregnancies. This indicates that at least some of the mosaic embryos are likely to arrest development. Indeed, the incidence of embryos carrying chromosomally abnormal cells was found to decrease during development from the eight-cell to the periimplantation blastocyst stage. This indicates that a proportion of mosaic embryos undergo developmental arrest between compaction and blastocyst formation.

However, not all mosaic embryos will elicit a full embryonic arrest and a significant number of mosaic embryos continue to develop until Day 8 after fertilization, and may have continued development if transferred. Through growth advantage of normal cells or elimination of abnormal cells, some of the mosaic embryos may even become normal or will show limited mosaicism that allows further development. Their fate may then depend on the abnormality involved or on yet unknown factors such as distribution of abnormal cells over the different compartments of placenta and fetus, or on possible irregular shapes of the mosaic embryos due to different growth velocities of normal and abnormal cells. Subsequently, a (pre)clinical pregnancy loss may occur or mosaicism (CPM or generalized) may be encountered prenatally in CV or AF cells.

The incidence of chromosomal mosaicism postnatally is estimated to be about 1% [2]. However, little is known about the presence of chromosomal mosaicism in different organs in children and adults, as only blood is routinely investigated in postnatal cytogenetic diagnosis. Chromosomal mosaicism is increasingly recognized to play a role in brain development and disease [29]. Due to the high incidence as encountered in preimplantation embryos, chromosomal mosaicism may be underestimated as the cause of human disease. Therefore, important biological questions remain concerning the origin and impact of chromosomal mosaicism in embryo development.

References

1. Nagaoka SI, Hassold TJ, Hunt PA. Human aneuploidy: mechanisms and new insights into an age-old problem. *Nat Rev Genet* 2012; 13: 493–504.

2. Mantzouratou A, Delhanty JD. Aneuploidy in the human cleavage stage embryo. *Cytogenet Genome Res* 2011; 133: 141–8.

3. van Echten-Arends J, Mastenbroek S, Sikkema-Raddatz B *et al.* Chromosomal mosaicism in human preimplantation embryos: a systematic review. *Human Reprod Update* 2011; 17: 620–7.

4. Capalbo A, Bono S, Spizzichino L *et al.* Sequential comprehensive chromosome analysis on polar bodies, blastomeres and trophoblast: insights into female meiotic errors and chromosomal segregation in the preimplantation window of embryo development. *Hum Reprod* 2013; 28: 509–18.

5. Santos MA, Teklenburg G, Macklon NS *et al.* The fate of the mosaic embryo: chromosomal constitution and development of Day 4, 5 and 8 human embryos. *Hum Reprod* 2010; 25: 1916–26.

6. Kops GJ, Weaver BA, Cleveland DW. On the road to cancer: aneuploidy and the mitotic checkpoint. *Nat Rev Cancer* 2005; 5: 773–85.

7. Mantikou E, Wong KM, Repping S *et al.* Molecular origin of mitotic aneuploidies in preimplantation embryos. *Biochim Biophys Acta* 2012; 1822: 1921–30.

8. Mertzanidou A, Spits C, Nguyen HT *et al.* Evolution of aneuploidy up to Day 4 of human preimplantation development. *Hum Reprod* 2013; 28: 1716–24.

9. Vassena R, Boue S, Gonzalez-Roca E et al. Waves of early transcriptional activation and pluripotency program initiation during human preimplantation development. *Development* 2011; 138: 3699–709.

10. Schatten H, Sun QY. New insights into the role of centrosomes in mammalian fertilization and implications for ART. *Reproduction* 2011; 142: 793–801.

11. Avo Santos M, van de Werken C, de Vries M et al. A role for Aurora C in the chromosomal passenger complex during human preimplantation embryo development. *Human Reprod* 2011; 26: 1868–81.

12. Dupont C, Harvey AJ, Armant DR et al. Expression profiles of cohesins, shugoshins and spindle assembly checkpoint genes in rhesus macaque oocytes predict their susceptibility for aneuploidy during embryonic development. *Cell Cycle* 2012; 11: 740–8.

13. Lampson MA, Cheeseman IM. Sensing centromere tension: Aurora B and the regulation of kinetochore function. *Trends Cell Biol* 2011; 21: 133–40.

14. Fadloun A, Eid A, Torres-Padilla ME. Mechanisms and dynamics of heterochromatin formation during mammalian development: closed paths and open questions. *Curr Top Dev Biol* 2013; 104: 1–45.

15. Fragouli E, Wells D. Aneuploidy screening for embryo selection. *Semin Reprod Med* 2012; 30: 289–301.

16. van den Berg C, Van Opstal D, Polak-Knook J et al. (Potential) false-negative diagnoses in chorionic villi and a review of the literature. *Prenat Diagn* 2006; 26: 401–8.

17. Bianchi DW, Wilkins-Haug LE, Enders AC et al. Origin of extraembryonic mesoderm in experimental animals: relevance to chorionic mosaicism in humans. *Am J Med Genet* 1993; 46: 542–50.

18. Pittalis MC, Dalpra L, Torricelli F et al. The predictive value of cytogenetic diagnosis after CVS based on 4860 cases with both direct and culture methods. *Prenat Diagn* 1994; 14: 267–78.

19. Wolstenholme J. Confined placental mosaicism for trisomies 2, 3, 7, 8, 9, 16, and 22: their incidence, likely origins, and mechanisms for cell lineage compartmentalization. *Prenat Diagn* 1996; 16: 511–24.

20. Van Opstal D, Van den Berg C, Deelen WH et al. Prospective prenatal investigations on potential uniparental disomy in cases of confined placental trisomy. *Prenat Diagn* 1998; 18: 35–44.

21. Hsu LY, Perlis TE. United States survey on chromosome mosaicism and pseudomosaicism in prenatal diagnosis. *Prenat Diagn* 1984; 4: 97–130.

22. Jacod BC, Lichtenbelt KD, Schuring-Blom GH et al. Does confined placental mosaicism account for adverse perinatal outcomes in IVF pregnancies? *Hum Reprod* 2008; 23: 1107–12.

23. van den Berg MM, van Maarle MC, van Wely M et al. Genetics of early miscarriage. *Biochim Biophys Acta* 2012; 1822: 1951–9.

24. Lebedev I. Mosaic aneuploidy in early fetal losses. *Cytogenet Genome Res* 2011; 133: 169–83.

25. Scott SA, Cohen N, Brandt T et al. Detection of low-level mosaicism and placental mosaicism by oligonucleotide array comparative genomic hybridization. *Genet Med* 2010; 12: 85–92.

26. Conlin LK, Thiel BD, Bonnemann CG et al. Mechanisms of mosaicism, chimerism and uniparental disomy identified by single nucleotide polymorphism array analysis. *Hum Mol Genet* 2010; 19: 1263–75.

27. Li G, Liu Y, He NN et al. Molecular karyotype single nucleotide polymorphism analysis of early fetal demise. *Syst Biol Reprod Med* 2013; 59: 227–31.

28. Kalousek DK, Barrett IJ, Gartner AB. Spontaneous abortion and confined chromosomal mosaicism. *Hum Genet* 1992; 88: 642–6.

29. Devalle S, Sartore RC, Paulsen BS et al. Implications of aneuploidy for stem cell biology and brain therapeutics. *Front Cell Neurosci* 2012; 6: 36.

DNA is not the whole story

Transgenerational epigenesis and imprinting

Ashwini Balakrishnan and J. Richard Chaillet

Introduction

There are two types of genomic information accurately inherited or maintained following DNA replication: the entire genomic DNA sequence and epigenetic information in the form of patterns of CpG methylation on a subset of the genome. These DNA methylation patterns are crucially important for mammalian development, primarily because they regulate gene transcription. There are cyclical declines and increases in DNA methylation during gametogenesis and embryogenesis, and the oscillations in methylation occurring across generations must depend on *de novo* methylation and demethylation processes to rearrange the existing methylation patterns. Within any single reproductive cycle, changes in genomic methylation are the outcome of a linked sequence of active and passive processes that rearrange genomic methylation to generate epigenetic milestones, each with a defined future role. For example, genomic imprints are established during gametogenesis by *de novo* methylation to generate mature gametes with complete complements of paternal methylation imprints in sperm and maternal methylation imprints in oocytes. The establishment of a collective set of imprints within a sperm and an oocyte is an epigenetic milestone, whose purpose after sperm–oocyte fusion is to ensure monoallelic expression of imprinted genes during fetal development. We postulate that another essential epigenetic milestone is found in the blastocyst-stage embryo; this milestone is achieved at the generation, through the poorly understood process of epigenetic reprogramming, of pluripotent embryo stem cells, whose role is to contribute to the development of the conceptus. Primordial germ cells (PGCs), largely devoid of genomic methylation and poised to differentiate into gametes with sex-specific imprints, and adult stem cells, poised

to differentiate into organs, would be other possible epigenetic milestones. The developmental locations of three fundamental milestones (gametes, blastocyst, and PGCs), and the epigenetic processes by which they are crafted, are depicted in Fig. 5.1.

In this chapter, we describe the molecular processes underlying generation of epigenetic milestones, and discuss how these processes define much of what we know about transgenerational epigenesis. We will focus on genomic imprinting because much is known about the molecular mechanisms of genomic imprinting, and these mechanisms involve two critically important milestones, the gamete and the blastocyst. We will also discuss abnormalities in the processes of generating epigenetic milestones, and how these abnormalities can reduce or possibly even enhance transgenerational epigenesis.

DNA is not the whole story

The non-equivalence of the genome inherited from the mother versus the father was convincingly demonstrated in the early 1980s. Pronuclear transfer experiments in mice were performed to create embryos that contained either two copies of the maternal genome (gynogenotes) or two copies of the paternal genome (androgenotes) [1]. Both gynogenetic and androgenetic uniparental embryos were not viable and had opposing phenotypes. Gynogenetic embryos displayed more advanced embryonic development than androgenetic embryos whereas androgenetic embryos emphasized well-developed extraembryonic tissues. These observations indicated that the chromosomes inherited from the male and female parents are functionally different, and importantly, since this difference is independent of the embryo's sex, the genome differences must reside in the autosomes.

Textbook of Human Reproductive Genetics, eds Karen Sermon and Stéphane Viville. Published by Cambridge University Press.
© Cambridge University Press 2014.

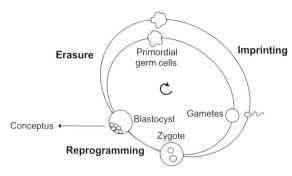

Figure 5.1 Depiction of the developmental locations of the fundamental epigenetic milestones. Erasure, imprinting, and reprogramming are three processes involving major rearrangement of CpG methylation patterns in the genome.

Mouse embryos with uniparental disomies, in which each conceptus inherits both copies of a particular chromosome from just one parent, beautifully validated the theory that functional differences exist between maternal and paternal versions of one or more autosomes. For example, mouse embryos with uniparental disomies of chromosome 11 had very different phenotypes depending on whether the chromosome was inherited maternally or paternally. Maternal disomic mice for chromosome 11 (and nullisomic for paternal chromosome 11) were smaller than their chromosomally normal littermates while paternal disomic mice for chromosome 11 (and nullisomic for maternal chromosome 11) were larger than their normal littermates [2]. This sex-specific inheritance effect indicated that the maternal alleles of one or more genes on chromosome 11 function differently than the opposite paternal alleles. We now know that the functional difference between maternal and paternal alleles of particular genes on chromosome 11 is because one allele of each of these genes is expressed (transcribed) and the other is not expressed. Assuming that the DNA sequence of these genes was not reversibly altered after passage through spermatogenesis and oogenesis, the two parental alleles of each gene must be epigenetically distinguished so that one parental allele is expressed and the other allele is silent. Many genes whose parental alleles function differently due to a parent-specific epigenetic footprint have now been definitively identified. They are known as imprinted genes and they are located on those chromosomes found to exhibit developmental abnormalities when inherited as maternal and/or paternal uniparental disomies. Moreover, the parental alleles exhibit unambiguous differences in DNA methylation,

a heritable form of genome modification. A list of mouse imprinted genes and their chromosomal location can be found on the MouseBook website [3].

Establishment of genomic imprints

Nature of an imprint

If functions of the two haploid genomes during embryogenesis are truly strictly determined by their parental origins, then imprints should have certain inalienable features. They must mark two genetically identical alleles differently in mature gametes, and following fertilization imprints should be maintained long enough to affect development of the conceptus. Furthermore, because maternal chromosomes become paternal chromosomes during spermatogenesis and paternal chromosomes become maternal chromosomes during oogenesis, the perpetuation (inheritance) of imprints must be disrupted in every generation before germ cells commit to either the male or female lineage (i.e. in PGCs) to ensure a switch in parental form.

The patterns of DNA methylation observed during development fulfill all of the aforementioned features of the genomic imprinting process. Precise biochemical mechanisms are in place for both the establishment and maintenance of methylation (Fig. 5.2), which ensures the accurate formation and then perpetuation of patterns of genomic methylation following DNA replication. In this scheme, unmethylated symmetric CpGs in DNA are converted to fully methylated CpGs by *de novo* methyltransferases. The symmetric arrangement of methylated CpG dinucleotides on complementary strands of fully methylated DNA in a cell is reproduced in both daughter cells by DNA replication followed immediately thereafter by maintenance methylation, carried out by a maintenance methyltransferase enzyme.

There are tremendous cyclical changes in the average percentage of total genomic CpGs that are methylated during development (Fig. 5.3A). There are two prominent hiatuses in methylation, one in undifferentiated PGCs and the other in blastocyst-stage embryos. Between these two low points, pronounced and apparently monotonic increases in methylation occur during gametogenesis and post-implantation embryogenesis. Notably, any given methylation pattern or imprint that was established on just one parental allele during gametogenesis is maintained during the

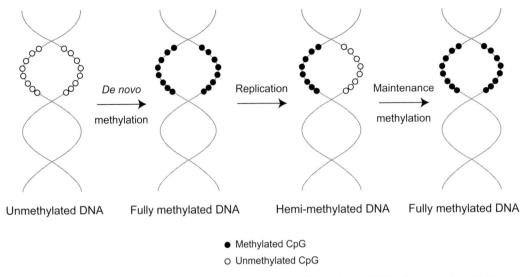

● Methylated CpG
○ Unmethylated CpG

Figure 5.2 Biochemical processes of *de novo* methylation (conversion of unmethylated DNA to fully methylated DNA) and maintenance methylation (conversion of hemi-methylated to fully methylated DNA) following DNA replication in a CpG-rich region.

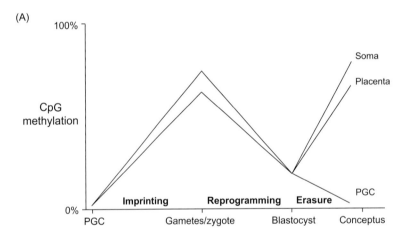

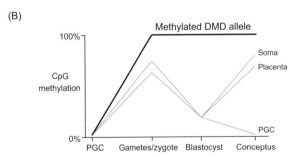

Figure 5.3 (**A**) Cyclical increases and decreases of genomic DNA methylation during gametogenesis and embryonic development. (**B**) Inheritance of methylation on differentially methylated domains (DMDs). Methylation is established on one parental allele during gametogenesis and this methylation is maintained (inherited) after fertilization. PGC, primordial germ cell.

fall in preimplantation genomic methylation (Fig. 5.3B). The important genomic locations of inherited imprinted methylation are called differentially methylated domains (DMDs) because one parental allele is highly methylated and the opposite allele is unmethylated.

In discussing the important correlations between genomic methylation and genomic imprinting, we will first address the way in which parent-specific methylation is acquired in the gametes. Thereafter, we will focus on the all-important mechanism whereby patterns of DNA methylation are faithfully inherited following fertilization.

Enzymes involved in imprint establishment

A ground state of an unmethylated diploid genome is present in undifferentiated PGCs. Although there are some quibbles about whether the PGC genome is completely stripped of methylation marks, it is clear that all maternal and paternal methylation imprints are absent [4, 5]. From this ground state, as the germ cells differentiate through spermatogenesis in males and oogenesis in females, new methylation of a large percentage (50–70%) of genomic CpG dinucleotides occurs (*de novo* methylation). Within this newly methylated DNA are the DMD sequences. It is important to realize that DMD methylation is a very minor component of methylation acquired during the entirety of both female and male gametogenesis. It is logical that parent-specific imprints are established during gametogenesis, as the two alleles are separated (in two organisms) where different processes specific to either female or male germ cells can act on the two otherwise identical parental alleles, methylating one but not the other. In this way, gametogenesis serves as the developmental stage for the establishment of parent-specific genomic imprints. Hence, during every developmental cycle, imprints are erased in PGCs (see below) and established during maturation of the male and female gametes [4].

What are the enzyme(s) that methylate unmethylated DMD sequences in one parental germ line but not in the opposite one and how specific are they? These enzymes are *de novo* DNA methyltransferases, whose specific function is to convert unmethylated DNA to fully methylated DNA, in which complementary CpG residues on both strands are methylated (Fig. 5.2). There are two known mammalian *de novo* DNA methyltransferases, DNMT3A and DNMT3B (Fig. 5.4A). Both are excellent candidates for establishing patterns of methylation because *in vitro* both enzymes exhibit primarily *de novo* methyltransferase activity, with little maintenance methyltransferase activity. A series of *in vivo* studies in the mouse indicated that DNMT3A is the active *de novo* methyltransferase during both male and female gametogenesis, and appears to be responsible for the acquisition of all DNA methy-

lation during these developmental stages. To elucidate the role of DNMT3A in imprinting, the *Dnmt3a* gene was eliminated specifically in male and female germ cells before Embryonic Day 14.5 (E14.5), i.e. in PGCs [6]. Embryos from female mice missing germ cell DNMT3A died around E10.5, while males without germ cell DNMT3A showed such impaired spermatogenesis that the effects of missing methylation marks on embryonic development in the next generation could not be studied in this model. Maternal imprints were lost in the embryos from the females lacking DNMT3A in their germ cells while spermatogonia from mutant males lacked DMD methylation at a subset of paternal imprints. DNMT3A is involved in methylation-induced transposon silencing at a subset of repetitive elements specifically in male PGCs [7]. Defective spermatogenesis in male PGCs without DNMT3A may be due to meiotic failure caused by partial retrotransposon reactivation (see also Chapter 6).

In the female germ line, genomic methylation occurs during the oocyte growth phase after the meiotic arrest, and a number of different sequence types, not just DMD sequences, become methylated by DNMT3A [6]. In contrast, in the male germ line, *de novo* methylation occurs premeiotically in fetal prospermatogonia and targets repetitive DNA of many different types. Because *de novo* methylation catalyzed by DNMT3A is established on many more sequences than just germline imprints, this enzyme itself does not provide the machinery for specifically directing methylation to the relevant imprinted regions. A similar approach was used to explore the role of *Dnmt3b* in genomic imprinting. Loss of DNMT3B in PGCs had no effect on the establishment of male or female imprints. Thus, DNMT3A and not DNMT3B is the *de novo* methyltransferase used to catalyze the addition of methylation to imprinted DMD sequences in germ cells.

Auxiliary factors

DNMT3L is a protein with homology to DNMT3 family members but lacking a functional catalytic domain (Fig. 5.4A). DNMT3L has been shown to interact with both DNMT3A and DNMT3B [8]. It is the interaction between DNMT3L and DNMT3A that is relevant to the establishment of parental imprints. Concomitant increases in DNMT3A and DNMT3L concentrations are seen in the embryonic

(A)

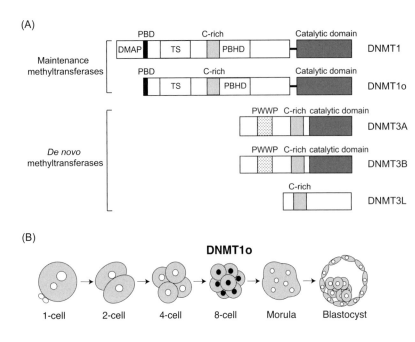

Figure 5.4 (**A**) Depiction of various domains in *de novo* and maintenance methyltransferases. Dnmt3L lacks the methyltransferase catalytic domain and DNMT1o (oocyte specific) lacks the N-terminal DNMT1 domain known to interact with DNMT1-associated protein 1 (DMAP1). DMAP = DMAP1-interaction domain; PBD = PCNA-binding domain; PBHD = Polybromo homology domain; PWWP motif = Proline–Tryptophan–Tryptophan–Proline motif; TS = Replication focus targeting sequence. (**B**) DNMT1o is synthesized in the oocyte and retained in the cytoplasm except at the 8-cell stage when it moves into the nuclei of all blastomeres. (**C**) Loss of DNMT1o at the 8-cell stage results in an abnormally unmethylated imprint in one-half of cells after the 16-cell stage. A representative maternally (M) imprinted chromosome is shown. The normally methylated (imprinted) and abnormally unmethylated chromosomes will segregate into different cells. DMD, differentially methylated domain.

(B)

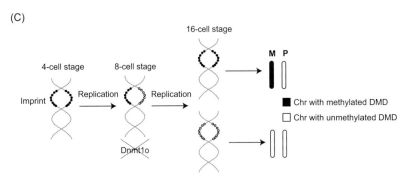

(C)

testis between E15.5 and E18.5 and their levels are down-regulated shortly after birth. In the ovary, levels of DNMT3A are relatively constant but the levels of DNMT3L peak sharply in the phase associated with rapid oocyte growth [9]. These results indicate that high levels of both DNMT3A and DNMT3L coincide with acquisition of sex-specific methylation in the ovary and testis. Importantly, these phases are associated with the establishment of functional genomic imprints [10–12].

Genetic experiments confirmed that germ cells are the sites where DNMT3L has biological functions. *Dnmt3l*−/− adult mice obtained from crosses between heterozygous *Dnmt3l*+/− female and male mice are viable and have normal genomic methylation, indicat-

ing that DNMT3L is not required for post-zygotic *de novo* methylation. There is, however, a strict requirement for DNMT3L in germ cells because *Dnmt3l*−/− males are sterile and embryos from *Dnmt3l*−/− females are phenotypically abnormal and die around mid gestation (E10.5) [13, 14]. The embryos from *Dnmt3l*−/− females show loss of DMD methylation at several maternally imprinted loci indicating that DNMT3L is needed to establish imprints in the oocyte. DNMT3L is also needed for the establishment of methylation in male germ cells. *Dnmt3l*−/− males are sterile with no germ cells present in the adult male. Paternally imprinted sequences are partially demethylated by the lack of DNMT3L in germ cells from 17-day-old male mice. However, there seems to be a complete loss of

(A)

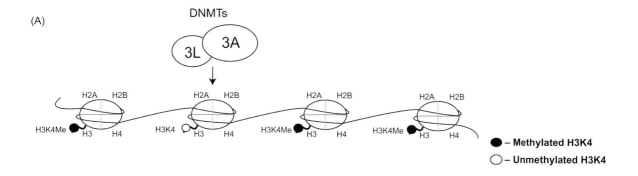

(B)

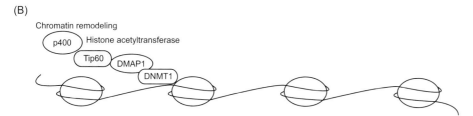

Figure 5.5 (**A**) *De novo* DNA methylation is directed to a region devoid of histone H3K4 methylation by DNMT3L, which interacts with unmethylated H3K4. (**B**) Chromatin remodeling by the Tip60-p400 complex and DNMT1-mediated maintenance methylation may be coordinated by interactions with DMAP1 during preimplantation reprogramming.

methylation at retrotransposon elements in the male germline, which are consequently transcribed at a high frequency causing meiotic failure [14]. The importance of DNA methylation as a mechanism of repression of retrotransposon transcription is discussed in Chapter 6.

The simultaneous germ-cell expression of DNMT3A and DNMT3L, as well as the similarities in phenotypes of mice with germ-cell deletions in the *Dnmt3a* and *Dnmt3l* genes, indicate that DNMT3L is an essential, albeit catalytically inactive, auxiliary factor for DNMT3A-mediated *de novo* methylation in female and male gametogenesis. Crystallographic studies have provided insight into the mechanism of imprint establishment by the DNMT3A–DNMT3L complex. DNMT3L and DNMT3A interact through the carboxy terminal region of DNMT3L and this complex forms a tetramer through interaction between two DNMT3A–DNMT3L dimers [15]. DNMT3L stabilizes the catalytic activity of DNMT3A, and mutations in interacting amino acids between DNMT3L and DNMT3A cause loss of DNMT3A catalytic function. Further experiments illustrated that the DNMT3A–DNMT3L complex methylates

CpG residues with an average spacing of 9.5 residues. This interval was observed in maternally imprinted genes, which had an average periodicity of 9.5 base pairs between them, but not in the DMDs of paternally imprinted genes. *Dnmt3a* and *Dnmt3l* knockout experiments also illustrated that maternally imprinted DMDs are more susceptible to the loss of these proteins than paternally imprinted DMDs.

Although there is a dual requirement for DNMT3A and DNMT3L in the establishment of maternal and paternal imprints, these two proteins together do not account for the specific establishment of genomic imprints. What other factors, if any, direct the DNMT3A/DNMT3L complex to sequences on which methylation imprints are deposited? One attribute of genomic structure that appears to be relevant is the chromatin makeup of target regions. DNMT3L binds to genomic sequences devoid of H3K4 methylation through its Plant Homeo Domain (PHD)-like domain (Fig. 5.5A). This interaction, as well as other similar ones may refine the targets of the DNMT3A/DMNT3L complex toward imprinted sequences [16]. Of course, there are likely to be limits to the specificity provided by such genome-wide post-translational modifications of histones, and the real specificity lies in some as yet unknown features of the DNA target sequences themselves.

Acquisition at different times

The different times at which imprints are established in the maternal and paternal germ lines is intriguing. Paternally imprinted DMDs such as the *H19/Igf2* DMD acquire methylation before the onset of meiosis in prospermatogonia during their mitotic proliferation in mice. These paternal methylation imprints are maintained through the remainder of male gametogenesis by maintenance methylation, and are present in haploid sperm. In contrast, maternal imprints are acquired postnatally, after mitotic expansion of oogonia and during the period of oocyte growth and meiotic arrest. The reason for the mitotic acquisition of paternal imprints and the meiotic acquisition of maternal imprints is not known. It is also not known why the acquisition of the different maternal imprints is a highly orchestrated process in which some imprints such as methylation of *Snurf/Snrpn* DMD sequences are established early in meiotic maturation whereas others such as methylation of *Peg1* DMD sequences are established just before completion of meiosis I in mice [10–12]. In humans, a similar pattern of imprint establishment is observed where paternal imprints are acquired prior to entry into meiosis and maternal imprints are established during oocyte growth after meiotic arrest. The timing of imprint establishment makes oocytes particularly vulnerable to artificial reproduction technologies that accelerate oocyte maturation (such as ovarian hyperstimulation with gonadotrophins) because immature oocytes with incomplete imprints may also be released. Furthermore, *in vitro* maturation of germ cells and preimplantation embryos can affect imprint establishment or maintenance as described in Chapter 12.

Inheritance and maintenance of genomic imprints

Enzymes involved in imprint maintenance

Maintenance methylation involves the methylation of cytosines in CpG residues of the newly synthesized DNA strand, but only in CpG dinucleotides complementary to methylated CpGs of the parent DNA strand. Therefore maintenance methyltransferases act on hemi-methylated DNA after each S phase to convert it to fully methylated DNA. The DNMT1 DNA cytosine methyltransferase is the only enzyme known to possess maintenance methyltransferase activity in mammals (Fig. 5.4A). DNMT1 has been shown to possess a high affinity for hemi-methylated DNA and is targeted to replication foci during S phase [1].

DNMT1 is required for the maintenance of overall genomic methylation. The catalytic methyltransferase activity of DNMT1 is located in the C-terminal domain, while the N-terminus contains domains specialized for nuclear translocation and other regulatory functions. Embryos developing in the absence of DNMT1 die around the middle of gestation, and have a severe reduction in the methylation of imprinted DMDs and repetitive DNA sequences. Several imprinted genes are expressed abnormally from both parental alleles (biallelic expression), consistent with the loss of parent-specific imprinted methylation. Because *Dnmt1*$^{-/-}$ embryos lack appropriate methylation marks at several sequences, it was not possible to determine the contribution of disrupted imprinted gene expression to the observed embryonic lethality.

DNMT1 has been shown to possess two main protein-coding isoforms – the longer somatic DNMT1s isoform and the short DNMT1o isoform expressed specifically in oocytes and preimplantation embryos (Fig. 5.4A). DNMT1s is expressed in all stages of preimplantation development including the pronuclear stage and is found in the nucleus from the two-cell stage of preimplantation development onward [17]. Translation of the DNMT1s protein is initiated from an AUG codon encoded in exon 1s of the *Dnmt1* gene, whereas translation of the oocyte-specific transcript is initiated from an AUG codon encoded in exon 4 of the gene. Mouse DNMT1o is a catalytically active maintenance methyltransferase, lacking the first 118 amino acids of mouse DNMT1s, but otherwise identical. DNMT1o is synthesized solely in the oocyte and is a maternal-effect protein found in high concentrations in the ooplasm and cytoplasm of early preimplantation mouse embryos. Cytoplasmic DNMT1o moves into the nucleus only at fourth embryonic S phase (eight-cell stage) (Fig. 5.4B). Homozygous *Dnmt1*$^{\Delta 1o/\Delta 1o}$ female mice and embryos derived from these lack DNMT1o in all cells.

Analysis of DNMT1o has provided important insights into the role of the *Dnmt1* gene in genomic imprinting [18]. Although DNMT1s (zygotically produced) is present in the nucleus at this stage, it is unable to compensate for a loss of eight-cell DNMT1o. Because embryos from $Dnmt1^{\Delta 1o/\Delta 1o}$ female mice are missing nuclear DNMT1o at the eight-cell stage, the hemi-methylated DNA at this stage is not converted to fully methylated DNA (Fig. 5.4C). After the next round of replication, the hemi-methylated DNA duplex gives rise to a hemi-methylated DNA duplex and an unmethylated DNA duplex. At this stage (16-cell) DNMT1s is present in the nucleus and it converts the hemi-methylated duplex into a fully methylated duplex. The unmethylated duplex, which is not a substrate for DNMT1s, remains unmethylated during future cell divisions. The net result is a reduction to 50% of the normal level of methylation. When E9.5 embryos from $Dnmt1^{\Delta 1o/\Delta 1o}$ mothers were examined, the loss of methylation was restricted to the genomic imprints. The global genomic methylation and methylation at repeats such as the intracisternal A particle (IAP) provirus were normal in E9.5 embryos from $Dnmt1^{\Delta 1o/\Delta 1o}$ females. These experiments indicate two possibilities: (1) DNMT1o has maintenance methyltransferase activity exclusive to genomic imprints, or (2) both imprinted and non-imprinted (for example IAP) sequences lose methylation in the absence of DNMT1o, but only the imprints are unable to regain methylation in later embryogenesis. Different chromosomes and embryo cells lost DMD methylation in this model depending on the random assortment of individual chromosomes (Fig. 5.4C). As a consequence, embryos derived from oocytes lacking DNMT1o showed a mosaic loss of imprints in different cells, causing a wide range of embryonic and placental defects. These findings clearly illustrate that perturbations in normally inherited imprinted DNA methylation can severely impact fetal growth and development.

Features of Imprinted DMDs

More than 100 imprinted genes have been identified in the mouse and they are organized into discrete clusters of two or more genes each [1]. Imprinted clusters can stretch for thousands of kilobases and they can consist of paternally and maternally imprinted protein-coding genes, often interspersed with imprinted untranslated genes, as well as non-imprinted genes. In general, each imprinted cluster contains a primary DMD, which serves as the imprinting control element (ICE) and whose methylation is established in the germ line. The importance of an ICE (primary DMD) can be shown by the effect of an ICE deletion on imprinted gene expression. For example, deletion of the ICE between the $Igf2$ and $H19$ genes results in abnormal expression of the normally silent paternal allele of the $H19$ gene (Fig. 5.6A). More details of the molecular function of this $H19/Igf2$ ICE will be discussed below. Secondary DMDs can also be present in the cluster, which acquire their methylation after fertilization due to cis-directed effects of a nearby primary DMD.

DMDs consist of a high density of CpGs, which are arranged as tandem repeats and imprinted genes require a minimum number of tandem repeats for differential methylation (Fig. 5.6B) [19]. Tandem repeats occur mostly in maternally imprinted genes at a frequency of 6–9 repeats of 18–170 base pairs in size. Paternally imprinted DMDs such as the $H19/Igf2$ DMD do not possess tandem repeats even though they possess a high density of CpG residues. It has also been found that DMDs of maternally imprinted genes contain imprinted promoters while paternally imprinted genes lack promoters in the DMD region. These differences indicate that maternally and paternally imprinted DMDs may be regulated differently. Maternally imprinted DMDs are predicted to have similar secondary structure even though they show considerable sequence divergence [1].

Other important features of DMDs were revealed in studies of DMD methylation in mouse embryonic stem (ES) cells. When imprinted sequences in ES cells lose their CpG methylation due to a transient loss of DNMT1, they are unable to recover these marks after DNMT1 is restored [20]. Importantly, this inability to recover DMD methylation occurs despite the expression of both DNMT3A and DNMT3L, two proteins that normally cooperate to establish methylation imprints in germ cells. These experiments indicate that imprinted DMDs have unique inheritance properties. First, they acquire methylation only during gametogenesis. Second, this germ-line methylation is normally continuously maintained (inherited) in the offspring's cells irrespective of changes in non-imprinted methylation. Lastly, after fertilization, the unmethylated DMD allele does not become methylated. In essence, DMD sequences evolved to maintain or inherit the methylation state established in the gamete, which is highly methylated on one parental allele and unmethylated on the opposite parental allele. Precisely how the sequence makeup of DMDs

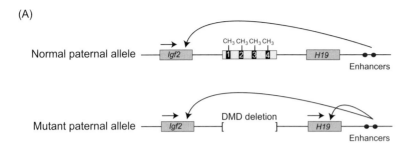

(A)

Normal paternal allele

Mutant paternal allele

Figure 5.6 (**A**) Deletion of the differentially methylated domain (DMD) from the paternal allele of the *H19/Igf2* cluster causes paternal *H19* expression and thus abnormal biallelic *H19* expression. (**B**) Structures of a maternally methylated DMD (overlapping the *Snrpn* gene) and a paternally imprinted DMD (near the *H19* gene) are shown. Gray rectangles = DMDs. Black arrowheads = tandem repeats. Arrows = transcription start sites. Solid ovals = CTCF binding sites.

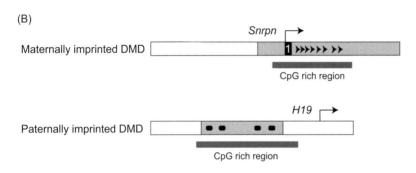

(B)

Maternally imprinted DMD

Paternally imprinted DMD

provides these important inheritance properties is not known.

Consequences of inherited methylation: monoallelic gene expression

Although a normal embryo has two alleles of each imprinted gene, only one parental allele of the gene is expressed. For each imprinted gene, monoallelic expression is determined by the presence of a nearby DMD. Some DMDs overlap a gene's promoter, and the parent-specific methylation directly suppresses transcription. Many regulatory DMDs however are quite distant (> 500 kilobase (kb)) from imprinted genes' promoters. How does the methylation of a DMD lead to transcriptional suppression of these genes? There are two main mechanisms that have been characterized to date, which describe how methylation of a DMD can lead to transcriptional suppression of genes in the entire imprinted cluster [21].

Insulator model: H19/Igf2 imprinting

The conserved *H19/Igf2* locus is located on mouse chromosome 7 and human chromosome 11. *H19* is a maternally expressed non-coding RNA, while

insulin-like growth factor 2 (*Igf2*) is a paternally expressed gene involved in promoting embryonic growth and development. The expression of these genes is reciprocally controlled by the methylation of the DMD located between them (Fig. 5.7A). Hypomethylation of both maternal and paternal DMD alleles leads to biallelic expression of the *H19* gene and corresponding silencing of *Igf2* expression. The mechanism for this regulation was elucidated by identification of binding sites of the insulator protein CCCTC-binding factor (CTCF) in the DMD region. On the maternally inherited chromosome, CTCF binds to the unmethylated DMD and acts as an insulator preventing enhancers 3' of the *H19* gene from activating *Igf2* expression. Instead, the enhancers activate *H19* expression. The DMD in the paternally inherited chromosome is methylated preventing CTCF binding, allowing the enhancer to activate its preferred target *Igf2*.

Non-coding RNA model: Kcnq1 locus

The other generally recognized mechanism of imprinted gene regulation shared by several clusters is through transcriptional suppression by a non-coding RNA (ncRNA). Most imprinted clusters are associated with at least one ncRNA. The *Kcnq1* cluster is regulated by a maternally methylated DMD (KvDMR1),

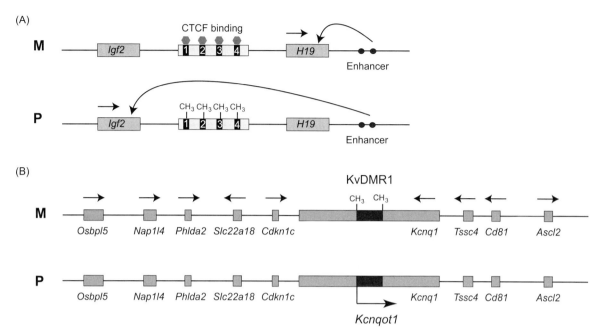

Figure 5.7 (**A**) Transcriptional regulation of *H19/Igf2* expression by imprinted DMD methylation mediated by CTCF binding at four sites causes selective enhancer activation of *H19*. (**B**) *Kcnq1* locus regulates monoallelic expression of several genes through expression of non-coding RNA *Kcnq1ot1*. Horizontal arrows indicate transcribed alleles.

which is located in an intron of the *Kcnq1* gene (Fig. 5.7B). When this DMD is unmethylated, which is the normal paternal allele, the long (>60 kb) *Kcnq1ot1* ncRNA, whose promoter lies within KvDMR1, is expressed. This expression in turn leads to the suppression of transcription of surrounding genes on the same chromosome. On the maternally inherited chromosome, the DMD is methylated, suppressing expression of *Kcnq1ot1* and allowing expression of the surrounding genes. The mechanism by which the long ncRNA is able to suppress gene expression is not known. Mechanisms of RNA interference may explain how *Kcnq1ot1* suppresses *Kcnq1* expression but not the expression of genes in the cluster, several kilobases away from KvDMR1. Truncation of the ncRNA *Kcnq1ot1* leads to de-repression of the genes on the paternal chromosome and biallelic expression, hence the length of the ncRNA seems to be important for the parent-specific expression. Coating of genes in the cluster by the ncRNA or transcription of the ncRNA itself has been postulated to recruit repressive chromatin marks leading to gene silencing. However, these hypothetical mechanisms have yet to be rigorously tested, and if correct, would not explain how certain genes in the cluster escape imprinting and exhibit non-imprinted, biallelic expression.

Interplay between chromatin modifications and DNA methylation

Recent studies have identified interactions between DNA methylation and other chromatin modifications that control transcription. Besides regulating ncRNA expression and the function of insulator sequences, DNA methylation in imprinted regions is observed to alter local chromatin states, which further result in suppression or activation of transcription of the surrounding genes. The interplay between DNA methylation and chromatin modifications is complex and interdependent and may vary between different imprinted genes. Studies have reported parent-specific differences in histone acetylation in differentially methylated regions of imprinted genes with the unmethylated allele being associated with a transcriptionally active chromatin state [22]. We will describe two well-documented interactions between DNA methylation and other chromatin features to understand how different chromatin processes may direct DNA methylation and consequently affect transcription.

As discussed above in the "Establishment of genomic imprints" section, the DNMT3A–DNMT3L complex mediates *de novo* methylation of imprinted genes in gametogenesis and loss of DNMT3L in females results in embryos without maternal imprints. DNMT3L was found to interact with histone H3 tails specifically when they were unmethylated on the lysine residue at position 4 (H3K4). Because methylation of H3K4 inhibited this interaction, DNMT3L is specifically directed to regions devoid of H3K4 methylation (Fig. 5.5A). This study demonstrates the mechanism by which chromatin modifications could contribute to the targeting of DNA methylation to specific regions [16].

The essential role of the Tip60-p400 chromatin remodeling complex in preimplantation development was shown by the failure to identify homozygous mutant preimplantation embryos from crosses between heterozygous mice that have engineered mutations in any one of a number of genes encoding components of the complex [23, 24]. These findings suggest that Tip60-p400 is involved in a process of remodeling the epigenetic makeup of the preimplantation genome, a process possibly associated with epigenetic reprogramming to a pluripotent cell state (see below). Interestingly, the DNMT1-associated protein DMAP1 is one of the essential components of Tip60-p400 [24], further suggesting that preimplantation functions of Tip60-p400 and DNMT1 may be coordinated through DMAP1. If so, we speculate that during preimplantation development, Tip60-p400 chromatin remodeling activity participates in a process of epigenetic reprogramming to rearrange genomic methylation (Fig. 5.5B). In this model, by the milestone blastocyst stage, a pattern of genome-wide methylation is established such that the blastocyst's pluripotent stem cells can contribute to normal and complete embryonic development.

Abnormalities of imprinting

Genomic imprinting has been shown to be vital for both prenatal and postnatal development and loss of imprinting on certain chromosomes can lead to congenital anomalies [25]. Abnormal imprinting in a region can occur due to deletion or duplication of the DMD region or failure to establish correct methylation patterns. A few of the well-characterized human diseases caused by loss of imprinting result in growth abnormalities or neurodevelopmental disorders. The Beckwith–Weidemann syndrome is characterized by somatic overgrowth, congenital malformations and embryonic neoplasia. About 60% of the sporadic Beckwith–Weidemann syndrome cases have abnormal methylation patterns in a 1-Megabase (Mb) region of chromosomal 11 at position 11p15.5. This region contains both the *H19/IGF2* and *KCNQ1* imprinted clusters, and abnormal CpG methylation results in biallelic expression of either the *IGF2* gene or the *KCNQOT1* transcript or both.

Loss of imprinting can also result in neurobehavioral disturbances in the Prader–Willi and Angelman syndromes. The Prader–Willi syndrome is caused either by maternal uniparental disomy, paternal deletion, or loss of methylation in a 2-Mb region on chromosome 15 at 15q11–13. The shortest region of overlap (SRO) of numerous Prader–Willi syndrome deletions is a 4.3-kb region containing the DMD (ICE) of a large cluster of imprinted genes. Angelman syndrome is due to loss of imprinting and deficiency of the normally maternally expressed gene *UBE3A*. Interestingly, although this gene is embedded in the Prader–Willi syndrome cluster, its imprinting is regulated by a unique ICE.

Genomic imprinting defects can occur during establishment of imprints in germ cells or during the maintenance of imprints in the early embryo. Because assisted reproductive technology (ART) such as intracytoplasmic sperm injection, superovulation of oocytes, sperm cryopreservation, and *in vitro* fertilization manipulate gametes and early embryos, it is not surprising that ART has been postulated to cause imprinting disorders. In this regard, certain imprinting diseases like the Beckwith–Weidemann syndrome have been reported to occur at a 6–9 times higher frequency in children from ART patients. The effect of various ART procedures on genomic imprinting is further described in Chapter 12.

Preimplantation reprogramming

Global DNA methylation and pluripotency

The role of the *Dnmt1* gene in maintenance of genomic imprints in preimplantation embryos is complex. After fertilization, both parental genomes undergo a general or global loss of genomic methylation in the presence of nuclear DNMT1 [4]. The notable exception to this demethylation is the continual retention of methylation on imprinted DMD sequences at each and every cleavage (replication) stage of preimplantation development [4, 26]. The clear difference between imprinted DMD sequences and global decline in methylation may be the most obvious feature of a complex molecular program whereby genomic methylation is rearranged on one but not the other allele during preimplantation development. A widely held view is that this complex epigenetic rearrangement is a central element in the important biological process of cellular reprogramming. In this process, the totipotent fertilized egg (zygote), a fusion of two highly differentiated gametes, undergoes a series of cleavages to produce a blastocyst containing small, pluripotent inner cell mass (ICM) cells. A programmed reduction in genomic methylation by the blastocyst stage may be required for the global reprogramming to pluripotency of the ICM cells. Following this period of preimplantation reprogramming, during post-implantation development, global methylation levels increase and the cells of the embryo become committed to various cell lineages. The importance of methylation at the blastocyst stage has been nicely illustrated in studies of mice lacking DNMT1; blastocysts lacking all forms of DNMT1 protein develop normally, but following implantation into the uterus, cells of these embryos fail to differentiate and instead undergo apoptosis, leading to embryonic death. Two distinct mechanisms for the programmed reduction in preimplantation methylation have been proposed. One mechanism is the active removal of methylated cytosine from the genome and the other mechanism is the passive loss of genomic methylation due to absence of maintenance methyltransferase activity following replication of the nuclear genome [27].

Model of active demethylation

Although both parental genomes lose a significant proportion of methylation during preimplantation development, the paternal genome in the mouse zygote appears to lose its methylation at a faster rate than does the maternal genome [27]. This observation suggests that active demethylation, or removal of methyl groups from cytosine bases outside the replication stage of the cell cycle, occurs during preimplantation. The molecular mechanism for putative demethylation proposes that demethylation occurs through the conversion of methylated cytosine (5mC) to a hydroxyl-methylated

cytosine (5hmC) intermediate by a family of dioxygenases called TET (ten-eleven-translocation) proteins [27]. Mouse ES cells express TET1 and TET2, while TET3 is expressed in early preimplantation embryos, and the activity of one or more of these dioxygenases to generate 5hmC might be followed by a mechanism to remove 5hmC and replace it with an unmethylated cytosine, possibly through activity of a base-excision repair pathway.

If active demethylation is responsible for the significant reduction in preimplantation genomic methylation, inherited, imprinted DMD methylation must be blocked from this activity. How might this occur? It might occur by specifically protecting sequences from active demethylation. This protective property has been attributed to the protein STELLA, a maternal-effect protein present in early embryos [27]. When $stella^{-/-}$ females are mated to wild-type males, the maternal genome in the resulting embryos shows a decrease in 5mC levels by immunofluorescence, at a stage when the maternal genome may be protected from active demethylation. Bisulfite sequencing analysis of genomic DNA in pronuclear-stage embryos revealed that some maternally imprinted genes, paternally imprinted genes, and IAP repeats show a decrease in methylation when derived from $stella^{-/-}$ mothers. The partial loss of methylation on the maternal genome and from imprinted DMDs due to the deficiency in STELLA reveals that they may be multiple molecular components that regulate the methylation status of the maternal genome and imprinted genes, possibly through interaction with DNMTs during various stages of embryonic development. Identification of these proteins and their interaction partners may help better understand the process of epigenetic reprogramming.

Model of passive demethylation

An alternative explanation for the loss of genomic methylation accompanying preimplantation development is passive demethylation, or the loss of methylation due to replication of the nuclear genome in the absence of DNMT1-mediated maintenance methylation. The mechanism by which DNMT1 is able to distinguish imprinted DMDs from other genomic CpGs is not known. However, such a discriminating feature of DNMT1 may reside in a recently identified mammal-specific region (amino acids ~190–350), located in the enzyme's N-terminal regulatory

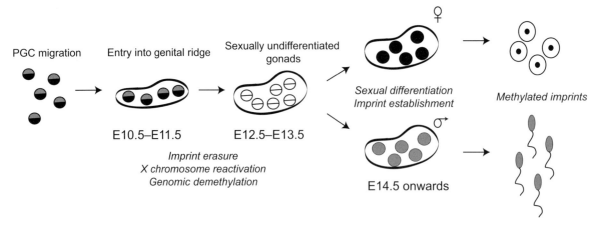

Figure 5.8 Erasure of both paternal (gray portion of circles) and maternal (black portion of circles) imprints in primordial germ cells (PGCs) following migration into the undifferentiated gonad. Imprints are established in maturing germ cells following differentiation of the gonad into an ovary or testis.

domain [20]. Deletion mutagenesis of the mammal-specific region of *Dnmt1* produced a series of mutants that either maintain DMD methylation but not non-imprinted methylation, maintain non-imprinted but not DMD methylation, or maintain neither non-imprinted nor DMD methylation *in vitro* in ES cells. At present, it is not known whether the mammal-specific region of DNMT1 plays a role in maintaining the high DMD methylation *in vivo* during the global decrease in methylation after fertilization. A plausible mechanism of passive demethylation would exclude DNMT1 from certain methylated regions of the genome and the regions would consequently become unmethylated over successive rounds of DNA replication.

Erasure of parent-specific imprints in primordial germ cells

After epigenetic reprogramming to generate blasto-cyst-stage embryos, the level of global genomic methylation, primarily defined by the large fraction of non-imprinted sequences, rapidly increases in all somatic cells of the conceptus (Fig. 5.3). This rise in methylation is due to the combined activities of *de novo* methyltransferases and DNMT1. Methylation of imprinted DMDs is maintained at a high level during the period of epigenetic reprogramming and thereafter in the developing post-implantation embryo. In contrast, PGCs in the embryo undergo erasure of their imprinted DMD methylation as prelude to the establishment of sex-specific genomic imprints (Fig. 5.8). The PGCs migrating to or residing in the fetal gonad

are the most logical site of imprint erasure because PGCs are permanently allocated to the germ lineage and this stage precedes establishment of sex-specific and functional imprints. Erasure of imprints completes the cycle of imprint establishment and maintenance allowing for transgenerational inheritance of the imprints established in the new gonad into the somatic cells of the developing embryo in the next generation.

Erasure of both maternal and paternal imprinted methylation patterns on DMD sequences takes place after the migration of the PGCs to the genital ridge, between E10.5 and E13.5 [5]. A few days before this, at E7.25, genomic imprints in PGCs are identical to those found in somatic cells. The timing of erasure differs somewhat for the different DMD sequences. However, analysis of cloned mouse embryos generated from E12.5 or E13.5 PGC nuclei showed biallelic expression of imprinted genes and reduced developmental potential [28], indicating that imprint erasure is complete by Day 12.5 of gestation. The enzymes involved in imprint erasure are currently unknown. It is also not known whether imprint erasure is an active demethylating or a passive demethylating process whereby the genome loses its methylation through rounds of DNA replication in the absence of DNMT1 maintenance methyltransferase activity. Moreover, erasure of methylation is not specific to imprints in the PGCs; methylation is also lost on all categories of non-imprinted DNA sequences. Knowledge of the kinetics of methylation loss on imprinted and non-imprinted sequences would lead to a better understanding of the mechanism of methylation loss – a rapid loss would suggest active demethylation, whereas a slow and steady decline would suggest passive demethylation.

Conclusions

This chapter illustrates how epigenetic modifications to the DNA sequence in the form of CpG methylation can serve as a heritable mark passed on from generation to generation. Genomic imprints are an excellent example of DNA sequences undergoing transgenerational inheritance of epigenetic modifications. Transmission of genomic imprints consists of an establishment phase mediated by *de novo* methyltransferases and a maintenance phase by maintenance methyltransferases. The methylation on imprinted DMDs is maintained during epigenetic reprogramming and is erased or reset only in PGCs. Imprinted sequences and DNA methylation are associated with transcription factors and histone modifications, which facilitate their actions on transcriptional control of genes in the imprinted cluster. Defects in imprinted genes have profound effects on development; hence accurate transgenerational inheritance of imprints during ART (see Chapter 12) or natural fertilization is vital to the survival of the embryo.

References

1. Reinhart B, Chaillet JR. Genomic imprinting: *cis*-acting sequences and regional control. *Int Rev Cytol* 2005; 243: 173–213.

2. Cattanach BM, Kirk M. Differential activity of maternally and paternally derived chromosome regions in mice. *Nature* 1985; 315: 496–8.

3. MouseBook: www.mousebook.org/catalog.php?catalog=imprinting

4. Chaillet JR, Vogt TF, Beier DR *et al*. Parental-specific methylation of an imprinted transgene is established during gametogenesis and progressively changes during embryogenesis. *Cell* 1991; 66: 77–83.

5. Hajkova P, Erhardt S, Lane N *et al*. Epigenetic reprogramming in mouse primordial germ cells. *Mech Dev* 2002; 117: 15–23.

6. Kaneda M, Okano M, Hata K *et al*. Essential role for *de novo* DNA methyltransferase Dnmt3a in paternal and maternal imprinting. *Nature* 2004; 429: 900–3.

7. Kato Y, Kaneda M, Hata K *et al*. Role of the Dnmt3 family in *de novo* methylation of imprinted and repetitive sequences during male germ cell

8. Hata K, Okano M, Lei H *et al*. Dnmt3L cooperates with the Dnmt3 family of *de novo* DNA methyltransferases to establish maternal imprints in mice. *Development* 2002; 129: 1983–93.

9. La Salle S, Mertineit C, Taketo T *et al*. Windows for sex-specific methylation marked by DNA methyltransferase expression profiles in mouse germ cells. *Dev Biol* 2004; 268: 403–15.

10. Kono T, Obata Y, Yoshimzu T *et al*. Epigenetic modifications during oocyte growth correlates with extended parthenogenetic development in the mouse. *Nat Genet* 1996; 13: 91–4.

11. Li JYY, Lees-Murdock DJ, Xu GLL *et al*. Timing of establishment of paternal methylation imprints in the mouse. *Genomics* 2004; 84: 952–60.

12. Lucifero D, Mann MR, Bartolomei MS *et al*. Gene-specific timing and epigenetic memory in oocyte imprinting. *Hum Mol Genet* 2004; 13: 839–49.

13. Bourc'his D, Xu GL, Lin CS *et al*. Dnmt3L and the establishment of maternal genomic imprints. *Science* 2001; 294: 2536–9.

14. Bourc'his D, Bestor TH. Meiotic catastrophe and retrotransposon reactivation in male germ cells lacking Dnmt3L. *Nature* 2004; 431: 96–9.

15. Jia D, Jurkowska RZ, Zhang X *et al*. Structure of Dnmt3a bound to Dnmt3L suggests a model for *de novo* DNA methylation. *Nature* 2007; 449: 248–51.

16. Ooi SK, Qiu C, Bernstein E *et al*. DNMT3L connects unmethylated lysine 4 of histone H3 to *de novo* methylation of DNA. *Nature* 2007; 448: 714–17.

17. Cirio MC, Ratnam S, Ding F *et al*. Preimplantation expression of the somatic form of Dnmt1 suggests a role in the inheritance of genomic imprints. *BMC Dev Biol* 2008; 25: 8–9.

18. Howell CY, Bestor TH, Ding F *et al*. Genomic imprinting disrupted by a maternal effect mutation in the *Dnmt1* gene. *Cell* 2001; 104: 829–38.

19. Reinhart B, Paoloni-Giacobino A, Chaillet JR. Specific differentially methylated domain sequences direct the maintenance of methylation at imprinted genes. *Mol Cell Biol* 2006; 26: 8347–56.

20. Borowczyk E, Mohan KN, D'Aiuto L *et al*. Identification of a region of the DNMT1 methyltransferase that regulates the maintenance of genomic imprints. *Proc Natl Acad Sci USA* 2009; 106: 20 806–11.

21. Ideraabdullah FY, Vigneau S, Bartolomei MS. Genomic imprinting mechanisms in mammals. *Mutat Res* 2008; 647: 77–85.

22. Singh P, Cho J, Tsai SY *et al.* Coordinated allele-specific histone acetylation at the differentially methylated regions of imprinted genes. *Nucleic Acids Res* 2010; 38: 7974–90.

23. Sapountzi V, Logan IR, Robson CN. Cellular functions of TIP60. *Int J Biochem Cell Biol* 2006; 38: 1496–509.

24. Mohan NK, Ding F, Chaillet JR. Distinct roles of DMAP1 in mouse development. *Mol Cell Biol* 2011; 31: 1861–9.

25. Paoloni-Giacobino A, Chaillet JR. Genomic imprinting and assisted reproduction. *Reprod Health* 2004; 1: 6.

26. Tremblay KD, Duran KL, Bartolomei MS. A 5′ 2-kilobase-pair region of the imprinted mouse *H19* gene exhibits exclusive paternal methylation throughout development. *Mol Cell Biol* 1997; 17: 4322–9.

27. Saitou M, Kagiwada S, Kurimoto K. Epigenetic reprogramming in mouse pre-implantation development and primordial germ cells. *Development* 2012; 139: 15–31.

28. Lee J, Inoue K, Ono R *et al.* Erasing genomic imprinting memory in mouse clone embryos produced from Day 11.5 primordial germ cells. *Development* 2002; 129: 1807–17.

Chapter

6

Genes are not the whole story

Retrotransposons as new determinants of male fertility

Patricia Fauque and Déborah Bourc'his

Introduction

The release of the human genome sequence has revealed that our genes represent only a minor fraction, with exons making up less than 2% of our DNA. In contrast, transposable elements represent some 45% of the genomic mass. Contrary to other species like *Drosophila* or plants, these elements are not clustered in specific chromosomal regions in mammals but are rather scattered throughout the genome, residing between but also inside genes. The transposon landscape of our genome reflects an evolutionary tug-of-war between integration and propagation events orchestrated by these elements, and counteracting defense mechanisms exerted by the host.

By providing raw material for genetic innovation and diversification, transposons have positively participated to genome shaping and speciation during evolution. However, on a short-term basis, transposon activity can adversely modify the function and the architecture of the genome [1]. They can induce damageable genetic changes by hopping into new genomic locations, or create some major chromosomal rearrangements by ectopic recombination between nonallelic copies. When occurring in somatic cells, cancer can ensue; when occurring in gametes, heritable mutations can be generated and lead to congenital disorders [2]. Their effect can also be non-genetic, by influencing the expression patterns of adjacent genes through their strong promoter sequences, or by inducing alternative splicing or premature transcriptional termination.

To ensure their propagation, transposons need to mobilize in cells destined for the next generation, the germ cells. Recent studies have highlighted the existence of specialized pathways acting in the germline for the lifelong repression of transposons and the

protection of the hereditary material [3]. Genetic impairment of this system in mice invariably leads to massive transposon reactivation and complete failure to produce spermatozoa in males [4]. Transposon control therefore appears as a major safeguard of male fertility in both mouse and in other animal species. Such a role is highly likely to be conserved in the human, but has drawn very little attention so far. The purpose of this review is to shed light onto these newly appreciated determinants of male reproductive fitness, the transposons. Improper control of these elements, of genetic or environmental origin, could be revealed as a major cause of male infertility.

Human transposable elements

Transposons, also known as mobile DNA elements or "jumping genes," are widespread in nature and comprise an estimated half of the human genome. This is likely an underestimation of the true proportion of genomic transposons, as their repetitive and divergent nature hampers efficient sequencing and annotation. Several classes of transposons have evolved in the human lineage and coexist in the current *Homo sapiens* genome, with some elements having expanded with more success than others (Fig. 6.1).

The transposons' mobilizing strategies allow a classification into two main classes, the DNA transposons and the retrotransposons. **DNA transposons** move by a "cut-and-paste" mechanism via an element-encoded transposase. They comprise ~3% of the human genome and are mostly inert remnants of ancient elements, which have accumulated deleterious mutations over the course of evolution. **Retrotransposons** on the other hand still have some active representatives, which have retained the ability to duplicate themselves via a "copy-and-paste" mechanism using

Textbook of Human Reproductive Genetics, eds Karen Sermon and Stéphane Viville. Published by Cambridge University Press. © Cambridge University Press 2014.

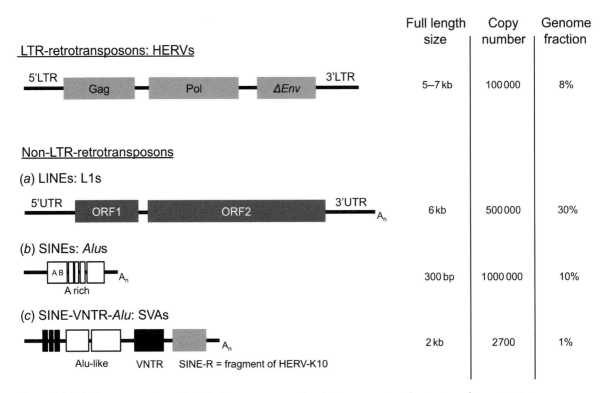

		Full length size	Copy number	Genome fraction
LTR-retrotransposons: HERVs				
5'LTR — Gag — Pol — ΔEnv — 3'LTR		5–7 kb	100 000	8%
Non-LTR-retrotransposons				
(a) LINEs: L1s				
5'UTR — ORF1 — ORF2 — 3'UTR A_n		6 kb	500 000	30%
(b) SINEs: Alus				
A B / A rich — A_n		300 bp	1 000 000	10%
(c) SINE-VNTR-Alu: SVAs				
Alu-like — VNTR — SINE-R = fragment of HERV-K10 — A_n		2 kb	2700	1%

Figure 6.1 Retrotransposon elements in the human genome. The retrotransposon type, the structure of representative retrotransposon elements and the size, copy number and contribution (percentage) to the human genome are reported in this figure. Abbreviations for human endogenous retrovirus (HERV): LTR (long terminal repeat), Gag (group specific antigen), Pol (polymerase), Env (envelope protein). For LINE (L1): UTR (untranslated region), ORF1 and ORF2 (Open Reading Frames). For Alu: A and B (component sequences of the RNA polymerase III promoter), A rich (adenosine-rich segment). For the SINE-R/VNTR/Alu (SVA): VNTR (variable number of tandem repeats), SINE-R (domain derived from a HERV-K). An: poly(A) tail.

an RNA intermediate converted into a complementary DNA (cDNA) by reverse transcription. While transposons have been largely ignored or even purposely discarded from genomic analyses for a long time, nowadays more and more technological and computational methods are specifically developed to allow accurate classification, evaluation of their activity, and mapping of new integration events.

So far three families of retrotransposons have been recognized as competent for mobilization in the human genome, the LINEs (Long INterspersed Elements), *Alu*, and SVA (SINE-R/VNTR/Alu) elements. They all rely on a combination of host-provided cellular factors and LINEs-encoded proteins to fulfill their life cycle. These mobile families belong to the non-LTR (long terminal repeats) class of retrotransposons. This is opposed to the LTR-class of retrotransposons, also known as human endogenous retroviruses (HERVs), which are considered to be mostly immobile.

LTR elements

The HERVs comprise 7–8% of the human genome. These elements evolved through the endogenization of infectious retroviruses, which became part of our genetic material after a non-lethal insertion of a viral particle in the germline, and passage of this integrated proviral sequence to the offspring by Mendelian inheritance. Further expansion in copy number occurred by several rounds of either reinfection or intracellular retrotransposition [5]. Among the four known retroviral genera, three have given rise to HERVs, the gamma, the beta, and the spuma retroviruses. Around 7–11 kilobases (kb) long, full-length HERVs resemble their retrovirus ancestors in their structure (Fig. 6.1): they are flanked on both 5′ and 3′ sides by LTR sequences, which contain binding motifs for cellular transcription factors, while the internal part encodes *gag* and *pol* proteins, which notably encode the reverse transcriptase and integrase activities necessary for retrotransposition. They usually lack a functional *envelope* (*env*) gene, which prevents most of the HERVs from assembling infectious particles and relegates them to an intracellular existence. Among the 100 000 HERV copies estimated to reside in the human genome, only 3500 more or less complete elements have been identified. Fragments of HERVs are more commonly found, usually in the form of "solo" LTRs, which result from the deletion of intervening sequences by recombination between LTR repeats.

Thirty-one individual groups of HERVs can be distinguished in the human genome, ranging in copy numbers from one to several thousands. The HERV nomenclature is traditionally based on the host transfer RNA (tRNA) species they use as a primer for reverse transcription [6]. For example, HERV-K members use a lysine tRNA, while the HERV-H group uses a histidine tRNA. However, this classification cannot apply when the tRNA primer sequence is not known at the time of the discovery of novel elements; in these cases, designation becomes arbitrary based on neighbor genes, the name of the probe used for cloning, the chromosomal location, or any type of discriminating information. More recently, efforts have been made towards the development of phylogenetic methods to cluster HERV subfamilies according to LTR sequence similarities [7].

Most groups of HERVs are also found in Old World monkey and ape genomes, suggesting that the majority of retroviral endogenization events occurred some 30 million years ago. There are nonetheless some species-specific ERVs, which have been identified in human and non-human primate genomes, demonstrating the continuous incorporation of new elements throughout evolution. Although numerous polymorphic HERVs were identified in the human population, they mostly consist in contractions from full-length elements into solo LTRs by recombination. There are very few insertional HERV polymorphisms, defined by alleles present in both the preintegration and the post-integration forms, which attests to the relative immobility of these elements in the recent era of modern humans. Less than a dozen of full-length HERVs are dimorphic, and they are all of the HERV-K type, the most recent retroviral species to have entered our genome. This situation is in striking contrast to the high rate of insertional polymorphisms of LTR retrotransposons in the mouse genome, or the

high frequency of non-LTR retrotransposon polymorphisms in the human genome. The relative dormancy of HERVs in the human genome may reflect either fast evolutionary erosion and/or the existence of potent restraining pathways acting specifically on these elements.

Because of this apparent immobility, HERVs are often just considered as fossilized versions of ancient retroviruses. Nonetheless, they can be transcriptionally active and produce retroviral proteins, which can be co-opted for useful physiological functions. Syncytin proteins provide a well-characterized example of endogenous retrovirus domestication. Encoded by the *env* gene of HERV-W and HERV-FRD elements, they play a key role in placentation, by promoting membrane fusion and syncytium formation [8]. Interestingly, high expression levels of other HERV types, such as HERV-R and HERV-K, have been reported in the human placenta, suggesting an evolutionary, regulatory, or functional connection between this short-lived mammalian-specific reproductive organ and HERV biology.

Non-LTR elements

The origin of non-LTR retrotransposons is unclear, as they do not resemble infectious retroviruses in their structure or their transposition cycle. They can be stratified into three subgroups: Long INterspersed Elements (LINEs), Short INterspersed Elements (SINEs), and SINE-R/VNTR/Alu (SVA) elements. These elements have nothing in common in terms of size and structure. The LINEs represent the most abundant retrotransposon family in humans and in all mammals in general. LINE-1 (L1) elements are considered to be the master retrotransposons, as they account for 30% of the genome, have self-propagating properties, and can provide in *trans* the machinery required for the mobilization of SINEs and SVAs [1].

Full-length L1 elements are ~6 kb in length and are flanked by 5′ and 3′ UTR sequences (Fig. 6.1). They are transcribed in an RNA polymerase II-dependent manner and translated into two open reading frames, ORF1 and ORF2, which encode the necessary machinery for mobilization. ORF1 is an RNA chaperone, which coats and protects L1 mRNAs, while ORF2 provides the enzymatic activities of an endonuclease and a reverse transcriptase. Contrary to LTR retrotransposons, the reverse transcription of L1 elements is

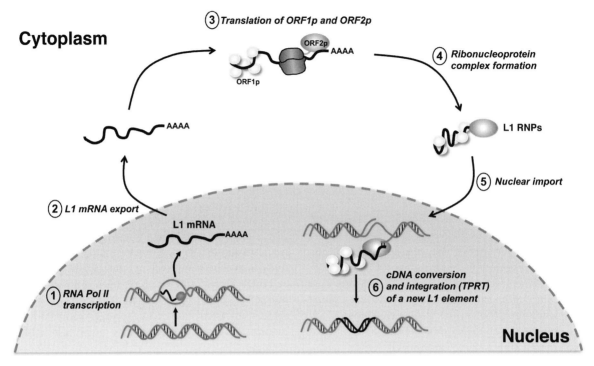

Figure 6.2 L1 retrotransposition cycle. (**1**) L1 life cycle starts with transcription of the element by RNA polymerase II (RNA Pol II). (**2**) The L1 mRNA is then exported to the cytoplasm. (**3**) L1-encoded proteins (ORF1p and ORF2p) are translated and assemble with the L1 mRNA into ribonucleic acid particles (L1 RNPs), which are then imported into the nucleus. (**4**) The ORF2p-encoded endonuclease nicks genomic DNA in the host genome and is responsible for the reverse transcription of the L1 mRNA. Reverse transcription occurs at the site of integration, in a process referred to as target-primed reverse transcription (TPRT) and is then integrated. The mechanism of second cDNA strand synthesis remains unclear.

coupled to chromosomal integration, therefore taking place in the nucleus and not in the cytoplasm, in a process known as target primed reverse transcription (TPRT) (Fig. 6.2).

From an evolutionary point of view, L1s are thought to have been part of our genome for hundreds of millions of years, meaning that they predated LTR retrotransposons. Several L1 subfamilies have succeeded each other, each replacing the last as the dominant active member. The majority of L1s are shared by human and chimpanzee genomes. Nowadays, these elements are inert, having accumulated mutations, truncations, and deleterious rearrangements. However, around 1000 L1s are specific to humans and among them, the Ta (transcribed, subset a) or L1PA1 subfamily has around 100 members, which have intact ORFs, can be expressed and are competent for mobilization, as shown in cellular retrotransposition assays and their involvement in interindividual insertional polymorphisms. Ta elements contain a sequence variant signature within their 3′ UTR, in the form of

an ACA instead of a GAG trinucleotide. The L1 Ta members seem to be the only autonomous L1s residing in the human genome, if not the only autonomous retrotransposons of any kind in our genome. Their active machinery allows not only their own retrotransposition but also the *trans*-mobilization of nonautonomous L1 elements that may be transcriptionally active, with an intact promoter, but deleted for ORF sequences. As mentioned earlier, L1s are also responsible for the mobility of other families of non-LTR retrotransposons, the SINEs, and the SVAs. Finally, they can promote the mobilization of cellular mRNAs and the creation of intron-less retroposed copies of genes into new genomic locations, which can degenerate into pseudogenes or develop novel functions under selective pressure.

Recent estimation inferred from high throughput sequencing approaches gave a total L1 retrotransposition rate of 1/100–1/150 births, with 1 in 20 of these births being associated with a disease phenotype. Since the first association of an hemophilia case with a *de novo* germline L1 insertion in 1988, approximately 65 disease-causing mutations have been attributed to L1-retrotransposition events [9]. They can act as mutagens by directly disrupting exons or inducing misexpression when they insert into introns, or at proximity of promoter or enhancer regions.

SINEs have no common history with LINEs, although they strictly rely upon L1-encoded proteins for their mobilization. Among them, *Alu* sequences are the most abundant, with an estimated copy number of 1 million, which accounts for ∼10% of human genomic mass [10]. Around 5500 are specific to humans and are not shared by the chimpanzee genome. *Alu*s evolved some 65 million years ago from the 7SL RNA, which serves in the ribosomal signal recognition particle for addressing nascent proteins to the endoplasmic reticulum. This sequence may be required for L1-mediated transposition, by placing the *Alu* mRNA in close proximity to the L1 ribonucleoprotein particles. Similar to their precursors, *Alu*s are around 300 nucleotides (nt) in length, contain an RNA polymerase III promoter and end with an A-rich tail (Fig. 6.1). Among thousands of *Alu* sequences that have an intact promoter and may be transcriptionally active in the human genome, the *Alu*Ya5/8 and *Alu*Yb8/9 subfamilies account for the vast majority of *de novo* insertions in humans. Comparisons between individuals in human and primate populations give an estimate of 1 *Alu de novo* insertion every 20 live births. They provide the highest number of all retrotransposon-derived insertional polymorphisms in the human genome.

The last family of active, although non-autonomous, retrotransposons in humans corresponds to the SVA elements. While LINEs and SINEs have colonized the genome of multiple animal species, vertebrate, and invertebrate, SVAs evolved uniquely in primate genomes, some 25 million years ago. They have a composite structure, combining from 5′ to 3′: an *Alu*-like segment consisting of two inverted *Alu* fragments; a variable number of tandem repeats (VNTR) region, which is made of copies presumably derived from the SVA2 element found in Rhesus macaques and humans; a fragment derived from an extinct HERV-K10 element (SINE-R); and a poly(A) tail (Fig. 6.1). The events which led to the emergence of this chimeric entity in the hominid lineage are unknown. Although quite convergent in terms of sequence identity, they are very heterogeneous in size, ranging from 700 base pairs to 4 kb, with a canonical 2 kb long element. SVA elements are likely to be transcribed by RNA polymerase II. They are mobilized by L1-encoded proteins, potentially with the help of their *Alu*-derived sequence, and *de novo* SVA insertions have been associated with several human diseases. In agreement with their evolutionarily young age, their genomic number is less than the other retrotransposon classes, estimated at 2700 copies, among which around 800 are specific to humans (subfamilies SVA_E and F), while the others are shared with chimpanzees (subfamilies SVA_A to D).

Control mechanisms of retrotransposon activity

As stressed above, derepression of individual retrotransposons can cause diseases, by generating insertional mutations or interfering with proper gene control. Massive derepression of retrotransposons has an even more dramatic outcome as it typically leads to lethality and sterility, depending on whether it occurs in the developing embryo or in germline cells, as exemplified from mouse mutant models [3]. To counteract, the host has evolved various defense mechanisms, which maintain retrotransposons under control.

The most potent control of retrotransposon activity is evolution. Inserted retrotransposon copies are subject to host pressures altering their DNA sequence, either by favoring the maintenance of an empty allele over an allele where the retrotransposon has inserted, or by allowing genetic drift. So, with time, unless they provide an important function for the host, retrotransposons are doomed to become inactive. But there is still a subset of transcriptionally and retrotranspositionally competent elements in our genome. These have to be dealt with on a short-term basis, and the cell uses a plethora of strategies to hit them at various stages of their life cycle (Fig. 6.2). Retrotransposon families are greatly diverse in sequence, in numbers, and evolutionary origins. Accordingly, these restricting pathways are usually based on proteins that are universal and flexible, and are used for other cellular functions, generally related to gene expression control. But there are also some examples of specialized proteins that are dedicated to either LTR or non-LTR elements.

Currently known host defense mechanisms target: (a) transcription of retrotransposons; (b) post-transcriptional processing of retrotransposon mRNAs; and (c) integration of new retrotransposon copies.

Most of the corresponding restraining factors have been identified and functionally studied in mammalian model organisms such as mice [3], but the same rules seem to apply to human retrotransposons. While not being directly considered as a host defense strategy, it is important to mention that cell division could be a strict requirement for the retrotransposition cycle. *In vitro* reporter assays notably showed that L1 retrotransposition is strongly reduced in G_0-arrested cells [11], implying that non-mitotic cells may be less sensitive to retrotransposon activity. This may be linked to the need of nuclear membrane breakdown to allow the nuclear import of L1 ribonucleic acid particles (RNPs) (Fig. 6.2).

Transcriptional control

Mobilization of a retrotransposon first requires its expression. The primary way to prevent retrotransposition is therefore to block the transcription of genomic copies of retrotransposons. Chromatin modifications, also referred as epigenetic modifications, locally modulate the compaction of the genome and its accessibility to transcription factors. Both the DNA and histone protein components of chromatin are subject to secondary biochemical modifications. Dense DNA methylation assembled at promoter regions is a known potent inhibitor of transcription. The majority of methylated cytosines in human genomic DNA are actually contained in retrotransposon sequences, and indeed it has been proposed that DNA methylation evolved primarily as a defense mechanism against transposable elements [12]. Notably L1, *Alu,* and SVA elements have all been shown to be methylated in human somatic tissues. The enzymes responsible for the DNA methylation reaction are the DNA methyltransferases (Dnmts) and among them, Dnmt1, Dnmt3A, and the cofactor Dnmt3L are cooperating in methylation-dependent transcriptional repression of retrotransposons of the LTR and non-LTR classes in mice. Similarly, chemical impairment of genomic methylation patterns with 5-azadeoxycytidine leads to retrotransposon reactivation in human cellular systems. In addition to members of the Dnmt family, proteins that assist the DNA methylation reaction also have a role in retrotransposon repression. Among them, Lsh (Lymphoid specific helicase) is a member of the SNF2 family of chromatin remodeling ATPases that facilitates the access of Dnmts to DNA, and is required for the methylation and repression of retrotransposons in mice.

Various repressive histone modifications have also been linked to transcriptional repression of retrotransposons. In particular, H3K9, H4K20, and H3K27 methylation are commonly found at 5'LTR or UTR sequences of retrotransposons, and genetic deletion of the enzymes driving these modifications can lead to retrotransposon reactivation [13]. Proteins that bind H3K9 methylated histones are also required for retrotransposon repression. Notably, in mouse embryonic stem cells, the TRIM28/KAP1 transcriptional repressor (KRAB-associated protein1) is recruited to and reinforces H3K9 methylation marks at ERVs only, and not at any non-LTR elements. Interestingly, TRIM28/KAP1 also silences infectious retroviruses. This example illustrates that repressors involved in innate immunity against retroviruses have a conserved function on endogenized retroviruses.

Post-transcriptional control

Retrotransposons have an RNA-centered mode of replication. Retrotransposon transcripts serve both as messengers to produce retroviral proteins following translation, but also as templates to generate new genomic copies, following reverse transcription. Accordingly, different defense strategies have been developed against their RNA phase, and at least two forms of RNA alteration, RNA editing and RNA interference, are known to target retrotransposon transcripts.

The term RNA editing refers to molecular processes that modify the information content of the RNA molecule, most often by nucleoside deamination. By altering RNAs and therefore promoter strength and/or amino acid sequence of encoded proteins, RNA editing enzymes can reduce the activity of new copies of retrotransposons. The ADAR family of RNA editases converts adenosine residues into inosines. Analysis of the human transcriptome has revealed that ADARs target double-stranded RNAs that are formed from inverted *Alu* and L1 repeats. The APOBEC proteins form another family, which catalyze the deamination of cytosine residues into uracils and have greatly expanded in the primate lineage. APOBEC3G was originally shown to reduce human immunodeficiency virus (HIV) replication, by inducing the accumulation of uracil mutations on the nascent retroviral cDNA strand and subsequently inactivating the newly integrated copy [14]. Retrotransposition assays have shown that APOBEC3A, 3B, 3C, and 3F enzymes are also potent restrictors of different classes of LTR- and non-LTR retrotransposons in human and mouse cells. However, retrotransposon restriction triggered by some of the APOBEC3 proteins does not involve C to U conversion. It has been hypothesized that these enzymes mediate cytoplasmic sequestration of L1 RNA and/or L1-encoded proteins, or directly inhibit L1 ORF activity [15]. Considering the master role of L1 in retrotransposition biology, this would not only impact on L1 activity but could also render the L1 machinery inaccessible to non-autonomous retrotransposons of other classes.

RNA interference (RNAi) represents another post-transcriptional mechanism of retrotransposon suppression [16]. In this case, small RNAs operate through homology-based recognition to induce the degradation of complementary retrotransposon transcripts, via the recruitment of the RNA-Induced Silencing Complex (RISC). The slicing activity in this complex is provided by the Argonaute protein family: the human genome encodes four classical Argonautes (AGO1 to 4), and four germline-restricted members named PIWI (PIWIL1 to 4). Only three PIWI genes are present in the mouse genome, which lacks the homolog of PIWIL3.

There are three classes of small RNAs in mammals. The microRNAs (miRNAs) and the endogenous small interfering RNAs (endo-siRNAs) require the DICER protein for their production and associate with the canonical AGO proteins. The PIWI-interacting RNAs (piRNAs) are specifically produced in the germline, where they require and associate with PIWIL proteins only, and are produced in a DICER-independent manner. They also differ in size, ranging from 25 to 30 nt, while miRNAs and endo-siRNAs are traditionally 22–24 nt long. So far, all these small RNA types have been linked to retrotransposon biology. DICER deficiency induces the cytoplasmic accumulation of *Alu* RNAs, whose toxic effects are responsible for the development of age-related macular degeneration [17]. PIWIL mutations in mouse compromise piRNA production and lead to global reactivation of LTR and non-LTR retrotransposons in the male germline, which completely compromises sperm production [3, 18, 19]. Interestingly, the female germline does not use piRNAs to target retrotransposons, but may rather rely on endo-siRNAs. Finally, any component of the RNAi pathway represents a potential candidate for retrotransposon restriction. Among them, the MOV10 RNA helicase, which helps RNA processing within the RISC complex, has been recently shown to severely reduce the retrotransposition rate of L1, *Alu*, and SVA elements in cellular assays.

Integration control

Finally, the last stage of the retrotransposon life cycle, the integration of the cDNA copy into a new genomic location, is also subject to restriction. The ERCC1/XPF heterodimer complex has endonuclease activity and is involved in DNA repair mostly through the nucleotide excision repair (NER) pathway. Reduction of XPF in human cell lines increases L1 retrotransposition, suggesting that intermediates of the L1 retrotransposition process may be cleaved by this enzyme. Interestingly, other DNA repair enzymes have an inverse effect on retrotransposition: the double-strand break repair protein ATM is indeed facilitating L1 integration [20], indicating that various DNA repair pathways may be able to recognize and process retrotransposon integration intermediates in a positive or negative manner.

Retrotransposons and fertility: what we learned from animal models

The only opportunity for retrotransposons to propagate is by generating new genomic copies in cells destined to the next generation, i.e. germ cells or early embryonic cells upstream from the formation of the germline. Accordingly, a large number of retrotransposon repressors are specifically expressed in the developing germline. Moreover, functional studies in mice have revealed that these germline factors act as major determinants of reproductive fitness, in particular in males [3, 4, 18, 19]. Genetic, cytological, and biochemical studies in mouse models have led to the elaboration of a molecular scenario taking place in male germ cells during fetal life for the lifelong protection of the genetic material against retrotransposons. This involves a relay between RNA interference mechanisms centered on piRNAs, and transcriptional control mediated by DNA methylation.

Primordial germ cells (PGCs), the progenitors of the germline, are set aside very early from the rest of the cell lineages of the developing embryo, around 6–7 days post-coïtum (dpc) in mice (Fig. 6.3). These specified germ cells undergo a massive reprogramming of

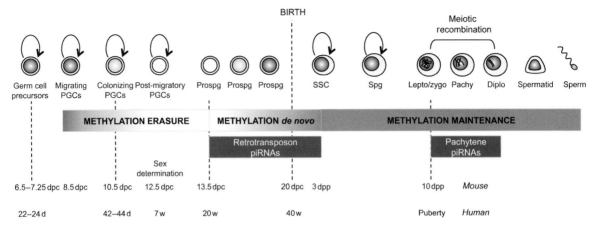

Figure 6.3 Kinetics of spermatogenesis and piRNA/DNA methylation pathway in mice and potential developmental equivalents in humans. Germ cell emergence occurs around 6.25–7.25 dpc in mouse (22–24 days in the human). Global erasure of genomic methylation starts during the migration phase of PGCs and culminates at the time of their incorporation into the genital ridges, at 10.5 dpc. At 12.5 dpc, sexual determination is initiated (7 weeks in the human). At 13.5 dpc, mouse PGCs become prospermatogonia, as they enter mitotic arrest (starts around 20 weeks in the human). This cellular change coincides with a wave of *de novo* methylation, which occurs in association with retrotransposon-derived piRNAs, and is completed before birth. Rapidly, the prospermatogonia differentiate into self-renewing SSCs, around 3 dpp in mouse. DNA methylation is stably maintained throughout the different phases of postnatal spermatogenesis, until the release of mature spermatozoa. At the time of entry into the prophase of meiosis I, a second population of piRNAs is produced, called pachytene piRNAs, whose function is not related to retrotransposon control. Methylation states are depicted here with increasing intensities of gray, representing increasing methylation levels. The timing of methylation erasure, establishment and production of various populations of piRNAs is not precisely known in humans. dpc, days post-coïtum; dpp, days post-partum; PGC, primordial germ cell; Prospg, prospermatogonia; SSC, spermatogonial stem cell; Spg, spermatogonia; Lepto, leptotene; Zygo, zygotene; Pachy, pachytene; Diplo, diplotene.

their epigenetic repertoire, which culminates at the time they colonize the fetal gonads, around 10 dpc. At 12.5 dpc, the expression of the Y-linked *Sry* gene determines a male fate in XY individuals, while its absence leads to female differentiation in XX animals. In males, this phase is immediately followed at 13.5 dpc by a mitotic arrest of germ cells, which take the name of prospermatogonia. Germline epigenetic reprogramming implies a genome-wide loss of DNA methylation, which leaves the retrotransposons unleashed [21]. However, fetal prospermatogonia are equipped with specialized slicing machinery, the PIWI proteins, which can cleave the retrotransposons transcripts into 25–30 nt piRNAs. In mouse, retrotransposons-derived piRNAs depend on Mili (PIWIL2) and Miwi2 (PIWIL4) proteins and feed what has been referred to as the "ping-pong" mechanism (Fig. 6.4), which relies on the hypothesis that both sense and antisense retrotransposon mRNAs are transcribed at the same time and can serve as substrates for sense and antisense piRNAs, respectively. In this model, the Mili protein loaded with sense piRNAs recognizes and degrades antisense retrotranscripts, generating antisense piRNAs that are loaded into Miwi2. The Miwi2-piRNAs can then target sense retrotransposon mRNAs, gen-

erating new sense piRNAs that will bind to Mili, therefore forming a positive amplification loop. This chain of events occurs in specialized cytoplasmic compartments, the pi- and piP-bodies, which gather general components of RNA biogenesis and processing [18]. Following this post-transcriptional degradation of retrotransposons, Miwi2 loaded with antisense piRNAs is able to translocate into the nucleus, where it triggers *de novo* methylation of genomic copies of retrotransposons, by recruiting, in an unknown manner, the DNA methyltransferase DNMT3A and its cofactor DNMT3L (Fig. 6.4). DNA methylation is completed before birth, and then maintained in postnatal germ cells as they undergo spermatogonial proliferation, meiosis, and maturation into spermatids and finally spermatozoa (Fig. 6.3), allowing the stable repression of retrotransposons for the rest of the reproductive lifetime of the male mouse.

As an illustration of the importance of this pathway for spermatogenesis, some 17 genes have been so far involved in the relay between piRNA and DNA methylation in mouse, for the purpose of stable repression of retrotransposons in the male germline (Table 6.1). As an example, various Tudor domain containing proteins (TDRD) are responsible for organizing

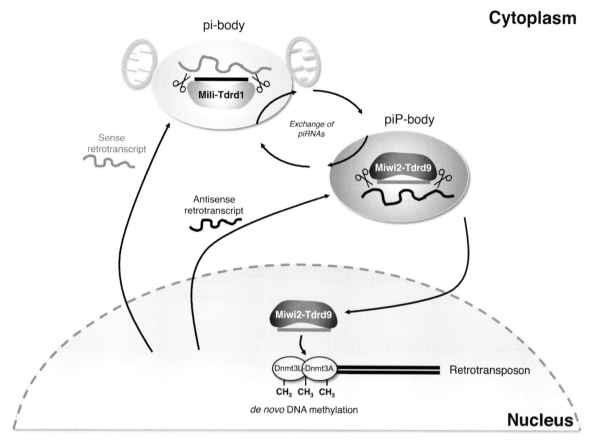

Figure 6.4 piRNA/DNA methylation pathway acting in mammalian germ cells for the repression of retrotransposons. This pathway is active in fetal male germ cells, the prospermatogonia, present from 13.5 dpc to birth in mouse. Sense (gray line) and antisense (black line) mRNAs (retrotranscripts) are produced from genomic retrotransposon sequences interspersed within the nucleus. These mRNAs get cleaved into sense and antisense piRNAs, respectively. Two Piwi proteins, Mili and Miwi2, interacting with Tudor domain-containing (Tdrd) proteins -1 and -9, respectively, localize to different cytoplasmic granules (pi- or piP-bodies). Sense and antisense piRNAs associate with Mili-Tdrd1 and Miwi2-Tdrd9 complexes, respectively, where they will further lead to the recognition and cleavage of retrotransposon mRNAs in opposite orientation, and promote amplification for post-transcriptional degradation of retrotranscripts through the so-called "ping-pong" loop. The relay beween post-transcriptional and transcriptional control is achieved by the translocation of the Miwi2-piRNA complex into the nucleus, where it facilitates de novo DNA methylation (by the recruitment of the Dnmt3L/Dnmt3A machinery), to stably silence retrotransposons. Once established, DNA methylation patterns are then stably maintained throughout the end of spermatogenesis.

the pi and piP bodies, through the recognition of arginine modifications carried by Mili and Miwi2 proteins [18]. Various RNA helicases, such as the Mouse Vasa Homolog (Mvh) and Mov10L1, are also required. Single inactivation of any of these 17 genes leads to retrotransposon reactivation in fetal germ cells, which profoundly affects spermatogenesis after birth in the form of a complete interruption in the prophase of meiosis I and a rapid exhaustion of the pool of spermatogonial stem cells (SSCs), which normally sustain spermatogenesis throughout life [3]. Retrotransposon reactivation seems therefore deleterious for the process of homologous recombination and germline stem cell renewal.

As a result, mutant males do not produce any spermatozoa and exhibit a Sertoli-only testicular phenotype after a few weeks. Interestingly, the female germline seems more tolerant to alteration of the piRNA pathway, as none of the aforementioned genes has an effect on oocyte production in mouse mutant models.

It should be mentioned that a second class of piRNAs is produced in postnatal spermatogenesis, during the prophase of meiosis I (Fig. 6.3). These so-called "pachytene piRNAs" do not originate from retrotransposons but are rather produced from large, poorly annotated genomic clusters, mostly through the control of a third PIWI protein, Miwi (PIWIL1).

Table 6.1 Germline repressors of retrotransposon activity in mouse

Gene	Biochemical function/role
Dnmt3A	DNA methyltransferase/*de novo* methylation
Dnmt3L	Cofactor of Dnmt3A/*de novo* methylation
Fkbp6	FK-506 binding protein 6/supports piRNA biogenesis
Gasz	Unknown/supports piRNA biogenesis
Gtsf1	Unknown/likely to support piRNA pathway
MitoPLD	Lipid signaling/supports piRNA biogenesis
Miwi2	RNaseH (Piwi family)/piRNA biogenesis
Mili	RNaseH (Piwi family)/piRNA biogenesis
Maelstrom	Unknown/supports piRNA pathway
Mov10L1	RNA helicase/supports piRNA pathway
Mvh	RNA helicase/supports piRNA pathway
Tdrd1	Tudor protein, binds to Mili/supports piRNA pathway
Tdrd5	Tudor protein/supports piRNA pathway
Tdrd6	Tudor protein/supports piRNA pathway
Tdrd7	Tudor protein/supports piRNA pathway
Tdrd9	Tudor protein/binds to Miwi2/supports piRNA pathway
Tex19.1	Unknown/supports piRNA pathway?

Although Miwi is required for spermiogenesis, the function of pachytene piRNAs on genome control is currently unknown.

Transposons and fertility in humans: what we suppose and what we really know

The number of genes involved in the piRNA/DNA methylation pathway of retrotransposon control and the dramatic consequences of their inactivation provide strong bases for considering retrotransposon repressors as major guardians of fertility in males. Moreover, the piRNA pathway has been shown to be conserved in the germline of all animals: PIWI homologs have been identified and genetically analyzed in *Drosophila*, *Caenorhabditis elegans*, and zebrafish, and they are systematically required for fertility through retrotransposon silencing. What is the evidence so far that the piRNA/DNA methylation pathway may play a similar role in human reproduction?

Developmental kinetics of human spermatogenesis

As a first step towards involving retrotransposons as important determinants of male fertility, it is important to anticipate at which stage the piRNA/DNA methylation pathway may be active during human development. The main actors of this pathway are all conserved between mouse and human, from the PIWI proteins to the DNMT3A-DNMT3L *de novo* methylation complex. There are even four PIWI genes in humans, while the mouse genome contains three of them. Although high-throughput sequencing analyses have confirmed to existence of pachytene piRNAs in testis samples of adult men, retrotransposon-derived piRNAs have not been observed in humans so far. This does not imply that they do not exist. It may rather reflect their restricted access linked to their fetal origin, estimated to span the time of prospermatogonia existence in the mouse, from their emergence at 13.5 dpc to their conversion into dividing SSCs at birth (Fig. 6.4). Developmental equivalences would therefore suggest that the piRNA machinery may be active starting around 20 weeks post-conception in human male fetuses, at the time when PGCs initiate their differentiation into prospermatogonia. Fundamental differences exist though: in mouse, PGC to prospermatogonia conversion occurs in a synchronous manner and prospermatogonia then become SSC right at birth. In the human, prospermatogonia appear throughout the duration of fetal gonad development and are maintained until puberty. Retrotransposon-piRNAs may therefore continue being produced after birth in humans.

Cycles of DNA methylation erasure and establishment occur in the developing germline of all mammalian species examined so far. Not only retrotransposons undergo this process, but also, notably, genes subject to genomic imprinting, that is the imprinted genes as described in Chapter 5. Although the dynamics of retrotransposon methylation has not been specifically studied in human spermatogenesis, analyses of paternally imprinted loci have allowed dating the completion of DNA methylation patterns to occur sometime postnatally, before puberty. While a large number of studies have tried to make a correlation between methylation anomalies at imprinted genes and fertility in humans, very few have focused on the relationship between retrotransposon control and sperm criteria.

Table 6.2 Retrotransposon methylation and sperm parameters in humans

Refs	Studied population (N)	Analyses	Transposable elements	Results
El Hajj *et al.* [22]	NZ men (28) OA and/or T men (106)	Bisulfite-pyrosequencing	Alu and L1 elements	*Alu* methylation was lower in sperm samples from OA±T vs NZ men and higher in sperm samples leading to live birth
Boissonnas *et al.* [23]	NZ men (17) OAT men (22)	Bisulfite-pyrosequencing	L1 elements	OAT patients displayed a tendency to lower methylation levels (46 ± 3.8% in NZ vs 44 ± 4.1% in OAT)
Marques *et al.* [24]	NZ men (1) OAT men (4)	Bisulfite-sequencing	L1 elements	Ratio of the methylation showed no significant differences
Kobayashi *et al.* [25]	NZ men (14) OAT men (10)	Bisulphite–PCR restriction	L1 and *Alu* elements	Ratio of the methylation showed no significant differences

NZ, normal semen parameters (normozoospermia); OAT, abnormal sperm parameters (O: oligozoospermia; A: asthenozoospermia; T: teratozoospermia); PCR, polymerase chain reaction.

Transposon control and sperm criteria

There are two main approaches to link retrotransposons to abnormal spermatogenesis: by showing altered repression of these elements, or by identifying genetic mutations in retrotransposon repressors.

Only four studies have been carried out so far to assess the methylation levels of retrotransposons in relationship to sperm quality. Concerning *Alu* sequences, lower methylation levels were observed in the sperm of patients with abnormal semen parameters, including oligozoospermia, asthenozoospermia, and teratozoospermia, compared to normospermic men. However, reported differences are very subtle, with 23.1% and 24.2% of *Alu* methylation measured in altered versus normal sperm, respectively [22] (Table 6.2 [22–25]). This tendency was nonetheless associated with decreased pregnancy success and live-birth rate after assisted reproductive technologies (24.1% of methylation in sperm samples leading to birth as compared to 22.7% in those that did not). Concerning L1 methylation, while a tendency to lower average methylation was reported in one study of a small cohort of patients with abnormal sperm parameters [23], others failed to provide evidence for abnormal L1 methylation in the sperm of infertile men [22, 24, 25]. Further studies are clearly needed to allow definite conclusions about the relationship between abnormal retrotransposon methylation and altered sperm criteria. Moreover, conclusions should be tempered, as abnormal retrotransposon methylation in infertile patients may be equally a cause or a consequence of altered spermatogenesis. Additionally, gamete manipulation inherent to human sperm studies may be a cause of abnormal retrotransposon control. Of note, a recent study has concluded that spermatozoa cryopreservation, one of the main sperm manipulations, is safe in terms of *Alu* and L1 methylation [26].

Although functional studies in mice have led to a list of 17 proteins involved in safeguarding fertility (Table 6.1), this pathway has drawn very little attention in the field of human reproductive genetics so far. In mice, complete inactivation of these repressors invariably results in azoospermia. Two main spermatogenetic processes are affected: an interruption at meiosis I, and a rapid exhaustion of SSCs that eventually leads to a complete lack of germ cells (Sertoli-cell-only phenotype). By analogy, mutations in retrotransposon repressors are expected to be associated with non-obstructive azoospermia (NOA) with a block of spermatogenesis at meiosis I, and Sertoli-cell only syndrome (SCOS) in men. However, causal genetic mutations are more often hypo- than nullimorphic in humans, so a wider range of infertility phenotypes could be expected. In this regard, a SNP (single nucleotide polymorphism) located in the 3'UTR of the *PIWIL2* gene and a nonsynonymous SNP in the *PIWIL3* gene have been associated with a reduced risk of oligozoospermia in a Chinese population of patients recruited in an infertility clinic [27]. However, the biological significance of these polymorphic variants on retrotransposon control is unknown.

Although genetic mutations were not investigated, another study has identified lower expression of genes encoding germline retrotransposon repressors in the testes of cryptorchid boys, a condition leading to a high risk of infertility [28]. These included *PIWIL2*, *PIWIL4*, *MAELSTROM*, *TDRD9*, and the RNA helicases *VASA* and *MOV10L1*. Although being an interesting result, the lower expression of these germline genes may just be a consequence of germ cell depletion in the testes of these cryptorchid boys. Similarly, a recent study reported a gain of methylation at the promoters of *PIWIL2* and *TDRD1*, along with transcript level downregulation, in adult infertile patients suffering various degrees of secretory spermatogenic failure [29]. Once again, as the analysis was performed on whole testis biopsies, this may rather reflect a more somatic-like pattern due to germ cell depletion rather than direct alteration of these *PIWI*-related genes. However, interestingly, a slight defect in LINE1 methylation was specifically observed in some cases of early spermatogenetic interruption, at the spermatogonia or spermatocyte stages. This type of investigation may set the stage for further analysis of retrotransposon control in altered spermatogenesis, performed on cellular fractions or in a more genome-wide manner.

Situations at risk: endocrine disruptors and synthetic gametes

Environmental factors could also alter retrotransposon control and lead to altered gamete integrity. Exposure to endocrine disruptors has been linked to abnormal gonadal development and gametogenesis, both in animal models and human epidemiologic studies. These molecules are more and more widely represented in our industrial environments. To cite a few, bisphenol A, phtalates, and perfluorinated substances are found in a variety of household consumables such as plastics, cosmetics, pesticides, and cleaning products, etc. These chemicals have the ability to interfere with the metabolism of endogenous hormones and to impact on their downstream targets, which include the epigenetic setting of the germline. The fetal window of development has been highlighted as particularly susceptible to these compounds, in agreement with the major phases of sexual determination and germline development occurring before birth. Notably, DNA methylation anomalies have been sporadically reported to occur in response to endocrine disruptor exposure during fetal male germ cell development, mostly in rodent models [30]. However, no study has been dedicated so far to the analysis of

retrotransposon control following exposure to these factors. Considering the short- and long-term consequences that retrotransposon reactivation can have on gamete production and the development of the next generation, this appears as an area of utmost importance to investigate, to document the origin of transgenerational effects induced by endocrine disruptor exposure.

The recent development of induced pluripotent stem cells (iPSC), which consists in the forced reversion of a somatic cell (such as a fibroblast) into an embryonic-like state of pluripotency, holds great promise for regenerative medicine, including regenerative reproductive medicine. Consequently, attempts have been made towards producing "synthetic" gametes from the differentiation of these iPSC cells in a Petri dish, as an unlimited source of reproductive cells for infertile patients [31]. Protocols are currently being optimized, converging towards an obligate transplantation step into a gonad to promote full gametogenesis. However, a recent study has raised awareness about the potential risk of this method of iPSC-derived gametes by showing that human iPSC derivation induces a dramatic relaxation of L1 control. These cells exhibit a loss of DNA methylation, increased expression, and even more worryingly, a high rate of retrotransposition of L1 elements, when compared to parental fibroblasts [32]. Considering the ability of L1-encoded proteins to also promote the mobilization of other retrotransposon classes, the number of L1-mediated insertional mutations has probably been underestimated. This observation seriously questions the safety of using iPS cells as a source of gametes, as their altered genetic integrity induced by L1 reactivation is likely to promote abnormal phenotypes in children conceived by this extreme technique of medically assisted reproduction.

Concluding remarks

Studies dedicated to the biology of retrotransposons are of utmost importance to understand the life cycle of retrotransposons in the germline, the defense routes preventing their activity, and the impact they have on the production of gametes and the quality of the genetic information that will pass to subsequent generations. Retrotransposon repressors appear to represent major determinants of mammalian reproduction and human fertility. Further researches exploring the world of retrotransposons in human spermatogenesis, in both normal and pathological contexts, may be helpful in increasing our understanding of the etiology of male infertility and, eventually, to consider new therapeutic approaches in the human.

Acknowledgements

We would like to thank the members of our teams for useful discussion and specially Natasha Zamudio.

References

1. Ostertag EM, Kazazian HH, Jr. Twin priming: a proposed mechanism for the creation of inversions in L1 retrotransposition. *Genome Res* 2001; 11: 2059–65.

2. Cordaux R, Batzer MA. The impact of retrotransposons on human genome evolution. *Nat Rev Genet* 2009; 10: 691–703.

3. Zamudio N, Bourc'his D. Transposable elements in the mammalian germline: a comfortable niche or a deadly trap? *Heredity* 2010; 105: 92–104.

4. Bourc'his D, Bestor TH. Meiotic catastrophe and retrotransposon reactivation in male germ cells lacking Dnmt3L. *Nature* 2004; 431: 96–9.

5. Feschotte C, Gilbert C. Endogenous viruses: insights into viral evolution and impact on host biology. *Nat Rev Genet* 2012; 13: 283–96.

6. Burns KH, Boeke JD. Human transposon tectonics. *Cell* 2012; 149: 740–52.

7. Stoye JP. Studies of endogenous retroviruses reveal a continuing evolutionary saga. *Nat Rev Microbiol* 2012; 10: 395–406.

8. Esnault C, Priet S, Ribet D *et al*. A placenta-specific receptor for the fusogenic, endogenous retrovirus-derived, human syncytin-2. *Proc Natl Acad Sci U S A* 2008; 105: 17 532–7.

9. Goodier JL, Kazazian HH, Jr. Retrotransposons revisited: the restraint and rehabilitation of parasites. *Cell* 2008; 135: 23–35.

10. Lander ES, Linton LM, Birren B *et al*. Initial sequencing and analysis of the human genome. *Nature* 2001; 409: 860–921.

11. Shi X, Seluanov A, Gorbunova V. Cell divisions are required for L1 retrotransposition. *Mol Cell Biol* 2007; 27: 1264–70.

12. Yoder JA, Walsh CP, Bestor TH. Cytosine methylation and the ecology of intragenomic parasites. *Trends Genet* 1997; 13: 335–40.

13. Matsui T, Leung D, Miyashita H *et al*. Proviral silencing in embryonic stem cells requires the histone methyltransferase ESET. *Nature* 2010; 464: 927–31.

14. Bishop KN, Holmes RK, Sheehy AM *et al*. Cytidine deamination of retroviral DNA by diverse APOBEC proteins. *Curr Biol* 2004; 14: 1392–6.

15. Beauregard A, Curcio MJ, Belfort M. The take and give between retrotransposable elements and their hosts. *Annu Rev Genet* 2008; 42: 587–617.

16. Obbard DJ, Gordon KH, Buck AH, Jiggins FM. The evolution of RNAi as a defence against viruses and transposable elements. *Philos Trans R Soc Lond B Biol Sci* 2009; 364: 99–115.

17. Kaneko H, Dridi S, Tarallo V *et al*. DICER1 deficit induces Alu RNA toxicity in age-related macular degeneration. *Nature* 2011; 471: 325–30.

18. Aravin AA, van der Heijden GW, Castaneda J *et al*. Cytoplasmic compartmentalization of the fetal piRNA pathway in mice. *PLoS Genet* 2009; 5: e1000764.

19. Carmell MA, Girard A, van de Kant HJ *et al*. MIWI2 is essential for spermatogenesis and repression of transposons in the mouse male germline. *Dev Cell* 2007; 12: 503–14.

20. Gasior SL, Wakeman TP, Xu B, Deininger PL. The human LINE-1 retrotransposon creates DNA double-strand breaks. *J Mol Biol* 2006; 357: 1383–93.

21. Popp C, Dean W, Feng S *et al*. Genome-wide erasure of DNA methylation in mouse primordial germ cells is affected by AID deficiency. *Nature* 2010; 463: 1101–5.

22. El Hajj N, Zechner U, Schneider E *et al*. Methylation status of imprinted genes and repetitive elements in sperm DNA from infertile males. *Sex Dev* 2011; 5: 60–9.

23. Boissonnas CC, Abdalaoui HE, Haelewyn V *et al*. Specific epigenetic alterations of IGF2-H19 locus in spermatozoa from infertile men. *Eur J Hum Genet* 2010; 18: 73–80.

24. Marques CJ, Costa P, Vaz B *et al*. Abnormal methylation of imprinted genes in human sperm is associated with oligozoospermia. *Mol Hum Reprod* 2008;14: 67–74.

25. Kobayashi H, Hiura H, John RM *et al*. DNA methylation errors at imprinted loci after assisted conception originate in the parental sperm. *Eur J Hum Genet* 2009; 17: 1582–91.

26. Klaver R, Bleiziffer A, Redmann K *et al*. Routine cryopreservation of spermatozoa is safe – Evidence from the DNA methylation pattern of nine spermatozoa genes. *J Assist Reprod Genet* 2012; 29: 943–50.

27. Gu A, Ji G, Shi X *et al*. Genetic variants in Piwi-interacting RNA pathway genes confer susceptibility to spermatogenic failure in a Chinese population. *Hum Reprod* 2010; 25: 2955–61.

28. Hadziselimovic F, Hadziselimovic NO, Demougin P, Krey G, Oakeley EJ. Deficient expression of genes involved in the endogenous defense system against transposons in cryptorchid boys with impaired mini-puberty. *Sex Dev* 2011; 5: 287–93.

29. Heyn H, Ferreira HJ, Bassas L *et al.* Epigenetic Disruption of the PIWI Pathway in Human Spermatogenic Disorders. *PLoS One* 2012; 7: e47892.

30. Bromer JG, Zhou Y, Taylor MB, Doherty L, Taylor HS. Bisphenol-A exposure in utero leads to epigenetic alterations in the developmental programming of uterine estrogen response. *FASEB J* 2010; 24: 2273–80.

31. Yang S, Bo J, Hu H *et al.* Derivation of male germ cells from induced pluripotent stem cells *in vitro* and in reconstituted seminiferous tubules. *Cell Prolif* 2012; 45: 91–100.

32. Wissing S, Munoz-Lopez M, Macia A *et al.* Reprogramming somatic cells into iPS cells activates LINE-1 retroelement mobility. *Hum Mol Genet* 2012; 21: 208–18.

Chromosomal causes of infertility
The story continues

Svetlana A. Yatsenko and Aleksandar Rajkovic

Chromosomal causes of male infertility

The genetic causes of male infertility are highly heterogeneous, and a large portion of these causes remains unexplained. More than 2300 testes-specific genes may contribute to male infertility [1]. Primary testicular disorders affecting spermatogenesis are commonly associated with abnormal semen parameters, including sperm concentration (oligo- or azoospermia), morphology, motility, and vitality. Studies in infertile men demonstrated that up to 20% carry constitutional chromosome aberrations [2–5]. Genomic aberrations found in these patients include numerical abnormalities, such as Klinefelter syndrome and its variants; XYY karyotype; testicular disorders of sex development, such as XX males; structural chromosome rearrangements, including Robertsonian translocations, balanced reciprocal translocations and inversions; as well as submicroscopic DNA copy number alterations (microdeletions and microduplications) encompassing genes associated with spermatogenesis or gonadal development.

Sex chromosome abnormalities

Klinefelter syndrome

Klinefelter syndrome (KS) is the most common chromosomal aberration among infertile men, accounting for 14% of azoospermia patients [6]. Klinefelter syndrome is characterized by the presence of one or more extra X chromosomes in a normal male karyotype (Fig. 7.1). The most common variant, the 47,XXY karyotype (Fig. 7.1B), is seen in about 90% of KS men [6]. Klinefelter syndrome variants such as 48,XXXY; 48,XXYY, or 49,XXXXY are much less frequent. The extra X chromosome in KS usually arises from meiotic nondisjunction, when the X chromosome fails to separate during the first or second meiotic division in male or female gametogenesis [5]. About 10% of males with KS are mosaic (47,XXY/46,XY). The extra X chromosome in a portion of cells is due to the mitotic nondisjunction in the developing zygote [6].

Due to the variability of the phenotype, KS is underdiagnosed, with only 10% of KS patients recognized prepubertally and an additional 15% identified after puberty [2, 3, 7]. In childhood, KS boys may present with language delay, learning, and behavioral problems. Boys with KS have a normal number and morphology of Sertoli and Leydig cells; a reduced number of spermatogonia; and normal serum levels of testosterone, follicle-stimulating hormone (FSH), luteinizing hormone (LH), and inhibin B during the prepubertal period [4, 6, 7]. The degenerative process in testes is accelerated with a decline in testosterone and a gradual increase in FSH and LH concentrations after the onset of puberty. Infertility and small testes are the most prevalent characteristics in adult KS patients. The testes in adult KS males are characterized by extensive fibrosis and hyalinization of the seminiferous tubules and impaired spermatogenesis, with azoospermia or severe oligozoospermia [3–7]. Although most KS patients are infertile, testicular spermatozoa can be identified and recovered from at least 50% of men with the non-mosaic 47,XXY karyotype [3, 4, 7]. In mosaic and rare non-mosaic KS cases, mature spermatozoa can be found in ejaculates [4, 7]. Testicular sperm extraction (TESE) combined with intracytoplasmic sperm injection (ICSI) allows over 50% of patients with KS to father their own biological children [3, 4, 6–8].

Sperm from KS men usually have a normal 23,X or 23,Y haploid chromosome complement. Despite this,

Textbook of Human Reproductive Genetics, eds Karen Sermon and Stéphane Viville. Published by Cambridge University Press. © Cambridge University Press 2014.

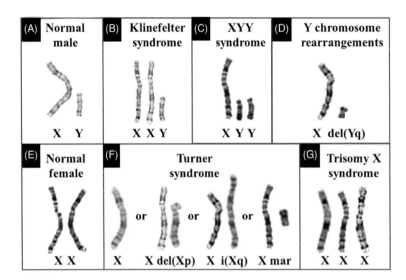

Figure 7.1 Sex chromosome numerical and structural abnormalities associated with human infertility. Normal male (**A**) and normal female (**E**) chromosomal complement is shown. The common sex chromosome aneuploidies detected by classical karyotype analyses are shown for (**B**) Klinefelter syndrome (47,XXY), (**C**) XYY men, (**F**) Turner syndrome (45,X), and (**G**) trisomy X women (47,XXX). (**F**) Gross structural X and Y chromosome rearrangements include deletions of the short arm of chromosome X (del(Xp)), isochromosome composed of the two long arms of chromosome X (i(Xq)), small marker (mar) chromosome containing X-specific or Y-specific DNA. The X- and Y-chromosome structural rearrangements can be observed by chromosome analysis, such as deletions of the long arm (del(Yq)) (**D**). However, high resolution techniques (fluorescence *in situ* hybridization (FISH) or chromosomal microarray analyses) are essential for better characterization.

an increased frequency for both autosomal and sex chromosome aneuploidy has been reported in fetuses [2, 3, 8, 9].

47,XYY karyotype

An extra copy of the Y chromosome is present in 47,XYY males (Fig. 7.1C). This chromosomal aneuploidy occurs in 1/1000 live male births in the general population, and is seen more frequently in the infertile population [2, 6]. Men with the 47,XYY karyotype have a normal phenotype. With regards to fertility, semen analyses may show oligozoospermia or azoospermia in some patients, while the majority of 47,XYY males are fertile with normal semen parameters, and produce normal haploid spermatozoa [8]. The extra Y chromosome is eliminated via apoptosis of the cells carrying two Y chromosomes during the premeiotic stage of spermatogenesis, although the frequency of aneuploidy for the sex chromosomes is slightly increased in mature sperm [6]. Testes biopsies demonstrate that perturbation during meiotic pairing may contribute to sperm apoptosis and subsequent oligozoospermia and infertility in men with the 47,XYY karyotype [2, 8].

Y chromosome microdeletions

The human Y chromosome contains many genes that are essential for male sex determination and spermatogenesis [1, 5, 10]. Based on observation of cytogenetically visible deletions, the azoospermia factor (AZF) region has been established within the Yq and

extensively studied during the last decade. Microdeletions involving the long arm of chromosome Y (Yq) are one of the most significant pathogenic defects in infertile males, found in about 10% of men with oligozoospermia and in up to 15% of azoospermic patients [2, 4, 6]. The AZF region consists of three genetic domains in the long arm of the human Y chromosome: *AZFa*, which is located within Yq11.21, *AZFb*, and *AZFc*. *AZFb* and *AZFc* overlap and map within bands Yq11.22 and Yq11.23, respectively (Fig. 7.2). Overall, these three regions contain gene families for 27 distinct proteins [10, 11]. Microdeletions involving *AZFa*, *AZFb*, and *AZFc* result in disruption of spermatogenesis at three different stages. *AZFa* deletions cause Sertoli-cell-only syndrome with a complete absence of germ cells. Arrest at the spermatocyte stage (normal population of spermatogonia and primary spermocytes, but no post-meiotic germ cells) was observed in the testes of all patients with the *AZFb* region deletion. *AZFc* deletions affect the post-meiotic spermatid maturation process, resulting in a decreased number of mature germ cells [10, 11]. Microdeletions encompassing other genes located on the Y chromosome have been proposed to influence spermatogenesis, although their role remains to be elucidated.

Gross structural abnormalities of the Yq chromosome (Fig. 7.1D), such as whole long arm deletions (del(Y)(q11.2)), isochromosome Yp (i(Yp)), and dicentric Yp (dic(Yp)), occur less frequently than microdeletions and result in complete absence of germ cells [3, 8].

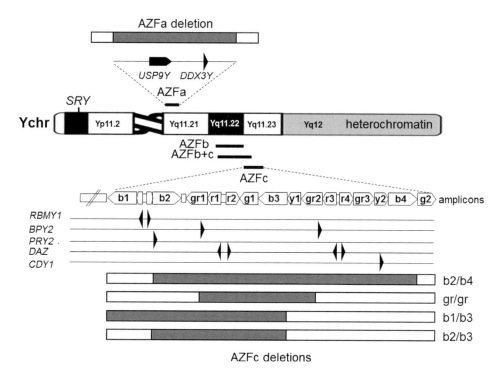

Figure 7.2 The AZF regions of the Y chromosome. Y chromosome (Ychr) schema details the location of the *SRY* gene at Yp11.31, as well as *AZFa*, *AZFb*, and *AZFc* deletion regions. The three AZF regions map to the Yq11.21, Yq.11.22, and Yq11.23 bands. Above the Ychr, the *AZFa* chromosome region is magnified to show the *USP9Y* and *DDX3Y* genes. Below the Y chromosome, complex genomic organization within the *AZFc* region is shown. *AZFb* and *AZFc* regions are formed by amplicons (nearly identical stretches of DNA). Amplicons consist of five sequence families: b, gr, r, g, and y, originally named as blue, green, red, gray, and yellow, respectively. Nearly identical segments within the same sequence family are differentiated by numbers (b1, b2, b3, etc.). Sequence orientation is shown by black arrowheads. Functional genes and their 5'–3' orientation are indicated by black-filled triangles; pseudogenes are not shown. *AZFc* deletions associated with azoospermia are shown in gray.

AZFa

The *AZFa* region, a segment of 792 kilobases (kb) in size, is located at the proximal Yq (chromosome position: ~12.9–13.7) (Fig. 7.2) [3, 4, 11]. This region is flanked by two repetitive DNA elements that are about 10 kb each in size and share 94% sequence identity. Non allelic homologous recombination between these repeats results in a complete *AZFa* deletion (OMIM #400042), a fairly rare but recurrent event. This deletion removes two genes that are located in the *AZFa* region, *USP9Y* (OMIM #400005) and *DBY* (OMIM #400010) (also called *DDX3Y*), and is associated with Sertoli-cell-only syndrome, a condition characterized by the presence of Sertoli cells in the testes but a lack of spermatozoa in the ejaculate [3, 4, 11]. A testicular biopsy shows degeneration of germ cells within tubules due to a failure of differentiation and maturation of spermatocytes and spermatids [2, 11]. Partial *AZFa* deletions encompassing either *USP9Y* or *DBY*

genes are rarely identified. Deletions involving only the *USP9Y* gene have been found among infertile men with azoospermia, oligozoospermia, or oligoasthenozoospermia, as well as in fertile men, suggesting that the gene might not be critical for sperm production [3, 4]. Small, 98-kb deletions encompassing only the *DBY* gene, have been reported in multiple infertile patients; however, this was in a single population study and requires future replications.

AZFb

Deletions involving the *AZFb* region account for about 30% of all AZF deletions [6, 11]. The *AZFb* region spans a 6.2-Megabase (Mb) segment between ~18.1 and 24.7 Mb of the Y chromosome. *AZFb* has a complex genomic structure (Fig. 7.2), and contains multiple highly identical sequences organized in opposite orientation to each other (palindromic amplicons) [4]. Similar amplicons are also present distally to

AZFb, within the *AZFc* region [4, 10]. The outcome of non-allelic homologous recombination between these amplicons results in deletion of a 6.2-Mb or 7.7-Mb segment. Therefore, deletions spanning the *AZFb* region are variable in size, have different proximal and distal breakpoints, and may include both *AZFb* and *AZFc* regions (Fig. 7.2). Complete *AZFb* microdeletion is 6.2 Mb in size. There are a number of testis-specific genes located within the *AZFb* region (Fig. 7.2). Four main gene families (*CDY*, *HSFY*, *RBMY*, and *PRY*) are present in more than one copy in the *AZFb* deletion interval. A combined *AZFb + c* deletion additionally removes a 1.5-Mb part of the *AZFc* region, and is therefore 7.7-Mb in size. Patients with *AZFb* or *AZFb + c* deletions present with azoospermia due to maturation arrest at the primary spermatocyte stage [11].

AZFc

The *AZFc* region is located at the distal long arm of the Y chromosome at band Yq11.23 and encompasses a segment of about 3.5-Mb in size (Fig. 7.2). The region where recurrent *AZFc* deletions occur consists of five large DNA sequences (amplicons) ranging from 115 to 678 kb that are repeated several times and are arranged in either direct or inverted orientation to each other [10]. Such complex genomic structure makes *AZFc* susceptible to genomic rearrangements, including deletions, duplications, and inversions. Complete and partial *AZFc* deletions that affect the dosage of genes implicated in spermatogenesis can cause spermatogenic impairment and infertility [4, 10, 11]. The *AZFc* region contains at least four protein-coding germline-specific gene families: *BPY2*, *PRY2*, *DAZ*, and *CDY1* [10]. There are four functional copies of the *DAZ* gene, three copies of *BPY2*, two copies of *CDY1*, and a single copy of the *PRY2* gene, as well as their inactive copies (pseudogenes) in the reference human genome (Fig. 7.2).

The *DAZ* (deleted in azoospermia, OMIM #400003) genes (*DAZ1–DAZ4*) encode four RNA-binding proteins that are expressed exclusively in the adult testis in all stages of germ cell development. *DAZ* genes regulate translation, are involved in control of meiosis and maintenance of the primordial germ cell population, and are therefore thought to be critical genes in the *AZFc* region [10]. Despite sequence homology, the four DAZ proteins have variability in their number of functional domains,

and may have overlapping, but not identical, roles in spermatogenesis.

A complete 3.5-Mb *AZFc* deletion, also known as a b2/b4 deletion (Fig. 7.2), is the product of intrachromosomal homologous recombination between the b2 and b4 amplicons, and is the most frequent deletion among infertile men with Y chromosome microdeletions. Men with complete *AZFc* deletions have reduced spermatogenesis ranging from azoospermia to severe oligozoospermia. *AZFc* deletions cause approximately 12% of non-obstructive azoospermia and 6% of severe oligozoospermia [10, 11].

Additionally, four recurrent rearrangements involving a part of the *AZFc* region have been described: b1/b3, b2/b3, gr/gr partial deletions, and gr/gr duplication (Fig. 7.2). Partial deletions remove 1.6–1.8 Mb of *AZFc* and reduce the copy number of several testis-specific *AZFc* genes; however, only the gr/gr deletions are associated with increased risk of spermatogenic failure. Men with a gr/gr deletion show significant phenotypic variability ranging from normozoospermia to azoospermia, likely due to a complex interaction of many factors including the influence of ethnic and environmental backgrounds. Deletions b2/b3 and b1/b3, and complete or partial *AZFc* duplications, do not seem to have an effect on semen parameters [3, 4, 6, 10].

The vast majority of complete *AZFc* microdeletions occur *de novo* (i.e. are not present in the patient's father); however, rare cases of natural transmission have been reported. Partial gr/gr deletions can be passed from father to son [6, 11]. It has also been shown that the presence of a partial *AZFc* deletion in a father can increase the risk of a complete *AZFc* deletion in his sons [3, 4].

46,XX male syndrome or testicular disorder of sex development

The XX male syndrome, or testicular disorder of sex development (testicular DSD) is a rare condition with a frequency of 1/25 000 male newborns, and is characterized by the presence of a 46,XX karyotype and male genitalia [12]. Approximately 20% of boys with testicular DSD have ambiguous genitalia at birth, whereas the remaining 80% present with steroidogenic and spermatogenic dysfunction after puberty.

The majority of males with the 46,XX karyotype are *SRY* positive by fluorescence *in situ* hybridization (FISH) or polymerase chain reaction (PCR)

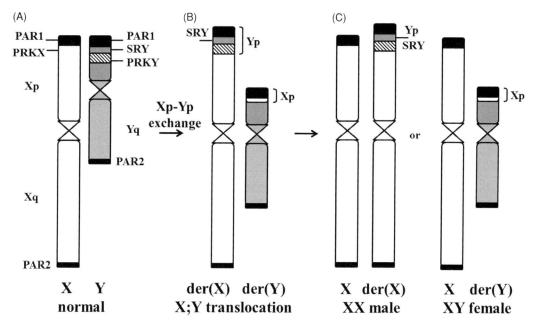

Figure 7.3 X;Y chromosomes translocation. During male meiosis (**A**), X and Y chromosomes normally pair and recombine within the two homologous regions (pseudoautosomal regions, PAR1 and PAR2) located at the distal short and long arms of sex chromosomes. Aberrant recombination involving highly homologous DNA sequences such as the *PRKX* and *PRKY* genes results in exchange of X-specific and Y-specific DNA segments. The X;Y translocation causes transposition of the *SRY* gene from the Y to the X chromosome resulting in derivative chromosome X (derX), comprising *SRY*, and derivative chromosome Y (derY), deleted for the *SRY* gene (**B**). Fertilization by a sperm containing the derivative X chromosome will conceive an *SRY*-positive XX male, whereas sperm carrying derivative Y chromosome, deleted for *SRY*, will conceive an XY female (**C**).

amplification [6, 12]. The *SRY* gene, also known as the testis-determining factor (located on the Y chromosome at Yp11.31, Fig. 7.3), encodes for the sex-determining Y protein, which activates a cascade of male-specific transcription factors essential for male development. In most instances, 46,XX male syndrome is caused by an exchange of segments between the short arms of the X and Y chromosomes (X;Y translocation) during paternal meiosis (Fig. 7.3A), resulting in the derivative chromosome X containing the *SRY* gene (Fig. 7.3B,C), and the derivative chromosome Y deleted for *SRY*. Fertilization with an abnormal gamete, containing either the *SRY*-positive X chromosome or the Y chromosome with the *SRY* gene deletion, will result in a sterile XX male or XY female, respectively. Translocations between the Y and autosomal chromosomes can also give rise to *SRY*-positive XX males, where the *SRY* gene is located on the autosomal chromosome [12] (Fig. 7.4). *SRY*-positive males with 46,XX testicular DSD and normal male genitalia have small testes with severe atrophy and absent spermatogenesis, azoospermia, and hypergonadotropic hypogonadism [12].

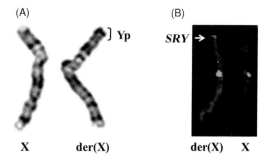

Figure 7.4 Partial karyotype and fluorescence *in situ* hybridization (FISH) analysis in the XX male. (**A**) Chromosome analysis detected a derivative chromosome X containing the Yp segment at the distal short arm of X chromosome. (**B**) FISH analysis with *SRY* specific probe (red signal, arrow) shows that the *SRY* gene is present in the derivative X chromosome. The centromere of the X chromosome is colored in green. See plate section for color version.

About 10% of 46,XX men are *SRY*-negative and can present with ambiguous genitalia at birth. *SRY*-negative, 46,XX infertile men can also have normal external genitalia [13]. *SRY* normally triggers testes formation by activating expression of *SOX9*, located at 17q24.3. Like *SRY*, *SOX9* is necessary for testis

Table 7.1 Genomic imbalances associated with complete gonadal dysgenesis (CGD) in 46,XX males

Locus	Genomic abnormality	Gene	Molecular mechanism	Phenotype	OMIM #
1p34.3	Disruption	RSPO1	Loss of function	CGD, palmoplantar hyperkeratosis	610644
17q24	Duplication	Regulatory region SOX9	Gain of function	CGD	613080
Xq26	Duplication, deletion	SOX3	Gain of function	CGD	300833
Yp11	Presence	SRY	X;Y or Yp-autosome translocation	CGD	400044

differentiation, and its overexpression can lead to male development in the absence of *SRY*. *SOX9* expression is regulated by testis-specific transcriptional enhancer elements mapped within a 1-Mb non-coding region upstream of the *SOX9* gene [13]. Submicroscopic chromosome 17q24.3 duplications and triplications detected by array comparative genomic hybridization (aCGH) analysis, as well as balanced translocations upstream of *SOX9*, have been identified in some infertile XX males that are *SRY* negative [12]. In addition to *SRY*, genes encoding steroidogenic factor 1 (*NR5A1*, 9q33.3) and *SOX3* (Xq27.1) can upregulate expression of *SOX9* [12]. Genomic rearrangements that cause *SOX3* gain-of-function have been identified among *SRY*-negative XX males (Table 7.1). Disruption of the gene encoding R-spondin 1 (*RSPO1*, 1p34.3) is also a rare cause of the XX male phenotype. Genetic etiology in many other XX male *SRY*-negative individuals remains unknown.

Balanced chromosome rearrangements

Structural chromosomal abnormalities are frequent in infertile men, with an overall incidence of about 5%, a percentage that is 10-fold higher than the 0.5% prevalence in the general population [3, 4, 6, 14]. Chromosome rearrangements are found in approximately 14% of azoospermic and 4.5% of oligozoospermic patients. Autosomal aberrations (3%) are more commonly associated with oligozoospermia, whereas sex chromosome defects (12.6%) predominate among azoospermic men [14, 15]. Structural chromosome rearrangements may cause impaired spermatogenesis by adversely affecting chromosome synapsis during meiosis [2, 15]. Alternatively, chromosome breaks may result in disruption/inactivation of a single dosage-sensitive gene involved in spermatogenesis, thus resulting in the arrest of abnormal male germ cell development [14, 15].

Balanced chromosome rearrangements may be classified as reciprocal translocations, inversions, complex chromosome rearrangements (CCRs), or Robertsonian translocations (see Chapter 1 for detailed information) (Fig. 7.5).

Reciprocal translocations occur when segments are exchanged between two chromosomes with no apparent loss or gain of genetic material at the breakpoint sites. Carriers of balanced chromosome rearrangements usually have a normal phenotype and are often diagnosed during evaluation of their infertility problem, or following the birth of a child with an unbalanced chromosome complement [2, 14, 15]. In balanced translocation carriers, meiotic pairing results in the formation of a quadrivalent structure between translocated chromosomes and their normal homologs. Chromosome segregation analyses demonstrate a high proportion (up to 80%) of unbalanced spermatozoa among carriers of reciprocal translocations [14, 15]. Fertility problems in male carriers can be attributed to disturbance of the meiotic process and various degrees of sperm defects. However, the presence of a balanced chromosome rearrangement is not necessarily associated with spermatogenic failure and infertility [2, 15]. Fertilization by an unbalanced gamete does occur, but many resulting embryos do not survive. Therefore, individuals carrying balanced rearrangements benefit from preimplantation genetic diagnosis (PGD) to identify and implant embryos with normal or balanced chromosome complement (see Chapter 11).

Individuals who carry chromosome inversions (see Chapter 3) are healthy in general, but infertility, recurrent pregnancy losses, and chromosomally abnormal offspring have been reported [2, 14, 15]. During meiosis, pairing of inverted segments is achieved by the formation of an inversion loop. The size of the inverted segment and position of the crossover determine the outcome of meiotic pairing. In carriers of paracentric

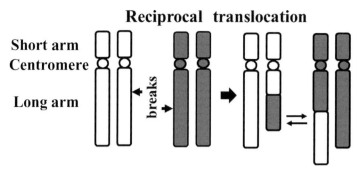

Reciprocal translocation

Short arm
Centromere

Long arm

breaks

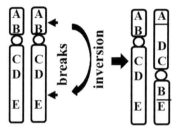

Pericentric inversion

breaks

inversion

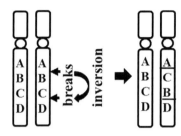

Paracentric inversion

breaks

inversion

Figure 7.5 Balanced structural chromosome rearrangements. Reciprocal translocations can occur between non-homologous chromosomes. Breaks in the DNA (arrowheads) at two different chromosomes, followed by exchange of chromosomal segments distal to the break, will lead to two derivative chromosomes. Paracentric and pericentric inversions are associated with two breakpoints on a single chromosome (arrowheads). Balanced rearrangements may disrupt gene functions at the translocation breakpoints and cause chromosomally abnormal offspring and recurrent miscarriages.

inversions, unbalanced chromosomal complements have been reported in about 1% of spermatozoa; however, such studies have been performed on a limited number of individuals [15]. In contrast, carriers of pericentric inversions may have a high proportion (up to 54%) of spermatozoa with unbalanced recombinant chromosomes [2, 8]. In general, large pericentric inversions (encompassing more than half of the chromosome length) are more likely to produce unbalanced chromosomes and are therefore more frequently observed among infertile men [8, 15].

Complex chromosome rearrangements, structural aberrations with at least three breakpoints and an exchange of genetic material between two or more chromosomes, occur in around 0.5% of newborns [16]. Unbalanced CCRs are often associated with intellectual disability and congenital abnormalities. Balanced CCRs are seen in phenotypically normal individuals with a history of recurrent abortions and infertility. Molecular studies using high resolution aCGH and analysis of breakpoint sequences demonstrate that many genomic rearrangements are complex events; however, neither the complexity nor the number of breaks can be used to predict infertility in men with complex chromosome rearrangements. General risk of spontaneous abortion for CCR carriers is estimated to be approximately 50% and about 20% for affected offspring. Each CCR is unique and reproductive risks will depend upon multiple factors such as

chromosome origin, location of breakpoints, number of chromosomes involved, and overall breaks, genome content, rearrangement type, and complexity [15, 16]. There are 64 possible combinations of chromosomes in spermatozoa of a carrier for CCR with three breaks involving three chromosomes. The number of combinations increases with the involvement of additional chromosomes and/or breakpoints. Because of the low proportion of balanced sperm available (~10–20%), ICSI is not recommended in male CCR carriers [15, 16].

Robertsonian translocations are the most common structural chromosomal rearrangement in humans, resulting in a derivative chromosome composed of the long arms of two acrocentric chromosomes (13, 14, 15, 21, and 22) (Fig. 7.6; for more information see Chapter 1). The most frequent Robertsonian translocations are der(13;14) and der(14;21) with incidences of about 1 in 1000 and 1 in 5000, respectively [2, 4, 8, 17, 18]. Carriers of Robertsonian translocations have an increased risk for infertility, chromosomally unbalanced offspring, and spontaneous abortions, but are otherwise healthy. Studies involving male carriers of der(13;14) showed that in about 80% of cases the partners had spontaneous pregnancies, while in 20% of cases the male carriers were infertile [18]. Carriers of Robertsonian translocations account for about 1.6% of infertile male patients. The cause of infertility in these individuals has been associated with

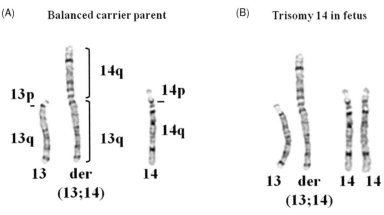

(A) Balanced carrier parent

14q
13p
14p
13q   13q   14q
13   der   14
(13;14)

(B) Trisomy 14 in fetus

13   der   14   14
(13;14)

Figure 7.6 Robertsonian translocation between chromosomes 13 and 14. (A) Balanced carrier of the Robertsonian translocation has a derivative chromosome der(13;14) composed of the long arms of chromosome 13 and 14, as well as one normal homolog of chromosomes 13 and 14. The derivative (13;14) is formed by fusion of two acrocentric chromosomes at the centromere, with accompanying loss of the short arms 13p and 14p. **(B)** Trisomy 14 in the fetus is due to the inherited Robertsonian translocation. Fertilization with gametes containing both the der(13;14) and normal chromosome 13 or 14 can lead to either trisomy 13 (Patau) syndrome or trisomy 14.

meiotic disturbances of rearranged chromosomes and subsequent meiotic arrest, resulting in oligozoospermia or azoospermia [17, 18]. During meiosis, pairing of the translocated chromosomes gives rise to a trivalent configuration. Most of the mature spermatozoa (75–90%) are normal or balanced as a result of alternate segregation; however, certain variability exists among patients [17]. It is remarkable that in the mature spermatozoa a much higher proportion of nullisomies versus disomies has been found for chromosomes 13, 14, 15, and 22. These findings correlate with a higher incidence of monosomic embryos detected by PGD [17, 18]. Monosomic embryos are usually lost during early pregnancy. In rare cases these embryos may survive due to the maternal uniparental disomy (UPD). In contrast, male carriers of a Robertsonian translocation involving chromosome 21 are more likely to produce disomic as opposed to nullisomic gametes. Such gametes are more likely to produce trisomy 21 offspring rather than monosomic embryos. However, male carriers of Robertsonian translocations are subfertile due to low sperm counts, and the overall chance of such a male producing trisomy 21 offspring is very low. In addition, some carriers demonstrate an increased risk for aneuploidy of the sex chromosomes in the spermatozoa produced, suggesting an interchromosomal effect [19].

Infertile men are found to have significantly increased levels of chromosome abnormalities in their sperm, despite the fact that the majority of them have a normal constitutional karyotype [8]. Increased aneuploidy frequencies have been reported for all chromosomes; however, chromosomes 21, 22, X, and Y are more prone to nondisjunction [2, 8]. High aneuploidy levels have been associated with abnormal semen profiles including azo-, oligo-,

astheno-, and teratozoospermia [20]. To date, chromosomal causes have been identified only in about 20% of infertile men. However, it is clear that disturbances in male meiosis, particularly in chromosome pairing, synapses, and meiotic recombination, are associated with male infertility, and a number of genes involved in this process remain to be discovered.

Chromosomal causes of female infertility

Female infertility is often attributed to an impairment of ovarian function that can result from several different genetic mechanisms – numerical X chromosome abnormalities, including Turner and triple X karyotype; balanced structural chromosomal rearrangements; genomic imbalances involving the X chromosome and autosomes; XY gonadal dysgenesis and single gene alterations leading to ovarian dysgenesis; premature ovarian failure; and reproductive dysfunction. X chromosome-linked aberrations play a major role among currently known genetic defects. Here, we review chromosomal and genomic alterations that result in ovarian insufficiency and present in syndromic and non-syndromic forms.

Sex chromosome abnormalities

Turner syndrome

Turner syndrome is a common genetic disorder that results from loss of a sex chromosome (45,X or monosomy X) in a phenotypic female (Fig. 7.1F). Turner syndrome occurs in approximately 1/2000–3000 female live births as a result of chromosome nondisjunction during meiosis [5]. Monosomy X is a common abnormality among spontaneous abortions and only 1–3% of fetuses survive to term. Clinical manifestations are variable in affected females and include short stature, skeletal abnormalities, congenital heart and kidney anomalies, characteristic physical features such as a wide and webbed neck, a low hairline at the back of the neck, flat chest, lymphedema in infancy, and gonadal dysgenesis with primary amenorrhea [21]. Most women with Turner syndrome have normal intelligence, although cognitive deficits, developmental delays, non-verbal learning disabilities, and behavioral problems are possible.

Approximately half of females diagnosed with Turner syndrome have 45,X chromosome complement, whereas the other half have mosaicism for the 45,X cell line or 46 chromosomes with one normal X and a structurally abnormal X or Y chromosome [21]. Other X chromosome abnormalities associated with Turner syndrome include deletion of the short arm (46,X,del(Xp)), isochromosome Xq (46,X,i(Xq)), ring X chromosome (46,X,r(X)), derivative X chromosome (46,X,der(X)), and small marker chromosome, which usually contains an X chromosome centromere and pericentromeric DNA sequences (Fig. 7.1F). Mosaicism for multiple abnormal cell lines can also be found. The chromosome constitution and level of mosaicism influence the resulting phenotype in Turner syndrome patients. Deletions in the distal short arm of chromosome X involving the *SHOX* gene are associated with short stature and skeletal anomalies, whereas variable deletions in the proximal Xp and deletions in the long arm of X chromosome have been observed in patients with gonadal dysgenesis and premature ovarian insufficiency (POI) [21]. An abnormal X chromosome is preferentially inactivated, unless rearrangement involves the X inactivation center (*XIST* gene) [5, 21]. Lack of the X inactivation center on the aberrant X chromosome causes a much more severe phenotype. In 80% of females with the 45,X karyotype, the X chromosome is maternal in origin and the paternal sex chromosome has been lost. In 20% of 45,X cases, the paternally derived X is present; however, there is no difference in the phenotype based on the X chromosome parent of origin [5, 21].

Patients with Turner syndrome do not undergo puberty, have infantile internal and external genitalia, and fail to develop secondary sexual characteristics unless they receive hormone therapy. Early diagnosis is important to initiate appropriate therapy with growth hormone and estrogen. Girls with short stature should be karyotyped to rule out Turner syndrome. In

Turner girls, primordial germ cells form but are lost rapidly, and hypoplastic "streak" gonads, composed of fibrous tissue, are detected at the time of puberty [21]. In females, one X chromosome in every cell is inactivated; however, gene expression from both X chromosomes in oocytes is necessary for normal ovarian development [5]. Haploinsufficiency for the X-linked genes is likely responsible for gonadal dysgenesis and infertility in 45,X individuals.

A combination of a 45,X (Turner syndrome) cell line and a normal 46,XX chromosome complement is the most common form of mosaicism in Turner syndrome individuals. Many patients with mosaicism for monosomy X are mildly affected, undergo breast development, menstruate, and may present in clinic only due to infertility or POI as a major concern [21]. 45,X/47,XXX mosaicism occurs less frequently, but clinical manifestations are similar to those in 45,X/46,XX. The ovaries of teenage girls who have Turner syndrome with X chromosome mosaicism contain follicles that secrete estrogen but their ovarian function rapidly declines [21, 22].

47,XXX karyotype

Trisomy X, triple X, or 47,XXX karyotype (Fig. 7.1G) is a fairly common chromosome aneuploidy condition caused by a nondisjunction event of the X chromosome, either during gametogenesis or after conception [5, 23]. Trisomy X affects approximately 1 in 1000 girls. It is estimated that only 10% of cases are diagnosed, as a majority of these women are normal. Some women with 47,XXX can be taller than average, may present with learning disabilities, delayed development of motor skills, and speech and language problems. Most females with trisomy X syndrome have normal pubertal onset and sexual development, and are fertile [23]. However, some individuals are not able to conceive due to POI or genitourinary malformations. Trisomy X syndrome is found in approximately 3% of females with POI [23].

A majority of trisomy X is maternal in origin, derived from meiosis I (~60%) or meiosis II (~17%) errors, and results in non-mosaic 47,XXX karyotypes [5]. Mosaicism occurs in about 20% of cases due to X chromosome nondisjunction during the early development of an embryo. Overall phenotype and fertility is affected by the presence of abnormal cells such as 45,X (Turner) or 48,XXXX (tetrasomy X). Polysomy X (48,XXXX or 49,XXXXX) is associated with more severe developmental retardation and multiple congenital defects [23]. The risk of trisomy X, similar to other chromosome trisomies, significantly increases with advanced maternal age. Fertile females with trisomy X produce normal haploid gametes, with no particularly increased risk for a 47,XXX or 47,XXY child [5, 23].

X-chromosome structural rearrangements

Structural abnormalities of the X chromosome, including deletions, duplications, inversions, complex rearrangements, and balanced and unbalanced X-autosome translocations, are frequently correlated with a normal or mild phenotype in females, but are associated with infertility, repeated miscarriages, and chromosomal imbalances in offspring [21, 22]. In females, X inactivation is established early during the embryo development at the late blastocyst stage, and is maintained in all somatic cells and transmitted to the daughter cells during mitosis. Therefore, one X chromosome is randomly inactivated in each cell [5]. Thus, each female has two cell populations; one with the paternal and another with the maternal functional X chromosome. When one of the X chromosomes is abnormal, the X inactivation pattern is usually skewed towards the unbalanced clone as a result of cell selection. Derivative X chromosomes resulting from unbalanced X autosomal translocation, isochromosome, and the X chromosome carrying deletions or duplications, are typically inactive.

In contrast to somatic cells, the inactive X chromosome is reactivated in female germ cells so that mature oocytes have two active X chromosomes; therefore, X chromosome rearrangements are more likely to affect oogenesis [5, 22]. Based on analysis of partial X chromosome monosomies in women with a Turner syndrome phenotype or isolated ovarian failure, four regions critical for ovarian function have been delineated. Deletions and translocations detected within Xp11–p13.1 (POF4), Xq13.3–q22 (POF2), Xq22–q25, and Xq27–q28 (POF1), are associated with POI. Deletions involving the Xq13 region are associated with primary amenorrhea, lack of breast development, and ovarian failure in the majority of patients [21, 22]. Women with an Xq21–q24 deletion have a less severe phenotype than individuals with Xq13 deletions. Premature ovarian insufficiency is more commonly associated with Xq25–q28 deletions [21, 22].

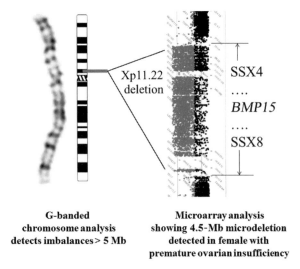

G-banded chromosome analysis detects imbalances > 5 Mb

Microarray analysis showing 4.5-Mb microdeletion detected in female with premature ovarian insufficiency

Figure 7.7 Array comparative genomic hybridization can detect submicroscopic Xp deletion. Partial high resolution G-banded karyotype and ideogram of the X chromosome shows a normal X chromosome in a woman with premature ovarian insufficiency. Array comparative genomic hybridization detected a 4.5-Mb deletion in the Xp11.22 region encompassing the *BMP15* gene. See plate section for color version.

To date, the number and precise location of genes relevant to X-linked POI are still under investigation. Despite a wealth of evidence implicating X chromosome in ovarian reserves, alterations in only few X-linked genes such as *BMP15*, *DIAPH2*, and the premutation *FMR1* alleles have been associated with POI [21, 22]. The *BMP15* gene (bone morphogenetic protein 15, OMIM #300247), is a member of the transforming growth factor-β superfamily, and maps to the Xp11.2 region. Submicroscopic deletions (Fig. 7.7) and mutations of the *BMP15* gene are observed in women with premature ovarian failure or primary amenorrhea [24]. Disruption of the *DIAPH2* gene (POF2A, Xq21.33, OMIM #300108) has been identified in mother and daughter with POI and a balanced translocation t(X;12). These data demonstrate that haploinsufficiency of ovary-specific genes is one of the molecular mechanisms responsible for X-linked POI [21, 22, 24]. Premutation FMR1 alleles account for 2–3% of sporadic POI cases and 10–15% of familial POI cases [22]. Other X-linked genes such as *USP9X*, *ZFX*, *XPNPEP2*, *XIST*, and *SPANX* have been proposed as candidate genes for POI, but their role remains to be elucidated [24, 25]. The application of the high resolution aCGH analyses of the X chromosome, as well as the whole exome/genome-sequencing technologies, is likely to uncover new X-linked genes involved in POI [26].

In order to identify novel candidate genes, mapping of the breakpoints has been performed for a significant number of patients with POI and balanced X-autosome translocations [21, 22]. However, in some patients, X chromosome breakpoints were identified within the genomic regions free of transcribed sequences (so-called gene deserts), suggesting an alternative molecular mechanism for POI, such as positional effects of the X chromosome on autosomal genes. Gene expression can be greatly influenced by regulatory elements that can be located far from the actual gene. It is also possible that integrity of the X chromosome influences expression of key autosomal genes required for proper oogenesis.

Autosomal structural rearrangements

About 1 in 500 people in the general population is a balanced chromosome rearrangement carrier. Phenotypically normal carriers of balanced chromosomal rearrangements (translocations and inversions; see Chapter 1), have an increased risk of infertility and cytogenetically abnormal offspring [21, 27]. Beside sex chromosome abnormalities, rearrangements involving autosomes are common in infertile patients. Several mechanisms may account for gonadal insufficiency and infertility in carriers of autosomal structural rearrangements: (1) rearrangement may disrupt expression of an ovary-specific gene at the breakpoint by reducing dosage or causing abnormal expression; (2) rearrangement may cause "position effect" by disrupting regulatory elements that influence expression of genes near the breakpoint; (3) rearrangement may cause high predisposition to form chromosomally unbalanced gametes with low survival rate. *FOXL2* (OMIM #605597), *NOBOX* (OMIM #610934), *FIGLA* (OMIM #612310), and *NR5A1* (OMIM #612964) genes are representative subset of autosomal genes required for normal ovarian development, differentiation and oogenesis [21, 24, 25]. Disruption of any of these genes by structural rearrangements, may adversely affect ovarian function. Disruption of an ovary-specific gene by a translocation breakpoint is a rare cause of infertility, and can be associated with syndromic or non-syndromic POI. Women who carry a balanced chromosomal abnormality have a much higher risk for infertility due to early pregnancy loss or miscarriage of an unrecognized pregnancy [27].

The reproduction outcomes greatly depend on the chromosome involved, breakpoint location, gene content, and the complexity of the rearrangement in each individual case. However, on average, about half of the pregnancies in a person carrying a balanced chromosome rearrangement will be lost in miscarriage [14, 16, 18, 27]. Both male and female carriers of constitutional structural chromosomal rearrangements are likely to produce genetically unbalanced gametes, resulting in partial monosomy or trisomy in the embryo [14–18, 27]. In males, numerous studies have been performed to determine meiotic segregation patterns in spermatozoa [14–18], whereas the cytogenetic analysis of female gametes and embryos remains extremely difficult to study in humans. In cases of balanced chromosome rearrangements, most imbalances at birth result from a rearrangement carried by the mother [27]. In male gametogenesis unbalanced segregation of structurally abnormal chromosomes results in oligo/azoospermia, male infertility, and much reduced likelihood of transmission to the offspring [14–18]. Female gametogenesis on the other hand, has a less stringent meiotic quality control, and oocyte maturation is less affected by autosomal genomic imbalances. Successful pregnancy in these families can be achieved with IVF and PGD to transfer embryos with normal or balanced chromosome complements (see Chapter 11 for detailed information).

46,XY female (Swyer syndrome)

In mammals, the gonads in both sexes have the potential to develop into either ovaries or testes. Normal male sexual differentiation in 46,XY individuals depends on a proper function and complex interaction of numerous testis-determining genes, including *SRY*, *SOX9*, *NR5A1/SF1*, *NR0B1*, *AR*, *DHH*, and *CBX2* [12]. Failure in the normal male sex differentiation process can cause complete or partial 46,XY gonadal dysgenesis. Partial 46,XY gonadal dysgenesis is characterized by impaired testicular development and ambiguous external genitalia, whereas individuals with complete 46,XY gonadal dysgenesis, or Swyer syndrome, have normal female external genitalia and internal organs, but also have bilateral streak gonads [12, 21, 28]. Swyer syndrome has been estimated to occur in approximately 1/30 000 individuals. Affected females are typically tall, lack secondary sexual characteristics, may have mild clitoromegaly, and are infertile. This condition commonly remains undiagnosed until adolescence, when puberty fails to occur. Females with a 46,XY karyotype (Fig. 7.3A) have the increased risk of developing gonadoblastoma or dysgerminoma; therefore, streak gonads are usually removed shortly after diagnosis. Women with Swyer syndrome cannot produce eggs, but successful pregnancies have been achieved in some patients using donated eggs or embryos [21, 28].

Complete 46,XY gonadal dysgenesis is a heterogeneous disorder that results from chromosomal abnormalities (deletions, duplications, structural rearrangements) or point mutations of genes implicated in sexual differentiation [12, 21, 28]. Despite considerable advances in understanding the genetic factors involved in gonadal determination and differentiation, a molecular diagnosis is made in only about 20% of cases with complete 46,XY gonadal dysgenesis. Mutations and deletions of the *SRY* gene are the cause of complete 46,XY gonadal dysgenesis in approximately 10–15% of patients with Swyer syndrome [28]. The *SRY* gene is located on the short arm of the Y chromosome, within a 35-kb sequence proximal to the pseudoautosomal region boundary (Fig. 7.2). Structural Y chromosome rearrangements resulting in the loss of the *SRY* gene include Yp deletion, dicentric Y isochromosomes composed of the long arm (idic(Yq)), ring Y chromosomes (r(Y)), small marker Y chromosomes, and Y autosome translocations [21, 28]. Structurally abnormal Y chromosomes can be detected by conventional G-band chromosome analysis in some cases; however, molecular cytogenetic studies such as FISH and aCGH analyses are essential for accurate diagnosis. Y chromosome rearrangements are frequently accompanied with mosaicism for multiple Y chromosome-containing abnormal cell lines or 45,X chromosome complement [21].

X chromosomal rearrangements in 46,XY females have led to the identification of a dosage-sensitive sex locus at the Xp21 region containing the *NR0B1* (*DAX1*) gene. Patients with cytogenetically visible Xp21 duplications, containing multiple genes in addition to *NR0B1*, have a complex phenotype with congenital anomalies, dysmorphic features, intellectual disability, and gonadal dysgenesis (Table 7.2). Isolated 46,XY gonadal dysgenesis has been reported in two siblings carrying an Xp21.2 duplication of 637 kb in size that encompasses *DAX1* as well as four *MAGEB* genes. A submicroscopic 257-kb deletion upstream of *DAX1* has been described in a

Table 7.2 Genomic imbalances associated with complete gonadal dysgenesis in 46,XY females

Locus	Genomic abnormality	Gene	Molecular mechanism	OMIM #
1p36.12	Duplication	*WNT4*	Gain of function	603490
5q11.2	Deletion	*MAP3K1*	Loss of function	613762
8p23.1	Deletion downstream	*GATA4*	Regulatory region	600576
9p24.3	Deletion	*DMRT1, DMRT2*	Loss of function	154230
9q33.3	Deletion	*NR5A1/SF1*	Loss of function	612965
12q13.1	Homozygous deletion	*DHH*	Loss of function	233420
Xp21	Duplication deletion upstream	*NR0B1/ DAX1*	Gain-of-function regulatory region	300018
Yp11.31	Deletion	*SRY*	Loss of function	400044

46,XY female with primary amenorrhea and gonadal dysgenesis. This deletion likely affects regulatory sequences leading to altered *DAX1* expression and 46,XY gonadal dysgenesis.

Many autosomal genes are implicated in disorders of sexual development in humans. Cytogenetically visible chromosome abnormalities including deletions of 9p22, 9q33, 10q25, 11p13, 13q32–q34, and 17q24; duplication of 1p34; and balanced translocations involving 17q24 have been identified in patients with XY gonadal dysgenesis (Table 7.2). These rearrangements comprise multiple genes and usually are associated with multiple congenital anomalies and intellectual disabilities (syndromic XY gonadal dysgenesis) [12, 21, 26]. Isolated or non-syndromic forms of XY gonadal dysgenesis are most probably due to a singl gene defect and are unlikely to be detected by classical karyotype. Detection of small deletions and duplications, encompassing a single gene, are beyond the resolution of classical G-band chromosome and FISH analyses, and require application of a high resolution genome analysis technique such as aCGH [26]. Table 7.2 summarizes several genes that are known to cause non-syndromic XY gonadal dysgenesis, including those with microdeletions or microduplications affecting the gene or its regulatory regions. Using high resolution whole genome and sex chromosome aCGH analyses, the cause of 46,XY gonadal dysgenesis can be elucidated in up to 30% of affected individuals, while the remaining patients will benefit from next generation sequencing (NGS) or exome sequencing tests.

Submicroscopic DNA copy number alterations

Cytogenetically visible numerical and structural chromosomal rearrangements are already known to cause a substantial number of human diseases. These abnormalities are commonly identified by conventional karyotype analysis (see Chapter 1), a low resolution technique that has limited ability to detect genomic imbalances less than 4–10 Mb in size (Fig. 7.7). With the development of microarray technology, aCGH- and SNP-array platforms can be used to detect genomic deletions and duplications (losses and gains) as small as 1 kb (1000 base pairs) in size [26]. Submicroscopic chromosomal imbalances or DNA copy number variations (CNVs) are present in the genome of each individual and can be classified as benign, pathogenic, or variants of unknown clinical significance. It is now established that CNVs cause genetic syndromes, isolated congenital defects, disease susceptibility, miscarriages, or reproductive failure [24–26]. In addition, CNVs can also result in the unmasking of a recessive mutation, functional polymorphism, epigenetic, or environmental interactions. Many CNVs are benign and exist in healthy individuals. Databases of genomic variants (see [29]) can help distinguish normal variation from pathogenic; however, reproductive history of individuals in these databases is rarely known.

Application of microarray technology in basic research and clinical diagnosis of male and female infertility has led to the identification of multiple autosomal loci implicated in POI, male infertility, abnormal fetal development, and placental dysfunction [24–26]. Remarkably, such genomic imbalances contain many genes involved in meiosis, DNA repair, and ovarian folliculogenesis [24–26].

The advent of high-resolution genome analyses such as aCGH and high-throughput sequencing will enable identification of many genes implicated in human sex determination, differentiation, and reproduction. These new powerful tools will revolutionize clinical diagnosis and personalized reproductive management in the future.

Practical clinical approach

Identification of genetic causes underlying male and female infertility is an essential part of the clinical evaluation, genetic counseling, and successful treatment of the infertile couple. Accurate genetic diagnosis presents the couple with an opportunity to guide treatment options, to achieve natural conception with their own gametes, and provides important information regarding the health and reproductive potential of an affected individual. Moreover, genetic counseling of the couple is essential to provide information about the risk of transmitting a genetic abnormality to the offspring. Genetic evaluation is indicated for couples that fail to achieve pregnancy after 12 months of regular unprotected intercourse, as well as for patients with a clinical diagnosis or medical history of a chromosomal or genetic disorder. Careful family history is necessary to determine if there is a clear familial pattern of infertility, miscarriages, skewed gender ratios (e.g. complete androgen insensitivity syndrome), rapid aging, and/or syndromic causes associated with infertility (Fanconi anemia, Bloom syndrome, ataxia telangiectasia). However, negative family history does not rule out any genetic contribution as *de novo* genetic events likely account for a substantial number of sporadic cases. Examples include most chromosomal abnormalities such as KS. Karyotype analysis of peripheral blood samples should be performed as an initial component of evaluation for male or female infertility to identify sex chromosome aneuploidy and gross structural chromosome rearrangements (Fig. 7.8). Despite gonadal failure in most affected patients with Klinefelter or Turner syndrome, 5–20% of individuals with sex chromosome aneuploidy may have a limited number of mature germ cells, enabling the live birth of biological children. The number of available germ cells significantly decreases with age. Cryopreservation of ovarian follicles or retrieved testicular spermatozoa as an infertility treatment option may be feasible for some patients with Turner or Klinefelter syndrome, respectively [5, 7, 22]. Spontaneous pregnancy in Turner syndrome is reported to be possible in about 2% of patients with mosaic monosomy X chromosome constitution [22]. Pregnancy and delivery, either spontaneous or more commonly from donor oocytes, are associated with a 2% risk of death in non-mosaic Turner syndrome due to the dissection and rupture of the aorta [22]. Pregnancy is a relative contraindication in women with Turner syndrome who have a

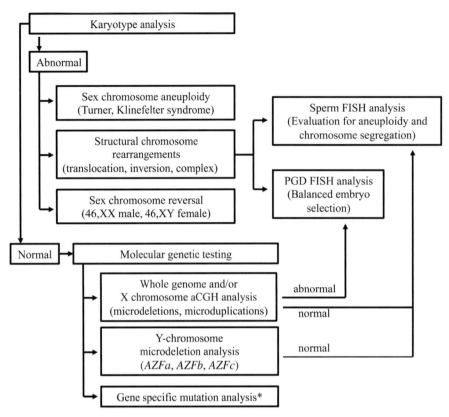

Figure 7.8 Genetic evaluation in patients with infertility.
* See Chapter 8 for implicated genes.

negative preconception cardiac evaluation but an absolute contraindication in those with documented cardiac anomaly.

Structural chromosome abnormalities detected by karyotype analysis confer an increased risk for spermatogenic failure, miscarriages, stillbirth, and live born children with congenital defects and chromosomal aberrations. In some patients balanced chromosome abnormalities are present but they are below the resolution of detection by conventional cytogenetic analysis. Microarray analysis should be considered on DNA from spontaneous abortions and stillbirth, if available. Fluorescence *in situ* hybridization analysis on sperm cells from a male carrier of structural chromosome rearrangement will help determine chromosome segregation patterns, the likelihood of abnormal chromosome complement in the embryo, as well as find best approach to PGD (Fig. 7.8). For couples undergoing IVF, PGD should be performed to discover suitable embryos with normal or balanced chromosome complement for transfer.

In the case of a normal karyotype, expanded genetic testing should include microarray analysis to detect submicroscopic chromosome abnormalities, Y chromosome microdeletions, and, depending on gathered clinical information, a possible individual gene mutation analysis (Fig. 7.8). It is critical that men with non-obstructive azoospermia undergo molecular and cytogenetics analyses for Y chromosome rearrangements and microdeletions in order to receive accurate diagnosis and proper genetic counseling prior to assisted reproduction. The Y chromosome microdeletions are not associated with health problems; however, male offspring will inherit the AZF microdeletion from infertile fathers in pregnancies achieved by assisted reproduction.

High-resolution whole genome and the X chromosome microarray analyses are recommended as a part of genetic evaluation of infertility in patients with normal karyotype (Fig. 7.8). Gonadal failure and recurrent pregnancy losses of male fetuses have been associated with submicroscopic X chromosome deletions and duplications [5, 24–26]. *FMR1* testing for the CGG repeat in the 5′ untranslated region of the gene is essential to rule out premutation carrier status, and is now recommended for all women with cessation of menses and elevated gonadotropin levels prior to age 40. Women found to have the *FMR1* premutation are at risk for POI and for fragile X associated tremor and ataxia syndrome, while their offspring is at risk for the mental retardation syndrome. It is important to note that negative genetic testing does not exclude genetic pathology, as there are other, presently unknown, genes that are implicated in normal gametogenesis. To date, mutations have been found in approximately 300 genes, of which 70 syndromes are known to be associated with reproductive disorders, and this list will continue to grow. Massive parallel sequencing is now a logical extension of molecular karyotyping to define genetic pathology at the nucleotide level.

Genetic counseling should be ideally provided before a genetic test is offered, so that the couple understands the pros and cons of genetic testing. Post-test genetic counseling is necessary for the couple to understand the significance of each possible outcome: normal results, pathological test findings, and findings of unknown clinical significance. It is essential that fertility specialists be engaged with clinical genetic experts, including those in the genomic laboratories, in order to provide the most optimal and appropriate testing to their patients.

References

1. Schultz N, Hamra FK, Garbers DL. A multitude of genes expressed solely in meiotic or postmeiotic spermatogenic cells offers a myriad of contraceptive targets. *Proc Natl Acad Sci USA* 2003; 100: 12 201–6.

2. Harton GL, Tempest HG. Chromosomal disorders and male infertility. *Asian J Androl* 2012; 14: 32–9.

3. McLachlan RI, O'Bryan MK. Clinical review: state of the art for genetic testing of infertile men. *J Clin Endocrinol Metab* 2010; 95: 1013–24.

4. O'Flynn O'Brien KL, Varghese AC, Agarwal A. The genetic causes of male factor infertility: a review. *Fertil Steril* 2010; 93: 1–12.

5. Heard E, Turner J. Function of the sex chromosomes in mammalian fertility. *Cold Spring Harb Perspect Biol* 2011; 3: a002675.

6. Walsh TJ, Pera RR, Turek PJ. The genetics of male infertility. *Semin Reprod Med* 2009; 27: 124–36.

7. Wikström AM, Dunkel L. Testicular function in Klinefelter syndrome. *Horm Res* 2008; 69: 317–26.

8. Martin RH. Cytogenetic determinants of male fertility. *Hum Reprod Update* 2008; 14: 379–90.

9. Hennebicq S, Pelletier R, Bergues U *et al*. Risk of trisomy 21 in offspring of patients with Klinefelter's syndrome. *Lancet* 2001; 357: 2104–5.

10. Kuroda-Kawaguchi T, Skaletsky H, Brown LG *et al*. The *AZFc* region of the Y chromosome features massive palindromes and uniform recurrent deletions in infertile men. *Nat Genet* 2001; 29: 279–86.

11. Sadeghi-Nejad H, Oates RD. The Y chromosome and male infertility. *Curr Opin Urol* 2008; 18: 628–32.

12. Kousta E, Papathanasiou A, Skordis N. Sex determination and disorders of sex development according to the revised nomenclature and classification in 46,XX individuals. *Hormones (Athens)* 2010; 9: 218–31.

13. Vetro A, Ciccone R, Giorda R *et al*. XX males SRY negative: a confirmed cause of infertility. *J Med Genet* 2011; 48: 710–12.

14. Hann MC, Lau PE, Tempest HG. Meiotic recombination and male infertility: from basic science to clinical reality? *Asian J Androl* 2011; 13: 212–18.

15. Marchetti F, Wyrobek AJ. Mechanisms and consequences of paternally-transmitted chromosomal abnormalities. *Birth Defects Res C Embryo Today* 2005; 75: 112–29.

16. Madan K. Balanced complex chromosome rearrangements: reproductive aspects. A review. *Am J Med Genet A* 2012; 158A: 947–63.

17. Roux C, Tripogney C, Morel F *et al*. Segregation of chromosomes in sperm of Robertsonian translocation carriers. *Cytogenet Genome Res* 2005; 111: 291–6.

18. Engels H, Eggermann T, Caliebe A *et al*. Genetic counseling in Robertsonian translocations der(13;14): frequencies of reproductive outcomes and infertility in 101 pedigrees. *Am J Med Genet A* 2008; 146A: 2611–16.

19. Machev N, Gosset P, Warter S *et al*. Fluorescence *in situ* hybridization sperm analysis of six translocation carriers provides evidences of an interchromosomal effect. *Fert Steril* 2005; 84: 365–73.

20. Viville S, Mollard R, Bach M-L *et al*. Do morphological anomalies reflect chromosomal aneuploidies? *Hum Reprod* 2000; 15: 2563–6.

21. Simpson JL, Rajkovic A. Ovarian differentiation and gonadal failure. *Am J Med Genet* 1999; 89:186–200.

22. Toniolo D, Rizzolio F. X chromosome and ovarian failure. *Semin Reprod Med* 2007; 25: 264–71.

111

23. Tartaglia NR, Howell S, Sutherland A *et al.* A review of trisomy X (47,XXX). *Orphanet J Rare Dis* 2010; 5: 8.

24. McGuire MM, Bowden W, Engel NJ *et al.* Genomic analysis using high-resolution single-nucleotide polymorphism arrays reveals novel microdeletions associated with premature ovarian failure. *Fertil Steril* 2011; 95: 1595–600.

25. Aboura A, Dupas C, Tachdjian G *et al.* Array comparative genomic hybridization profiling analysis reveals deoxyribonucleic acid copy number variations associated with premature ovarian failure. *J Clin Endocrinol Metab* 2009; 94: 4540–6.

26. Rajcan-Separovic E. Chromosome microarrays in human reproduction. *Hum Reprod Update* 2012; 18: 555–67.

27. Desjardins MK, Stephenson MD. "Information-rich" reproductive outcomes in carriers of a structural chromosome rearrangement ascertained on the basis of recurrent pregnancy loss. *Fertil Steril* 2012; 97: 894–903.

28. Jorgensen PB, Kjartansdóttir KR, Fedder J. Care of women with XY karyotype: a clinical practice guideline. *Fertil Steril* 2010; 94: 105–13.

29. Database of Genomic Variants: dgv.tcag.ca/dgv/app/home

Genes and infertility

Inge Liebaers, Elias El Inati, Willy Lissens, and Stéphane Viville

Introduction

The prevalence of infertility, i.e. the inability to conceive within 12 months despite regular unprotected intercourse, is estimated to be 9%. This represents more than 70 million infertile women worldwide, of whom more than 40 million are seeking infertility treatment [1, 2]. To indicate that infertility may be a reversible condition, the term subfertility is preferred by many experts in the field of reproductive medicine. Infertility can be primary, when there is no pregnancy in the reproductive history, or secondary, when a previous pregnancy has occurred. Infertility leads to reproductive failure as do recurrent miscarriages, but the causes and pathogenic mechanisms of both conditions are different. If not acquired or functional, infertility is mainly the result of abnormal gametogenesis, aberrant embryogenesis, and implantation failure, while recurrent miscarriages result from fetal wastage.

The causes of male and female infertility are heterogeneous; they may be acquired, caused by infectious or toxic agents, functional, such as erectile dysfunction or ejaculatory failure, or genetic. Genetic causes may be numerical chromosomal anomalies often of the sex chromosomes, or structural anomalies such as reciprocal or Robertsonian translocations (discussed in Chapter 7).

The present chapter is dedicated to monogenic causes of female and male infertility, of which little is known so far. In the first section, monogenic mutations causing infertility in the female or in the male as discovered over the last decade will be described and discussed. Some of these mutated genes may very specifically cause absent or abnormal gametogenesis without any other problem and are called non-syndromic forms of infertility. Others cause diseases or syndromes that include infertility as a major or minor feature. A practical approach to the infertile couple in the clinic will be proposed. In the final section, the way to perform studies allowing the identification of more genes involved in female and male infertility will be described and illustrated with some examples.

Genes involved in female infertility

Monogenetic defects leading to female infertility are characterized by amenorrhea and may be due to abnormal sex development, a disturbed hypothalamic–pituitary–gonadal axis leading to hypogonadotrophic hypogonadism, or primary ovarian insufficiency leading to hypergonadotrophic hypogonadism. The condition can occur before puberty and result in primary amenorrhea or later in life resulting in secondary amenorrhea. Amenorrhea is a consequence of the absence of production and maturation of oocytes, or of a severe decrease, or even a stop, in production.

Abnormal sexual development

In an embryo a sequence of events has to take place at the right time to develop from the chromosomal sex (XX or XY), to the gonadal sex (ovaries or testes), and finally to the phenotypical sex (female or male) with the correct primary and secondary sexual characteristics. Chromosomal as well as monogenic defects causing disorders of sexual development or differentiation (DSD) are known, and many of these rather rare conditions will be diagnosed at birth or shortly thereafter because of sexual ambiguity. Others will be diagnosed at puberty, and some patients will only be diagnosed because they are amenorrheic, infertile, or both. In this section only conditions

Textbook of Human Reproductive Genetics, eds Karen Sermon and Stéphane Viville. Published by Cambridge University Press.
© Cambridge University Press 2014.

leading to patients with a female phenotype that may be encountered at the fertility clinic will be described. Recently a revised preferred nomenclature has been proposed [3].

Monogenic disorders of sexual development in an XX or XY fetus leading to a female phenotype may be grouped into gonadal developmental anomalies, called gonadal dysgenesis, and conditions which are the result of impaired androgen production or action.

The term "gonadal dysgenesis" not only denotes a phenotypic female with a male karyotype as described in this section, but conversely also a phenotypic male with a female karyotype described later in this chapter.

46,XY complete gonadal dysgenesis (previously XY sex reversal)

XY gonadal dysgenesis is characterized by amenorrhea in otherwise phenotypically normal female patients. These patients have either no ovaries, streak ovaries, or non-functional testes. Besides the Turner patients who have a 45,X or related karyotype, as well as some other features, females with gonadal dysgenesis may have a 46,XY or a 46,XX karyotype. In the case of XY gonadal dysgenesis, 10% or even more of the patients have a *SRY* gene deletion or inactivating mutation. In the past these patients were known as patients with Swyer syndrome or male pseudohermaphroditism [4]. These patients have delayed sexual maturation, amenorrhea, normal pubic hair, as well as female internal (notably a normal uterus) and external characteristics. Hormone replacement therapy as well as gonadectomy, due to the risk of cancer in the dysgenic gonad, are indicated. These patients can become pregnant using donated oocytes and *in vitro* fertilization (IVF).

In the other patients with pure XY gonadal dysgenesis, autosomal gene defects involved in SRY action or in the testis-determining pathway have been reported, but in most of the cases the cause – most probably genetic – has still to be uncovered. In cases of XX gonadal dysgenesis in female patients, autosomal monogenic causes are also involved and mentioned below as causes of primary ovarian insufficiency. In cases of true hermaphroditism, a very rare condition, ovotestes are present in the patient who can have a female phenotype and an XX karyotype. So far one patient with a homozygous mutation in the *RSOP1* gene has been reported [5].

Androgen deficiency or impaired androgen action and androgen excess

Androgen insensitivity is an X-linked recessive syndrome affecting 46,XY individuals who present phenotypically as females. Mutations in the androgen receptor gene cause insensitivity to dihydrotestosterone, which normally triggers the development of the male external genitalia. Individuals with complete androgen insensitivity (CAIS) are infertile and present with amenorrhea at adolescence. They have no ovaries but have testes, which may be palpable in the labia majora or mimic inguinal hernia, and they have no uterus. The testes should be removed when sexual development is completed and hormonal replacement therapy started. At disclosure of the diagnosis, psychological support is strongly advised for the parents, if informed, and later for the proband. Genetic counseling to the family is important especially to at-risk carrier females with the XX karyotype since they have a one in four risk of having an affected child. Prenatal or preimplantation genetic diagnosis (PGD) can be offered. Some patients with partial androgen insensitivity (PAIS) may still present as females; genitalia are usually ambiguous or even predominantly male; these patients are also infertile. Genotype and phenotype are correlated to a certain extent especially in CAIS [6]. Mild androgen insensitivity (MAIS) will lead to a male phenotype, presenting with undervirilization, gynecomastia, and impaired spermatogenesis [7]. Expanded trinucleotide mutations in the same gene may lead to impaired sperm quality among other symptoms leading to Kennedy's disease (as discussed below).

Inactivating luteinizing hormone receptor (LHR) mutations in XY individuals cause Leydig cell hypoplasia, and may result in a female phenotype from birth because of lack of androgen synthesis. Secondary sexual characteristics remain infantile and the patients are amenorrheic. They also have no female internal sexual organs. Other genes, such as *StAR*, *CYP11A1*, *CYP17A1*, and *17HSD3*, encoding enzymes active in testosterone synthesis, may if mutated result in a female phenotype in an XY individual [8].

Congenital adrenal hyperplasia (CAH) due to mutations in the *CYP21A2* gene responsible for 21-hydroxylase activity is an autosomal recessive disorder affecting both sexes with a different phenotypic expression in girls compared to boys. Two forms of the condition exist: the classical form showing simple virilization sometimes associated with salt losing due to excess of steroid hormone production, and the non-classical, late-onset form. Salt-losing symptoms appear early in life in both boys and girls and have to be treated urgently with glucocorticoids. Virilizing symptoms are seen only in girls, who are often born with ambiguous genitalia; however, the extent of virilization can vary from clitoromegaly only to a nearly male appearance. Around 12 mutations account for most of the classical forms with total or partial enzyme deficiency. About 1 in 60 in the Caucasian population is a healthy carrier. Other mutations or combinations of mutations are responsible for the non-classical form. Regardless of the form of the disease or the treatment with glucocorticoids, affected female children, adolescents, and adults may present with premature pubarche often combined with a growth spurt and advanced skeletal maturation and hirsutism, acne, alopecia, amenorrhea or oligomenorrhea, and decreased fertility due to anovulation or dysovulation. The symptoms of women with CAH may resemble polycystic ovary syndrome (PCOS) patients. Clinical diagnosis or suspicion of CAH should be confirmed by measuring the concentration of 17-OH-progesterone as such or after stimulation with adrenocorticotropic hormone (ACTH) as a first test. Genetic testing of the patient, the family, and the partner of the patient should be performed in order to be able to deliver adequate reproductive counseling, including recurrence risks. Affected women who do not want to become pregnant may benefit from oral contraceptives and anti-androgens. Infertile female CAH patients who want to reproduce should receive adequate treatment: they may need ovulatory stimulating agents, while concomitant use of glucocorticoids may reduce the risk of miscarriage. If the partner is a carrier of a CAH-causing mutation, this will result in a 50% risk of the couple having an affected child (of which half will be affected females). For these couples, the following options are available. In the case of pregnancy, high doses of dexamethasone may be administered in early gestation until the sex of the child is known by chorionic villus sampling (CVS) or non-invasive prenatal diagnosis. Only if it is a girl, treatment should be continued. This treatment is however not without risks for the mother, and little is known about possible adverse effects on the child. Therefore, another option for such couples is to opt for PGD.

Other, less frequent enzyme deficiencies in the adrenal–cortisol synthesis pathway (11-β-hydroxylase deficiency – *CYP11B1*; 3-β-hydroxysteroid dehydrogenase – *HSD3B2*) may lead to androgen excess and, as a consequence, to a clinical picture similar to the one caused by 21-hydroxylase deficiency in XX individuals. Here, too, the patients may present with symptoms similar to PCOS [9].

An overview of genetic sexual disorders is given in Table 8.1 [2–19].

Hypothalamic–pituitary–gonadal deficiencies

Isolated gonadotropin-releasing hormone (GnRH) deficiency (IGD), also called isolated hypogonadotropic hypogonadism (IHH), is the result of impaired gonadotropin release leading to low concentrations of luteinizing hormone (LH) and follicle-stimulating hormone (FSH). This causes hypogonadism in both females and males with an otherwise normally functioning pituitary gland. This condition may be caused by dominant as well as recessive mutations, but is usually non-genetic, meaning that secondary causes like brain pathology, medication, and systemic diseases, such as hemochromatosis or chronic systemic illness, should first be excluded. When associated with anosmia, and sometimes other developmental anomalies such as synkinesia of the digits, unilateral renal agenesis, hearing loss, cleft lip and palate, the condition is known as Kallmann syndrome (KS). In women, GnRH deficiency will lead to low gonadotropin levels causing incomplete sexual maturation with little or no breast development as well as anovulation and amennorhea. Diagnosis is most often established at puberty. The *KAL1* gene on the X chromosome was the first gene to be discovered as being linked to the X-linked recessive form of this syndrome. Although this form, called KS1, mainly affects males, carrier females are at risk for affected sons. Mutations in *FGFR1* (KS2), *PROKR2* (KS3), *PROK2* (KS4), *CHD7* (KS5), and *FGF8* (KS6) were shown to be responsible for autosomal dominant forms of KS. Both *PROKR2* and *PROK2* have also been found in autosomal recessive forms of the syndrome and digenic inheritance has also been reported. Mutated autosomal recessive genes leading to IHH and not reported in KS are *GNRHR*, *KISS1R*, *TACR3*, *TAC3*, and *GNRH1*. Family history may help to determine the mode of inheritance but cases are often sporadic. Although not all gene defects are known, genetic testing may help to properly counsel patient and

Table 8.1 Overview of sexual disorders

Disease	Transmission	OMIM #	Locus/gene	Major symptoms	Karyotype	Ref(s)
46,XY complete gonadal dygenesis (sex reversal; Swyer syndrome)	Y-linked	400044	*SRY*	Female phenotype gonadal dysgenesis	46,XY	[2–4]
46,XX complete gonadal dygenesis (sex reversal; Swyer syndrome)	Y-linked	400045	*SRY*	Male phenotype, sterile	46,XX	[10]
True hermaphroditism	AR	610644	*RSPO1*	Female phenotype, ovotestis, hyperkeratosis	46,XX	[3–5]
Androgen insensitivity	X-linked	300068	*AR*	Female phenotype, testis, no uterus	46,XY	[4–7]
Leydig cell hypoplasia	AR	288320	*LHR*	Female phenotype, no uterus	46,XY	[6–8]
Congenital adrenal hypoplasia	AR	201910	*CYP21A2*	Non-classical, late-onset form virilization	46,XX	[7–9]
Testicular regression	AR?	273250		Male phenotype, uni- or bilateral cryptorchidy, absent gonads	46, XY	[10]
5α-reductase deficiency	AR	264600	*SRD5A2*	Masculinization	46,XY	[8, 9, 11–17]
LHB and LHR defects	AR	238320	*LHR, LHB*	Undervirilization	46,XY	[9, 11–18]
Persistant Müllerian duct syndrome	AR	261550	*AMHR2*	Male phenotype, inguinal hernia	46,XY	[11–19]
Androgen insensitivity (PAIS) and (MAIS)	X-linked	300068	Androgen receptor	Undervirilization, gynecomastia, OAT	46,XY	[5–7]
Isolated GnRH deficiency and Kallmann syndrome	AD/AR	147950	*FGFR1* and other genes	Hypogonadotropic hypogonadism with/without anosmia	46,XY	[11–13]

AD, autosomal dominant; AR, autosomal recessive; GnRH, gonadotropin-releasing hormone; LHB, luteinizing hormone beta; LHR, luteinizing hormone receptor; MAIS, mild androgen insensitivity; OAT, oligoastenoteratospermia; PAIS, partial androgen insensitivity.

family by informing them about recurrence risks and the possibility of prenatal or preimplantation genetic diagnosis, especially if IVF is needed [11].

Altogether, no gene defects have been found so far in at least 50% of IGD patients, even if family history shows several affected family members. Adequate hormonal treatment will trigger sexual maturation and may reverse infertility.

Primary ovarian insufficiency

Primary ovarian insufficiency, previously called premature ovarian failure, is characterized by amenorrhea for at least four months along with increased FSH concentrations and low estrogen levels in women under 40 years of age. Recently, anti-Müllerian hormone (AMH) concentration determination is considered to be useful in measuring the ovarian reserve [12–14].

Syndromic primary ovarian insufficiency

This term is used when the ovarian insufficiency is part of a known monogenic condition presenting with multiple symptoms.

Female fragile X syndrome carriers with a CGG expansion in the premutation range between 55 and 200 repeats in the *FMR1* gene may present with premature ovarian insufficiency, which is also referred to as premature menopause. At a young age, infertility may be the only problem in some of these women. The fragile X syndrome is, however, a common X-linked form of mental retardation and is present in all males with a full mutation, i.e. a large CGG expansion of 200 repeats or more, and in half of the women that carry a full mutation. It is now clear that male premutation carriers who do not present with mental retardation may present with neurological problems at a later age such as ataxia. The same is true for premutation female carriers although less frequently. Female premutation carriers may learn about their genetic status either because of infertility or because of their family history. In the latter case, it is important to timely counsel them about the possible premature ovarian insufficiency so that they can make the adequate reproductive choices. In any case, genetic counseling is mandatory but not easy. Of course, if still fertile, prenatal diagnosis possibly followed by termination of pregnancy is an option. However, difficult choices may have to be made if the result is a female fetus with a full mutation or a female or male fetus with a premutation, while counseling is simpler if the result is a male fetus with a clear-cut full mutation. At least, theoretically, PGD may be the more suitable option, even if the patient is fertile, because only XX or XY embryos without a pre- or full mutation can be chosen for transfer. However, premutation carriers may have to turn to oocyte donation if they do not respond to ovarian stimulation. The prevalence of female premutation carriers seems to be high but the percentage of these individuals with ovarian insufficiency is unclear. Conversely, 4–6% of patients with primary ovarian insufficiency carry the *FMR1* premutation [15].

Blepharophimosis, ptosis, and epicanthus inversus syndrome (BPES type 1) is an autosomal dominant condition caused by mutations in the *FOXL2* gene. Women with such mutations present with ovarian insufficiency; however, because of their typical face with very small palpebral fissures this rare condition should be recognized. A family history can be taken and genetic testing performed. Menarche is usually normal but is followed by oligomenorrhea and, finally, amenorrhea. The patient should be informed about possible surgical interventions, the possibility to preserve oocytes or ovarian tissue as long as possible, the need for hormone replacement therapy as soon as necessary, and the possibility to still become pregnant with donor oocytes. Male patients are not infertile but can have daughters who will present with ovarian insufficiency later in life. They should know about the possibility of PGD if they want children free of the condition [11, 12].

Galactosemia is a rare inherited autosomal recessive metabolic disease that is life-threatening because of liver failure if not immediately treated with a lactose/galactose-restricted diet. Even then these patients often have a developmental delay and decreased intellectual functioning. Moreover, in adult females primary or secondary ovarian insufficiency may occur and they may seek help to become pregnant. Enzyme testing and molecular analysis of the *GALT* gene allow confirmation of the clinical diagnosis and/or the neonatal screening result. Moreover, the degree of enzyme deficiency and the type of mutations have been reported to predict to a certain extent the probability of developing ovarian insufficiency. Genetic counseling to both the patient and their family should be offered [12, 13].

More monogenic syndromes with ovarian insufficiency as one of many symptoms exist, but usually affected patients will not reproduce because of the severity of the condition [13].

Non-syndromic primary ovarian insufficiency

Here the ovarian insufficiency is due to ovarian dysgenesis or insufficiency with primary or secondary amenorrhea as the major symptom.

BMP15 mutations on chromosome Xp resulting in abnormal folliculogenesis have been found in several women with ovarian insufficiency. Inactivating *LH*, *LHR* and *FSH* and *FSHR* mutations as well as *PSMC3IP* mutations, *CYP17*, and *CYP19* mutations are known to cause ovarian insufficiency, but most of these patients have been described as case reports. More single case reports of causal gene mutations or putative genes that may play a role in ovarian function have been reported and should be further explored [15]. A mutation in the *NR5A1* gene has been linked to ovarian insufficiency as well as to azoospermia, as discussed below [12].

An overview of genes involved in female infertility is given in Table 8.2 [15–17].

Genes involved in male infertility

Male infertility due to genetic defects may, as in females, be due to abnormalities in the sexual development, deficiencies of the hypothalamic–pituitary–gonadal axis, or impaired spermatogenesis as well as other anomalies leading to obstructive or non-obstructive azoospermia or oligoasthenoteratospermia [16]. Here, too, infertility due to sperm anomalies may be the only or the major symptom, while in other conditions they are part of a broader condition; nevertheless, categorizing the conditions into syndromic or non-syndromic is not always obvious.

Table 8.2 Genes involved in female infertility

	Disease	Transmission	OMIM #	Locus/gene	Major symptoms	Karyotype	Ref(s)
Syndromic	Fragile X syndrome	X-linked	31136	*FMR1*	Ovarian insufficiency with premature menopause	46,XX	[4–17]
	Blepharophimosis, ptosis, epicathus inversus	AD	110100 608996	*FOXL2*	Small palpebral fissures, gonadal insufficiency	46,XX	[10]
	Galactosemia	AR	230400	*GALT*	Developmental delay, ovarian insufficiency	46,XX	[10]
Non-syndromic	Premature ovarian failure, ovarian dysgenesis	X-linked	300510	*BMP15*	Primary ovarian insufficiency	46,XX	[10]
	Primary ovarian insufficiency	X-linked	300624	*LH, LHR, FSH, FSHR, PSMC3IP, NR5A1*	Primary ovarian insufficiency	46,XX	[10]

AD, autosomal dominant; AR, autosomal recessive.

Abnormal sexual development

Monogenic disorders of sexual development in an XY or XX fetus leading to a male phenotype may be grouped into gonadal developmental anomalies, called gonadal dysgenesis, and conditions which are the result of impaired androgen production or action.

46,XX testicular disorder of sexual development (previously XX male or XX sex reversal)

This type of gonadal dysgenesis is characterized by azoospermia in phenotypically normal males. They are categorized as *SRY* positive or *SRY* negative.

The presence of the *SRY* gene in XX males can cause sex reversal and is due to an aberrant recombination event during paternal spermatogenesis. The *SRY* gene normally present on the short arm of the Y chromosome is translocated to the short arm of the X chromosome in the spermatozoon. After fertilization this generates an XX embryo containing an *SRY* gene. The presence of the *SRY* gene in an embryo is sufficient to drive further development towards a male phenotype but with abnormal spermatogenesis due to the absence of other genes on the Y chromosome. This condition is clinically comparable to Klinefelter patients but its incidence is much lower (1/20 000). Moreover, in Klinefelter patients with a 47,XXY karyotype, spermatogenesis is severely impaired while in XX males spermatogenesis is absent and therefore these individuals are infertile. Other known and yet unknown genes

with a function in sexual development exist since in 10% of XX males the *SRY* gene is absent. These patients can only become a father with sperm from a donor. The so-called true hermaphrodites with XY or XY/XX karyotypes and ovotestis may also present as infertile males with testicular regression syndrome. These patients are phenotypic males with unilateral or bilateral cryptorchidy, and are therefore without testicular tissue and thus azoospermic.

Androgen deficiency or impaired androgen action

Androgen deficiency due to enzyme deficiencies in the biosynthesis pathway are usually recognized in childhood or at puberty because of ambiguous genitalia; however, undervirilized males may also be diagnosed with one of these deficiencies. Steroid 5α-reductase deficiency, an autosomal recessive condition in an XY individual, is peculiar in that at birth the genitalia are usually ambiguous but at puberty these individuals virilize. At puberty, female patients may also present with amenorrhea [17].

Autosomal recessive LH and LHR mutations may be found in XY individuals presenting as males with undervirilization [18]. Autosomal recessive mutations in AMH or its receptor AMHR2 will lead to individuals with normal male primary and secondary sexual characteristics but with an inguinal hernia containing differentiated Müllerian duct structures. It is therefore called persistent Müllerian duct syndrome (PMDS) [19].

More yet unknown genetic defects causing DSD in XY individuals, characterized by hypospadias, cryptorchidism, and/or bifid scrotum at birth, must exist, and these individuals are at high risk of developing testicular insufficiency later in life [20].

Some patients with PAIS may still present as females; genitalia are usually ambiguous or even predominantly male. These patients are also infertile. Genotype and phenotype are correlated to a certain extent, especially in CAIS [6]. MAIS will lead to a male phenotype, who will present with undervirilization, gynecomastia, and impaired spermatogenesis [7]. Expanded trinucleotide mutations in the same gene may lead to impaired sperm quality among other symptoms leading to Kennedy's disease, which is discussed below.

Hypothalamic–pituitary–gonadal axis

Men with IGD are characterized by the absence of secondary sexual characteristics, a diminished libido, infertility due to azoospermia, and by erectile dysfunction. These symptoms are also present in primary hypogonadism characterized by an impaired gonadal function but with elevated LH and FSH concentrations. As in females, the condition is much rarer than secondary acquired hypogonadotropic hypogonadism (HH). Acquired causes have to be excluded first, but if anosmia or hyposmia and possibly other associated anomalies are reported the diagnosis is most probably KS. Typically for the male, KS1 caused by mutations in the X-linked *KAL1* gene. Besides, the same genes as in females, as well as mutations in the X-linked *DAX1* gene, may be responsible for KS or IGD in the male. However, in half of IGD patients no gene defects have been found so far. In the clinic, IGD may be considered as a minor problem by the physician and by the patient because adequate hormone treatment is available. Only if major associated symptoms are present, like in CHARGE syndrome, does management become more problematic [11].

Kallmann syndrome may be the cause of reversible non-obstructive azoospermia. Affected patients present in childhood or as adolescents, because of delayed puberty sometimes with cryptorchidism and micropenis, or later in life when they want to reproduce. Hormonal treatment will result in sperm production and reverse infertility. Autosomal dominant and recessive KS also occurs in both sexes as described previously.

Azoospermia or oligoasthenoteratospermia

Syndromic azoospermia or oligoasthenoteratospermia

Gene defects causing obstructive or non-obstructive azoospermia or oligospermia, or asthenospermia or teratospermia are most of the time syndromic.

Congenital bilateral absence of the vas deferens (CBAVD) leads to obstructive azoospermia in otherwise healthy males [21]. In this situation, spermatogenesis is normal but the spermatozoa do not reach the ejaculate. In about 80–90% of these males, CBAVD is caused by mutations in the *CFTR* gene, the gene defective in the autosomal recessive disease cystic fibrosis (CF). In males with CF, CBAVD is present in up to 99% of patients. Therefore, CBAVD in males without other clinical signs of CF but with mutations in the *CFTR* gene is considered a genital form of CF. The other 10–20% of patients with isolated CBAVD suffer from urogenital and renal abnormalities, and in these patients CBAVD is not caused by mutations in the *CFTR* gene.

In CF-related CBAVD patients, the frequency of *CFTR* mutations is high [21]. In general, two mutations, either one severe and one mild, or two mild mutations, or one severe mutation and the so-called 5T variant, and adjacent TG repeat are found upon genetic testing. One of both mutations is mostly typical for isolated CBAVD, and is not found in CF. However, two mutations cannot always be identified, possibly because of lack of standardized scanning strategies for mutation analysis. However, if these patients want to reproduce, it is very important to screen their partner for *CFTR* mutations at least in European countries and in the USA where the carrier frequency of CF is high (around 1/20–1/30). If the partner is indeed a carrier, the couple should be informed about the recurrence risk for CBAVD or even more so for CF which can be 25 or even 50%. The couple may then opt for PGD as they will need IVF and intracytoplasmic sperm injection (ICSI) to conceive. Selection of embryos carrying the normal *CFTR* allele of the female might be indicated.

Primary ciliary dyskinesia, also called immotile cilia syndrome, is an autosomal recessive condition causing infertility in about half of the male patients due to asthenozoospermia; other symptoms often already present in neonates or children are chronic respiratory tract disease, rhinitis, and sinusitis. Partial or total situs inversus (a mirror-image reversal of visceral organs such as heart and liver) is present in half of the patients and is often referred to as Kartagener syndrome. So far 12 causal genes with different mutations, duplications, or deletions are known with *DNAH5* and *DNAI1* being the most frequently involved followed by *DNAI2*, *DNAAF2*, *DNAAF1*, *CCDC39*, *CCDC40*, *DNAH11*, *RSPH4A*, *RSPH9*, *NME8*, and *DNAL1* covering the molecular defects in less than 50% of the patients so far known. The azoospermia is the result of the same ultrastructural defects at the base of the flagellae as in the respiratory epithelium. These defects in the epithelium from the nose or bronchus can be analyzed if the expertise is available and allow confirmation of a clinical diagnosis, and the type of abnormality may point to specific gene defects. Genetic counseling to both patient and their family should be offered, especially if a gene defect has been identified. Confronted with male patients who want to reproduce, the risk of having a healthy carrier partner is related to the disease incidence in a particular population. Taking a prevalence of 1 in 16 000 in Norway and Japan, the carrier frequency of this autosomal recessive condition is 1 in 63. This means that without any further testing the risk of an affected child to a couple with an affected male is $1 \times 1/63 \times 1/2 = 1/126$. With further genetic testing, still limited today but certainly possible in the rather near future, more accurate risks can be given and in case of treatment with IVF and ICSI, PGD can be offered.

Dystrophia myotonica type 1 (DM1), also known as Steinert's disease, is an autosomal dominant condition with variable expression. Its cause is a CTG trinucleotide repeat expansion in the *DMPK* gene. The size of the expansion is correlated with the severity of the disease, typically characterized by myotonia or muscular cramps, and a sad facial expression often only recognized by experts. Often, it is only after the birth of a child with the very severe congenital form due to a large expansion of the CTG repeat that the diagnosis is established in the mother who is the carrier of a much smaller repeat. Further testing of the family will reveal many more asymptomatic and mildly symptomatic members who should then be counseled. Male patients may present with infertility due to oligoasthenoteratospermia and they may need IVF and ICSI to achieve pregnancy. Preimplantation genetic diagnosis can then be offered, which would avoid transmission of the condition, especially because of the risk of increased severity of the disease in subsequent generations resulting from further expansion of the triplet repeat [22].

Kennedy's disease or spinal and bulbar muscular atrophy (SBMA) is a late-onset X-linked recessive disorder characterized by slow progressive muscular weakness and testicular atrophy leading to oligospermia or azoospermia. Its cause is an expanded CAG trinucleotide repeat sequence in the androgen receptor gene. Point mutations in the same gene cause androgen insensitivity syndrome, as discussed earlier. A clinical diagnosis of Kennedy's disease based on a personal and familial history and a physical/neurological examination will be confirmed by increased creatine kinase (CK) levels as well as elevated concentrations of LH, FSH, testosterone, and progesterone. The analysis of the androgen receptor gene will show the CAG expansion. Usually enough sperm can be obtained to propose IVF with ICSI to couples in which the partner is affected. Taking into consideration that the female partner is not a carrier, children of this couple will not be affected; however, girls will always be carriers, who in turn have a risk of 25% of having an affected child. Prenatal or preimplantation genetic diagnosis may be offered to them.

Noonan syndrome is an autosomal dominant disease with variable expressivity characterized by a short stature and a typical mild facial dysmorphism more pronounced in childhood than later in life. It is characterized also by other congenital anomalies such as a cardiopathy in a high percentage of cases, cryptorchidism, and delayed puberty resulting in progressively deteriorating sperm quality. Developmental delay and intellectual disability may be present in up to 30% of patients. In up to 70–80% of the cases, the syndrome, not always recognized by non-experts, is caused by mutations in the *PTPN11* gene (50%) or in one of the other genes known today such as *SOS1* (13%), *RAF1* (3–17%), *KRAS* (<5%), *NRAS* (<1%), *BRAF* (<1%), and *MAP2K1* (<1%). Mainly because of the high incidence of severe cardiac problems, diagnosis in these patients is primordial and counseling concerning the 50% recurrence risk before considering any fertility treatment such as IVF with ICSI, including PGD, should be offered [23].

Aarskog–Scott syndrome is a very rare X-linked recessive disease characterized by short stature, facial abnormalities, and skeletal and genital anomalies. It is known also as faciodigitogenital syndrome with typical anomalies such as facial dysmorphism becoming less pronounced with age, digital particularities described as the swan neck deformity of the fingers resulting from hyperextension of the proximal interphalangeal joints and flexion of the distal interphalangeal joints. The physical phenotype is characterized also by a shawl scrotum obvious in 80% of children as well as mild intellectual deficiency in about 30% of the patients. These patients may be seen in the clinic because of cryptorchidism, delayed puberty, and infertility due to acrosomal sperm defects as a result of mutations in the *FGD1* gene responsible for this syndrome. Again genetic counseling should be available to the patient and his family taking into account that affected males will never have affected children but daughters will all be carriers.

Beckwith–Wiedemann syndrome is the most frequent overgrowth syndrome with a cancer predisposition and is reported in at least 1 of every 13 000 live births. It is an autosomal dominant disease with extremely variable expressivity including more or less obvious dysmorphic features of the face and the ears, such as macroglossia, ear creases, and pits. It is characterized also by omphalocele or umbilical hernia, hemi-hyperplasia, visceromegaly, renal anomalies, and cryptorchidism possibly causing infertility. It is an imprinting disorder related to abnormal methylation of the imprinted genes *CDKN1C*, *NSD1*, *H19*, and *KCNQ1* at the 11p15.5 locus which can also be deleted or duplicated. Because of its extreme variability, infertile male patients may first present at the clinic. Genetic work-up prior to treatment is necessary. The syndrome is known in reproductive medicine because it is reported among children born after IVF, with or without ICSI, due to a methylation defect (see Chapters 5 and 12).

Other monogenic diseases primarily show developmental anomalies such as mental retardation as well as azoospermia or oligospermia. Affected patients will not be seen at the fertility clinic because their other symptoms will preclude them from reproduction.

Reduced sperm motility has been documented in mitochondrial diseases of which several also cause severe encephalopathies. Patients with a proven mitochondrial disease may be referred to a fertility clinic by other specialists who established the diagnosis. In this case IVF treatment is safe if the genetic defect is located in the mitochondrial DNA, since DNA present in the mitochondria of the sperm will not be transmitted to the embryo. Of course if the genetic defect is of nuclear origin, classical Mendelian inheritance has to be taken into account. Despite the observation that male patients with these mitochondrial diseases may have impaired sperm function, searching for mitochondrial DNA mutations in men with disturbed sperm motility has not yielded any clear-cut results [24].

Non-syndromic azoospermia or oligoasthenoteratospermia

These are gene defects resulting in obstructive or non-obstructive azoospermia or oligoasthenoteratozoospermia as the only symptom.

Genes in the *AZFa*, *b*, and *c* region on the long arm of the Y chromosome, more specifically the Yq11 locus, have been shown to play a role in spermatogenesis. It has been known for some time that males with deletions in this region are either azoospermic or severely oligospermic [25]. Mutations in the *AZFc* region are most commonly found (69%), and this condition causes a heterogeneous phenotype ranging from azoospermia to severe oligozoospermia. In about 70% of these patients sperm cells for ICSI are found in either the ejaculate or the testis, and these patients can have their own genetically related children. Appropriate genetic counseling should be given to these couples because the transmission of the defective Y chromosome will probably be associated with impaired spermatogenesis in their sons. As far as we know, daughters will have no problems, and the couple might opt for PGD to avoid the transmission of the Y chromosome by selecting female embryos [26]. *AZFb* (14%) and *AZFa* (6%) deletions are less common; the remaining 11% of patients have combined deletions, *AZFa* + *b*, *AZFb* + *c*, or *AZFa* + *b* + *c*. Most patients with an *AZFa* deletion have Sertoli cell-only syndrome; *AZFb* patients present with maturation arrest of spermatogenesis. In both of these patient groups no sperm cells can be found in the testis, and consequently a testicular biopsy in view of ICSI is unnecessary. This is also true for combined deletions. Molecular detection of these microdeletions should be offered to males with fertility problems resulting from non-obstructive azoospermia with severely impaired spermatogenesis.

Partial deletions of the *AZFc* region, so-called gr/gr deletions, show an increased frequency in males with fertility problems, but are also found in men with normal sperm parameters. Therefore these deletions should be considered as a risk factor for male infertility and not as a causative factor. These deletions are not screened for routinely in infertile males, and their prognostic value needs to be better defined in the future.

Recently, genes with mutations responsible for two types of teratozoospermia, namely globozoospermia and macrocephaly, as well as for asthenozoospermia, have been identified.

Globozoospermia is a rare and severe autosomal recessive type of teratozoospermia characterized by round-headed spermatozoa lacking an acrosome. Patients suffering from globozoospermia are infertile because of the incapacity of their spermatozoa to breach through the zona pellucida. This means that ICSI may help them. Mutations in three genes, *SPATA16*, *PICK1*, and *DPY19L2*, have been identified so far as responsible for globozoospermia [27–29]. Out of these three genes, *DPY19L2* is the most frequently found mutated since almost 70% of globozoospermic patients are found mutated for *DPY19L2*. As the most common mutation is the deletion of the whole gene, globozoospermia can be considered as a new genomic disorder [29]. Because of the lack of acrosome and consecutively the lack of the phospholipase C-zeta (PLCζ) oocyte activation factor, ICSI attempts give poor results except when artificial oocyte activation is applied to the injected oocytes [30].

Macrocephalia or large-headed spermatozoa is another autosomal recessive type of teratozoospermia resulting in infertility or rather sterility. Recently the gene *AURKC* on chromosome 19 was identified in 10 infertile men with macrocephalia, and *AURKC* is highly expressed in testes [31]. Little is known about *AURKC*'s function. In mice, *AURKC* is involved in chromosome segregation and cytokenesis during spermatogenesis, which fits well with the human phenotype. Indeed, it was shown that all the spermatozoa of these patients are tetraploid, strongly suggesting the implication of *AURKC* in the segregation of chromosomes and/or meiotic cytokinesis, explaining the large size of the gametes. This study also established a frequency of heterozygotes of over 1/50, implying an expected prevalence of 1 in 10 000 men. Such a high frequency is surprising since it makes *AURKC*-related infertility among the most frequent genetic causes of infertility in this population. This information is important for consanguineous couples or if sperm donation is used and preconceptional screening should be offered. Interestingly, the authors identified two fertile homozygous females, excluding a fundamental role of *AURKC* in female meiosis and confirming the differences between male and female meiotic mechanisms. Recently, the same group described other mutations in *AURKC* [32].

Mutations in *CATSPER1* and *SLC26A8* genes have also been identified: both proteins are required for the membrane flux of anion and cation and the hyperactivation of the sperm [33].

An overview is given in Table 8.3 [10–13, 18–21, 22–24, 27–33].

A practical clinical approach to the infertile couple

Today's knowledge about the genetic causes of infertility should be integrated in reproductive care when confronted with an infertile couple. A careful personal history, recording problems at birth, in childhood or puberty, as well as a familial history (i.e. mental retardation, CF) has to be taken in combination with a thorough physical examination, especially of the external genitals, of both partners in order to guide further testing. Medical reports from colleagues who possibly took care of the patients as a child or adolescent should be collected. Immediate basic tests are needed in almost all cases to be able to establish a diagnosis or a differential diagnosis. In women, the required tests are FSH, AMH, estrogen levels, and a karyotype. In men, the tests needed are FSH, LH, testosterone levels, a karyotype, and a semen analysis. If at the first consultation a specific diagnosis is suspected additional tests can be added, such as *FMR1* testing in a female with premature ovarian insufficiency and mental retardation in the family or *CFTR* testing in a male patient presenting with CBAVD. Yq11 deletions should be tested for if non-obstructive azoospermia or oligoastenoteratospermia has been observed in the male. More sophisticated diagnostic genetic tests may be performed when a female is diagnosed with hypergonadotrophic hypogonadism or hypogonadotrophic hypogonadism. The same holds true for the male if globozoospermia or macrocephalic sperm is observed. If a genetic cause is established or suspected, expert advice for further evaluation and testing should be provided. For all of the above-mentioned genetic causes of infertility, genetic testing is readily available with a variable but reasonable turnaround time. As already mentioned, it is important to inform the couple and their families about these diseases or syndromes with their recurrence risks and the available options to fulfill their child wish and to prevent recurrence. For instance, in case of male infertility due to abnormal spermatozoa, today ICSI is often a possibility for these men to have a genetically

Table 8.3 Genes involved in male infertility

	Disease	Transmission	OMIM #	Locus/gene	Major symptoms	Karyotype	Ref(s)
Syndromic	Kallmann syndrome	X-linked	308700	KAL1	Asthenozoospermia	46,XY	[11–13]
	Cystic fibrosis	AR	219700	CFTR	Obstructive azoospermia, CBAVD	46,XY	[18–21]
	Primary ciliary dyskinesia	AR	608644	DNAH5	Asthenozoospermia	46,XY	[10]
	Kartagener syndrome		244400	DNAI1			
	Myotonic dystrophy	AD	160900	DMPK1	OAT progressive	46,XY	[19–22]
	Kennedy syndrome	X-linked	313200	Androgen receptor	Oligo- to azoospermia progressive	46,XY	[10]
	Noonan syndrome	AD	163950	PTPN11	Cryptorchidy, OAT progressive	46,XY	[20–23]
	Aarskog–Scott syndrome	X-linked	305400	FGD1	Acrosomal defect	46,XY	[10]
	Beckwith–Wiedemann	Imprinting disorder	130650	Several	Cryptorchidy	46,XY	[10]
	Mitochondrial disease	mtDNA, nDNA	Many	Several	OAT?	46,XY	[21–24]
Non-syndromic	Globozoospermia	AR	102530 613958	SPATA16, PICK1, DPY19L2	Acrosomal defects	46,XY	[23;24; 27–29]
	Macrocephalic sperm	AR	243060	AURKC	Polyploidy, multiflagellar sperm	46,XY	[28–32]
	Astenospermia	AR	606389	CATSPER	Immotile sperm	46,XY	[30–33]

AD, autosomal dominant; AR, autosomal recessive; CBAVD, congenital absence of vas deferens; mtDNA, mitochondrial DNA; nDNA, nuclear DNA; OAT, oligoastenoteratospermia.

related child. However, available knowledge should be taken into account before embarking on ICSI. As an example, in the case of a Yq11 deletion, especially in the *AZFc* region, spermatozoa may be available but the defect will be transmitted and will result in infertile male children. Preimplantation diagnosis with sex selection against XY embryos may therefore be proposed. However, ICSI will not solve the problem of patients with large-headed spermatozoa, due to a mutation in *AURKC* because all their gametes are tetraploid. For them donor sperm could be a solution. In contrast, it is reasonable to propose ICSI treatment for globozoospermic patients, since round-headed spermatozoa do not present a higher rate of chromosomal abnormalities [30]. For many couples with an established genetic cause of their infertility, PGD has helped them to conceive an unaffected child [34]. Unfortunately, for many couples, no specific diagnosis of their infertility problem can be established. Nevertheless, the worldwide efforts devoted to the field of genetics of infertility are expected to provide new genetic tests in the near future allowing for more accurate diagnoses and treatment.

How to find new genes involved in infertility

To unravel the pathophysiology of diseases, proper clinical and basic research is needed. Genetic studies aiming at identifying genes causing diseases or playing a role in disease development have already taught us a great deal about normal and aberrant molecular mechanisms resulting in functional or structural abnormalities. More such studies are needed, not the least in the field of infertility which today is still very poorly understood. Moreover, not all pathologies have a genetic origin, but understanding the ones which have opens avenues to understand most of the non-genetic causes. This is obviously true for infertility, affecting the female or the male, through gonad formation, hormonal production, or gametogenesis.

Patient selection

As for any other study in search of new genes or gene defects, material from affected patients is needed in the first place, next to samples from well-selected control individuals. It is needless to say that a correct clinical diagnosis is of utmost importance because any incorrect diagnosis will introduce a bias in the patient recruitment and render the genetic analysis void. This means that a close collaboration between the clinicians and the scientists is necessary. Before embarking on a research project, together they should decide about careful selection and work-up of the patients to be recruited. Usually, at least, the classical tests to establish a diagnosis will be performed, and possibly additional tests according to the scientific hypothesis can be added. For instance, in the case of non-obstructive azoospermia it is important if not mandatory to have information on testes histology. This is necessary to define the defect in terms of sperm number (absence or decreased number; azoospermia or oligozoospermia), the motility of the sperm cells present (normal or inadequate; asthenozoospermia) and the morphology (normal or not; teratozoospermia), or of a combination of these. This analysis will also provide information on the developmental stage of the sperm cells, and thus on the stage at which development is arrested in immature sperm cells.

Furthermore, geneticists need informative patients, who are those that will allow identification of a genetic causative mutation. Informative patients will differ according to the expected mode of transmission of the condition studied, being X- or Y-linked, autosomal dominant, or autosomal recessive. For instance, so far, in the case of non-syndromic spermatogenic failure the mode of transmission, with the exception of the microdeletion of the Yq11 locus, has been autosomal recessive in most cases. In this context, recruited patients will preferentially be part of: (1) families with some degree of consanguinity; or (2) a large group of patients from a restricted area or living in a limited sociocultural enclave where the abnormality seems to have a quite high occurrence, which should correspond to a founder effect.

Approaches to identify genes involved in human infertility

Classically, geneticists use two main approaches to identify genetic causes of pathologies, but technologies are rapidly evolving and new approaches are more often used. All of these can also be applied to the genetics of infertility. The two classic strategies are reverse and forward genetics. The reverse approach, also known as the candidate gene approach, is initiated by selecting genes from infertile animals,

mainly mice models, assuming that the gene function is conserved through evolution. Forward genetics, also known as positional cloning or descent studies, benefit from technical improvement facilitating the identification of recessive autosomal mutations. The main approach, homozygosity mapping, is based on genotyping studies and aims to investigate, for a single patient, thousands of single nucleotide polymorphisms (SNPs) simultaneously on a microarray. The success of homozygosity mapping studies strictly depends on the availability of patients and their rigorous selection.

Recently, a new method has promised to speed up discovery of the genetic causes of disease by allowing the parallel sequencing of millions of sequences at high throughput (see Chapter 2): next generation sequencing (NGS). A popular variant of NGS combined with enrichment technologies is used to sequence the exome (the set of all coding exons representing 3% of the human genome) in order to discover variations in exons which represent most of the disease-related mutations [35]. In other words, this technique allows the identification of protein-coding mutations, including missense, nonsense, splice site, and small deletion or insertion mutations. Exome sequencing has become a powerful and efficient strategy for identifying the genes responsible for Mendelian disorders and complex diseases [36] and may be applicable in the case of infertility.

The combination of homozygosity mapping with genome sequencing may lead to rapid identification of the causative mutation for a disease [37]. The technical locks of whole genome genotyping and sequencing have now been broken and we believe that the key to successfully identifying causative mutations by descent studies depends on the adequate recruitment of patients. Some caution is necessary here, as the bioinformatics employed in NGS are of a high level of complexity and the data obtained often contain so much noise that reliable identification of causative mutations is not possible. Several success stories can be found in the literature, but failures exist as well but remain hidden. The failure for instance to identify causative genes in PCOS and endometriosis, so frequently encountered, can be explained by the fact that human gametogenesis is a complex process and infertility may be the result of multigenic and multifactorial causes.

Several examples of successful identification of mutations causing male infertility can be found in El Inati *et al.* [38]. The same technology and approaches have been used to find new genes causing primary ovarian insufficiency [15].

Conclusions

In this chapter known gene defects causing infertility have been discussed. Besides monogenic defects leading to non-syndromic or syndromic infertility, numerical or structural chromosomal anomalies are also known to cause infertility. Moreover, acquired causes of infertility are also known or are under investigation. However, in the clinic today for many couples the final diagnosis remains idiopathic infertility. This means that more research is necessary to identify the unknown, most probably genetic, causes. Therefore, further studies are of tremendous importance in different ways: they represent a unique way to study human gametogenesis and to decipher the underlying mechanisms, which in turn will have clinical and fundamental repercussions. First, patients will benefit by having a molecular diagnosis followed by appropriate counseling and care. Secondly, the findings will contribute to a better understanding of the physiopathological process of human reproduction. Thirdly, in the longer term, a better understanding of the genes involved in spermatogenesis will help to identify the extrinsic factors that compromise spermatogenesis and prevent the deterioration of fecundity. Indeed, a general decline in fertility or rather sperm quality has been observed, which is obviously not due to genetic causes but is rather caused, at least in part, by increased concentrations of environmental endocrine disruptors, such as environmental estrogen-like molecules. We believe that a better understanding of spermatogenesis, starting with an in-depth knowledge of all the genes involved, will eventually be instrumental in identifying and understanding the effects of these toxic chemicals and in finding solutions to stop their adverse effects. Taken together, this should also improve the practice of artificial reproductive technologies, not only for infertile couples due to a genetic defect, but for all couples.

In other words, the development of new analytical technologies like whole genome sequencing will certainly speed up the discovery of more genes that may cause infertility. Well-described patients will remain central in this research. New technology combined with the ever-growing knowledge concerning genome structure and gene regulation will explain impaired gametogenesis, embryogenesis, and implantation as well as miscarriages and help to find solutions to infertile couples who want children.

References

1. Zegers-Hochschild F, Adamson GD, de Mouzon J et al. The International Committee for Monitoring Assisted Reproductive Technology (ICMART) and the World Health Organization (WHO) Revised Glossary on ART Terminology, 2009. Hum Reprod 2009; 24: 2683–7.

2. Boivin J, Bunting L, Collins JA, Nygren KG. International estimates of infertility prevalence and treatment-seeking: potential need and demand for infertility medical care. Hum Reprod 2007; 22: 1506–12.

3. Lee PA, Houk CP, Ahmed SF, Hughes IA. Consensus statement on management of intersex disorders. International Consensus Conference on Intersex. Pediatrics 2006; 118: e488–500.

4. Rocha VB, Guerra-Junior G, Marques-de-Faria AP, de Mello MP, Maciel-Guerra AT. Complete gonadal dysgenesis in clinical practice: the 46,XY karyotype accounts for more than one third of cases. Fertil Steril 2007; 96: 1431–4.

5. Tomaselli S, Megiorni F, De Bernardo C et al. Syndromic true hermaphroditism due to an R-spondin1 (RSPO1) homozygous mutation. Hum Mutat 2008; 29: 220–6.

6. Gottlieb B, Beitel KL, Trifiro MA. Androgen insensitivity syndrome. In GeneReviews [Internet]. NCBI bookshelf: www.ncbi.nlm.nih.gov/books/ NBK1429/

7. Hellmann P, Christiansen P, Johannsen TH et al. Male patients with partial androgen insensitivity syndrome: a longitudinal follow-up of growth, reproductive hormones and the development of gynaecomastia. Arch Dis Child 2012; 97: 403–9.

8. Mendonca BB, Costa EM, Belgorosky A et al. 46,XY DSD due to impaired androgen production. Best Pract Res Clin Endocrinol Metab 2010; 24: 243–62.

9. Krone N, Arlt W. Genetics of congenital adrenal hyperplasia. Best Pract Res Clin Endocrinol Metab 2009; 23: 181–92.

10. Online Medelian Inheritance in Man (OMIM) online: www.omim.org

11. Pallais JC, Au M, Pitteloud N, Seminara S, Growley WF. Kallmann syndrome. In GeneReviews [Internet]. NCBI bookshelf: www.ncbi.nlm.nih.gov/books/ NBK1334/

12. Visser JA, Schipper I, Laven JS, Themmen AP. Anti-Müllerian hormone: an ovarian reserve marker

in primary ovarian insufficiency. *Nat Rev Endocrinol* 2012; 8: 331–41.

13. De Vos M, Devroey P, Fauser BC. Primary ovarian insufficiency. *Lancet* 2010; 376: 911–21.

14. Simpson JL. Genetic and phenotypic heterogeneity in ovarian failure: overview of selected candidate genes. *Ann N Y Acad Sci* 2008; 1135: 146–54.

15. Saul RA, Tarleton JC. *FMR1*-related disorders. In *GeneReviews* [Internet]. NCBI bookshelf: www.ncbi.nlm.nih.gov/books/NBK1384

16. Gordon UD. Assisted conception in the azoospermic male. *Hum Fertil (Camb)* 2002; 5: S9–14.

17. Skordis N, Shammas C, Efstathiou E *et al.* Late diagnosis of 5-α steroid-reductase deficiency due to IVS12A>G mutation of the *SRD5a2* gene in an adolescent girl presented with primary amenorrhea. *Hormones (Athens)* 2011; 10: 230–5.

18. Lofrano-Porto A, Barra GB, Giacomini LA *et al.* Luteinizing hormone beta mutation and hypogonadism in men and women. *N Engl J Med* 2007; 357: 897–904.

19. Mazen I, Abdel Hamid MS, El-Gammal M, Aref A, Amr K. *AMH* gene mutations in two Egyptian families with persistent Müllerian duct syndrome. *Sex Dev* 2011; 5: 277–80.

20. Blanc T, Ayedi A, El-Ghoneimi A *et al.* Testicular function and physical outcome in young adult males diagnosed with idiopathic 46 XY disorders of sex development during childhood. *Eur J Endocrinol* 2011; 165: 907–15.

21. Yu J, Chen Z, Ni Y, Li Z. CFTR mutations in men with congenital bilateral absence of the vas deferens (CBAVD): a systemic review and meta-analysis. *Hum Reprod* 2012; 27: 25–35.

22. Verpoest W, De Rademaeker M, Sermon K *et al.* Real and expected delivery rates of patients with myotonic dystrophy undergoing intracytoplasmic sperm injection and preimplantation genetic diagnosis. *Hum Reprod* 2008; 23: 1654–60.

23. Ankarberg-Lindgren C, Westphal O, Dahlgren J. Testicular size development and reproductive hormones in boys and adult males with Noonan syndrome: a longitudinal study. *Eur J Endocrinol* 2011; 165: 137–44.

24. Rajender S, Rahul P, Mahdi AA. Mitochondria, spermatogenesis and male infertility. *Mitochondrion* 2010; 10: 419–28.

25. Massart A, Lissens W, Tournaye H, Stouffs K. Genetic causes of spermatogenic failure. *Asian J Androl* 2012; 14: 40–8.

26. Stouffs K, Lissens W, Tournaye H, Van Steirteghem A, Liebaers I. The choice and outcome of the fertility treatment of 38 couples in whom the male partner has a Yq microdeletion. *Hum Reprod* 2005; 20: 1887–96.

27. Dam AH, Koscinski I, Kremer JA *et al.* Homozygous mutation in SPATA16 is associated with male infertility in human globozoospermia. *Am J Hum Genet* 2007; 81: 813–20.

28. Liu G, Shi QW, Lu GX. A newly discovered mutation in PICK1 in a human with globozoospermia. *Asian J Androl* 2010; 12: 556–60.

29. Elinati E, Kuentz P, Redin C *et al.* Globozoospermia is mainly due to DPY19L2 deletion via non-allelic homologous recombination involving two recombination hotspots. *Hum Mol Genet* 2012; 21: 3695–702.

30. Kuentz P, Vanden Meerschaut F, Elinati E *et al.* Assisted oocyte activation overcomes fertilization failure in globozoospermic patients regardless of the DPY19L2 status. *Hum Reprod* 2013; 28: 1054–61.

31. Dieterich K, Soto Rifo R, Faure AK *et al.* Homozygous mutation of AURKC yields large-headed polyploid spermatozoa and causes male infertility. *Nat Genet* 2007; 39: 661–5.

32. Ben Khelifa M, Zouari R, Harbuz R *et al.* A new AURKC mutation causing macrozoospermia: implications for human spermatogenesis and clinical diagnosis. *Mol Hum Reprod* 2011; 17: 762–8.

33. Avenarius MR, Hildebrand MS, Zhang Y *et al.* Human male infertility caused by mutations in the CATSPER1 channel protein. *Am J Hum Genet* 2009; 84: 505–10.

34. Goossens V, Traeger-Synodinos J, Coonen E *et al.* ESHRE PGD Consortium data collection XI: cycles from January to December 2008 with pregnancy follow-up to October 2009. *Hum Reprod* 2012; 27: 1887–911.

35. Metzker ML. Sequencing technologies – the next generation. *Nat Rev Genet* 2010; 11: 31–46.

36. Krawitz PM, Schweiger MR, Rodelsperger C *et al.* Identity-by-descent filtering of exome sequence data identifies PIGV mutations in hyperphosphatasia mental retardation syndrome. *Nat Genet* 2010; 42: 827–9.

37. Nielsen R, Paul JS, Albrechtsen A, Song YS. Genotype and SNP calling from next-generation sequencing data. *Nat Rev Genet* 2011; 12: 443–51.

38. El Inati E, Muller J, Viville S. Autosomal mutations and human spermatogenic failure. *Biochim Biophys Acta* 2012; 1822: 1873–9.

Chapter

9

Genetic counseling and gamete donation in assisted reproductive treatment

Alison Lashwood and Alison Bagshawe

Introduction

Increasing knowledge and understanding of the genetic basis of health and disease has lead to major changes in clinical practice. Competent professionals working within reproductive medicine will increasingly need to understand basic genetic principles and how they contribute to the diagnosis and treatment of their reproductive medicine patients. It would be unreasonable to expect reproductive medicine specialists to adopt an additional role as genetic counselor, but an understanding of the basis of genetic disorders and risks is essential to ensure that relevant at-risk patients are referred to the appropriate health professionals for genetic counseling and testing in a timely manner when required. An awareness of the impact of genetic testing on individuals and families and the unique issues that arise in the context of genetic diagnoses will help the reproductive medicine specialist understand the difficulties some patients may encounter and how they can be helped.

Couples requiring assisted reproductive technology will do so for a number of reasons, including clearly diagnosed functional or structural abnormalities or infertility of unknown cause. A subgroup of this population will present with a genetic condition and possible reproductive risk. These include:

- Infertile/subfertile couples where one or other is affected by or a carrier of a known unrelated single gene disorder or chromosome rearrangement.
- A single gene disorder or chromosome abnormality has contributed to the fertility problem. For example, a male with cystic fibrosis [1] who has congenital bilateral absence of the vas deferens or an anovulatory female with Turner syndrome [2].

- A chromosome rearrangement in a male has resulted in suboptimal sperm parameters or is linked to recurrent miscarriages in a couple.
- Incidental findings of genetic risk are detected during preparatory reproductive medicine clinical tests. For example, where a couple or an individual gamete donor is found to be an hemoglobinopathy carrier.
- A couple is at risk of having a child affected with a specific genetic disorder and they wish to use preimplantation genetic diagnosis (discussed in Chapter 11).

The aim of this chapter is to provide an overview of genetic counseling and how it is relevant to reproductive medicine practice. It will address different forms of genetic testing, how genetic risks are presented and understood and what they mean for the patients, the options available for dealing with reproductive genetic risk, the psychosocial impact of genetic risk, and the complexities of genetic testing. It will provide the reproductive medicine specialist with a practical reference tool to know when to make appropriate referrals accompanied with relevant clinical details to a genetic counseling service.

Gamete donation is an option for couples with a genetic risk and the discovery of such risk is sometimes a by-product of screening potential gamete donors. The second part of the chapter will address the need for gamete donors and surrogacy, the types of donation, and the options available to couples with a genetic diagnosis or who have a reproductive risk. Internationally most countries have regulatory frameworks which protect donors, recipients, and the donor-conceived children. The legal position and ethical framework in relation to gamete donation is fundamental to such

Textbook of Human Reproductive Genetics, eds Karen Sermon and Stéphane Viville. Published by Cambridge University Press.
© Cambridge University Press 2014.

services and consideration of the impact of gamete donation is essential to address the complex needs of donors and recipients.

Genetic counseling

Who offers it and why genetic specialists are required?

If we take the case of a couple who have a child with cystic fibrosis, genetic counseling will first aim to ensure that they understand the diagnosis and the implications and assess how the couple feels about this. The couple will need to understand the genetic basis of cystic fibrosis and the risk of recurrence. If they wish to extend their family they may require information about options to aid their reproductive choice and possibly proceed with prenatal diagnosis (PND) or preimplantation genetic diagnosis (PGD), for example, where they may require ongoing support following the outcome.

Genetic disorders will affect individuals, couples, and families over successive generations and genetic diagnoses, testing, and options for treatment may change over time. This makes the dynamics of genetic counseling quite unique as the information and support offered to patients will often extend to wider family members over an extensive time frame. Other family members may have different needs and views about the implications of a genetic condition. As a result genetic counselors must be cognizant of the potential variation in family dynamics, the ability of family members to communicate with each other, and the potential risk of breaching confidentiality. These issues are further discussed in the "Impact of genetic testing" section below.

It is important not to confuse genetic counseling, which employs the use of "counseling skills," with therapeutic counseling that is long term and undertaken by recognized accredited counselors. However, all health professionals should at least be aware of basic counseling skills as health and psychosocial issues are closely related [3]. Those clinicians consulting with patients should be aware of the need to:

- Ask open questions
- Notice non-verbal communication
- Allow periods of silence
- Clarify understanding as consultation proceeds
- Summarize and paraphrase what the patient has said
- Challenge if things are unclear

One of the essential tenets of genetic counseling is that it is "non-directive." Patients are provided with the information they require to make an informed decision, but the clinician avoids directing them towards a certain course of action. This does not mean that the clinician cannot offer the patient support in their decision making. Appropriate support for a couple making a decision indicating their choice that appears to be the best way forward for them in their circumstances, gives the patients control over their actions.

In 1975 the American Society of Human Genetics provided a useful definition of genetic counseling and, although the scope has changed over four decades, the basis of the description is still relevant [4]:

> Genetic counseling is a communication process which deals with the human problems associated with the occurrence, or risk of occurrence, of a genetic disorder in a family. It involves an attempt to help the individual or family:
>
> Comprehend the medical facts about a disorder
>
> Appreciate the way in which heredity contributes to the disorder and to the risk of recurrence
>
> Understand the options for dealing with the risk of recurrence
>
> Choose the course of action which seems most appropriate to them
>
> Make the best possible adjustment to the disorder in an affected family member.

Of perhaps greatest importance is that the genetic counseling is patient-centered and Biesecker and Peters in 2001 reinforced the individual nature of genetic counseling and that it needs to be tailored to the individual [5]:

> A dynamic psycho-educational process centred on genetic information. ...Clients are helped to personalise technical and probabilistic genetic information, to promote self-determination and to enhance their ability to adapt over time. The goal is to facilitate clients' ability to use genetic information in a personally meaningful way that minimizes psychological distress and increases personal control.

Although genetic counseling does not include long-term therapeutic counseling, it does build on basic counseling skills that should be used by all health professionals [3].

Professionals offering genetic counseling may be medically qualified clinical geneticists or genetic counselors. For the purposes of this chapter the authors do not make a distinction and the genetics health professional will be referred to as "genetic counselor." Genetic counseling is a recognized accredited profession with differing regulatory frameworks across the world. Internationally the availability, extent, and quality of genetic counseling will vary.

Referrals for genetic counseling

Clinical genetics historically has been practiced as an independent medical speciality. However, as the genetic etiology of disease is increasingly recognized, more integrated pathways are now commonplace in the management of disease and the scope of clinical genetics is likely to change and become more integrated within general medicine.

Commonly, referrals to genetic counseling would include those:

- With a known family history of a genetic condition
- Who are affected with a genetic condition
- Who have a child with a genetic condition
- Who are seeking a diagnostic opinion about a child with dysmorphic features and/or developmental delay
- Who are in consanguineous relationships
- Whose ethnic background indicates an increased genetic risk

At the time of referral some of these couples may be pregnant or due to commence fertility treatment. This can create a sense of urgency and additional patient anxiety, especially in relation to trying to establish a molecular or chromosomal basis for the condition in question. As some couples may consider PND as an option during pregnancy, the time frame for confirming the diagnosis is limited if PND is to be made available at the optimal time, usually between 12 and 16 weeks gestation. Due to the specialist nature of genetic testing, it may not be possible to complete some genetic tests within the usual time frame for PND. Other couples, who discover a genetic risk during the process of fertility treatment, may wish to consider PGD instead of embarking upon fertility treatment alone. In most cases this will invoke a delay in starting treatment

whilst molecular or chromosomal laboratory analysis is completed. Avoiding such a delay to treatment may limit the testing options for couples and therefore there is a great benefit to those at risk being referred for genetic consultation prior to pregnancy or fertility treatment.

Outcome of genetic counseling

Success of treatment is measured by outcome. Measuring the benefits of genetic counseling has been hampered by a poor understanding of what outcome measures should be used. Measuring patient satisfaction or a simple cost–benefit analysis without taking account of the greater social impact of genetic counseling is of limited use. However, McAllister *et al.* through qualitative research have now developed a patient-reported outcome measure (PROM) for measuring outcomes in a validated and reliable manner [6]. The score is called the Genetic Counseling Outcome Scale (GCOS-24) and provides a reliable tool for further studies.

Prior to the GCOS-24 score it was clear that one of the key elements for patients' understanding and satisfaction following genetic counseling was whether or not their perceived needs were met at the consultation. Therefore, a key tenet of genetic counseling (and could be argued any medical discipline) is to ask the patient to explain what information they want from the consultation. This will enable the health professional to address the issues that may be of greatest importance to them and prevent any misunderstanding of their needs.

Process of genetic counseling

Good history taking is an essential aid to making a genetic diagnosis and defining probable risk and this can be further clarified by the availability of a correctly recorded family pedigree. Practically based genetic counseling textbooks exist to aide the clinician in creating an accurate efficient family pedigree [7]. Electronic pedigree programs exist, but are probably not relevant to clinicians outside the specialist genetics arena. An accurate pedigree can demonstrate that the risk to a patient is negligible and offers immediate reassurance, or may clearly indicate that there is a risk and referral to the appropriate professional is warranted. Figure 9.1 demonstrates how complete and incomplete family history details can affect the potential risk information given to a couple.

129

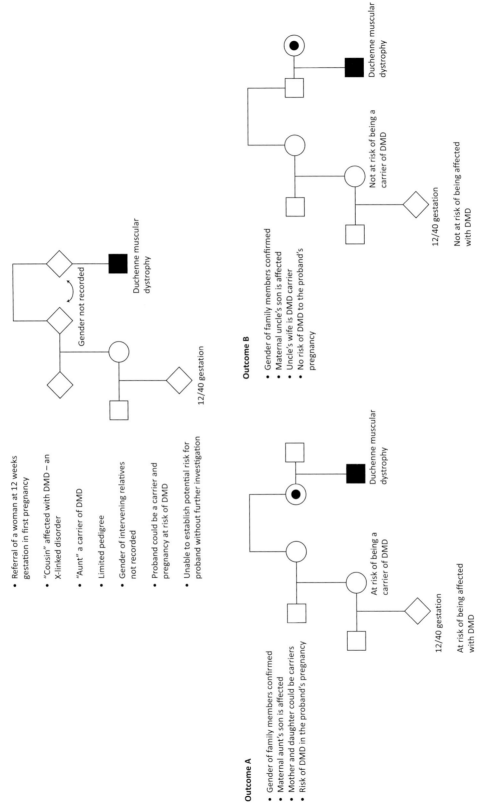

- Referral of a woman at 12 weeks gestation in first pregnancy
- "Cousin" affected with DMD – an X-linked disorder
- "Aunt" a carrier of DMD
- Limited pedigree
- Gender of intervening relatives not recorded
- Proband could be a carrier and pregnancy at risk of DMD
- Unable to establish potential risk for proband without further investigation

Gender not recorded

Duchenne muscular dystrophy

12/40 gestation

Outcome A

- Gender of family members confirmed
- Maternal aunt's son is affected
- Mother and daughter could be carriers
- Risk of DMD in the proband's pregnancy

Duchenne muscular dystrophy

12/40 gestation

At risk of being a carrier of DMD

At risk of being affected with DMD

Outcome B

- Gender of family members confirmed
- Maternal uncle's son is affected
- Uncle's wife is DMD carrier
- No risk of DMD to the proband's pregnancy

Duchenne muscular dystrophy

Not at risk of being a carrier of DMD

12/40 gestation

Not at risk of being affected with DMD

Figure 9.1 The value of recording detailed family history. DMD, Duchenne muscular dystrophy.

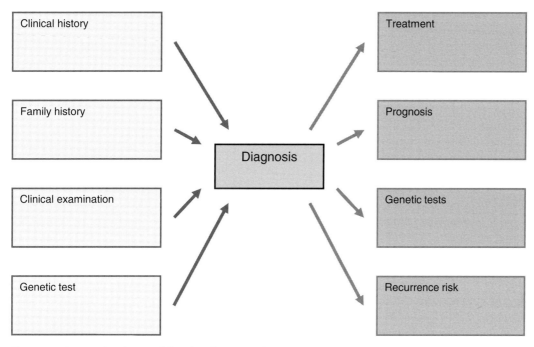

Figure 9.2 Process of reaching, and the value of, a genetic diagnosis.

During a genetic counseling consultation the key questions for patients will broadly fall into the following categories:

- What is the diagnosis?
- Why did it happen to me/us?
- Will it happen again?
- Is there a genetic test?
- Can we prevent passing on the genetic condition to our children?
- Will this affect other family members?

The value of a diagnosis

Confirmation of a genetic diagnosis is pivotal to the discussions about subsequent testing, treatment, and risks (Fig. 9.2). A medical diagnosis can be confirmed by molecular or cytogenetic testing. Additional benefits of genetic testing may avoid the need for invasive tests such as electromyogram (EMG) or muscle biopsies, which were traditionally used to confirm diagnoses of congenital muscular dystrophies, for example [8]. Molecular diagnosis of *BRCA1* and *BRCA2* mutations in breast cancer patients may inform prognosis and surgical management of the condition. If they have a mutation that increases the risk of cancer recurrence, some women may opt for complete mastectomy (instead of simple excision), possibly prophylactic mastectomy of the second breast or oophorectomy [9]. For those of reproductive age an understanding of the molecular or cytogenetic basis of the disorder will clarify recurrence risk and potential reproductive options.

Accurate information and dealing with risk

It is essential that couples are aware of current information in relation to the genetic disorder itself. Some individuals may have consulted with clinical genetics professionals several years previously, when they were tested for their carrier status using older technology. Advances in the molecular characterization of genetic conditions by next generation sequencing and microarray analysis means that more accurate defining of carrier status may be possible, and could even alter previous genetic results. For example, a woman with a family history of X-linked Duchenne muscular dystrophy, caused by a mutation in the dystrophin gene [10] requested carrier testing. Initially, no mutation was detected in her affected brother, so polymorphic markers in the region of the dystrophin gene on Xp21 were used to establish whether or not she had inherited the same maternal X chromosome and would thus be a carrier. As she carried the same X chromosome she was given a high carrier risk (95%), with a small risk of error due to recombination and therefore given a 50% risk of having an affected son. Subsequent sequencing determined a molecular deletion in her brother but not in her; therefore, she was not a carrier and would not have affected children.

In addition, some chromosomal rearrangements initially believed to carry reproductive risk in the form of miscarriage or physical or mental disability, where family members may have considered prenatal testing, may be reevaluated and thus now represent normal variants without reproductive risk [11].

Explaining risks

One of the aims of genetic counseling is to explain the risk associated with a genetic condition. It is not only important for the patient to understand this, but the patient will be responsible for forwarding this information to other family members (see "Communication and confidentiality within the family" section below). In most cases an individual or couple will have a clear understanding of the medical aspects of the condition diagnosed as this will have been addressed by the referring medical specialist; for example, by the pediatrician, neurologist, or breast surgeon.

Explaining genetic risk is an essential component of a genetic counseling consultation and information about risk must be presented in a way that is understood by the patients. Factors which may influence understanding should be acknowledged and considered. There may be marked differences in perceived risk and actual risk, as described by Marteau *et al.* looking at women's uptake of amniocentesis for raised maternal age [12]. McAllister found that some individuals may even construct a theory as to the background of their inheritance, which may help them to cope with their risk but may be a barrier to their understanding of risk [13]. Pilarski describes risk perception as "A complex and incompletely understood concept which seeks to capture the myriad meanings that an individual attaches to the experience of being at increased risk" [14]. Further exploration of such beliefs and an awareness of such behavior can help to ensure genetic risks are understood.

The presentation of risk in either numerical or descriptive terms has been reviewed in several studies (see references in [15, 16]) and the overall conclusion is that recall and understanding is better if a numerical odds risk is given. It is therefore better to give the risk as 1 in 400, for example, rather than a descriptive "low chance." Not all patients will understand risks if

given in percentages, and so when applying a numerical risk it is helpful to give both a percentage and an odds ratio, and give the chance of being affected and unaffected. For example, in the case of a couple with a recessive condition present the risk figures as either:

- A 25% chance of having an affected child against a 75% chance of having an unaffected child.

Or

- A 1 in 4 chance of having an affected child versus a 3 in 4 chance of an unaffected child.

However, Pilarski also noted that risk is not a simple numerical value, "but rather it is an evolving, subjective, experienced reality" [14]. Therefore it should be within the scope of genetic counseling practice to focus not solely on risk figures, but more how the patient perceives and will act on that risk. For those who may struggle with understanding risk, context can be an alternative option.

Genetic testing

Screening

Newborn screening for a range of medical conditions is available in many countries internationally. The extent of the screening will vary, but, for example, the UK Newborn Screening Programme [17] currently offers testing for congenital hypothyroidism, medium-chain acyl-CoA dehydrogenase deficiency (MCAD; OMIM #607008), cystic fibrosis, sickle cell disease, and phenylketonuria. The latter four are all genetic conditions and were integrated into the test program as they met the criteria for a clinical efficacious service. These conditions are relatively common, have high specificity rates, and if detected medical intervention is beneficial. In addition, MCAD is linked to sudden infant death in response to hypoglycemia and can be prevented if diagnosis is determined neonatally. Screening programs also exist for ethnicity-related risks such as the hemoglobinopathies and Tay–Sachs disease. However, population screening for genetic disease is not currently available at a National Health Service level in the UK and in standard health care services in many other countries, although "direct to consumer testing" (DTC) is available on a private basis. Set up on the basis that individuals have an interest in their personal genetic information and want to take some control over this, companies have developed a range of DTC tests. These include diagnostic tests; for example, breast and ovarian cancer genes (*BRCA1/2*), and predisposition to common conditions such as heart disease and addictions. The DTC tests have proven highly controversial as they are offered outside standard healthcare frameworks where the pretest counseling may not be informative and not provided by an appropriately qualified health professional. Although no overarching policies exist in relation to DTC tests, both the USA and European Union have investigated the legislative frameworks that exist and acknowledged the need for legislation [18].

Policies have been developed in both Europe and the USA to aid interpretation of such results. The current view is that appropriate pretest counseling and informed consent must be a prerequisite for such a service. The Human Genetics Commission has recommended that high standards could be achieved by international companies offering DTC by the development of codes of practice that cover: marketing, patient information, counseling and support, data protection, and laboratory analysis [19].

Assisted reproductive medicine health professionals should be aware of relevant screening tests available in their region. In most cases this will be based on the ethnicity of the patient only. However in some cases, where there is a family history of a genetic disorder, cascade screening may be appropriate (see "Carrier testing" section below).

Diagnostic testing

Clinical examination continues to be the most valuable tool for determining a diagnosis. However, molecular or cytogenetic testing is now often the first additional test of choice to help confirm a diagnosis. As above, congenital muscular dystrophies, for example, are a heterogeneous group of disorders with differing levels of severity and prognosis. At least nine genes are now recognized as being associated with the subtypes and the presence of a mutation may negate the need to perform invasive clinical tests and offer some degree of prognostic value [8]. The case for diagnostic genetic testing in the presence of symptoms is generally accepted as a clinical necessity to benefit the patient.

Genetic testing also provides confirmation of the mode of inheritance which enables an individual at risk to understand the risks to offspring. Retinitis pigmentosa (RP) [20], a group of degenerative retinal disorders leading to severe visual impairment, can be inherited in an autosomal dominant, recessive, or X-linked manner. To accurately advise a woman with a family history where only males have been affected, yet the molecular basis of the disorder is not known, one would need evidence that the causative mutation was on the X chromosome. It is possible that the RP is an autosomal dominant form and it is by chance that females in this family have been unaffected.

Carrier testing

Carrier testing refers to the testing for the heterozygous state of an autosomal recessive, X-linked gene or a balanced chromosome rearrangement in a healthy individual. Carrier testing usually arises as a result of one of the following:

- New diagnosis of a recessive or X-linked disorder in a child or adult.
- Genetic screening on the basis of ethnicity which determines carrier status for common recessive conditions in specific populations; for example, sickle cell anemia, Tay–Sachs disease, and beta-thalassemia.
- Newborn screening tests, now widely implemented, detect neonates with recessive conditions that lead to carrier testing of parents.
- A genetic diagnosis in a family member may initiate cascade screening whereby multiple family members present for testing in a structured manner.
- Consanguineous couples who have an increased risk of shared recessive genes.

As there are few health implications associated with carrier testing this is usually done in the context of reproductive decision making. The impact on patients will vary depending upon the mode of inheritance; the risk to a child with an autosomal recessive disorder is shared between the parents whereas the risk of an X-linked disorder is related to the mother only. James *et al.*, in their study of X-linked carrier women, found that being such a carrier was perceived as more stigmatizing with associated increased guilt compared with those who were carriers of recessive conditions, probably as in the latter scenario the burden of guilt is shared [21].

Presymptomatic testing

A number of genetic conditions will present in adulthood with no clinical manifestations in childhood;

for example, Huntington's disease (HD) [22], and spinocerebellar ataxia type 1 (SCA1) [23]. Some individuals at risk wish to know whether or not they are gene carriers ahead of the onset of symptoms and with appropriate clinical input can be tested. This is known as presymptomatic testing.

Huntington's disease and SCA1 are both inherited in an autosomal dominant manner giving the at-risk individuals a 50% risk of inheriting the gene. Huntington's disease is a later-onset, degenerative, neuropsychiatric disorder with an average age of onset between 35 and 50 years and the disease course is about 20 years' duration. Both HD and SCA1 are fully penetrant so those inheriting the mutation will develop symptoms at some stage, although predictions as to the exact age of onset are not possible. International guidelines exist [24] to manage this form of testing and generally the management of presymptomatic testing is considered best addressed by clinical genetics specialists.

Those at risk will request testing because they wish to end the uncertainty about genetic status, are considering their reproductive options, or they wish to inform their offspring of the risk. In a few situations at-risk individuals may have concerns about their clinical status and request testing to establish whether symptoms have started; however, the most efficient and reliable way of establishing disease status remains clinical examination. Further discussion about the impact of predictive testing is discussed in the "Late-onset diseases and predictive testing" section below.

Childhood testing

Whilst the reproductive medicine specialist is unlikely to be involved in the genetic testing of children, it does raise several issues that require careful consideration. The complexity of childhood testing is such that guidelines exist to help clinician and parents consider the issues and make the best decision for the child [25, 26]. Diagnostic testing to confirm a suspected disorder is likely to benefit the child and the family as the genetic basis of the condition is then understood and any relevant treatment can be initiated or inappropriate further investigations excluded. Carrier testing for the sake of making reproductive choices is not considered necessary in childhood and may have negative implications for the child. Recommendations are that such carrier testing is delayed until a child is of an age where they can give fully informed consent about testing.

Testing for late-onset disease is generally not recommended at an international level. There are limited benefits to a child knowing whether or not they will carry the gene for a late-onset disorder like HD, the impact of which may not be relevant for 40–50 years. Children should have the right to make their own decision about such testing and therefore testing during childhood would compromise the individual rights of that child.

In the context of genetic testing in childhood there are tensions where health professionals and perhaps parents or others compete for what is felt to be in the "best interests of the child." For example, adoption agencies may request testing of a child so that they can be placed for adoption and believe that this will be an easier task if the genetic status of the child is known. The American Society of Human Genetics and American College of Medical Genetics [27] issued a joint statement in 2000, which is reflected in the British Society for Genetic Medicine guidelines, that testing of children for the adoption process should equal the testing and limitations of testing all children. Once again their recommendation was that genetic testing should only be undertaken for diseases with a childhood onset and a proven clinical benefit of knowing gene status. Newson and Leonard state that if testing is to be considered in adoption cases then it is imperative that prospective adoptive parents have a consultation with a clinical geneticist to understand the full implications of testing [28].

Some parents believe that they are in the best position to decide when testing should be offered to their child and that their parental responsibility permits them to make decisions on behalf of their offspring. Whilst professionals involved in childhood testing will refer to the existing guidelines, specific family relationships and situations should be considered. If it is felt appropriate to test a child then the child should be engaged in the decision where possible [29].

Whilst guidelines exist, challenges will occur and the role of genetic counseling is to explain the guidelines and the implications of testing and to work with the parents to reach an acceptable outcome.

Reproductive options

Once the diagnosis of a genetic condition is confirmed and the molecular or cytogenetic basis determined, the offspring risk can be clarified. For those of childbearing age the issue of reproductive choice may require consideration. In keeping with the aims of genetic counseling, those at risk should be presented with accurate contemporaneous and complete information about the options and then supported through the decision making process. Social and religious values, prior experience of the condition, family relationships, and support systems will all contribute to the decisions made. In some circumstances, national regulation may dictate the extent of options available. Generally the main options for consideration will include:

- Accepting the risk and taking the chance with a pregnancy
- Making a decision against having children
- Adoption
- Gamete donation
- Prenatal diagnosis
- Preimplantation genetic diagnosis

Reproductive decision making for couples at risk of genetic conditions is complex. Due to the nature of genetic inheritance couples often only discover their genetic risk after the loss of a pregnancy or the birth of an affected child. They then become aware of the diagnosis, prognosis, and recurrence risk for future pregnancies. These pregnancies often were planned and wanted, and therefore to decide against having further children may be an unacceptable option for such couples.

Many couples will have experienced the loss of a child or a pregnancy and possibly had PND in subsequent pregnancies. These may have ended in the termination of an affected pregnancy. Termination of pregnancy for fetal abnormality or "genetic termination" carries with it potentially serious psychological consequences in both the short and long term [30]. Many women requesting termination for an abnormality will have reached the second trimester. In one study of 84 women having undergone termination in the second trimester, 20% reported psychological difficulties affecting their general well being 2 years after the termination [31]. Korenromp et al. found more adverse outcomes where there was less support from partners, if the abnormality was not necessarily lethal, and when the gestation of pregnancy was advanced [32]. It is clear that termination for an abnormality in a supportive environment has benefits for longer term coping mechanisms [33, 34].

The sense of responsibility for the outcome is a factor in the decision making in relation to PND and Rapp noted that a family history of disability often leaves individuals feeling that the responsible option is to have a prenatal test and termination [35]. Guilt and responsibility are emotions that are closely associated with the decision. McCoyd discovered in her study that women broadly felt they needed to consider the details of the abnormality they were faced with, the social impact this would have on their family, and their own capacity to cope with an affected child before deciding about PND and possible termination of pregnancy [36].

The variability of the phenotype or the late stage of onset of a condition adds other complex dimensions to the decision about the reproductive option of choice. Neurofibromatosis type 1 (NF1) [37] is one such condition where genotype confers no correlation of severity. Affected individuals will range from those with minor neurofibromas to children with plexiform neurofibromas and severe developmental delay. A prenatal result indicating the presence of NF1 in the fetus will not confer information about the likely severity in the child. If a mild phenotype exists in the family, couples may feel less able to terminate a pregnancy. For those at risk of late-onset disease like HD, the hope for a cure is a prevalent issue as is concern of terminating a pregnancy when a resultant child would not be affected until the fourth decade of life [38].

Couples facing the option of PND will, in the majority of cases, have been aware of the genetic risk for some time and have a clear understanding of the disorder and the impact that this would have on their offspring. However, there will be a cohort of patients where a genetic diagnosis is recent and they have no experience of the disorder. For those who opt for PND, a number of options exist, but counseling prior to testing is essential to ensure that the impact of the outcome has been considered. The process of counseling prior to testing should be individualized and requires close communication between the genetic counselor, obstetrician, and parents [39]. Those considering PND may find it helpful to speak to specialist health professionals with extensive experience of the disorder; for example, a pediatrician or patient support groups.

Given that adverse prenatal results will often result in termination of pregnancy, support around making this decision and in the immediate aftermath and long term may be available through support networks such as Antenatal Results and Choices (UK) [40] or A Heartbreaking Choice (USA) [41].

It is important not to assume that all affected pregnancies will be terminated and the ongoing support for couples with affected pregnancies is paramount. Hickerton *et al.* found that whilst parents were coping with their own thoughts about the diagnosis and future loss of their baby, the positive and negative responses of others had a major impact on their experience [42]. In understanding this, health professionals can play a major supportive role. A further important point to consider for parents continuing with an affected pregnancy is that if the genetic condition is not associated with neonatal onset then the genetic status of the child may be known to parents before the manifestations of symptoms. This is not recommended in the case of adult-onset disorders as it breaches the child's right to make a choice about testing (see the "Childhood testing" section above). In the case of conditions manifesting later in infancy or childhood, it may create considerable anxiety for the parents whilst they anticipate the onset of symptoms.

Non-invasive prenatal diagnosis

The identification of cell-free fetal DNA in the maternal circulation was first described by Lo in 1997 [43]. The development of this technology now offers a risk-free test to establish fetal genotype. A maternal blood sample is analyzed for cell-free fetal DNA (cffDNA) from around nine weeks gestation for establishing fetal sex, RhD status, some paternally inherited single gene disorders, and Down syndrome [44, 45]. The sensitivity and specificity of the testing is still being established so non-invasive prenatal diagnosis (NIPND) is not available universally. The benefit is that it reduces the need for invasive PND however there are controversial issues in relation to the extent of its use in establishing fetal sex for non genetic reasons, paternity testing and new technology that could determine single gene disorders which may have implications for future health and other family members. It is likely that this form of testing will continue to develop although invasive PND will still be required in the foreseeable future.

Invasive prenatal diagnosis

Chorionic villus sampling, amniocentesis and fetal blood sampling procedures are widely available and continue to be the main choice for couples who wish to have fetal genotyping [46]. As the risk of abnormality is high, most women have PND with the intention of terminating an affected pregnancy. Prior discussion

about what a woman should expect of the procedure and termination are vital to ensure she can make a fully informed decision. Specialist fetal medicine centers will provide the appropriate technology and the support for women undergoing PND. Others may seek PND as a source of information and if the fetus is affected will continue the pregnancy. The confirmation of the genotype helps them to prepare for the birth of an affected child. Decisions around PND require health professionals to act in a supportive and non-directive manner.

Preimplantation genetic diagnosis

For couples who wish to conceive their own biological children who are unaffected by the disorder in the family, PGD could be considered. In most cases this choice is made to avoid termination of pregnancy or repeated high-risk pregnancies. However, the decision to undertake PGD is complex and requires consideration of religious beliefs, past reproductive experience, fertility status of the couple, genetic risk, severity of the genetic condition within the family, and desire to have their own biological child [47–50]. Whilst most couples undertaking PGD will do so in an assisted reproductive medicine center, high quality genetic counseling prior to treatment will ensure that patients' expectations of PGD are achievable. It is essential that accurate contemporary genetic testing has been completed, correct genetic risks have been attributed, alternative reproductive options have been fully discussed, and the success and scope of testing is understood. The details of the procedure are covered in Chapter 11.

Gamete donation presents an option to couples with a genetic risk and this will be discussed in the "Gamete donation" section below.

Impact of genetic testing

Bereavement and guilt

In 2002, Skirton and Patch said, "Psychological care of adult patients is as important as genetic information, as guilt, blame, anxiety and hopelessness may accompany the feeling of risk in any of these situations" [3]. For many, this means they have been bereaved by the loss of a child, pregnancy, or another family member. However, additionally it can signify the loss of

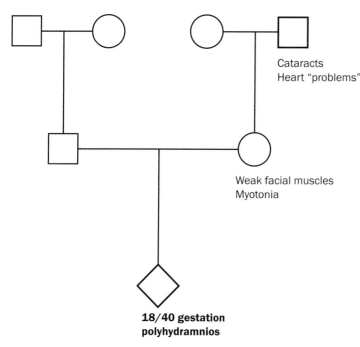

Cataracts
Heart "problems"

- First pregnancy, polyhydramnios detected at 18/40 gestation
- Mother noted to have myopathic features and hand myotonia
- Her father had a history of cataracts and cardiac arrhythmia
- Amniocentesis confirms that the fetus has congenital myotonic dystrophy

Multiple bereavements:
- Loss of pregnancy
- Loss of own health
- Loss of reproductive freedom
- Impact of diagnosis for other family members

Weak facial muscles
Myotonia

18/40 gestation polyhydramnios

Figure 9.3 Genetic results and multiple bereavements.

reproductive freedom or the loss of health of that individual. Multiple bereavements in the genetic context are commonplace. A woman, for example, was referred in her first pregnancy to the fetal medicine team with polyhydramnios (Fig. 9.3). A diagnosis of congenital myotonic dystrophy [51] was subsequently made following amniocentesis. Further examination of the patient herself confirms that she has myopathic features, hand myotonia, and a family history of cataracts, cardiac arrhythmia, early balding in her father, and developmental delay in a niece. Molecular analysis detects a mutation in the *DMPK* gene and thus confirms that she is also affected with myotonic dystrophy. She opts for termination of pregnancy. Within a minimal time frame she loses her pregnancy, her own health, her reproductive freedom, and is aware of the impact of the diagnosis for other family members.

During the genetic counseling process, revisiting the history is important to allow a couple to express their feelings and have the significance of their loss recognized. Telling one's personal story was recognized by Brock as a therapeutic process that helps adaptation to bereavement in the long term [52].

The impact of the history and the effect this has had on the couple will depend upon many issues, and so

it is important for the genetic counselor to consider how long ago a couple lost their child, for example, or how many times they have terminated a pregnancy. Alternatively, the couple may recently have experienced the death of another relative, and together these factors may have implications for the timing of any treatment or their coping mechanisms. Anniversaries of loss are important and can be incredibly difficult periods for those coping with grief. It may be in the interests of a couple or individual not to have specific genetic or prenatal testing that may coincide with a time when they may expect to have to face specific memories or acute grief such as the date of their child's death.

Some couples or individuals will experience feelings of guilt associated with their family history, apportioning blame to the carrier of the single gene disorder or chromosome rearrangement. The feelings of guilt and blame may differ with the disorder and mode of inheritance (see the "Carrier testing" section above). While investigating attitudes in women with dominant conditions, Faulkner and Kingston found that those with myotonic dystrophy reported high levels of guilt relating to the risk to their offspring, which, in turn, affected their reproductive decisions [53]. Although such thoughts are frequent and recognized, if a couple or individual do not adapt to the situation this may also indicate a need for referral for therapeutic counseling.

Communication and confidentiality within the family

The detection of a single gene alteration or chromosome rearrangement may be a *de novo* event and therefore relevant only in relation to the reproductive risk for that individual or couple. However, often the genetic result will have implications for wider family members and the need to communicate this becomes paramount.

The responsibility for communicating this information within the family lies with the proband (the individual presenting for genetic counseling) and genetic counselors will endeavor to help such individuals raise the subject and explain the need for specialist referral. The uptake of subsequent genetic testing may be determined by the communication within the family. Family members are crucial to the dissemination of genetic information and multiple studies have investigated family communication and particularly the potential barriers to this. The level of genetic risk, proximity of the relative to the proband, sex of the affected individual, family experience of the disorder, and the family culture will all contribute to the communication process. Wiseman *et al.*, in their meta-analysis, reviewed 33 papers looking at the communication of genetic risk within families, most relating to cancer genetics [54]. The studies confirmed the impact of the factors mentioned above and the importance of the proband who would deliver the information about risk to close relatives. However, these relatives were then tasked with both emotionally supporting the proband and forwarding this risk information to their own close relatives. Overall the meta-analysis concluded that the impact of this on these relatives is poorly studied. Further research is needed to establish how communication works for other genetic disorders, whether the gender of affected relatives, the age of onset of the condition, and the prognosis and severity is significant to the success of communication. From a practical point of view in the genetic counseling arena, the use of an introductory "to whom it may concern" letter explaining the results, risks, and details of how to obtain help and advice, coupled with patient information leaflets can aid this process.

The question arises as to whether the responsibility for this sharing of information shifts to the clinician if the family is unable or wilfully refuses to share the results. Reluctance to share genetic information is usually secondary to fear of causing distress, concern over what to say, or a belief that the risk is not relevant to other family members [55]. In most difficult cases with detailed discussion and exploration of the issues that may be causing a barrier to communication, reluctance to share information can be overcome [56]. However, ethical dilemmas can arise for clinicians if they believe that important risk information is being wilfully withheld from relevant family members. The ethical principles of maleficence and non-maleficence will need to be considered and direct contact with other family members may be justified. In UK case law, for example, clinicians can breach confidentiality if considered to be in the public interest, and there is debate over whether the privacy rights of an individual in genetic medicine supersede the needs of family members at risk. In genetic medical practice most contentious family situations can be successfully addressed if time is taken to review the context of the problem, explain the risks to other family members, and offer support in communicating the information and reassurance that genetic counseling will be accessible.

Complex issues

Late-onset disorders and predictive testing

Genetic conditions with an adult onset present health professionals and patients with a unique set of issues that require special consideration. Predictive testing is available for adult onset disorders such as HD, familial Alzheimer's disease, or cancer-susceptibility genes such as *BRCA1* and *BRCA2*. Those requesting testing will do so invariably as they "need to know," but others will consider testing to help with reproductive decisions, lifestyle choices, planning for the future, for the sake of children, and a few may have concerns that symptoms are already present. With the availability of predictive testing for HD from the mid 1980s, international guidelines were created as professionals were concerned about the impact of such testing. The guidelines have since been updated, but largely the principles remain [24]. Those who opt not to undergo testing often state the overriding reason behind non-participation is concern about their ability to cope with a bad news result [57]. The aim of genetic counseling in predictive testing is to ensure that the at-risk individual is well informed and certain about knowing their genetic status, as they may receive this several decades ahead of the onset of symptoms. Pretest genetic consultations are usually offered over an extended time frame and include discussions about the rationale for testing, expectations of result, coping mechanisms, family and friends support network, and implications for employment and insurance.

In a number of adult-onset genetic disorders the phenomenon of "survivor guilt" has been observed in individuals testing negative, when other family members have tested positive [58]. The genetic counselor needs to consider this especially when multiple siblings are tested.

Predictive testing for *BRCA1* or *BRCA2* genes presents another dimension to genetic counseling. Such pathogenic mutations in monogenic disorders are said to be non-fully penetrant and carrier status confers a lifetime risk of breast cancer of 60–80% or of ovarian cancer of 5–60% [59]. Coping with the uncertainty of carrier status is a significant counseling issue given that many women gene carriers will opt for prophylactic mastectomy or oophorectomy. The complex needs of such patients may be better addressed by a multidisciplinary team including geneticists, surgeons, and oncologists.

Inconclusive results

Molecular genetic testing for known, fully characterized mutations provides a clearly informative confirmation of the diagnosis. That notwithstanding, the predictive value of the mutation in terms of age of onset as in the case of HD or the severity of the disorder, as in NF1, may not be useful. Such limitations of testing are considered during the genetic counseling process to ensure that patient's expectations of the test are met.

With the introduction of full genome and exome sequencing and SNP microarray analysis (see Chapter 2) results of unknown significance are increasing. Such outcomes – copy number variants (CNVs) or variants of unknown significance (VUS) – are seen in both adult, pediatric, and prenatal diagnostic medical settings. Microarray platforms are now used to target specific groups of disorders like childhood developmental delay or multiple fetal anomalies. The issue that exercises clinicians responsible for interpreting the results

is the phenotypic relevance and the potential discovery of genetic susceptibility genes or other abnormalities unrelated to the indication for testing [60].

Welfare of the child

The potential for future ill health in a prospective parent warrants some consideration during genetic counseling around reproductive options. When the prospective parent either has a genetic disorder or may become symptomatic at a future stage, an open discussion with the couple is required. It is recognized that children of parents with dominant genetic conditions are more adversely affected than normal controls given the nature of the diseases and potential early death of a parent [61]. This is clearly a sensitive topic, but addressing issues about the future care of the affected partner in addition to the care of any children born as a result of spontaneous pregnancy or PGD may help a couple to consider how they would cope in such circumstances and what practical sources of support are accessible to them.

Gamete donation

In the context of genetics, the use of donated gametes serves two principal purposes. Firstly it enables people who have a genetic disorder to avoid passing on the gene to their children, and secondly it enables those who have a genetic disorder that directly impacts on their fertility, to become parents.

Uses of gamete donation

Gamete donation may be an acceptable alternative for:

- Fertile couples with a genetic risk who wish to avoid having an affected child, but will not consider PND, PGD, or adoption.
- Fertile couples who have experienced the repeated loss of a pregnancy or child(ren) the cause of which is suspected to be a genetic condition, but one that has not been identified.
- Couples who would consider PGD, but the female partner will not or does not produce sufficient eggs, or the male partner is azoospermic; when technically PGD is not possible; or when state or personal funding is not available.
- Couples with genetic conditions which cause infertility in themselves; for example, men who

have Klinefelter syndrome and women who have Turner syndrome.

- Couples with genetic conditions which cause infertility and also increase the risk of having an affected child; for example, a man with congenital bilateral absence of the vas deferens (CBAVD) secondary to a cystic fibrosis related disorder, where his partner is also a cystic fibrosis carrier.

Sperm and egg donation

Sperm donation is a minimally invasive procedure and has been recorded as a way for an infertile partnership to have a child since the eighteenth century. The developments of sperm freezing techniques and the creation of sperm banks in the 1950s allowed access to those wanting medical assistance with such a procedure [62]. Since then social attitudes and legislation have influenced (or reflected) how sperm donation is viewed and managed throughout the world. This varies widely, with some countries and religions forbidding its use whilst others are quite open to the practice. In doing so this draws criticism that restrictions are too great and deny many couples the opportunity of having a child [63].

Egg donation became a viable option in the mid 1980s, and for women who have experienced repeated miscarriages, neonatal death, or (a) child(ren) born with a serious health condition, it offers the chance to have a live healthy child.

Egg donation not only provides an older woman with an opportunity to have a child without the increased risks of age-related aneuploidy, but for those who have undergone premature ovarian failure, receiving donated eggs offers a solution. Improving cryopreservation techniques for the storage of eggs has extended the possibilities of egg banking although ethical discussions around this will continue [64].

Surrogacy using gamete donation

Women who have repeat miscarriages, an absent uterus, or a medical condition where pregnancy is contraindicated may benefit from the use of a surrogate to carry a child on their behalf. Surrogacy can be offered in conjunction with either egg or sperm donation and is a viable alternative when the female partner is unable to carry a child and a gamete donor is required to prevent a genetic condition being passed to the next generation. In the UK at least one of the commissioning parents has to be the biological parent.

As such, a woman unable to use her own eggs could not use a sperm donor in a surrogacy arrangement without going through adoption procedures. Internationally surrogacy is a complex process for couples to navigate due to the variation in practice and legal requirements making it a difficult and at times stressful option for couples [65].

Processes and access to donors: known, altruistic, and commercial donors

Gamete donation has elicited throughout the world a myriad of judgments, attitudes, and perceptions in response to the mores of religion, heritage, and culture. This significantly affects the ability to access donors, and the recruitment process of donors varies widely from country to country. Donors are recruited through personal contact (family or friend), altruistic anonymous donation, or as a paid donor in some countries where payment is permitted.

It is illegal in the UK to pay for eggs or sperm, although the regulatory body permits compensation to cover expenses and "inconvenience" [66]. However, there is no effective control over private arrangements and cross-border gamete donation [67]. Heng argued that the cross-border nature of obtaining donor eggs undermines local principles (where they exist) of the altruistic requirements of donation and limits the traceability of donors, which is relevant potentially for both the emotional welfare of donor-conceived children and their health (see below) [68].

Many donors empathize with the desire of the childless to have a family, and an understanding of their situation is evident. Relative donation to avoid genetic disease has the added necessity of ensuring that the prospective donor is not also a carrier of the monogenic or chromosome disorder in the family.

Legal position and rights of donors, recipients, and donor-conceived children

In the UK the legal position on a range of matters, including the rights of donors, recipients, and donor-conceived children, and the storage of gametes, are clearly laid out in the Human Fertilisation and Embryology Acts of 1990 and 2008. Clinic practices are regulated by the Human Fertilisation and Embryology Authority (HFEA), which was established in 1991 and which produces a Code of Practice that includes the relevant statutory requirements together with Guidance.

The HFE Act of 1990 also required the establishment of a central Register of Information to be held by the HFEA. This records all treatment procedures carried out under licence and their outcomes together with details of all donors, recipients, and children born through donor conception. Subsequent Regulations set out the rights of the different parties affected by donor conception to request information from the Register, both identifying and non-identifying. The HFEA determines policy as to the limits on children or families that are permitted to result from the use of any one gamete donor, which is currently 10 families.

The laws relating to the identity release of gamete donors again will vary internationally. Where donation is only permitted if identifying information about a donor is available, this is generally determined by its recognition as a human right for a child to have access to its genetic and biographical history. In Sweden donor identity has been in effect since 1985, whereas in the UK this did not occur until 2005 and has limitations of access to donor identity within a set time frame.

Internationally, generally, donors do not have any legal rights, claims, or responsibilities over a donor-conceived child, and a child has none on the donor. The legal parent of a child conceived through donation is the recipient parent(s) provided that they gave legal consent to treatment.

Counseling and ethical issues of gamete donation

Donors

During the screening process of a donor, it might become evident that the donor is a carrier of a previously unknown genetic condition which has considerable consequences. This can create potentially difficult dilemmas for the donor, the donor's family, and for the clinical team.

Usually a donor comes forward to donate with the confidence of assumed health and fitness. Screening for genetic disorders is variable [69] and can sometimes expose serious inherited health issues which have to be addressed by donors. It is recognized that a number of donors, especially sperm donors, do not inform members of their family of their intention to donate. A donor who in the course of screening is found to have a genetic condition will inevitably face a number of issues, not only about the condition itself but also about how, and if, such knowledge can be dealt with within the family unit. The situation might have serious implications for siblings of the donor if they too are likely to carry the condition. Genetic counseling is essential in such events and will usually be extended to the donor's family and partner (if they have one) since the impact of the diagnosis will affect all concerned.

Genetic screening

The genetic history of a donor is established during the initial screening process and medical consultations, supported by a detailed questionnaire which specifically asks whether or not they know of any genetic or inherited conditions that exist within the family. Further checks are made with their family doctor about their familial history, and donors undergo testing for the more usual genetic conditions. To safeguard future children and the recipients, donors are also informed of the Congenital Disabilities Act 1976, which apportions liability for a child born with a congenital or inherited disability. If donors know of a preexisting condition in the family yet fail to disclose this and continue to donate, and a child is born with this condition, then the child could sue the donor for failure to disclose the information. It is incumbent on the donor to prove that they were unaware that the condition existed and had not therefore wilfully withheld the information.

The extent of genetic screening of donors will vary. The USA (American Society for Reproductive Medicine, ASRM) and UK (HFEA) have developed guidelines for testing, but many argue that screening needs to be more extensive. Reports of donors developing or being carriers of genetic conditions have been described. The impact of this on the donors and recipients of donor treatment has lead to greater discussion about the need to extend screening and the management of such information. Maron *et al.* advocated extending donor-screening protocols and the development of a register of donor information that would facilitate identification and notification if a genetic disorder occurred [70]. However, the impact of such genetic screening on both donors and recipients necessitates careful counseling to ensure that the effects, expectations, and limitations of testing are understood [71].

Recipients

Welfare of the child

Gamete donation may be preferred to facing the uncertainty of having a biological child born with a severe disability or health condition. Some couples may already be parents to severely disabled child(ren), who require significant time and care and are now seeking to extend their family through gamete donation with or without PGD. Ethical issues are inevitably raised within the professional team about the welfare of both sets of children in such circumstances due to their differing needs and demands on the family as a whole. The process of assisted reproductive technology or PGD is complex and time consuming with associated female health risks. Discussion about the impact of treatment on family life in the event, for example, of ovarian hyperstimulation syndrome or the birth of premature twins, must form part of responsible informed counseling prior to the start of any treatment.

Telling the children

Donor-conceived children will generally rely on their parents to inform them of their biological inheritance. If the recipient couple decide not to tell the child, despite her/his right to know, that s/he has been conceived through donation they may deny her/him information about her/his genetic background and the reasons why the familial disorder does not put her/him at risk. Readings et al. in 2011 reported on a study of 101 families with 7-year-old children born following sperm donation, egg donation, or surrogacy [72]. "Surrogate" children were generally aware of the origin of their conception, whereas 50% and 75% of those conceived by egg and sperm donation respectively had not been informed. A number planned not to tell their children at all although this information had been shared with others in the majority of these cases. Another study in Sweden looking at intention to disclose in families with younger children demonstrated a 78% intention, with 16% having already done so [73]. However, even with legal guidance requiring that children are informed, 6% of families did not plan to tell their children.

The reasons for non-disclosure are complex and varied, but studies have indicated that the burden of non-disclosure on the patients is significant and many who delay informing their children until adulthood regret their decision to do so [74]. In support of this, Golombok et al. looked at mother and child relationships in donor-conceived and normally conceived 7-year-old children [75]. They found that there was less positive interaction from mothers who had not disclosed gamete donation to the child and suggested that such parents and children may benefit from a more open dialogue.

Some parents may want to disclose the information to their children, but just do not know how to do this and what words to use. Internationally there are internet forums and many countries will have established support groups like the Donor Conception Network in the UK [76]. Such groups are likely to help couples with these issues and may offer support meetings and workshops.

References

1. Online Mendelian Inheritance in Man (OMIM) #602421. Cystic fibrosis transmembrane conductance regulator; CFTR. Updated 6/20/2012: www.omim.org/entry/602421

2. Pinsker JE. Clincal review: Turner syndrome: updating the paradigm of clinical care. *J Clin Endocrinology Metab* 2012;97: 994–1003.

3. Skirton H, Patch C. *Genetics for Healthcare Professionals. A Lifestage Approach.* Oxford, UK: BIOS Scientific, 2002.

4. Ad Hoc Committee on Genetic Counseling American Society for Human Genetics. Genetic counseling. *Am J Hum Genet* 1975; 27: 240–2.

5. Biesecker BB, Peters KF. Process studies in genetic counseling: peering into the black box. *Am J Hum Genet* 2001; 106: 191–8.

6. McAllister M, Wood AM, Dunn G, Shiloh S, Todd C. The Genetic Counseling Outcome Scale: a new patient-reported outcome measure for clinical genetic services. *Clin Genet* 2011; 79: 413–24.

7. Harper PS. *Practical Genetic Counselling*, 6th edn. London, UK: Arnold, 2004.

8. Sparks S, Quijano S, Harper A et al. Congenital muscular dystrophy overview. Last revision August 23, 2012. In *GeneReviews* [Internet]. NCBI bookshelf: www.ncbi.nlm.nih.gov/books/NBK1291

9. Paradiso A, Formenti S. Hereditary breast cancer: clinical features and risk reduction strategies. *Ann Oncol* 2011; 22(Suppl 1): i31–6.

10. Online Mendelian Inheritance in Man (OMIM) #310200. Muscular dystrophy, duchenne type; DMD. Last updated 8/5/2012: www.omim.org/entry/310200

11. Gardner RJ, Sutherland GR. *Chromosome Abnormalities and Genetic Counselling*, 3rd edition. Oxford, UK: Oxford University Press, 2004.

12. Marteau TM, Kidd J, Cook R *et al*. Perceived risk not actual risk predicts uptake of amniocentesis. *Br J Obstet Gynaecol* 1991; 98: 282–6.

13. McAllister M. Personal theories of inheritance, coping strategies, risk perception and engagement in hereditary non-polyposis colon cancer families offered genetic testing. *Clin Genet* 2003; 64: 179–89.

14. Pilarski, R. Risk perception among women at risk for hereditary breast and ovarian cancer. *J Genet Couns* 2009; 18: 303–12.

15. Hopwood P, Howell A, Lalloo F, Evans G. Do women understand the odds? Risk perceptions and recall of risk information in women with a history of breast cancer. *Community Genet* 2003; 6: 214–23.

16. Marteau TM, Saidi G, Goodburn S *et al*. Numbers or words? A randomized controlled trial presenting screen negative results to pregnant women. *Prenat Diagn* 2000; 20: 714–8.

17. UK Newborn Screening Programme Centre. Why do we offer and recommend newborn blood spot screening? May 2012 update: www.newbornbloodspot. screening.nhs.uk/education2012pptx

18. Borry P, van Hellemondt RE, Sprumont D *et al*. Legislation on direct to consumer genetic testing in seven European countries. *Eur J Hum Genet* 2012; 20: 715–21.

19. Human Genetics Commission. A common framework of principles for direct-to-consumer genetic testing services, July 2010: www.sashg.org/documents/ HGC-UK-Policy-on-DTC-testing.pdf

20. Roberta A, Pagon, Stephen P Daiger. Retinitis pigmentosa overview. Last update, September 2005. In *GeneReviews* [Internet]. NCBI bookshelf: www.ncbi. nlm.nih.gov/books/NBK1417/

21. James CA, Hadley DW, Holtzman NA, Winkelstein JA. How does the mode of inheritance of a genetic condition influence families? A study of guilt, blame, stigma, and understanding of inheritance and reproductive risks in families with X-linked and autosomal recessive diseases. *Genet Med* 2006; 8: 234–42.

22. Online Mendelain Inheritance in Man (OMIM) #143100. Huntington disease; HD. Last updated 1/12/2011:www.omim.org/entry/143100? search=huntington%20disease&highlight= huntington%20disease

23. Spinocerebellar ataxia: www.ncbi.nlm.nih.gov/sites/ GeneTests/review/disease/spinocerebellar%20ataxia? db=genetests&search_param=contains

24. Macleod R, Tibben A, Frontali M *et al*. Recommendations for the predictive genetic test in Huntington's disease. *Clin Genet* 2013; 83: 221–31.

25. Borry P. Genetic testing in asymptomatic minors: recommendations of the European Society of Human Genetics. *Eur J Hum Genet* 2009; 17: 720–1.

26. British Society of Human Genetics. Report on the Genetic Testing of Children 2010: www.bsgm.org.uk/ media/678741/gtoc_booklet_final_new.pdf

27. The American Society of Human Genetics Social Issues Committee and The American College of Medical Genetics Social, Ethics and Legal Issues Committee. Genetic testing in adoption. *Am J Hum Genet* 2000; 66: 761–7.

28. Newson AJ, Leonard SJ. Childhood testing for familial cancer: should adoption make a difference? *Fam Cancer* 2010; 9: 37–42.

29. Parker M. Genetic testing in children and young people. *Fam Cancer* 2010; 9: 15–8.

30. Kersting A, Wagner B. Complicated grief after perinatal loss. *Dialogues Clin Neurosci* 2012; 14: 187–94.

31. White-Van Mourik MC, Connor JM, Ferguson-Smith MA. The psychosocial sequelae of a second trimester termination of pregnancy for fetal abnormality over a two year period. *Birth Defects Orig Artic Ser* 1992; 28: 61–74.

32. Korenromp MJ, Page-Christiaens GC, van den Bout J *et al*. Psychological consequences of termination of pregnancy for fetal anomaly: similarities and differences between partners. *Prenat Diagn* 2005; 25: 1226–33.

33. Hunt K, France E, Ziebland S, Filed K, Wyke S. "My brain couldn't move from planning a birth to planning a funeral": qualitative study of parents' experiences of decisions after ending a pregnancy for fetal abnormality. *Int J Nurs Stud* 2009; 46: 1111–21.

34. Fisher J. Termination of pregnancy for fetal abnormality: the perspective of a parent support organization. *Reprod Health Matters* 2008; 16(Suppl): 57–65.

35. Rapp R. *Testing Women, Testing the Fetus. The Social Impact of Amniocentesis in America*. New York, NY: Routledge, 2000.

36. McCoyd JL. "I'm not a saint.": Burden assessment as an unrecognised factor in prenatal decision making. *Qual Health Res* 2008; 18: 1489–500.

37. Online Mendelain Inheritance in Man (OMIM) #162200. Neurofibromatosis, type 1; NF1. Last updated 3/18/2010: www.omim.org/entry/162200

38. Decruyenaere M, Evers-Kiebooms G, Boogaerts A *et al.* The complexity of reproductive decision-making in asymptomatic carriers of the Huntington mutation, *Eur J Hum Genet* 2007; 15: 453–62.

39. Pergament E, Pergament D. Reproductive decisions after fetal genetic counseling. *Best Pract Res Clin Obstet Gynaecol* 2012; 26: 517–29.

40. Antenatal Results and Choices: www.arc-uk.org

41. A Heartbreaking Choice: www.aheartbreakingchoice.com

42. Hickerton CL, Aitken M, Hodgson J, Delatycki MB. "Did you find that out in time?": New life trajectories of parents who choose to continue a pregnancy where a genetic disorder is diagnosed or likely. *Am J Med Genet A* 2012; 158A: 373–83.

43. Lo YM, Corbetta N, Chamberlain PF *et al.* Presence of fetal DNA in maternal plasma and serum. *Lancet* 1997; 350: 485–7.

44. Hill M, Barrett AN, White H, Chitty LS. Uses of cell free fetal DNA in maternal circulation. *Best Pract Res Clin Obstet Gynaecol* 2012; 26: 639–54.

45. Liao GJ, Chiu RW, Lo YM. Prenatal assessment of fetal chromosomal and genetic disorders through maternal plasma DNA analysis. *Pathology* 2012; 44: 69–72.

46. Collins SL, Impney L. Prenatal diagnosis: types and techniques. *Early Hum Develop* 2012; 88: 3–8.

47. Palomba ML, Monni G, Lai R *et al.* Psychological implications and acceptability of preimplantation diagnosis. *Hum Reprod* 1994; 9: 360–2.

48. Pergament E. Preimplantation diagnosis: a patient perspective. *Prenat Diagn* 1991; 11: 493–500.

49. Farra C, Nassar AH, Usta IM *et al.* Acceptance of preimplantation genetic diagnosis for beta-thalassemia in Lebanese women with previously affected children. *Prenat Diagn* 2008; 28: 828–32.

50. Snowden C, Green JM. Preimplantation diagnosis and other reproductive options: attitudes of male and female carriers of recessive disorders. *Hum Reprod* 1997; 12: 341–50.

51. Online Mendelain Inheritance in Man (OMIM) #160900. Myotonic Dystrophy 1; DM1. Last updated 2/5/2012: www.omim.org/entry/160900

52. Brock SC. Narrative and medical genetics: on ethics and therapeutics. *Quality of Health Research* 1995; 5: 150–68.

53. Faulkner CL, Kingston HM. Knowledge, views, and experience of 25 women with myotonic dystrophy. *J Med Genet* 1998; 35: 1020–5.

54. Wiseman M, Dancyger C, Michie S. Communicating genetic risk information within families: a review. *Fam Cancer* 2010; 9: 691–703.

55. Gallo AM, Angst DB, Knafi KA. Disclosure of genetic information within families. *Am J Nurs* 2009; 109: 65–9.

56. Clarke A, Richards M, Halliday J *et al.* Genetic professional reports of non disclosure of genetic risk information within families. *Eur J Hum Genet* 2005; 13: 556–62.

57. Tibben A, Frets P, van de Kamp J *et al.* On attitudes and appreciation 6 months after predictive DNA testing for Huntington's disease in the Dutch program. *Am J Med Genet B Neuropsychiatr Genet* 1993; 43: 103–11.

58. Murakami Y, Gondo N, Okamura H, Akechi T, Uchitomi Y. Guilt from negative genetic test findings. *Am J Psychiatry* 2001; 158: 1929.

59. Ford D, Easton DF, Stratton M *et al.* Genetic heterogeneity and penetrance analysis of the *BRCA1* and *BRCA2* genes in breast cancer families. The Breast Cancer Linkage Consortium. *Am J Hum Genet* 1998; 62: 676–89.

60. Wapner RJ, Driscoll DA, Simpson JL. Integration of microarray technology into prenatal diagnosis: counselling issues generated during the NICHD clinical trial. *Prenat Diagn* 2012; 32: 396–400.

61. van der Meer LB, van Duijn E, Wolterbeek R, Tibben A. Adverse childhood experiences of persons at risk for Huntington's disease or *BRCA1/2* hereditary breast/ovarian cancer. *Clin Genet* 2012; 81: 18–23.

62. Sherman JK. Synopsis of the use of frozen human semen since 1964: state of the art of human semen banking. *Fertil Steril* 1973; 24: 397–412.

63. Cheng M. "Fertility treatment bans in Europe draw criticism." Associated Press, April 13, 2012: www.usatoday.com/news/health/story/2012-04-13/Europe-fertility-bans-limits/54250984/1

64. Klein JU, Sauer MV. Ethics in egg donation: past, present, and future. *Semin Reprod Med* 2010; 28: 322–8.

65. Armour KL. An overview of surrogacy around the world: trends, questions and ethical issues. *Nurs Womens Health* 2012; 16: 231–6.

66. Human Fertilisation and Embryology Authority. Payments for donors: www.hfea.gov.uk/500.html?fldSearchFor=donorexpenses9

67. ASRM Practice Committee. Recommendations for gamete and embryo donation: www.asrm.org/uploadedFiles/ASRM_Content/News_and_Publications/Practice_Guidelines/Guidelines_and_Minimum_Standards/2008_Guidelines_for_gamete(1).pdf

68. Heng BC. Legal and ethical issues in the international transaction of donor sperm and eggs. *J Assist Reprod Genet* 2007; 24: 107–9.

69. Sims CA, Callum P, Ray M, Iger J, Falk RE.Genetic testing of sperm donors: survey of current practices. *Fertil Steril* 2010; 94: 126–9.

70. Maron BJ, Lesser JR, Schiller NB *et al.* Implications of hypertrophic cardiomyopathy transmitted by sperm donation. *JAMA* 2009; 302: 1681–4.

71. Daar JF, Brzyski RG. Genetic screening of sperm and oocyte donors. Ethical and policy implications. *JAMA* 2009; 302: 1702–4.

72. Readings J, Blake L, Casey P, Jadva V, Golombok S. Secrecy, disclosure and everything in-between: decisions of parents of children conceived by donor insemination, egg donation and surrogacy. *Reprod Biomed Online* 2011; 22: 485–95.

73. Isaksson S, Sydsjö G, Skoog Svanberg A, Lampic C. Disclosure behaviour and intentions among 111 couples following treatment with oocytes or sperm from identity-release donors: follow-up at offspring age 1–4 years. *Hum Reprod* 2012; 27: 2998–3007.

74. Daniels KR, Grace VM, Gillett WR. Factors associated with parents' decisions to tell their adult offspring about the offspring's donor conception. *Hum Reprod* 2011; 26: 2783–90.

75. Golombok S, Readings J, Blake L *et al.* Children conceived by gamete donation: psychological adjustment and mother–child relationships at age 7. *J Fam Psychol* 2011; 25:230–9.

76. Donor Conception Network. Telling and Talking Workshops: www.donor-conception-network.org/telltalkpubs.htm

Genetic testing for infertile patients

Willem Verpoest

Introduction

It is generally accepted that 15% of couples trying to conceive are documented as having a fertility problem. The aim of this chapter is to describe the indications for genetic testing in these patients/couples, alongside other tests that will be performed to identify the cause of infertility.

The main benefit of genetic testing for patients presenting with a fertility problem is the potential identification of the cause of infertility and the associated reproductive prognosis that can be estimated on the basis of the genetic defect, if present. Other benefits include the information it provides to patients allowing them to make an informed decision on the use of *in vitro* fertilization (IVF) or intracytoplasmic sperm injection (ICSI), in association with preimplantation genetic diagnosis (PGD) where possible, or the use of alternative reproductive treatment including the use of donor gametes or zygotes. Information on the genetic status of the patient provides the basis for better understanding from both the physician's and the patient's point of view [1], allowing appropriate further medical and psychological guidance. However, with the advent of new techniques of genetic testing, including microarray analysis and next generation sequencing, both genetic and reproductive clinicians are challenged to interpret the results correctly in the light of the abundance of information that is gathered by these techniques, and to convey this information to the patient in a correct manner.

The disadvantages of genetic testing of infertile patients or couples include the cost of the testing, the implications for the individual and familial relationships (see Chapter 9 on counseling), moral and ethical objections to routine genetic testing, and the limitations in therapeutic options. Preimplantation genetic diagnosis (PGD) and prenatal diagnosis (PND) offer the patient or couple affected by or at risk of a genetic disorder the possibility to proceed to embryo selection or termination of pregnancy. However, PGD is not universally available, technically complex, expensive, and provokes moral, ethical, or religious discussion if not controversy. For those patients who consider it acceptable to perform PGD, the technique has now evolved to an established alternative for PND and is available for virtually all identifiable monogenic disorders or structural and numerical chromosomal abnormalities, similar to PND and subject to technical facilities. It is however still unclear what the exact risk is of unbalanced offspring in those patients carrying a balanced translocation. Furthermore, it is not entirely clear which translocations are at risk of or have been documented to give rise to unbalanced offspring, hence the benefit of PGD for these indications is still under debate [2].

In this chapter we aim to describe for which patients genetic testing is considered appropriate on a theoretical basis and using evidence provided in literature. It is necessary to take a thorough personal and family history of the possible presence of congenital malformations and/or chromosomal aberrations of all patients presenting at a fertility clinic. Couples should be referred for genetic advice if any hereditary condition is present, and in order to specify the appropriate genetic analyses and to counsel the patients on the diagnostic and therapeutic options. A complete clinical examination is useful in order to identify dysmorphic features, and in men to assess clinical features such as small testicular size, as found in Klinefelter syndrome, cystic fibrosis (CF), or associated congenital bilateral absence of the vasa deferens (CBAVD). Clinical examination and ultrasound of the

Textbook of Human Reproductive Genetics, eds Karen Sermon and Stéphane Viville. Published by Cambridge University Press.
© Cambridge University Press 2014.

uterus and adnexae can reveal dysmorphic features in females that are potentially secondary to hereditary conditions, such as streak ovaries in Turner syndrome or Müllerian abnormalities of the renal and genital system in women with Beckwith–Wiedemann syndrome. If in doubt, advice by a clinical geneticist is essential.

Karyotyping

Karyotyping of infertile females

The prevalence of chromosomal abnormalities in women with regular ovulation, as reflected by a regular menstrual cycle, is reported to be 0.58% [3]. This compares well with a background prevalence of chromosome abnormalities of 0.79%, as observed in a population of newborn females [4]. Surprisingly, Papanikolaou *et al.* found a higher incidence of chromosomal abnormalities in women who had conceived before (multigravida) compared to women who had never conceived (nulligravida). The sample size and the absolute risk of chromosomal abnormalities in this study were too limited to allow any clinical conclusions [3].

One needs to take into account that a higher detection rate of chromosome abnormalities can be caused by different techniques; for example, when low-level sex chromosome mosaicism is included in the analysis, karyotype abnormalities increase from normal to 9.8% in females enrolled in an ICSI program [5].

The prevalence of chromosome abnormalities is considered to be higher in women with primary amenorrhea, premature ovarian insufficiency (POI), and recurrent pregnancy loss; hence, for these women, karyotyping is commonly requested [6]. A number of publications suggest a comparable prevalence of karyotype abnormalities in different treatment groups. The prevalence of karyotype abnormalities ranges from 2.0% in women undergoing intrauterine insemination (IUI) [7] to 1.8–2.4% in women undergoing IVF [8, 9], and in female patients enrolled in an ICSI program the prevalence ranges from 1.1% to 9.8%, including low-level sex chromosome mosaicism, as previously mentioned [5]. A more recent analysis showed a prevalence of 1.92% karyotype abnormalities in women at intake and prior to IVF/ICSI treatment, the prevalence being higher in multiparous women compared to nulliparous women [10].

Fetal wastage is increased in couples where one of the partners is carrying a balanced reciprocal or Robertsonian chromosomal translocation. It is unclear whether female carriers of balanced autosomal translocations carry an increased risk of reduced ovarian response [11]. Specified autosomal translocations associated with POI have not been published. Ovarian insufficiency in these patients is rare. On the other hand, defective follicular production or excessive apoptosis has been reported in patients with a balanced translocation involving the long arm of the X chromosome, referred to as the critical region [12]. Patients with structural abnormalities should be counseled carefully about the risk of passing on unbalanced translocations at conception: typically the risk of finding an unbalanced translocation is around 56% [13] in carriers of a Robertsonian translocation and 80% [14] in carriers of a reciprocal translocation. For more information on the molecular mechanisms of infertility in carriers of chromosomal abnormalities, see Chapter 7.

Women carrying extra X chromosomes are at risk of reduced ovarian reserve and POI. Assessment of ovarian reserve is essential whenever numerical chromosomal translocations are involved. Women lacking an X chromosome (Turner syndrome) are known to be infertile with streak ovaries [15, 16]. In these women, analysis of the ovarian reserve is important in order to assess whether any ovarian response is to be expected, either spontaneously or by exogenous ovarian stimulation. The most sensitive test currently available is analysis of serum anti-Müllerian hormone, which is produced by the granulosa cells surrounding the oocytes and is quantitively related to the number of oocytes available [17]. Alternative testing includes early follicular phase serum follicle-stimulating hormone (FSH) analysis, early follicular phase antral follicle count on ultrasound, and ovarian challenge tests by short exogenous gonadotrophin stimulation. In cases where the ovarian reserve cannot be accurately estimated, ovarian biopsy via endoscopy can be performed in order to perform histological analysis for the presence of primordial follicles.

Premature ovarian failure (POF) is diagnosed when the ovaries become non-responsive in terms of developing mature oocytes by either endogenous or exogenous gonadotrophins before the age of 40 years. Whereas menopause is a comparable ovarian status, POF is not uniformly associated with side-effects, such as skin dryness and hot flushes, and menstrual cycles may rarely be ovulatory. The etiology of POF is diverse. Pathogenic mechanisms that may lead to the development of this heterogeneous disorder include genetic, autoimmune, metabolic, infectious, and iatrogenic causes. Among genetic causes of POF, chromosome abnormalities are the most common. Between 2.5 and 13% of the women with POF have an abnormal karyotype. Premature ovarian failure has most commonly been linked to X-chromosome abnormalities, ranging from numerical defects, deletions, and X-autosome translocations to isochromosomes. A higher frequency of X-chromosome aneuploidy in POF patients compared to the general population group is reported, in particular with Turner syndrome, XO/XX mosaics, deletions, inversions, and X-autosomal translocations. These findings confirm the importance of the X chromosome in POF etiology. In addition, many gene mutations have also been found to be involved in POF development, among them mutations in *FMR1/2, FSHR, BMP15, LHR, INHA, FOXL2, FOXO3, ERα, SF1, Erβ*, and *CYP19A1* genes. Despite the description of several candidate genes, the cause of POF remains undetermined in most women with POF. A genetic factor is a non-reversible cause of POF and so karyotyping is an important part of the diagnostic work-up for women with POF [18].

In summary, the prevalence of chromosome abnormalities may be increased in female patients enrolled in fertility treatment, but not necessarily in those with normal ovulation and normal ovarian reserve test results. There is still an ongoing debate as to whether karyotyping should be part of the comprehensive work-up of patients presenting with a fertility problem, taking into account therapeutic options such as PGD and PND. However, in the absence of strong literature data and because of health care cost issues, karyotyping for female patients suffering with infertility is currently not indicated for normoovulatory women or women with an obvious cause for ovulatory irregularity such as hypothalamic pituitary insufficiency or polycystic ovarian syndrome. Karyotyping is justified for couples suffering with recurrent miscarriage (see below), recurrent implantation failure (see below), primary amenorrhea, POF, poor ovarian reserve, or with a personal or family history of numerical or structural chromosomal abnormalities.

Karyotyping in recurrent miscarriage

To provide guidance on the investigation of couples with recurrent miscarriage (RM), the use of well-described definitions is essential. The World Health Organization (WHO) defines miscarriage as the spontaneous loss of a clinical pregnancy before 20 completed weeks of gestational age or the loss of an embryo/fetus weighing less than 400 g. However, this definition can vary between different countries where a spontaneous abortion is stated to occur before the 20th week or up to weeks 24, 26, or 28 of pregnancy. Very importantly, a lower threshold for defining a clinical pregnancy is set by most authorities at the level of an early ultrasound, and requires the ultrasonographic or histopathologic evidence [19].

Recurrent miscarriage is defined as two or more consecutive failed pregnancies by the American Congress of Obstetricians and Gynecologists (ACOG) [20]. The European Society of Human Reproduction and Embryology (ESHRE) [21] and the Royal College of Obstetricians and Gynaecologists (RCOG) [22] use three or more consecutive miscarriages as the criterion for defining RM. The guidelines of the Dutch Society of Obstetrics and Gynecology (NVOG) [23] and the American Society for Reproductive Medicine (ASRM) [24] define RM as "two or more failed pregnancies," and do not include "consecutive" in their definition. As a result of this discrepancy, it is unclear in daily clinical practice which couples should be diagnosed with RM and when to start the diagnostic work-up [25]. The incidence of RM reported in literature largely depends on the use of these aforementioned criteria, and therefore varies widely from less than 5% for two consecutive miscarriages to 1% for three or more miscarriages.

Very importantly, the apparent causes of RM do not appear more prevalent after three or more miscarriages than after two miscarriages [26]. Therefore, it is generally accepted to start diagnostic investigations following two miscarriages. With regards to genetic testing in both partners, there is an ongoing debate on age limits in relation to RM and the value of karyotyping with respect to the incidence of abnormalities. Franssen *et al.* identified additional factors influencing the probability of carrier status in couples with two or more miscarriages [27]. Four factors, namely low maternal age at second miscarriage, a history of three or more miscarriages, and a history of two or more miscarriages in a brother or sister or the parents of either partner increase the probability of carrier status. The prevalence of structural balanced chromosomal abnormalities in either partner of a couple experiencing RM increases according to the number of miscarriages; 2.2% after one miscarriage, 4.8% after two miscarriages, and 5.2% after three miscarriages. However, the frequency of structural chromosomal abnormalities did not differ between those patients suffering consecutive versus those patients suffering non-consecutive miscarriages [25]. A decision-analytic model into the health/economic value of karyotyping couples with RM shows that selective karyotyping after two miscarriages (i.e. when the second miscarriage tissue had a normal karyotype or balanced structural chromosomal abnormality) rather than universal karyotyping after two miscarriages is a cost-saving strategy, with increasing cost savings as maternal age advances [28]. This is the result of the increasing frequency of numerical chromosomal abnormalities in miscarriages with advancing age, hence more embryonic aneuploidy not related to parental chromosomal abnormalities.

In the absence of an identified cause of miscarriage, including structural or numerical chromosomal abnormalities, the risk of another miscarriage is not significantly increased. It is therefore of importance to perform karyotyping in order to seek reassurance for the couple [29]. On the other hand, a number of authors have argued that the cumulative chance of having a healthy child is equal for couples carrying a structural or numerical chromosomal abnormality, and that PGD is not universally indicated [30].

Karyotyping in recurrent implantation failure

Recurrent implantation failure is by definition the failure of embryo implantation in three or more consecutive treatment cycles with IVF/ICSI and embryo transfer. There is an ongoing debate on the exact definition of recurrent implantation failure and the question of whether or not to accept a number of embryos that failed to implant as the threshold (e.g. 10 embryos failed to implant) [31]. In couples presenting with recurrent implantation failure the prevalence of chromosome abnormalities on karyotyping is 2.11%, more specifically 2.73% in women with recurrent implantation failure compared to 1.89% in male partners of women suffering from recurrent implantation failure [32]. This is comparable to older data by Stern *et al.* who described chromosome abnormality rates of 2.53%, 2.73%, and 2.26% respectively in couples, females, and male partners experiencing recurrent implantation failure in IVF/ICSI [31]. The

prevalence of chromosomal abnormalities increases even more when additional explanatory factors are taken into account. In women with recurrent implantation failure with known secondary infertility and RM, the chromosomal abnormality rate is as high as 9.1%. In women with documented infertility and recurrent implantation failure the prevalence of chromosomal abnormalities is reported to be 6.1% [32]. In analogy to RM and because of a high prevalence of chromosomal abnormalities in these couples, karyotyping is justified following recurrent implantation failure of good quality embryos, a threshold for the number of failed embryo implantations being under debate.

Karyotyping in infertile males

Chromosomal abnormalities are reported in 2.1–8.9% of males attending a fertility clinic [33]. This compares to approximately 1% chromosomal abnormalities in the general population, as mentioned before, and even 0% in a population of men with normospermia studied by Stegen *et al.* [34]. Van der Ven *et al.* report a prevalence of chromosomal abnormalities of 2.0–3.3% in males undergoing ICSI treatment [35]. The prevalence of constitutional chromosomal aberrations increases overall in infertile males as sperm counts decrease. Sex chromosome abnormalities such as 47,XXY and 47,XYY are proportionally more prevalent in males with azoospermia than males with oligospermia, whereas autosomal aberrations such as Robertsonian and reciprocal translocations are more frequent in oligospermic males, see also Chapter 7.

Robertsonian and reciprocal translocations in men are associated with oligospermia [36]. The spermatogenic defect in these men varies widely, ranging from extreme oligospermia and even azoospermia to normozoospermia. The reduced reproductive potential is characterized by failed conception based on a low sperm count, in contrast with female carriers of balanced translocations in whom RM is the predominant feature.

In oligozoospermia, chromosomal abnormality rates vary between 1.5% and 4.6% and seem to be directly related to the sperm concentration [34, 36]. The prevalence of chromosomal abnormalities in men with extreme oligozoospermia and azoospermia in couples requesting ICSI was reported to be as high as 24% [37]. Other studies report karyotype abnormalities in 13.7–16.0% [36, 38, 39]. Chromosomal abnormalities are more prevalent in testicular sperm of men with azoospermia compared with ejaculated sperm, sex chromosome aneuploidy being the most prominent [40]. This increases the risk of chromosome abnormalities in offspring of these patients undergoing ICSI, especially when ICSI with non-ejaculated sperm is performed. This does not apply for Klinefelter patients [41].

Klinefelter syndrome is associated with testicular atrophy and is the most common genetic cause of non-obstructive azoospermia. Spermatogenesis may be preserved to some extent in these patients, explaining why in Klinefelter patients undergoing ICSI and testicular sperm extraction (TESE) spermatozoa were obtained in 48% [42]. The clinical reproductive outcome per treatment cycle is hard to estimate in view of the rarity of reports, but is estimated not to exceed 10% [43]. Clinical examination by orchidometry remains important in these patients in order to determine feasibility of testicular biopsy, in spite of the fact that testicular volume and/or serum FSH levels are not reliable predictors of spermatogenesis [42]. Spontaneous conception is rare but has been reported [41]. In spite of a reported increased aneuploidy rate of embryos conceived after ICSI/TESE in Klinefelter patients [44], abnormal karyotypes in the children conceived by these techniques are uncommon [43]. The value of PGD and PND for these patients is therefore questionable.

In men with azoospermia, sex chromosome abnormalities (for example, 47,XXY, mosaics of 46,XY/47,XXX) were present in 1.9–22.1%, while autosomal abnormalities were found in only 0.6–3.7% of such men. Among oligozoospermic men, sex and autosomal abnormalities are found in 0.9–3.6% and 0.9–4.9%, respectively [36].

Karyotyping is not routinely recommended in men presenting at an infertility clinic. However, in men with reduced sperm quality the prevalence of chromosomal abnormalities is increased, which may have significant implications for future family planning, reproductive treatment, and risk of inheriting a chromosomal abnormality in the offspring. The debate is still ongoing as to what threshold level of sperm concentration, motility, and/or morphology ought to be used in order to advise karyotyping and to what extent this may be justified from a health/economic point of view. Abnormal results of genetic analysis may have a major impact on the choice and outcome of treatment.

In some cases the genotype may present a very poor prognosis for sperm recovery. If the male partner is a carrier of an autosomal structural chromosomal aberration, the success rate of ICSI is lowered. In cases of a sex chromosome aneuploidy the success rate of the treatment is variable. The implications are variable but may involve alternative treatment options such as the use of donor gametes or PGD. The use of donor gametes may avoid costly IVF/ICSI treatments that carry a minimum chance of succeeding, hence saving both the patients and society unnecessary expenses. On the counterside, the risk of conceiving a child with an unbalanced autosomal chromosome problem or sex chromosome abnormality is very limited. It is currently unknown whether and which chromosomal abnormalities affect male fertility significantly, and there is a fierce debate on the pros and cons of PGD for structural or numerical chromosomal abnormalities [30]. By extrapolation, the cost-effectiveness of karyotyping from this angle is not clearly justified.

The American Society for Reproductive Medicine (ASRM) currently recommends karyotyping and analysis for Yq deletion in men with non-obstructive azoospermia. In addition, men with azoospermia as a result of testicular failure, such as in bilateral testicular atrophy, elevated serum FSH and normal or low serum testosterone), karyotyping is advised. As to oligospermic men there is no consensus. A study by Dull et al. confirms that karyotype abnormalities are most prevalent in men with non-obstructive azoospermia, especially if associated with hypergonadotrophism, but that non-azoospermic men are at low risk (2.3% (CI 1.4–3.9)) of having an abnormality [45].

DNA analysis

Analysis for CF gene mutations

Cystic fibrosis is the most common autosomal recessive condition in northern Europeans with a carrier rate of 1 in 25 Caucasians. It is caused by a mutation in the CF transmembrane conductance regulator (*CFTR*) gene, a gene that is widely expressed in the epithelial cells of a number of organs, including the reproductive tract. At present it is possible to identify up to 90% of CF carriers in the Caucasian population. Congenital absence of the vas deferens (CBAVD) is a type of obstructive azoospermia in which both vasa deferentia are absent, and the seminal vesicles are atrophic or absent as are large portions of the epididymis. This condition is most commonly found following the diagnosis of azoospermia in otherwise normal men, either on clinical examination or by ultrasound of the scrotum. In men with homozygous CF, 97–98% are found to have CBAVD. Conversely, in men that have been diagnosed with CBAVD and who are not known with clinical CF, the prevalence of a mutation for the *CFTR* gene is 78.9%, and in those cases where no mutation is identified, there remains a suspicion of a yet unknown mutation or combination of alleles. Seventy-one percent of CBAVD patients are reported to carry a mutation on both *CTFR* genes, 15.9% on one *CFTR* gene, and in 13.5% of CBAVD patients no mutation was found on either *CTFR* gene according to a study by Claustres *et al.* [46]. Most CBAVD patients do not have lung or pancreatic disease because the mutation(s) they carry may be milder and they may have a different tissue-specific effect [47]. Spermatogenesis is normal in most cases. However, a mutation in the *CFTR* gene has also been associated with non-obstructive spermatogenesis problems, including oligospermia, teratospermia, and asthenospermia [48]. Cystic fibrosis testing is indicated in men with both obstructive and non-obstructive azoospermia, and in view of its association with impaired sperm quality, also in men with oligo-, astheno-, and teratozoospermia.

Men with normozoospermia do not routinely need CF testing. Donors of sperm need CF testing, on the basis of the high prevalence of carriership in the general population and to avoid transmission to offspring. This advice is subject to ethic and moral debate, and some countries will not accept routine testing for CF in infertility patients or gamete donors. Couples that are entering into IVF treatment are allowed to request CF testing of one of the partners, in order to identify couples at risk and offer counseling for PGD or PND if and where appropriate. Men with azoospermia that is not attributable to mechanical factors or secondary to chemotherapy or radiotherapy are to be offered testing for CF in order to: (1) confirm for obvious reasons CF status when CBAVD is diagnosed; and (2) identify those men that are at risk of transmitting CF to their offspring in reproductive treatment and justify CF testing in the female, hence allowing to propose PGD or PND to these patients. When these conditions are known or suspected appropriate genetic counseling should be offered, as discussed in Chapter 9.

Analysis for fragile X mental retardation 1 (*FMR1*) gene mutation (fragile X syndrome; FXS)

Fragile X syndrome (FXS; OMIM #309550) has a prevalence of 1 in 4000 males and 1 in 6000 females and is the most common cause of mental retardation in men. It is caused by a dynamic CGG repeat expansion in the 5′ untranslated region of the *FMR1* gene that codes for the fragile X mental retardation protein (FMRP) [49]. A premutation is defined as more than 55 and less than 200 CGG repeats. In female carriers of the *FMR1* gene premutation, the *FMR1* gene remains transciptionally active and FMRP is produced; however, above a certain critical threshold of unstable expansion of CGG repeat in this gene there is an increased risk of POF [50, 51] that is non-linear in effect and is a result of a *FMR1* mRNA gain-of-function toxicity [52]. The lower limit of the premutation above which there is a clinical risk for POF remains under discussion. The average age at menopause is 47.87 years for premutation carriers and 52.96 years for non-carriers, which is important data in the counseling of these patients. A number of studies have suggested a relationship between triplet repeats on the *FMR1* gene and ovarian response, and have even suggested DNA analysis for the *FMR1* gene mutation as a screening test for ovarian response. Women with an expansion of repeats on the *FMR1* gene – when other ovarian reserve tests are considered suboptimal and, as a deduction of this, the risk of POI may be increased – may be eligible to cryopreserve eggs as a way of fertility preservation [53]. This approach is still very much under debate. It is clear, however, that in the comprehensive clinical approach of women with reduced ovarian reserve, or poor ovarian response at ovarian stimulation, DNA analysis for the *FMR1* gene is important.

Analysis for azoospermia factor (AZF) deletion (Yq deletion)

A microdeletion of a DNA sequence in the long arm of the Y chromosome (Yq11; azoospermia factor (AZF) region), also known as Yq deletion, is associated with extreme oligoasthenoteratozoospermia (OAT) or azoospermia. This deletion cannot be traced by conventional karyotyping or fluoresence *in situ* hybridization (FISH) but requires molecular techniques such as polymerase chain reaction (PCR). The AZF region can be divided in *AZFa*, *AZFb*, and *AZFc*. Deletions occur most commonly in the *AZFc* region. Spermatozoa have not been found in men with large deletions including and extending beyond the *AZFc* region. The Y chromosome is an important carrier of genetic information for the control of spermatogenesis. The prevalence of a microdeletion is higher in azoospermic than oligospermic men. The incidence of microdeletions in these patients varies from 1 to 55% with a mean of 8% depending on the inclusion criteria and the applied diagnostic technology [54, 55]. *De novo* microdeletions in Yq have been reported with a prevalence of between 3 and 18% of men studied. There is a high likelihood of transmission of these deletions, and hence infertility, to male offspring by applying ICSI [56]; however, infertility is not an absolute finding for all Yq deletions [57]. Van Golde *et al.* report that Y-deleted men undergoing ICSI had a significantly lower fertilization rate when compared with a control group without this genetic disorder (55% (95% CI 41–69%) vs. 71% (95% CI 67–74%); $P < 0.01$); however, no significant differences in pregnancy, implantation, or live birth rates were found [55].

It has now been reported that single copy gene mutations on the X chromosome may be involved in male infertility as well. Any mutation or deletion, be it inherited or *de novo*, is potentially related to infertility in men. X-linked mutations causing male infertility will not spread through the population. Mutations causing infertility are expected to feature throughout the genome, and are *de novo* in a majority of cases. It is, however, difficult to distinguish between a polymorphism and a mutation [58]. Routine testing for deletions or mutations other than the Yq deletion is therefore not considered relevant in infertile men.

Other genetic tests

Gamete donors

In patients presenting for gamete donation, either oocyte or sperm donation, it is considered useful to request karyotyping, although this is not common practice in all fertility centers. In view of the risk of inheriting autosomal recessive disorders, testing for the most common recessive disorders should be considered.

The European Cell and Tissue Directives [59] do not explicitly request genetic testing for donors of reproductive cells, which includes patients starting a reproductive treatment with autologous reproductive cells/gametes. They advise:

That genetic screening for autosomal recessive genes known to be prevalent, according to international scientific evidence, in the donor's ethnic background and an assessment of the risk of transmission of inherited conditions known to be present in the family must be carried out, after consent is obtained. Complete information must be provided, in accordance with the requirements in force in Member States. Complete information on the associated risk and on the measures undertaken for its mitigation must be communicated and clearly explained to the recipient [59].

The American Society for Reproductive Medicine (ASRM) and the Society for Assisted Reproductive Technology (SART) issue Practice Committee Guidelines on the management of gamete and embryo donation including on genetic testing [60]. Genetic screening for heritable disorders is advised in potential sperm donors. Other genetic testing should be performed as indicated by the donor's ethnic background and after obtaining a medical and family history. The Practice Committees of the ASRM and the SART do not consider chromosomal analysis advisable for all donors [60]. They provide no specific advice with regard to oocyte donors except for screening for fragile X carrier status at the discretion of the individual program. However, and this applies logically to all gamete donors, the donor should not have any major Mendelian disorder, neither autosomal dominant including late-onset disorders such as Huntington disorder, X-linked, nor autosomal recessive disorders. Heterozygous recessive conditions can not necessarily be excluded if recipients are not carriers. There should not be a significant familial disease with a major genetic component, particularly in first-degree relatives. The donor should not carry an identified karyotypic abnormality, but karyotyping in otherwise healthy subjects is optional because of the small risk of abnormalities.

Donors that belong to a high-risk group should be tested to determine carrier status for those disorders they are at risk of carrying. Heterozygosity for these, often autosomal recessive, disorders is not necessarily an absolute contra-indication to gamete donation;

Table 10.1 Overview of prevalence of karyotype abnormalities in infertile patients

Indication	Prevalence of chromosomal abnormalities on karyotype	Ref. [no.]
Infertile females		
Unselected newborns	0.85%	Nielsen and Wohlert [4]
Normo-ovulatory women before IVF/ICSI	0.58%	Papanikolaou et al. [3]
Females at start of IVF/ICSI	1.92%	Clementini et al. [10]
Females undergoing IUI	2.0%	Mattei et al. [7]
Females undergoing IVF	1.8–2.4%	Hens et al. [8]; Schreurs et al. [9]
Females undergoing ICSI	1.1–9.8%	Gekas et al. [5]
Female partner ICSI couple	3.3–5.4%	Meschede et al. [62]
Infertile males		
Normospermia	0%	Stegen et al. [34]
General male population	1.0%	Testart et al. [63]
Moderate oligozoospermia	1.5%	Stegen et al. [34]
Oligozoospermia	4.6%	Van Assche et al. [36]
Extreme oligozoospermia	1.2%	Stegen et al. [34]
Severe oligozoospermia	2.2%	Stegen et al. [34]
Total ICSI men	1.5%	Stegen et al. [34]
Men attending fertility clinic	2.1–8.9%	Irvine [33]
Male partner ICSI couple	2.0–3.3%	van der Ven et al. [35]
Males at start of IVF/ICSI	2.02%	Clementini et al. [10]
Azoospermia	13.7%	Van Assche et al. [36]
Non-obstructive azoospermia	16%	Vincent et al. [38]; Kumtepe et al. [39]
Recurrent miscarriage		
After one miscarriage	2.2%	van den Boogaard et al. [25]
After two miscarriages	4.8%	van den Boogaard et al. [25]
After three miscarriages	5.2%	van den Boogaard et al. [25]
Recurrent implantation failure		
RIF women	2.73%	Stern et al. (1999) [31]
RIF women	2.52%	De Sutter et al. (2012) [32]
RIF men	2.26%	Stern et al. (1999) [31]
RIF men	1.89%	De Sutter et al. (2012) [32]
RIF couples	2.53%	Stern et al. (1999) [31]
RIF couples	2.11%	De Sutter et al. (2012) [32]
High order implantation failure	10.77%	Raziel et al. (2002) [64]

ICSI, intracytoplasmic sperm injection; IUI, intrauterine insemination; IVF, *in vitro* fertilization; RIF, recurrent implantation failure.

however, it may be inappropriate not only in relation to the gamete receptor but also for the genetic status of the future child. The American Congress of Obstetricians and Gynecologists (ACOG) issues a number of Committee Opinions on preconception testing for certain ethnic populations [20]. This logically includes gamete donors although carriership, as mentioned before, does not necessarily exclude gamete donation. Some ethnic groups may not agree to gamete donation for moral or religious reasons.

Genetic testing for specific populations

Certain autosomal recessive disorders are more prevalent in specific populations. Individuals of Eastern European Jewish (Ashkenazi) descent are recommended to be offered preconception carrier screening for Tay–Sachs disease, Canavan disease, CF, and familial dysautonomia, and, if available, these individuals can also apply for screening for mucolipidosis IV, Niemann–Pick disease type A, Fanconi anemia, Bloom syndrome, and Gaucher's disease.

Non-Hispanic Caucasians should be offered CF screening. Individuals of African, Mediterranean, and Southeast Asian origin should be offered screening for the thalassemias and sickle cell disease [20].

Direct genetic testing for specific disorders

Other genetic conditions may be responsible for fertility problems, but testing for these conditions is only indicated when strong clinical arguments exist.

In female infertility, renal and genital Müllerian abnormalities (abnormalities arising from embryological malformations in the Müllerian duct system) can be found in patients with various genetic syndromes, such as the Beckwith–Wiedemann syndrome or the Mayer–Rokitansky–Küster–Hauser (MRKH) syndrome. These cases are rare and are usually associated with other pathognomic clinical features that can be detected by experienced clinical geneticists. Primary amenorrhea associated with streak ovaries on ultrasound or laparoscopy can be found in women with Turner syndrome. The androgen insensitivity syndrome (a.k.a. testicular feminization) is caused by a mutation in the androgen receptor resulting in androgen insensitivity, causing a female phenotype and a male genotype.

In male infertility, poor sperm quality can be caused by uncommon hereditary conditions such as myotonic dystrophy. Hypogonadotrophic hypogonadism can be caused by Kallmann syndrome, which can be X-linked, autosomal recessive as well as autosomal dominant and can be responsible for primary amenorrhea and dysovulation in women on the basis of the same pathophysiology. Beckwith–Wiedemann syndrome in males is associated with cryptorchidism, as can be Noonan syndrome. Spinal bulbar muscular atrophy (SBMA) is an X-linked neuromuscular disorder leading to testicular atrophy secondary to muscular weakness.

Conclusion

An ESHRE consensus paper suggests performing karyotyping only for those couples with a threshold risk of over 2.2%, which is consistent with the risk of chromosomal abnormalities in parental karyotypes of couples having suffered one clinical miscarriage [61]. If the same threshold were to be used for males, karyotyping is advised in men with severe oligospermia and azoospermia (Table 10.1).

The decision to perform karyotyping in defined patient groups depends on: (1) the value of knowing whether a genetic problem is underlying infertility; and (2) the possibility of avoiding miscarriages or affected children by such techniques as PGD and PND.

Genetic testing for monogenic disorders is largely determined by the personal and family history of either partner of the couple presenting for preconceptional investigations, but in specific populations and subject to the incidence of certain monogenic conditions and the availability of laboratory experience, genetic testing is to be advised.

References

1. Hastings R, de Wert G, Fowler B et al. The challenging landscape of genetic testing and its impact on clinical and laboratory services and research in Europe. *Eur J Hum Genet* 2012; 20: 911–16.

2. Stephenson MD, Goddijn M. A critical look at the evidence does not support PGD for translocation carriers with a history of recurrent losses. *Fertil Steril* 2010; 95: e1.

3. Papanikolaou EG, Vernaeve V, Kolibianakis E et al. Is chromosome analysis mandatory in the initial investigation of normoovulatory women seeking infertility treatment? *Hum Reprod* 2005; 20: 2899–903.

4. Nielsen J, Wohlert M. Chromosome abnormalities among 34910 newborn children: results from 13-year incidence study in Arhus, Denmark. *Hum Genet* 1991; 87; 81–3.

5. Gekas J, Thepot F, Turleau C et al. Chromosomal factors of infertility in candidate couples for ICSI: an equal risk of constitutional aberrations in women and men. *Hum Reprod* 2001; 16: 82–90.

6. ESHRE Capri Workshop Group. Optimal use of infertility diagnostic tests and treatments. *Hum Reprod* 2000; 15: 723–32.

7. Mattei JF, Mattei MG, Moreau N et al. Chromosome studies in 1042 women before artificial insemination with donor semen. In *Human Artificial Insemination and Semen Preservation*, Eds G David, Price W S; New York, NY: Plenum Press, 1980.

8. Hens L, Bonduelle M, Liebaers I, Devroey P, Van Steirteghem, AC. Chromosome aberrations in 500 couples referred for *in-vitro* fertilization or related fertility treatment. *Hum Reprod* 1988; 3: 451–7.

9. Schreurs A, Legius E, Meuleman C, Fryns JP, D'Hooghe TM. Increased frequency of chromosomal abnormalities in female partners of couples undergoing *in vitro* fertilization or intracytoplasmic sperm injection. *Fertil Steril* 2000; 74: 94–6.

10. Clementini E, Palka C, Iezzi I *et al.* Prevalence of chromosomal abnormalities in 2078 infertile couples referred for assisted reproductive techniques. *Hum Reprod* 2005; 20: 437–42.

11. Chen SH, Escudero T, Cekleniak NA *et al.* Patterns of ovarian response to gonadotropin stimulation in female carriers of balanced translocation. *Fertil Steril* 2005; 83: 1504–9.

12. Schlessinger D, Herrera L, Crisponi L *et al.* Genes and translocations involved in POF. *Am J Med Genet* 2002; 111: 328–33.

13. Keymolen K, Staessen C, Verpoest W *et al.* A proposal for reproductive counselling in carriers of Robertsonian translocations: 10 years of experience with preimplantation genetic diagnosis. *Hum Reprod* 2009; 24: 2365–7.

14. Harper J, Boelaert K, Geraedts J *et al.* ESHRE PGD Consortium data collection V: Cycles from January to December 2002 with pregnancy follow-up to October 2003. *Hum Reprod* 2006; 21: 3–21.

15. Laml T, Preyer O, Umek W, Hegstschlager M, Hanzal H. Genetic disorders in premature ovarian failure. *Hum Reprod Update* 2002; 8: 483–91.

16. Sybert VP, McCauley E. Turner's syndrome. *N Engl J Med* 2004; 16; 351: 1227–38.

17. Lie Fong S, Visser JA, Welt CK *et al.* Serum anti-Müllerian hormone levels in healhy females: a nomogram raging from infancy to adulthood. *J Clin Endocrin Metab* 2012; 97: 4650–5.

18. Cordts EB, Christofolini DM, Dos Santos AA, Genetic aspects of premature ovarian failure: a literature review. *Arch Gynecol Obstet* 2011; 283: 635–43.

19. Zegers-Hochschild F, Adamson GD, de Mouzon J *et al.* International Committee for Monitoring Assisted Reproductive Technology (ICMART) and the World Health Organization (WHO) revised glossary of ART terminology. *Fertil Steril* 2009; 92: 1520–4.

20. American Congress of Obstetricians and Gynecologists: www.acog.org

21. European Society of Human Reproduction and Embryology: www.eshre.eu

22. Royal College of Obstetricans and Gynaecologists: www.rcog.org.uk

23. Dutch Society of Obstetrics and Gynecology: www.nvog.nl

24. American Society for Reproductive Medicine: www.asrm.org

25. van den Boogaard E, Hermens RPMG, Verhoeve HR *et al.* Selective karyotyping in recurrent miscarriage: are recommended guidelines adopted in daily practice? *Hum Reprod* 2011; 26: 1965–70.

26. Jaslow RJ, Carney JL, Kutteh WH. Diagnostic factors identified in 1020 women with two versus three or more recurrent pregnancy losses. *Fertil Steril* 2010; 93: 1234–43.

27. Franssen MT, Korevaar JC, Leschot NJ. Selective chromosome analysis in couples with two or more miscarriages: case-control study? *BMJ* 2005; 332: 759–63.

28. Bernardi LA, Plunkett BA, Stephenson MD. Is chromosome testing of the second miscarriage cost saving? A decision analysis of selective versus universal recurrent pregnancy loss evaluation. *Fertil Steril* 2012; 98: 156–61.

29. Saravelos SH, Li TC. Unexplained miscarriage: how can we explain it? *Hum Reprod* 2012; 27: 1882–6.

30. Stephenson M, Goddijn M. A critical look at the evidence does not support PGD for translocation carriers with a history of recurrent losses. *Fertil Steril* 2011; 95: e1.

31. Stern C, Pertile M, Norris H, Hale L, Baker HWG. Chromosome translocations in couples with in-vitro fertilization implantation failure. *Hum Reprod* 1999; 14: 2097–101.

32. De Sutter P, Stadhouders R, Dutré M, Gerris J, Dhont M. Prevalence of chromosomal abnormalities and timing of karyotype analysis in patients with recurrent implantation failure (RIF) following assisted reproduction. *Facts Views Vis ObGyn* 2012; 4: 59–65.

33. Irvine DS. Epidemiology and aetiology of male infertility. *Hum Reprod* 1998; 13(Suppl 1): 33–44.

34. Stegen C, van Rumste MME, Mol BWJ, Koks CAM. The value of chromosomal analysis in oligozoospermic men. *Fertil Steril* 2012; 98: 1438–42.

35. van der Ven K, Peschka B, Montag M *et al.* Increased frequency of congenital chromosomal aberrations in female partners of couples undergoing intracytoplasmic sperm injection. *Hum Reprod* 1998; 13: 48–54.

36. Van Assche E, Bonduelle M, Tournaye H *et al.* Cytogenetics of infertile men. *Hum Reprod* 1996; 11 (Suppl 4): 1–24.

37. Dohle GR, Halley DJ, Van Hemel JO *et al.* Genetic risk factors in infertile men with severe oligozoospermia and azoospermia. *Hum Reprod* 2002; 17: 13–16.

38. Vincent MC, Daudin M, De MP *et al.* Cytogenetic investigations of infertile men with low sperm counts: a 25-year experience. *J Androl* 2002; 23: 18–22; discussion 44–5.

39. Kumtepe Y, Beyazyurek C, Cinar C *et al.* A genetic survey of 1935 Turkish men with severe male factor infertility. *Reprod Biomed Online* 2009; 18: 465–74.

40. Palermo GD, Colombero LT, Hariprashad JJ, Schlegel PN, Rosenwaks Z. Chromosome analysis of epididymal and testicular sperm in azoospermic patients undergoing ICSI. *Hum Reprod* 2002; 17: 570–5.

41. Maiburg M, Repping S, Giltay J. The genetic origin of Klinefelter syndrome and its effect on spermatogenesis. *Fertil Steril* 2012; 98: 253–60.

42. Vernaeve V, Staessen C, Verheyen G *et al.* Can biological or clinical parameters predict testicular sperm recovery in 47, XXY Klinefelter's syndrome patients? *Hum Reprod* 2004; 19: 1135–9.

43. Fullerton G, Hamilton M, Maheshwari A. Should non-mosaic Klinefelter syndrome men be labeled as infertile in 2009? *Hum Reprod* 2010; 25: 588–97.

44. Staessen C, Tournaye H, Van Assche E *et al.* PGD in 47,XXY Klinefelter's syndrome patients. *Hum Reprod Update* 2003; 9: 319–30.

45. Dull EC, Groen H, van Ravenswaaij-Arts CMA *et al.* The prevalence of chromosomal abnormalities in subgroups of infertile men. *Hum Reprod* 2011; 27: 36–43.

46. Claustres M, Guittard C, Bozon D *et al.* Spectrum of CFTR mutations in cystic fibrosis and in congenital absence of the vas deferens in France. *Hum Mutat* 2000 16: 143–56.

47. Cuppens H, Cassiman JJ. CFTR mutations and polymorphisms in male infertility. *Int J Androl* 2004; 27: 251–6.

48. Chen H, Ruan YC, Xu WM, Chen J, Chan HC. Regulation of male fertility by CTFR and implications in male infertility. *Hum Reprod Update* 2012; 18: 703–13.

49. De Caro JJ, Dominguez C, Sherman SL. Reproductive health of adolescent girls who carry the FMR1 premutation: expected phenotype based on current knowledge of fragile X-associated primary ovarian insufficiency. *Ann NY Acad Sci* 2008; 11: 99–111.

50. Fryns P. The female and the fragile X. A study of 144 obligate female carriers. *Am J Med Genet* 1986; 23: 157–69.

51. Murray A, Ennis S, MacSwiney F, Webb J, Morton NE. Reproductive and menstrual history of females with fragile X expansions. *Eur J Hum Genet* 2000; 8: 247–52.

52. Wittenberger MD, Hagerman RJ, Sherman SL *et al.* The *FMR1* premutation and reproduction. *Fertil Steril* 2007; 87: 456–65.

53. Gleicher N, Weghofer A, Barad DH. Ovarian reserve determinations suggest new function of *FMR1* (fragile X gene) in regulating ovarian ageing. *Reprod Biomed Online* 2010; 20: 768–75.

54. Van Landuyt L, Lissens W, Stouffs K *et al.* Validation of a simple Yq deletion screening programme in an ICSI candidate population. *Mol Hum Reprod* 2000; 6: 291–7.

55. van Golde RJ, Wetzels AM, de Graaf R *et al.* Decreased fertilization rate and embryo quality after ICSI in oligozoospermic men with microdeletions in the azoospermia factor c region of the Y chromosome. *Hum Reprod* 2001; 16: 289–92.

56. Page DC, Silber S, Brown LG. Men with infertility caused by *AZFc* deletion can produce sons by intracytoplasmic sperm injection but are likely to transmit the deletion and infertility. *Hum Reprod* 1999; 14: 1722–6.

57. Saut N, Terriou P, Navarro A, Lévy N, Mitchell MJ. The human Y chromosome genes *BPY2*, *CDY1* and *DAZ* are not essential for sustained fertility. *Mol Hum Reprod* 2000; 6: 789–93.

58. Stouffs K, Tournaye H, Liebaers I, Lissens W. Male infertility and the involvement of the X chromosome. *Hum Reprod Update* 2009; 15: 623–37.

59. European Union Tissues and Cells Directive, 2006/17/EC, *Annex III Section* 3.6.

60. Practice Committee of the American Society for Reproductive Medicine and the Practice Committee of the Society for Assisted Reproductive Technology: www.asrm.org/uploadedFiles/ASRM_Content/News_ and_Publications/Practice_Guidelines/Guidelines_ and_Minimum_Standards/2008_Guidelines_for_ gamete(1).pdf

61. Jauniaux E, Farquharson RG, Christiansen OB, Exalto N. Evidence-based guidelines for the investigation and medical treatment of recurrent miscarriage. *Hum Reprod* 2006; 21: 2216–22.

62. Meschede D, Lemcke B, Exeler JR *et al.* Chromosome abnormalities in 447 couples undergoing. intracytoplasmic sperm injection – prevalence, types, sex distribution and reproductive relevance. *Hum Reprod* 1998; 13: 576–82.

63. Testart J, Gautier E, Brami C *et al.* Intracytoplasmic sperm injection in infertile patients with structural chromosome abnormalities. *Hum Reprod* 1996; 11: 2609–12.

64. Raziel A, Friedler S, Schachter M *et al.* Increased frequency of female partner chromosomal abnormalities in patients with high-order implantation failure after *in vitro* fertilization. *Fertil Steril* 2002; 78: 515–19.

Preimplantation genetic diagnosis

Jan Traeger-Synodinos and Catherine Staessen

Introduction

Preimplantation genetic diagnosis (PGD) is an early form of prenatal diagnosis for couples at high risk of transmitting an inherited disease to their offspring, either monogenic disorders or structural chromosomal abnormalities. Its intended goal is to diagnose a specific genetic disease in cells biopsied from oocytes/zygotes or embryos obtained *in vitro* through assisted reproductive technology (ART), and following analysis, to transfer to the uterus only those embryos identified as unaffected for the disease under consideration. The selective transfer of unaffected embryos to the uterus for implantation means that PGD avoids the need to terminate affected pregnancies. This advantage of PGD means that it has become a widely acceptable alternative to conventional prenatal diagnosis. Of course, PGD is not applied without some ethical concerns. In patients with high risk for transmitting inherited disorders to their offspring, including single gene disorders and chromosomal rearrangements, there is usually little ethical debate. However, the increased availability and emergence of new uses, such as PGD for autosomal dominant late-onset disorders, cancer predisposition syndromes, PGD for histocompatibility (HLA) typing, and mitochondrial DNA (mtDNA) mutations, are associated with greater ethical controversy and serious ethical questions (see Chapter 13)

The feasibility of PGD was facilitated by developments in reproductive medicine, genetics, and biotechnology methods. Edwards and Gardner successfully performed the first known embryo biopsy on rabbit embryos in 1968. In humans, the first clinical application of PGD was reported in 1990 and described the exclusion of an X-linked disease through polymerase chain reaction (PCR)-based sexing of embryos [1]. In

the mid 1990s, the use of *in situ* hybridization with chromosome-specific probes was adapted to be used on single interphase nuclei [2]. This method, termed fluorescence *in situ* hybridization (FISH), was initially used for gender determination. With the development of multicolor FISH, the simultaneous detection of several chromosomes in a single cell became possible. It was the latter technique that was introduced in the setting of ART to select for chromosomally normal embryos in an effort to increase the rates of implantation and successful pregnancy. The latter procedure has been designated as preimplantation genetic screening (PGS) (see Chapter 4).

A first step in clinical PGD is an extensive counseling and genetic work-up of the couple, often including other consenting family members if available and acceptable to the couple. In addition, a robust genetic test has to be developed at the single cell level, and for PGD applied to preclude rare (private) genetic conditions (monogenic or chromosomal) the tests themselves often have to be personalized. Furthermore, clinical PGD requires close collaboration between experts in ART and genetics and involves many stages, including evaluation and counseling relative to the genetic and reproductive status of the couple, all stages of ART, zygote/embryo biopsy, the genetic testing, and, if, following embryo transfer, implantation occurs, follow-up of pregnancy and baby (or babies) delivered. The stages of embryo biopsy and genetic analysis must be performed with the highest precision, and both aspects have been continuously improved over the years (Fig. 11.1).

Probably the most challenging step in PGD remains the stage of genetic analysis. Since the first report of PGD by Handyside *et al.* in 1990 [1], two major diagnostic methods have been widely applied

Textbook of Human Reproductive Genetics, eds Karen Sermon and Stéphane Viville. Published by Cambridge University Press.
© Cambridge University Press 2014.

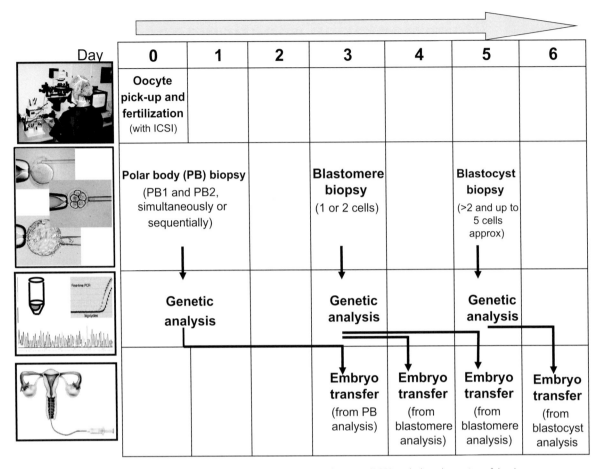

Day	0	1	2	3	4	5	6
	Oocyte pick-up and fertilization (with ICSI)						
	Polar body (PB) biopsy (PB1 and PB2, simultaneously or sequentially)			**Blastomere biopsy** (1 or 2 cells)		**Blastocyst biopsy** (>2 and up to 5 cells approx)	
	Genetic analysis			**Genetic analysis**		**Genetic analysis**	
				Embryo transfer (from PB analysis)	**Embryo transfer** (from blastomere analysis)	**Embryo transfer** (from blastomere analysis)	**Embryo transfer** (from blastocyst analysis

Figure 11.1 A representation of the procedure of preimplantation genetic diagnosis (PGD), including the option of the three developmental stages at which cells suitable for PGD analysis can be biopsied, and the timing of genetic analysis and embryo transfer. See plate section for color version.

in *in vitro* fertilization (IVF) and PGD centers around the world. They include PCR-based methods, mainly used for diagnosis in monogenic diseases, while FISH-based techniques are used to analyze chromosomes for patients carrying chromosome abnormalities or for embryo sexing for patients carrying X-linked diseases. Comparative genome hybridization (CGH), a relatively recent molecular cytogenetic technique that simultaneously evaluates all the chromosomes from a single cell, has been implemented since 2000. More recently, SNP arrays bring the simultaneous diagnosis for monogenic and chromosome abnormalities closer, and clinical validation studies are under way.

This chapter presents an overview which highlights many of the technical and practical issues associated with performing PGD as part of a clinical service to support couples at risk for transmitting a hereditary disorder to have healthy offspring.

ART and sources of genetic material for PGD

Assisted reproductive technology is an intrinsic part of PGD. With the exception of the procedure for oocyte/zygote or embryo biopsy, ART within PGD is essentially the same as for infertility treatment, irrespective of whether the couple is fertile or not. Controlled ovarian hyperstimulation supports the production of multiple mature oocytes to create sufficient zygotes/embryos and increases the chance of identifying embryos with the desired genetic status. For PGD methods involving a DNA amplification step, all cumulus cells should be removed from the aspirated oocytes. Furthermore fertilization should be through intracytoplasmic sperm injection (ICSI) rather than IVF to preclude contamination by residual sperm associated with the latter.

A prerequisite for the genetic analysis in PGD is the acquisition of genetic material for analysis through a biopsy step. Needless to say, this step should be performed by a highly skilled embryologist to ensure successful biopsy while maintaining embryo viability.

There are essentially three developmental stages at which cells suitable for PGD analysis can be biopsied. These include polar bodies (PBs) from the oocyte/zygote stage, blastomeres from cleavage-stage embryos, or trophectoderm cells from blastocysts. Both cleavage-stage biopsy and PB biopsy have been in use for over 20 years, whereas blastocyst biopsy has been more recently introduced. The first step of any biopsy procedure is to breach the zona pellucida that surrounds the oocyte or embryo until the expanded blastocyst stage, by either mechanical means, chemical means (with acid Tyrodes) or more recently with laser. Each zona breaching method and biopsy stage has relative advantages and disadvantages, and selection is made based on the indication for which PGD is to be performed. For zona breaching acid Tyrodes was initially most used, but since 2003 laser breaching has become the preferred method. The majority of PGD cycles performed to date have used cleavage-stage biopsy [3–5].

PB biopsy

Polar bodies are produced in the first and second meiotic division as oocytes complete maturation upon fertilization. In PGD the genotype status of the oocyte should be based on analysis of both the first and second PBs to preclude misdiagnosis which may arise from recombination or allele drop-out (ADO) (monogenic diseases), or by nondisjunction or meiotic errors (chromosomal analysis).

Timing of PB biopsy is critical to support optimal biopsy success and diagnostic result. Biopsy of both PBs may be done sequentially or simultaneously. Sequential biopsy disadvantageously requires two manipulations, whereas with simultaneous biopsy, the first PB may degenerate, precluding completion of an accurate diagnosis, and furthermore there may be difficulties distinguishing each PB. The optimal time for biopsy of the first PB is considered to be 4–12 hours after ICSI and 8–16 hours for the second PB [3].

For PB biopsy, zona breaching is performed using either mechanical or laser methods, since acid Tyrodes may adversely affect subsequent oocyte development. Although laser biopsy offers the advantage of speed, recent evidence indicates that it may have a negative effect on subsequent embryo quality. Relative to legal, ethical, and safety issues, PB biopsy is advantageous since manipulations involve oocytes rather than embryos, and moreover, the genetic material removed is not destined to become part of the developing embryo. In fact PB biopsy is the only option in countries where legislation prevents embryo biopsy. In addition PB biopsy allows more time to complete a genetic diagnosis. However, PB analysis is only useful for excluding mutations or aneuploidies of maternal origin, and the genetic contribution from the father remains unknown. Another practical disadvantage of PB biopsy for PGD is that diagnosis of both PBs doubles the number of samples for analysis. Furthermore, since some oocytes fail to fertilize or form embryos, analysis of all PBs may be considered a waste of time and resources, unless the biopsy samples are frozen/preserved until embryo development can be assessed, removing the time advantage of PB biopsy as compared to cleavage-stage embryo biopsy.

Cleavage-stage embryo biopsy

Biopsy of blastomeres from cleavage-stage embryos is performed on Day 3 about 66–72 hours following ICSI, when the early embryo has around 6–10 cells. On the third day post-insemination the cells are still totipotent and the cells of the embryos are usually not yet adhering to one another (compacting). In the event that compaction has started, brief exposure of the embryos to Ca^{2+}/Mg^{2+}-free media will reduce adherence between cells, facilitating the removal of a blastomere. Mechanical, chemical, and laser are all suitable for zona breaching when performing cleavage-stage biopsy [3, 5].

Preimplantation genetic diagnosis may be based on analysis of either one or two biopsied blastomeres from a single embryo. In the earlier years PGD analysis of two cells presented a means to potentially improve accuracy of diagnostic outcome. However, with remarkable improvements in single-cell genetic testing technologies, this is no longer an issue. Furthermore, results of recent studies confirm that removal of two cells at the cleavage stage is more detrimental to pregnancy outcome than removal of only a single cell [6].

The analysis of blastomeres is suitable for all PGD indications. The major disadvantage of cleavage-stage biopsy is the limited amount of material present in a single blastomere for analysis. In addition high rates of mosaicism are observed in embryos at this early stage of development, although for monogenic PGD, errors attributed to false positive or false negative results may be minimized by applying appropriate diagnostic strategies and interpretation of results.

Blastocyst-stage biopsy

The blastocyst develops about 5–6 days post-insemination and contains approximately 100 cells distinguished into the two cell lineages, the outer trophectoderm (TE) and the inner cell mass (ICM). Zona breaching may be performed by mechanical means or laser, and is usually done in the TE region furthest away (opposite) from the ICM.

With blastocyst biopsy several cells may be removed for analysis, a potential advantage compared to blastomere biopsy for subsequent diagnosis. However, many embryos fail to reach this stage of development. The fact that trophectoderm cells do not contribute to the embryo, but eventually form the placenta and other extra-embryonic tissue (comparable to an early chorionic villus sampling) partly reduces ethical considerations.

The first clinical PGD cycles based on blastocyst biopsy were reported in 2005 with high survival and pregnancy rates [7]. Blastocyst biopsy is becoming more widely used, supported by improvements in culture medium, although with current protocols only about 40–50% of preimplantation embryos develop to this stage *in vitro*, which limits the application of this biopsy method for PGD. In addition the time available to complete diagnosis based on blastocyst biopsy is very limited if fresh embryo transfer is to be performed by Day 6. The option of cryopreservation may address this issue, allowing transfer of embryos in a subsequent cycle.

Embryo cryopreservation in PGD

There are certain situations in PGD when it may be appropriate to freeze embryos. Besides cases when ovarian hyperstimulation syndrome has occurred, cryopreservation may provide more time to complete a diagnosis. In addition there are often "unaffected" supernumerary embryos in PGD cycles. Preimplantation genetic diagnosis embryos usually undergo biopsy prior to cryopreservation and thus do not have an intact zona pellucida, although current cryopreservation protocols do not generally differ between biopsied versus intact embryos [3, 5].

Reports of cycle outcomes for cryopreserved PGD embryos are not entirely conclusive [3, 5]. Generally intact embryos survive better, and vitrification generally shows higher survival rates compared to slow freezing. Since studies generally indicate a lower survival rate for biopsied embryos/blastocysts, it may be advantageous to perform the biopsy after thawing. On the other hand, if the biopsy for genetic analysis is done before cryopreservation then only embryos with an acceptable diagnosis need be cryopreserved, accelerating the procedures for transfer after thawing.

PGD for single-gene disorders (monogenic PGD)

Indications for monogenic PGD

To date PGD has been reported for almost 200 different genetic conditions, mainly severe autosomal recessive, autosomal dominant, or X-linked disorders [4]. Not surprisingly, the most PGD cycles have been reported for the common autosomal recessive disorders including cystic fibrosis and beta-hemoglobinopathies (beta-thalassemia major and sickle cell syndromes), followed by spinal muscular atrophy. For autosomal dominant disorders, the largest numbers of cycles have been reported for myotonic dystrophy type I and Huntington's disease (HD). For the X-linked disorders, fragile X syndrome is the most common indication, followed by Duchenne muscular dystrophy and hemophilia. Preimplantation genetic diagnosis for most other single-gene disorders is less frequently requested and performed.

The fact that PGD precludes pregnancy termination means that its application has been also adopted for many conditions which are not traditionally considered for conventional prenatal diagnosis. Besides late-onset disorders (e.g. HD) or high penetrance cancer predisposition such as familial adenomatous polyposis I, the use of PGD has also been extended to cancer predisposition syndromes with lower penetrance (e.g. breast cancer caused by *BRCA1* mutations), and even non-life threatening conditions such as non-syndromic deafness. Furthermore, the analysis of embryos for non-medical reasons is used for the selection of a histocompatible sibling to facilitate a bone marrow transplant in a sick child. This can be done for HLA matching alone (e.g. to treat a child affected with leukemia), or in combination with PGD to exclude the familial monogenic disease (for example to treat a child with beta-thalassemia major). For both applications, there was initially much ethical debate, but certainly HLA combined with PGD is now widely accepted, as evidenced by the steadily increasing number of requests and cycles each year for HLA-PGD [4]. Finally in the context of mitochondrial disorders, a non-Mendelian indication, PGD potentially offers a superior alternative to conventional prenatal diagnosis, apparently substantially reducing the risk of transmitting the mitochondrial disorder, although only a few cases have been reported to date [4].

Diagnostic strategies and protocol work-up

Preimplantation genetic diagnosis is feasible for any single-gene disorder, provided either the disease-causing mutation and/or the disease-associated phase within a family are confirmed. This information is mandatory to support the development of an appropriate protocol with a high diagnostic value. The molecular genetics associated with a disorder largely determines the strategy and method(s) selected for performing the PGD (see below). Factors that should be considered include the mode of inheritance within the family and the nature of the mutations involved; most single gene disorders are caused by variations of single or up to a few nucleotides and larger gene rearrangements (usually deletions) are rare. In the early years the strategies for PGD tended to focus on the detection (or exclusion) of the disease-causing mutation(s) alone, or for X-linked disorders the detection (or not) of Y-specific amplification products. With the evolution of molecular technologies, most notably improved Taq polymerases, instrumentation, and accumulated experience, current strategies tend to analyze multiple targets across the genomic region associated with the disease in the format of multiplex linkage analysis of polymorphic markers. In this way, linkage analysis, with or without concurrent analysis for the disease-causing mutation(s), supports confirmation of the diagnosis through results from more

than a single genomic region. The main disadvantage of this approach versus direct genotyping alone is the need to perform a family analysis.

Polymorphic markers include SNPs or microsatellite repeats, otherwise known as short tandem repeats (STRs). In PGD, STRs are more useful since they are usually highly polymorphic, providing an increased chance of being informative within the family, and also their analysis is easier than SNP analysis, through simply sizing the fluorescently labeled amplified repeats on an automated genome analyser (sequencer) (Fig. 11.2).

The first step in setting up a PGD protocol for any disorder involves locating the gene and/or disease-associated mutations *in silico* through any of the many databases for human genetic information available in the public domain (NCBI, Ensembl, UCSC, Blast). These databases will also support the identification of closely located STRs (ideally within 1 Megabase (Mb) distant from the disease-associated gene) and also facilitate the design of primer sets for direct mutation detection (if appropriate) and the amplification of the STRs. If possible, the STRs selected (ideally at least 2–4) should flank the disease mutation(s) to preclude misdiagnosis in the event of recombination.

During the work-up of a couple, informative STRs linked to the disease-causing gene are identified by testing appropriate family members with known genetic status, such that during the PGD application, embryo diagnosis can be based on the presence or absence of phase alleles at each linked STR (see Fig. 11.2) in the form of a mutiplex PCR (see "PCR-based protocols for monogenic PGD" section, below). For PGD to preclude transmission of dominant disorders, where one of the partners is the only family member affected, and the *de novo* germline mutation is known, the PGD protocol can be based on an assay for the mutation alone. However, to prevent misdiagnosis caused by allele drop-out, it is preferable to support the mutation diagnosis with linked markers. For *de novo* mutations that have arisen in the male partner, individual sperm can be tested to establish the phase, and if it has arisen in the female partner, then first and second polar bodies can be tested. This can be done as part of the first PGD cycle, with PB biopsy at Day 0 and embryo biopsy at Day 3 or 5.

The huge spectrum of disease indications, along with family-specific differences, even for the same disease indication, means that there are very few

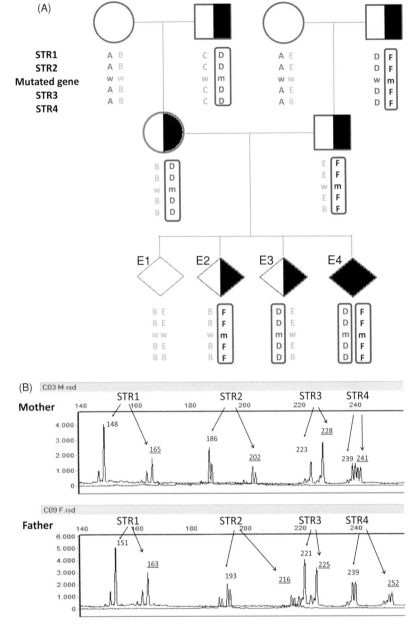

Figure 11.2 (**A**) The phase of informative short tandem repeats (STRs) syntenic to a disease locus in an imaginary family. (**B**) The sizing of the informative parental STRs following analysis on automatic sequencer. See plate section for color version.

completely generic PGD protocols, with the possible exception of those based on whole genome amplification (WGA) coupled with the analysis of large panels of STR markers [8] (see "Whole Genome Amplification" section, below).

Preimplantation genetic diagnosis for single-gene disorders requires an initial amplification step, essential with current technologies to facilitate the analysis of the tiny amount of sample, often no more than a single cell. The PCR constitutes the amplification step in most diagnostic protocols in PGD, although WGA may be appropriate for certain applications.

PCR-based protocols for monogenic PGD

Polymerase chain reaction from minimal sample quantity is associated with certain limitations and pitfalls. These include the occurrence of complete amplification failure, the chance that only one of the two target alleles will amplify to detectable levels, a phenomenon known as allele drop-out (ADO), and finally the likelihood of sample contamination. Total PCR failure may preclude a diagnostic result, something that is undesirable but which will not lead to transfer of an affected embryo. However, the occurrence of ADO and/or contamination may lead to an unacceptable misdiagnosis. It is paramount that PCR-based PGD protocols address and monitor these issues [9].

Both PCR failure and ADO can be minimized if protocols are stringently optimized prior to clinical application. To this end, it is general practice that work-up involves the design of robust primer sets, with potential for efficient coamplification in multiplex PCR formats (e.g. similar annealing temperatures, minimal cross-hybridization). Preclinical experiments are carried out to optimize the efficiency of amplification and minimize ADO for all amplicons included in the multiplex PCR protocol. To "model" the amounts of DNA in just a single cell (around 6 pg) it is general strategy to test genomic DNA diluted to a few genome equivalents, and then single-cells such as single lymphocytes, fibroblasts, or buccal cells, preferably from members of the family requesting the PGD. These model single-cells are considered acceptable in the light that single blastomeres from research embryos are rarely available, plus they are of uncertain quality and genotype.

The high number of amplification cycles required for analysis of a single or only a few cells leaves PCR-based PGD protocols extremely vulnerable to the accidental introduction of contaminating DNA at any of the many stages in PGD. Measures taken to preclude contamination during embryo fertilization have been mentioned above (see "ART and sources of genetic material for PGD" section, above). With respect to the genetic diagnosis, both operator contamination and amplicon carry-over contamination are a possibility, but these can be effectively precluded if all stages of PCR set-up are performed using stringent "single-cell analysis" conditions. It is extremely important to separate physically the pre-PCR steps from those of the PCR itself, and then finally any post-PCR steps. These include the set-up of PCR in dedicated ultraviolet (UV)-treated hoods, using exclusive UV-treated equipment, entirely separated from any post-PCR processing, and with operators wearing appropriate attire and employing correct handling procedures.

As an additional precaution, contamination during any PGD procedure should be monitored by the inclusion of negative controls and blanks at all stages. Additionally the inclusion of STRs supports the detection of likely contamination within each individual sample, such that identification of alleles not consistent with those expected from the parents implies the presence of contaminating DNA. The inclusion of several STRs linked to the disease-causing locus (gene) also monitors ADO and supports the accuracy of the genotyping.

The preclinical work-up required for PGD tests is challenging and time-consuming and is the major bottleneck within a clinical PGD service. The pioneering PGD cases for autosomal recessive disorders used non-fluorescent nested PCR and gel electrophoresis to identify the causative mutation, for example nested-PCR followed by restriction enzyme analysis or nested-PCR followed by denaturing gradient gel electrophoresis (DGGE). A major improvement in detecting PCR products from single cells came with the introduction of the labeling of PCR products by fluorescence. This lead to the development of more sensitive sophisticated assays and instruments, such as capillary electrophoresis for amplicon sizing or minisequencing, or alternatively real-time PCR for genotyping single nucleotide variants. Improved DNA polymerases and in silico PCR-primer design means that PCR-based protocols perform efficiently in multiplex formats to analyze many loci/markers directly in a single cell. However, they continue to be technically exacting, labor intensive, and must be preformed using highly stringent conditions [9].

Whole genome amplification

An emerging approach to overcome the limitations of testing single cells directly with PCR-based protocols is the possibility of performing WGA on the single (or few) cells prior to the genotyping step. Whole genome amplification methods can be grouped into those based on PCR (involving thermal cycling) or isothermal amplification.

The early PCR-WGA methods employed the use of Taq polymerases and degenerate or semi-degenerate primers, but they had limited success. They were usually very time-consuming, involving protocols that required around 16 hours to complete, and the multiple degenerate primers required were relatively costly. Current PCR-based methods for WGA consist of a DNA fragmentation step followed by a step to ligate adaptors to enable PCR amplification. Available as commercial kits, these protocols produce about 3–5 μg of DNA from a single cell, with fragment sizes up to 500 base pairs (bp) long.

Isothermal amplification techniques include multiple displacement amplification (MDA) which is based on the strand displacement amplification properties of Φ29 DNA polymerase in the presence of random exonuclease-resistant primers.

Both PCR-based and MDA WGA methods have been used for single-cell WGA in the context of PGD for monogenic diseases. However, both approaches have limitations; neither method usually amplifies the entire genome with equal efficiency, and a few regions may consistently fail to amplify. Both methods are vulnerable to high levels of ADO (up to around 30%), which means that the derivation of the genotype may require subsequent analysis of many disease-linked loci to support an accurate and reliable result.

Although the initial amplification step in WGA requires precautions to preclude contamination in the same way as PGD protocols based directly on PCR methods, all subsequent PCR-based assays do not require "single-cell analysis conditions" and almost any PCR-based method can be used for genotyping. This means that work-up for PGD involving WGA does not require optimization of the PGD-PCR protocol, but only work-up of the genetics within each family. Furthermore, once the sample has been subjected to WGA, it can be analyzed numerous times if needed. One successful strategy for PGD based on MDA WGA is known as preimplantation genetic haplotyping (PGH), which uses multiple STRs across the disease locus to derive the linked normal and affected haplotype [8].

Whole genome amplification (WGA) is also an essential step when performing PGD for structural chromosomal abnormalities using CGH or array-CGH (see "FISH-based PGD protocols for structural chromosomal abnormalities" section, below).

Monogenic PGD applications with special considerations

Some indications for PGD may require variation of classic strategies described above, and in addition, very rarely the genetic transmission within a family may not follow expected norms, for example in cases with mosaicism.

Amongst disorders that require a slightly different analytical approach are the trinucleotide-repeat disorders. Here, the disease-causing mutation is caused by expansion of a triplet-nucleotide repeat whereby the affected allele size may be refractory to amplification by PCR (although all normal alleles should be within the range that does amplify). Some trinucleotide-repeat disorders are autosomal dominant (e.g. myotonic dystrophy or HD) and others are X-linked (e.g. fragile X syndrome). In autosomal forms, normal embryos will be characterized by the amplification of the normal allele from the affected parent and one from the non-transmitting parent. In addition modified PCR protocols have been described which support amplification of both the expanded and non-expanded repeats, and distinguish embryos with an expansion from those without [10]. These protocols use a PCR with three primers in a semi-nested format, whereby one of the primers is complementary to the triplet-repeat sequence, and can be incorporated into the multiplex reaction alongside the informative STRs. In X-linked disorders, notably fragile X syndrome, affected males will give no amplification product from the primers used to amplify the triplet-repeat region, necessitating use of STRs to prevent misdiagnosis caused by ADO.

For the triplet disorder HD special considerations are associated with strategy ethics rather than technical issues. For individuals aware of their HD status, PGD can simply involve direct testing of the disease-causing expanded CAG repeat in exon 1 of the *HTT* gene (supported by linked STRs). Alternatively, for individuals at-risk of developing HD who do not wish to learn their risk status, two approaches for PGD exist: exclusion testing or non-disclosure testing. Exclusion testing is based on identifying the grandparental origin of the two *HTT* alleles and only embryos with an *HTT* allele from the non-affected grandparent are considered transferable. Disadvantage of exclusion testing include the requirement of DNA from family members with known disease status to support the derivation of phase, and also that statistically half of the rejected embryos are unaffected. For the non-disclosure approach, PGD embryos are analyzed directly for a CAG repeat, without revealing details of PGD results to the prospective parents. However, non-disclosure PGD remains controversial and is not widely accepted.

For gender-linked disorders, PCR was the original method used for sexing embryos [1]. However, it soon became apparent that the amplification of Y-chromosome-specific regions were susceptible to ADO, and thus FISH, a more robust technique, became the preferred method to determine gender. However, following marked improvements in PCR technologies, PCR-based methods have again become the preferred method for X-linked PGD cases, with the added advantage that they also support a specific diagnosis for X-linked disease. With this approach, more genetically transferable embryos are available, advantageous compared to gender analysis alone, whereby half of all male embryos were likely unaffected but discarded.

For families affected by mtDNA mutations, reproductive choices include prenatal diagnosis of a spontaneous conception, mtDNA replacement, the use of donor oocytes, and more recently PGD. However, the complicated pathobiology of genetic disorders caused by mtDNA mutations may limit the reliability of prenatal diagnosis and PGD. Mitochondria are maternally inherited and all cells have thousands of mitochondria, each containing many copies of the mitochondrial genome. A characteristic of disorders caused by mtDNA mutations is the coexistence of normal and mutated mtDNA within a single cell, known as heteroplasmy. The onset of clinical symptoms, as well as the variability in phenotype and penetrance of mtDNA diseases is influenced by factors including the threshold effect (whereby the mutational load in a cell has to exceed a certain level), mitotic segregation, clonal expansion, and the so-called bottleneck effect. Although the precise mechanism for the latter is still unclear, one prevalent theory is that there is a rapid reduction of mtDNA in early germ cell development followed by rapid expansion as the oocyte matures, causing some oocytes to have reduced mutation levels, which may sometimes be below the threshold level. The outcome of prenatal diagnosis when analyzing the proportion of mutant mtDNA in amniotic or trophoblast cells is unpredictable. However, it is possible to measure the ratio of mutated to normal mtDNA in an embryonic cell with a fair degree of accuracy and recent studies (for certain mtDNA mutations at least), have indicated that if the mutation load is low then there is a low chance

that this will lead to the development of an affected child. However, carriers of mtDNA mutations must be appropriately counselled, and although PGD for mtDNA disorders looks a promising option, further investigation and evaluation are required before wider clinical application [11].

Preimplantation genetic diagnosis for HLA-typing aims to establish a pregnancy that is HLA-compatible with a sibling who requires hematopoietic stem-cell transplantation. The HLA-typing alone can be performed when the affected child requires transplantation for treatment of a non-inherited disease, or simultaneously with PGD to exclude a familial inherited single gene disorder, as each offspring is also at-risk of being affected. Although initially considered ethically controversial, HLA-typing is now widely accepted as a valuable treatment option since transplantation success is strongly associated with the degree of HLA-match between the donor and recipient. The first combined PGD-HLA matching case was reported in 2001 for a case of Fanconi anemia [12], and since then the number of reported cases has been increasing every year [4]. According to data from the European Society of Human Reproduction and Embryology (ESHRE), the most common indication to date is for HLA matching combined with PGD for beta-thalassemia and/or sickle cell syndromes [4]. Fanconi anemia, Gaucher disease, adrenoleukodystrophy, and osteopetrosis are amongst other single gene disorders for which HLA-typing combined with PGD have been reported, and there are many reports of cycles for HLA typing for acquired diseases [4].

Reliable tests for HLA-typing of preimplantation embryos have to address several technical challenges, including the large size of the region (3.6 Mb), the large number of loci within the region, the high level of polymorphism, and the possibility of recombination within the HLA region. HLA haplotyping by linkage analysis of polymorphic STR markers located throughout the HLA region was first reported by Van de Velde et al. in 2004 [13], and has since become the preferred strategy for PGD-HLA, matching the haplotypes between the embryos and the affected sibling.

Genetic chance presents another limitation on the clinical utility of PGD for HLA-typing. The chance that two siblings will be HLA matched is 25%, amongst which only 75% will be unaffected for an autosomal recessive disroder (18.8%, or 3 of every 16 embryos) and 50% for an autosomal dominant or X-linked disorder (12.5% of all embryos fertilized in any cycle). As only approximately 25% of PGD cycles result in pregnancy and delivery, the overall success rate for HLA-PGD matching rarely surpasses about 10–15% for any cycle initiated, limiting the ultimate success, i.e. the birth of an unaffected histocompatible baby. As well as the advantages of HLA-PGD, couples should also be made aware of this limitation, before embarking on such a procedure.

PGD for chromosomal abnormalities

Indications: balanced translocations or Robertsonian translocations

It is estimated that 1 in 625 (0.16%) individuals carries a balanced chromosomal rearrangement, with translocations (reciprocal or Robertsonian) and inversions as the most frequent (see Chapters 1 and 7). An enormous number of reciprocal translocations have been described, with breakpoints scattered throughout all chromosomal regions. With few exceptions, the majority of reciprocal translocations are family-specific. Robertsonian translocations originate through centric fusion of the long arms of any two of the five acrocentric chromosomes (13, 14, 15, 21, and 22), with loss of the short arms. An inversion is a two-break event involving just one chromosome. Carriers of confirmed balanced chromosomal rearrangement are, most of the time, phenotypically normal. The production of unbalanced gametes, due to unfavorable meiotic segregation when the derivative chromosomes pair up at meiosis I, puts them at risk for repeated miscarriages, subfertility, or infertility, and unbalanced offspring. This explains why the incidence of balanced chromosomal rearrangement rises to about 3% in couples with reproductive problems. The theoretical chance of producing normal or balanced gametes is 4 out of 32 for reciprocal translocation carriers and 4 out of 16 for Robertsonian translocation carriers. However, the actual percentage depends on several factors, including which chromosomes are involved, the location of the breakpoints, and the gender of the carrier [14]. For carriers of an inversion the chromosomal imbalance occurs if there is, within the inverted segment, a crossover at the first meiotic division, between the inversion chromosome and the normal homolog resulting in a recombinant chromosome, which may produce four different segregates.

Analytical methods for structural chromosomal abnormalities

FISH-based PGD protocols for structural chromosomal abnormalities

Fluorescence *in situ* hybridization utilizes chromosome-specific DNA probes labeled with different colored fluorochromes that are hybridized to the target DNA (interphase or metaphase) fixed to a microscopic slide. As a result FISH detects a chromosome or a part of a chromosome, thereby allowing determination of the copy number of that region in a particular sample. Microscopic evaluation and computerized imaging systems enable fluorescent probe signals to be identified and counted.

Initial applications using FISH for diagnosing chromosomal translocations involved painting probes for metaphase chromosomes of polar bodies [15]. A major shortcoming of this method was that only translocations of the female could be examined. Subsequently, home-made probes, isolated from cosmid, YAC, or BAC libraries spanning or flanking the translocation breakpoints were applied on the interphase nucleus of a blastomere from cleavage-stage embryos. These probes gave very accurate results because they allowed the distinction between normal and balanced genotypes, but were very time-consuming to isolate [15]. The commercial availability of centromeric and subtelomeric probes opened completely new perspectives for PGD for translocation carriers. The PGD for Robertsonian translocations is relatively simple as dual-color FISH with one probe to enumerate each chromosome is sufficient. The situation is more complex for reciprocal translocations. Ideally the protocol should include a FISH probe for both centric segments and both the subtelomeric regions of the translocated segments. In this case two scoring errors would have to occur to misdiagnose an unbalanced product as normal/balanced. However, four suitable probes may not be available. Most centers performing PGD for reciprocal translocations use a combination of two subtelomeric probes distal to the breakpoint, along with a centromeric probe for one of the two chromosomes involved, to support the distinction between normal/balanced genotypes and unbalanced genotypes; all probes are labeled with different colors [14]. Carriers of reciprocal translocations and inversions usually have unique rearrangements, necessitating the development, preclinical testing, and optimization of the individualized probe-mixture for each couple.

The optimal outcome of the FISH method also depends on the step of cell fixation onto a microscope slide, a critical step that requires skill and experience. Another drawback of FISH for PGD includes failure of FISH probes to hybridize, and the accuracy of interpretation can be affected by signal overlap or split signals. Finally, the limited number of distinct fluorochromes available for labeling the DNA probes limits the number of chromosomes that can be assessed in a single analysis, although PGD for structural chromosomal abnormalities usually interrogates only the chromosomes involved in the translocation.

PCR-based PGD for structural chromosomal abnormalities

Polymerase chain reaction-based strategies have also been used to detect chromosome imbalances in embryos derived from carriers of chromosome rearrangements. Polymerase chain reaction-based protocols that utilize informative STRs on both segments (flanking the breakpoint) of the translocated chromosomes have been reported [16]. This approach offers the advantage of determining the inheritance of individual chromosomes, and allowing the detection of uniparental disomy.

Polymerase chain reaction-based PGD protocols for translocations have the potential to overcome several inherent limitations of FISH-based tests. They are not dependent on cell fixation and on microscopic signal interpretation, but on the other hand are subject to amplification failure, ADO, and contamination as discussed above. For the PCR-based methods also workup is necessary prior to any clinical case in order to identify which STR polymorphisms are informative. Similar to the FISH-based PGD for structural chromosome abnormalities, the number of chromosomes assessed remains limited, usually to the chromosomes involved in the translocation.

CGH-based PGD for structural chromosomal abnormalities

By contrast, genome-wide aneuploidy screening of a single cell can be performed by CGH. However, the DNA content of a single cell (about 5–10 pg) is insufficient for direct use in CGH, and therefore the method requires the use of WGA.

The CGH technique employs a competitive hybridization of differentially labeled DNA samples (DNA from the sample: green; chromosomally normal reference DNA: red) to normal metaphase chromosomes on a microscope slide. The principles of this technique are described in Chapters 1 and 2. With image-processing software, the metaphase chromosomes are evaluated. An excess of green fluorescence on a specific chromosome is indicative of a chromosomal gain, whereas an excess of red fluorescence is indicative of chromosome loss. This CGH technology has been applied with success in PGD cycles for aneuploidy screening [17]. The obvious advantage of CGH over FISH is that the copy number of all chromosomes can be determined. In addition, CGH provides a more detailed picture of the entire length of each chromosome, enabling the detection of imbalance of chromosomal segments. Using the CGH technique, Malmgren et al. [18] karyotyped 94 blastomeres of 28 embryos donated for research after PGD treatment with FISH. In 70% of the blastomeres a result was obtained. They found however that small deletions or duplications of the telomeric regions were difficult to interpret, and determined a resolution limit for CGH of 10–20 Mb.

Moreover, CGH is labor intensive and time-consuming, which limits its diagnostic potential for PGD.

Array-CGH PGD for structural chromosomal abnormalities

Array-CGH (aCGH) is a technique based on the same principle as CGH, but the competitive hybridization of differentially labeled test and reference DNA samples does not take place on metaphase spreads but on DNA probes fixed to a microcope slide (microarray). Each probe is specific to a different chromosomal region and occupies a discrete spot on a slide. After the labeling and hybridization procedure, a laser scanner is used to excite the hybridized fluorochromes and read and store the resulting images of the hybridization. Chromosomal loss or gain is revealed by the color adopted by each spot after hybridization based on software packages (i.e. ratio of fluorescence intensity for the two colors). Similar to CGH, an amplification step is required to increase the initial quantity of DNA. Different WGA procedures are available (see Whole genome amplification" section, above), but the one commonly used for aCGH applications is a WGA procedure based on random fragmentation of genomic

DNA, ligation of adaptors, and subsequent amplification by PCR (see section on WGA).

Over the last few years, a variety of single cells, including polar bodies, blastomeres, or trophectoderm biopsies have been successfully screened using aCGH on different platforms with the aim of aneuploidy screening. The commercial availability of different types of high-resolution microarrays opened new opportunities for clinical applications for translocation carriers and a validation study for PGD in couples with structural chromosome abnormalities has recently been published [19], which reported 28 cycles of PGD for chromosomal translocations. In this study paired comparison between aCGH and PCR-based PGD testing on 200 embryos from translocation carriers was performed. A high percentage of embryos (93%) were successfully diagnosed with the aCGH technique. Results were concordant between both diagnostic techniques for all embryos tested. Moreover, the study demonstrated that aCGH analysis can identify segmental aneusomy, as small as 2.5 Mb, from patients carrying a translocation. Only 30 embryos (16%) were found balanced/normal for the translocation as well as for the other chromosomes. A total of 22 embryos were transferred in 17 transfer procedures. A pregnancy was obtained in 12 patients, from which all were on-going at the time of publication. This demonstrates that aCGH can detect chromosome imbalances in embryos, also providing the added benefit of simultaneous aneuploidy screening for all 24 chromosomes [19]. Array-CGH potentially provides a generic solution which should be applicable to all translocations, avoiding the need for patient individualized tests.

Apart from errors directly related to the chromosomes involved in the translocation, it has been postulated that the segregation patterns could have an influence on meiotic synapsis and disjunction of other bivalents, causing aneuploidy in chromosomes not involved in the translocation. This phenomenon has been named interchromosomal effect [20], although its existence is controversial, and conflicting results have been reported in the literature. In the light of these findings, and with the technical feasibility offered by aCGH, aneuploidy screening, simultaneous to the PGD of translocations, could be considered to detect other possible post-zygotic chromosome errors. The number of patients involved in the study of Fiorentino *et al.* [19] is too small to speculate on the beneficial effect of testing for all the chromosomes.

Clinical outcomes of PGD for monogenic diseases and structural chromosome abnormalities

The ultimate goal of PGD is the birth of a healthy baby. To this end the optimization of every stage of PGD is important. To a great extent, the success of the stages of ART and embryology tend to be case-dependent, especially since a large percentage of cases undergoing PGD are also infertile (almost 40% of patients who undergo PGD for monogenic disorders, and over 50% for those who have PGD for structural abnormalities). It is really only the stage of genetic diagnosis which can be optimized and this has been facilitated by the continuous research efforts of PGD centers, along with improvements in reagents and instruments available for molecular analysis in single cells. According to the annual ESHRE PGD data collections for cycles performed between 1997 and 2008 inclusive, there have been over 6000 monogenic PGD cycles. These data clearly demonstrate an upward trend in the proportion of embryos with a successful diagnosis following testing for monogenic PCR; in earlier data sets successful diagnosis was achieved in just over 80% of embryos analyzed, whereas in the most recent data collection for cycles performed in 2008, diagnosis was achieved in over 90% of embryos [4]. If more embryos are successfully diagnosed, then the number of embryos available for transfer increases, supporting a higher chance of a successful PGD cycle. Overall, compared to all other indications, PGD for single-gene disorders demonstrates the highest pregnancy rates (23% per oocyte retrieval (OR) and 29% per embryo transfer (ET)).

With respect to PGD for chromosomal abnormalities, strategies based upon FISH have proved effective, resulting in thousands of successful cycles according to the data collected by the ESHRE PGD consortium. Between 1997 and 2008 [4] 4311 treatment cycles for inherited chromosome abnormalities were performed (male Robertsonian carriers: 905 cycles, female Robertsonian carriers: 535 cycles, male reciprocal carriers: 1394 cycles, female reciprocal carriers: 1477 cycles). Of the embryos successfully biopsied, 93% gave a diagnostic result. Consistent with the underlying abnormalities, a high number of embryos are not suitable for transfer due to chromosome imbalances detected in the embryos. Overall, amongst the embryos with diagnosis, only 24% were found normal for the chromosomes tested. As expected, the lowest percentage of transferable embryos was found in the reciprocal translocation group (20% and 19% transferable embryos for female or male reciprocal translocation carriers, respectively), whereas this rate was notably higher in cases with Robertsonian translocations (38% and 30% transferable embryos for male or female Robertsonian translocation carriers, respectively). As could be expected, 73% of the cycles for the Robertsonian carriers resulted in a transfer, versus 58% for the reciprocal translocation carriers.

The relatively low clinical pregnancy rate (17% per OR and 26% per ET) reflects the low proportion of embryos considered to be chromosomally normal and available for transfer. Robertsonian translocations (23% per OR and 31% per ET) had a higher pregnancy rate compared with reciprocal translocations (15% per OR and 25% per ET). The data demonstrate that there was little difference in outcome between male and female translocation carriers. However, there was a difference in outcome according to the type of translocation being tested, such that Robertsonian translocations showed a higher number of normal/balanced embryos available for transfer leading to a higher pregnancy rate compared with reciprocal translocations, irrespective of whether they were male or female carriers.

To date over 5000 children have been born following PGD, and so far no adverse outcomes are apparent. Several reports on children born after PGD have been published. In one such report that performed pediatric follow-up in a large series of children born after cleavage-stage biopsy and PGD, the data, collected on 581 post-PGD/PGS children, showed that term, birthweight, and major malformation rates were not statistically different from that of 2889 children born after fertility treatment involving ICSI [21]. The overall rates of major malformation among the post-PGD/PGS and ICSI children were 2.13 and 3.38%, respectively, and the authors concluded that embryo biopsy does not add risk factors to the health of singleton children born after PGD or PGS.

Accuracy and quality assurance in PGD

The absolute accuracy of PGD is difficult to estimate since it is impossible to confirm the diagnosis in every embryo. Pregnancy allows access for reanalysis (either during pregnancy or after birth), but most embryo transfers do not result in pregnancy and confirmatory testing is done on only a minority of untransferred embryos. Thus misdiagnosis is likely under-reported by PGD centers. Unacceptable misdiagnosis has serious consequences whereby the embryo transferred was characterized to be unaffected at PGD, but identified during pregnancy or after birth to be affected. Alternatively, benign misdiagnosis includes cases in which embryos diagnosed as negative for the hereditary mutation during PGD, result in an unaffected pregnancy or child who in fact carries a mutation (for a recessive disease). To date misdiagnosis rates have been estimated based on reporting (anonymously) to the ESHRE PGD consortium, and overall the rates are very low (0.16%). This includes 0.1% for FISH-based cycles, although rates are relatively higher (0.5%) for PCR-based cycles [22].

Audit through confirmatory testing on untransferred embryos (superfluous to reproductive needs of couples) is a good way to evaluate the diagnostic value of PGD protocols and highlight any pitfalls in methods and strategies used. Audit is also an important part of quality control, especially relevant for monogenic PGD since there are few universally standardized protocols, and most are case-specific "in-house" protocols, especially for rare monogenic diseases. The issues of quality control and quality assurance within PGD can be supported through some form of internationally or nationally recognized accreditation [23]. External quality assessment is also an important part of quality management and is an essential component of accreditation schemes [23]. External quality assessment provides an independent measure of service quality and a comparison against other laboratories. Assessment data gives service users (clinics, clinicians, and patients) a way to evaluate whether services reach the required standards. External quality assessment also has an educational element by highlighting variation between laboratories in testing protocols, and differences in interpretation and reporting of results. This information is important not only to support continual improvement of each laboratory but also for professional bodies responsible for providing the most relevant best practice guidelines.

Future developments in PGD

Even for fertile couples undergoing PGD, pregnancy rates rarely surpass 30–35%. Thus ideally a key objective associated with PGD is also the ability to select the best quality healthy embryo(s) most likely to implant.

Traditionally embryos are selected by morphological criteria which are, however, difficult to quantify. More recently the euploid status of an embryo by PGS has been introduced as a means of predicting potential embryo implantation and live birth, although there is still considerable controversy over its true clinical benefit [24].

However, the fast-emerging technologies of arrays and next generation sequencing for genome analysis do potentially offer generic approaches for simultaneous ploidy analysis (PGS) and PGD. In 2010, Handyside *et al.* [25] described a seminal approach coined "karyomapping," which is based on SNP arrays for embryo analysis, enabling, through family linkage, analysis of single-gene disorders, simultaneously with aneuploidy testing [25]. "Karyomapping" and analogous SNP array approaches can also potentially distinguish normal from balanced embryos in translocation cases, and identify uniparental disomy and parental origin of abnormalities. However, SNP array analysis of single cells is currently technically demanding, the data generated are complex, and the procedure is costly, although efforts are progressing to address these limitations.

Next generation sequencing in PGD may facilitate multiple-gene testing, the detection of SNPs, copy number variants, and chromosomal aneuploidies, as well as epigenetic profiling. Its use at a single-cell level is currently being explored for PGD. Besides providing a more holistic approach to PGD, next generation sequencing in patients undergoing ART may additionally support more "personalized" procedures to optimize pregnancy outcome. However, this technology awaits thorough validation and more knowledge to support interpretation of the hugely complex genetic information it generates. In addition there are many ethical issues foreseen; for example, with how to interpret and report all of the numerous genetic variants detected (see Chapter 13).

Although in the future PGD will likely incorporate many new technologies, it is mandatory to establish the safety and clear clinical benefit before they are incorporated within clinical practice. The innate biology of human reproduction will always limit the positive outcome of ART and thus PGD, while additional complex issues, such as the impact of epigenetics on embryos, remain unresolved. Ideally all developments in PGD should be based on hypothesis-driven research, and the exchange of expertise and knowledge through international forums, ensuring that PGD is always applied with the highest standards of laboratory, clinical, and ethical conduct.

References

1. Handyside AH, Kontogianni EH, Hardy K, Winston RML. Pregnancies from biopsied human preimplantation embryos sexed by Y-specific DNA amplification. *Nature* 1990; 244: 768–70.

2. Griffin DK, Wilton LJ, Handyside AH *et al.* Dual fluorescent *in situ* hybridization for simultaneous detection of X and Y chromosome-specific probes for the sexing of human preimplantation embryonic nuclei. *Hum Genet* 1992; 89: 18–22.

3. Xu K, Montag M. New perspectives on embryo biopsy: not how, but when and why? *Semin Reprod Med* 2012; 30: 259–66.

4. Goossens V, Traeger-Synodinos J, Coonen E *et al.* ESHRE PGD Consortium data collection XI: cycles from January to December 2008 with pregnancy follow-up to October 2009. *Hum Reprod* 2012; 27: 1887–911.

5. Harton GL, Magli MC, Lundin K *et al.* ESHRE PGD Consortium/Embryology Special Interest Group – best practice guidelines for polar body and embryo biopsy for preimplantation genetic diagnosis/screening (PGD/PGS). *Hum Reprod* 2011; 26: 41–6.

6. Haapaniemi Kouru K, Malmgren H, Nordenskjöld M *et al.* One-cell biopsy significantly improves the outcome of preimplantation genetic diagnosis (PGD) treatment: retrospective analysis of 569 PGD cycles at the Stockholm PGD centre. *Hum Reprod* 2012; 26: 2843–9.

7. Kokkali G, Vrettou C, Traeger-Synodinos J *et al.* Birth of a healthy infant following trophectoderm biopsy from blastocysts for PGD of beta-thalassaemia major. *Hum Reprod* 2005; 20: 1855–9.

8. Renwick PJ, Trussler J, Ostad-Saffari E *et al.* Proof of principle and first cases using preimplantation genetic haplotyping – a paradigm shift for embryo diagnosis. *Reprod Biomed Online* 2006; 13: 110–9.

9. Harton GL, De Rycke M, Fiorentino F *et al.* ESHRE PGD consortium best practice guidelines for amplification-based PGD. *Hum Reprod* 2011; 26: 33–40.

10. Kakourou G, Dhanjal S, Mamas T *et al.* Modification of the triplet repeat primed polymerase chain reaction method for detection of the CTG repeat expansion in myotonic dystrophy type 1: application in preimplantation genetic diagnosis. *Fertil Steril* 2010; 94: 1674–9.

11. Hellebrekers DM, Wolfe R, Hendrickx AT *et al.* PGD and heteroplasmic mitochondrial DNA point

mutations: a systematic review estimating the chance of healthy offspring. *Hum Reprod Update* 2012; 18: 341–9.

12. Verlinsky Y, Rechitsky S, Schoolcraft W, Strom C, Kuliev A. Preimplantation diagnosis for Fanconi anemia combined with HLA matching. *JAMA* 2001; 285: 3130–3.

13. Van de Velde H, Georgiou I, De Rycke M *et al.* Novel universal approach for preimplantation genetic diagnosis of beta-thalassaemia in combination with HLA matching of embryos. *Hum Reprod* 2004; 19: 700–8.

14. Scriven PN, Handyside AH, Ogilvie CM. Chromosome translocations: segregation modes and strategies for preimplantation genetic diagnosis. *Prenat Diagn* 1998; 18: 1437–49.

15. Munné S, Sandalinas M, Escudero T *et al.* Outcome of preimplantation genetic diagnosis of translocations. *Fertil Steril* 2000; 73: 1209–18.

16. Fiorentino F, Kokkali G, Biricik A *et al.* Polymerase chain reaction-based detection of chromosomal imbalances on embryos: evolution of preimplantation genetic diagnosis for chromosomal translocations. *Fertil Steril* 2010; 94: 2001–11.

17. Wilton L. Preimplantation genetic diagnosis and chromosome analysis of blastomeres using comparative genomic hybridization. *Hum Reprod Update* 2005; 11: 33–41.

18. Malmgren H, Sahlén S, Inzunza J *et al.* Single cell CGH analysis reveals a high degree of mosaicism in human embryos from patients with balanced structural chromosome aberrations. *Mol Hum Reprod* 2002; 8: 502–10.

19. Fiorentino F, Spizzichino L, Bono S *et al.* PGD for reciprocal and Robertsonian translocations using array comparative genomic hybridization. *Hum Reprod* 2011; 26: 1925–35.

20. Gianaroli L, Magli MC, Ferraretti AP *et al.* Possible interchromosomal effect in embryos generated by gametes from translocation carriers. *Hum Reprod* 2002; 17: 3201–07.

21. Liebaers I, Desmyttere S, Verpoest W *et al.* Report on a consecutive series of 581 children born after blastomere biopsy for preimplantation genetic diagnosis. *Hum Reprod* 2010; 25: 275–82.

22. Wilton L, Thornhill A, Traeger-Synodinos J *et al.* The causes of misdiagnosis and adverse outcomes in PGD. *Hum Reprod* 2009; 24: 1221–8.

23. Harper JC, Sengupta S, Vesela K *et al.* Accreditation of the PGD laboratory. *Hum Reprod* 2010; 25: 1051–65.

24. Harper J, Coonen E, De Rycke M *et al.* What next for preimplantation genetic screening (PGS)? A position statement from the ESHRE PGD Consortium Steering Committee. *Human Reprod* 2010; 25: 821–3.

25. Handyside AH, Harton GL, Mariani B *et al.* Karyomapping: a universal method for genome-wide analysis of genetic disease based on mapping crossovers between parental haplotypes. *J Med Genet* 2010; 47: 651–8.

Chapter 12

Epigenetics and assisted reproductive technology

Aafke P. A. van Montfoort

Introduction

Since the birth of the first *in vitro* fertilization (IVF) baby in 1978, there has been concern about the safety of IVF and other assisted reproduction technology (ART) procedures for the health of the ART-conceived children. Data show that ART singletons are at an increased risk for adverse perinatal outcomes like low birth weight and being small for gestational age, and congenital malformations [1]. The biological mechanism behind these risks is mainly unresolved. Since the publication of a few case reports on the incidence of rare imprinting disorders like Angelman syndrome and Beckwith–Wiedemann syndrome in ART-conceived children, epigenetic deregulation gained increasing attention as a possible common cause for the adverse outcomes. This led to an expansion of ART literature on epigenetic effects. In this chapter the focus will be on the current knowledge of epigenetic disturbances in humans, reported after ART in general and in relation to specific ART components. The subfertility of the population as a possible cause for the epigenetic deregulation will also be taken into consideration. Finally, it will be discussed whether epigenetic effects can be related to the reported health outcome in ART children and if these possible derangements can affect their health at adult age.

Epigenetics and gene–environment interactions

What is epigenetics?

An individual's susceptibility to disease is not only determined by the DNA sequence (with mutations or polymorphisms) inherited from both parents. Epi-genetic mechanisms also play a role. In the context of this chapter epigenetics is used to describe mitotically and/or meiotically heritable changes in gene expression without changing the DNA sequence. These changes are induced by an interplay of epigenetic chromatin modifications like DNA methylation, histone modifications, histone variants, and RNA-mediated chromatin modifications (see also Chapter 5). Mainly DNA methylation will be touched upon in this chapter.

Mammalian DNA can become methylated at the carbon 5 position of a cytosine in CpG dinucleotides. Most CpGs are methylated, including CpGs residing in genes, intergenic regions, and repetitive elements like transposons. Only CpG islands, that are often associated with gene promoters, remain unmethylated (with the exception of imprinted regions, see below). Methylation is regulated by DNA methyltransferases (DNMTs). DNMT3a and DNMT3b, together with the cofactor DNMT3L, are responsible for *de novo* methylation of unmethylated CpG sites. After DNA replication, the methylation mark is copied to the newly synthesized unmethylated strand by DNMT1. DNA methylation of promoter regions is generally associated with transcriptional repression, either directly by interfering with the binding of transcription factors or indirectly by recruitment of methyl CpG binding domain (MBD) proteins and their associated repressive chromatin remodeling activities [2].

Epigenetic regulation is instrumental in development and cell differentiation. All cells within an organism have the same genotype, but they can differ in phenotype due to epigenetically regulated changes in gene expression that are transmitted to daughter cells. Also chromosome stability, stable X chromosome inactivation in females, and sex-specific genomic imprinting

Textbook of Human Reproductive Genetics, eds Karen Sermon and Stéphane Viville. Published by Cambridge University Press. © Cambridge University Press 2014.

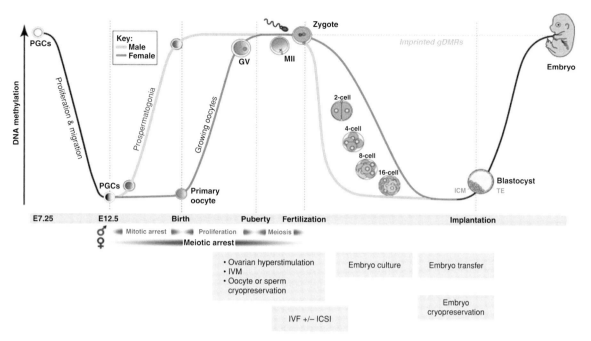

Figure 12.1 DNA methylation changes during developmental epigenetic reprogramming. The two phases of epigenetic reprogramming are schematically depicted. See text for an extensive description. The boxes below indicate the timing of ART procedures in relation to reprogramming events. gDMRs, germline differentially methylated region; ICM, inner cell mass; ICSI, intracytoplasmic sperm injection; IVF, *in vitro* fertilization; IVM, *in vitro* maturation; PGCs, primordial germ cells; TE, trophectoderm. Adapted with permission from Smallwood and Kelsey [2]. See plate section for color version.

are under epigenetic control. The latter is extensively described in Chapter 5. Briefly, in gametes, sex-specific epigenetic marks are deposited (mainly DNA methylation) that, after fertilization, result in parent-of-origin-specific gene expression of these genes. Given their role in placental and fetal growth and development and the increased risk for low birth weight in IVF children, these genes are often the targets of interest in ART-related epigenetic studies. Especially *H19*, *IGF2*, and the genes regulated by *KCNQ1OT1* imprinting control region (ICR, also called germline differentially methylated region or gDMR) draw attention since these are involved in Beckwith–Wiedemann and Silver–Russell syndromes that are characterized by overgrowth and growth retardation, respectively.

In order to acquire germ-cell specific imprints and to restore the totipotent state of an early preimplantation embryo after fusion of two differentiated germ cells, DNA methylation marks are erased and remodeled by two phases of epigenetic reprogramming; first at the primordial germ cell (PGC) stage and second after fertilization at the preimplantation embryo stage (see [2] for a review on this topic and

Fig. 12.1). Early in PGC development, global erasure of preexisting DNA methylation marks in differentially methylated regions (DMRs) of imprinted genes starts, together with the DNA demethylation of promoters, genic, intergenic and transposon sequences. This demethylation lasts until E13.5, preserving less than 10% methylation. Now, the female and male germ cells enter meiotic and mitotic arrest, respectively. The remethylation of imprinted loci in the male germ cells starts before birth at the prospermatogonial stage and is completed in the late spermatogonial stage. At the moment, three human paternally methylated gDMRs are known, all located at intergenic regions; between *H19* and *IGF2* (H19 DMR), between *DLK1* and *MEG3* (IG-DMR), and between *GPR1* and *ZDBF2*. In mice, a fourth DMR is located between *A19* and *RASGRF1*. In the female germ line, where the gDMRs are always located in promoter regions, remethylation starts after birth, around resumption of meiosis, and is completed just before ovulation for some loci. The second phase of reprogramming starts after fertilization with the active demethylation of the paternal genome. Shortly thereafter, the female genome passively loses methylation, generating a totipotent embryo. This continues until the morula stage, after which the inner cell mass becomes differentially methylated from the extra-embryonic lineages (Fig. 12.1). Both the paternally and maternally imprinted gDMRs maintain their methylation during this second reprogramming phase and in most cases during the rest of life.

Gene–environment interactions

Besides the developmentally induced epigenetic changes, the environment can also interfere with the epigenetic regulation. During pregnancy, particularly the periconceptional and preimplantation embryo stages are vulnerable. Epigenetic perturbations that arise during this period will be mitotically amplified and transmitted to the next cell generations, and therewith affect a large number of cells within an individual, while perturbations arising in more differentiated cells will only affect a (part of a) particular organ or tissue. As an example, a low protein diet in maternal rats restricted to the four days after mating, not only leads to altered expression levels of imprinted (*H19* and *Igf2*) and non-imprinted hepatic genes (phosphoenolpyruvate carboxykinase (*Pepck*) and 11β-hydroxysteroid dehydrogenase type 1 (*11βHsd1*)) in fetal liver but also to lower cell numbers in blastocysts, altered fetal and postnatal growth, changed organ weight, increased blood pressure, and anxiety-related behavior [3].

The importance of gestational environment in humans follows from studies highlighting that poor fetal growth (as a proxy for reduced fetal environment) leads to chronic diseases in adult life (known as the Barker theory). These findings led to the Developmental Origin of Health and Disease (DOHaD) paradigm, which is clearly exemplified by the adverse health outcomes reported in the people that were prenatally exposed to the Dutch Hunger Winter in World War II. During that period, which lasted for five months, food supplies to the northwestern part of the Netherlands were obstructed by the German occupying forces. The daily energy intake decreased rapidly, reaching 500 kcal/day at the end of this period. The neonates born after exposure to this famine during gestation had a lower birth weight, and at adult age these offspring were more susceptible to developing adverse metabolic and mental outcomes like obesity, diabetes, cardiovascular diseases, and schizophrenia when compared with subjects that were born before or conceived

after the famine. The early gestation period, including the periconceptional and early embryonic period, is extremely sensitive since most of the adverse outcomes that are reported after *in utero* exposure to famine during the Dutch Hunger Winter are related to exposure during this period. Moreover, the changes in methylation of several imprinted genes and loci involved in growth and metabolic disease found in blood from these adults are specific to the time of exposure. Exposure during early gestation has more effects than exposure late in gestation [4].

Epigenetic effects of ART

Considering the above, ART could be a risk for inducing epigenetic effects. Not only does ART lead to changes in environment during a sensitive period, ART procedures coincide with the major epigenetic reprogramming events during gameto- and embryogenesis (Fig. 12.1). During oogenesis, and coinciding with ovarian hyperstimulation, *in vitro* maturation and cryopreservation, the maternal-specific imprints are established. During spermatogenesis (cryopreservation) paternal imprints are established and should be maintained. After fertilization, non-imprinted genes get demethylated and imprinted ones should maintain their methylation, withstanding oocyte and sperm manipulation (IVF or intracytoplasmic sperm injection (ICSI), embryo culture, and cryopreservation). The current knowledge of ART-induced epigenetic alterations at these developmental stages as well as in IVF progeny is described below.

Imprinting disorders in ART offspring

Concern about epigenetic risks of ART in humans started with two case reports on children with the rare imprinting disorder Angelman syndrome (AS) that were born after ICSI (see [5] for review and Table 12.1). Angelman syndrome has an incidence of 1 in 15 000 births and is characterized by severe mental retardation, behavioral problems, and absence of speech (OMIM #105830). The defect lies in an imprinted region (*SNRPN* cluster) on chromosome 15 that leads to loss of maternal *UBE3A* expression. In more than 95% of the cases, the defect is genetic, i.e. a deletion or paternal uniparental disomy (UPD) of the chromosomal region or maternal *UBE3A* mutations. Less than 5% arise from a loss of maternal DNA methylation at *SNRPN*. Six cases of AS have been reported after ICSI (Table 12.1). Of these, the unexpected high

Table 12.1 Reports on the incidence of imprinting disorders after human IVF. See van Montfoort *et al.* [5] for a more extensive review of the studies

Studies	Type of study	N° cases	% IVF in cases	% IVF in studies	Estimated risk	Type of IVF	Molecular defect
Beckwith–Wiedemann syndrome							
DeBaun *et al.* (2003)	Case series	65	4.6%	0.76%	6.1[3]	IVF (N = 2) and ICSI (N = 5)	5/7 LOM KCNQ1OT1 gDMR 1/7 GOM H19 DMR 1/7 no imprint defect 1/7 not known
Maher *et al.* (2003)	Case series	149	4.0%	0.997%	4.0*	IVF (N = 3) and ICSI (N = 3)	2/6 LOM KCNQ1OT1 gDMR 4/6 not analyzed
Gicquel *et al.* (2003)	Case series	149	4.0%	1.3%	3.1*	IVF (N = 4) and ICSI (N = 2)	6/6 LOM KCNQ1OT1 gDMR (methylation levels range from 0–28%)
Halliday *et al.* (2004)	Case control	37	10.8%	0.67%	16.1*	IVF (N = 3) and ICSI (N = 1)	3/4 LOM KCNQ1OT1 gDMR 1/4 not analyzed
Chang *et al.* (2005)	Case series	341	5.6%[1]	–	–	IVF (N = 5) and ICSI (N = 5)[1]	NA
Sutcliffe *et al.* (2006)	Survey	209	2.9–7.6%[2]	0.8%	3.6–9.5[2],*	IVF (N = 1) and ICSI (N = 5)	6/6 LOM KCNQ1OT1 gDMR
Doornbos *et al.* (2007)	Survey	71	5.6%	0.92%	6.1*	IVF (N = 4)	4/4 LOM KCNQ1OT1 gDMR
Angelman syndrome							
Cox *et al.* (2002)	Case series	2	–	–	–	ICSI (N = 2)	2/2 LOM SNRPN (methylation level 0 and 10%)
Orstavik *et al.* (2003)	Case report	1	–	–	–	ICSI (N = 1)	1/1 LOM SNRPN
Ludwig *et al.* (2005)	Survey	79	3.8%	–	–	ICSI (N = 3)	1/3 LOM SNRPN 2/3 maternal deletion 15q11
Sutcliffe *et al.* (2006)	Survey	75	0%	0.8%	–	–	–
Doornbos *et al.* (2007)	Survey	63	0%	0.92%	–	–	–

Adapted with permission from van Montfoort *et al.* [5].
gDMR, germline differentially methylated region; GOM, gain of methylation; ICSI, intracytoplasmic sperm injection; IVF, *in vitro* fertilization; LOM, loss of methylation; – = not analyzed; NA, not applicable.
[1] All 19 ART cases are included, 10 after IVF (and ICSI), 2 after hormonal stimulation and insemination, and 7 for which no data on type of ART were available.
[2] Range takes into account the large number of lost to follow up by assuming that all non-responders conceived naturally.
[3] Seven ART-Beckwith–Wiedemann syndrome cases were identified in a database. Only three patients were from after 2001, when use of ART was systematically assessed. Only this period is included in the risk assessment.
* Risk is significantly increased in IVF compared to non-IVF pregnancies.

number of four cases showed a methylation defect. In one case there was a complete loss of methylation of the *SNRPN* region, while in another case only 10% of the alleles were methylated. This suggests that the demethylation finds its origin during oogenesis, or at least early in embryonic development by an error in imprint maintenance. In two other surveys covering 138 AS cases, none were conceived through IVF or ICSI. Instead, seven cases originated from ovula-tion induction and/or intrauterine insemination and of these one had a methylation defect at *SNRPN*.

Beckwith–Wiedemann syndrome (BWS, OMIM #130650), which has an incidence of 1 in 13 700, is a fetal and postnatal overgrowth disorder character-ized by a predisposition to tumor development and a variety of complications. The five most common fea-tures are macrosomia, macroglossia, abdominal wall defects, ear creases, and neonatal hypoglycemia, but some cases even lack these. The risk for BWS after IVF, expressed as the relative abundance of IVF in a BWS population compared with the relative abundance of IVF in the general population, is estimated at between 3.1 and 16.1 (Table 12.1). Beckwith–Wiedemann syndrome occurred irrespective of the cause of subfertility and ART characteristics like level of hormonal stimulation, mode of fertilization, fresh or frozen embryo transfer, or day of embryo transfer. Beckwith–Wiedemann syndrome cases have also been reported after intrauterine inseminations with or without ovulation induction, or after the use of fertility drugs alone. It should be kept in mind that the variability in clinical features makes it sometimes hard to identify BWS cases, especially since BWS children grow up as adults of normal size with normal intelligence. This might introduce a bias of over-identification of BWS in ART offspring since these tend to be followed-up more thoroughly. Nevertheless, it is appearing that after IVF almost all cases are related to a loss of maternal methylation at *KCNQ1OT1*, while in the general BWS population around 50% is caused by an epigenetic defect. In six of the ART-BWS cases, the actual level of methylation at the *KCNQ1OT1* locus was measured and ranged from 0 to 28%. Since most of the cases had some maternal methylation a post-fertilization imprint maintenance effect is likely to be the cause.

Retinoblastoma (RB) and Prader–Willi Syndrome (PWS) are two other disorders involving imprinted regions. The molecular defects are mostly (point) mutations or deletions, just as in three out of four PWS and three out of seven RB cases reported after IVF. For the remaining cases, the defect is unknown. In cases of the Silver–Russell syndrome (SRS) that are reported after ART, the defect is also often unknown. The numbers are too small, and the incidence of the disease too low to indicate a relation between SRS and ART.

Epigenetic effects in oocytes

In humans, studies on epigenetic reprogramming of imprinted genes during oogenesis are very limited for ethical reasons. Moreover, the analysis of the effect of hormonal priming or *in vitro* maturation on imprinting in oocytes might be confounded by maternal age and/or suboptimal oogenesis related to the subfertility and often lacks proper controls. Only one study used immature oocytes from non-stimulated fertile patients obtained after laparoscopy and compared these with superovulated germinal vesicle (GV) and metaphase I

(MI) oocytes from IVF treatments [6]. In oocytes with fully grown GVs, the methylation of *MEST* was almost complete, while after ovarian stimulation only 10 of the 16 GV/MI oocytes were methylated. The demethylation of the paternal imprint of *H19* DMR was not yet completed at the antral follicle stage of unstimulated follicles, leaving a remnant of around 12.5%. In superovulated GV/MI oocytes, two out of six were still erroneously methylated [6]. Since the cause of subfertility of the donating couples was male or tubal obstruction, the effects are likely to be attributed to superovulation.

From studies in mice it seems as if superovulation does not directly affect methylation at the oocyte stage, but that it exerts its effects indirectly resulting in a response at blastocyst stage or even at a later stage by temporarily changing the environment in the female reproductive tract. Although no causal effects are reported in superovulated mouse oocytes, a superovulation dose-dependent disturbance of CpG methylation in some imprinted loci in blastocysts was found [7]. Fortier *et al.* analyzed the effect of hormonal stimulation on the expression of *Snrpn*, *Kcnq1ot1*, and *H19* in embryos and placentas at Embryonic Day 9.5 and found that *Snrpn* and *H19* (but not *Kcnq1ot1*) showed biallelic expression in the placenta [8]. This effect vanished for *Snrpn* and was reduced for *H19* when embryos were transplanted to the uterus of non-stimulated foster mothers.

By culturing GV and MI oocytes that remain after an IVF treatment with hormonal stimulation, the effect of *in vitro* maturation (IVM) of human oocytes is investigated. After an overnight culture, all *in vitro* matured metaphase II (MII) oocytes display correct methylation at maternal (*KCNQ1OT1* and *SNRPN*) and paternal (IG-DMR) imprinted genes. However, in a study comparing *in vivo* and *in vitro*-derived MII oocytes, the methylation level of *KCNQ1OT1* was lower after IVM. *H19* is also vulnerable to the maturation environment. In two out of six patients, the pool of MII oocytes derived from IVM of GV oocytes displayed methylation in all or part of the oocytes [5].

The demand for cryopreservation of oocytes to preserve fertility is growing and the vitrification technique is gaining ground as the method of choice. Germinal vesicle-stage oocytes that were vitrified and, after thawing, matured *in vitro* to MII oocytes, showed a similar methylated and demethylated pattern in *KCNQ1OT1* and *H19* DMR, respectively, as compared to non-cryopreserved *in vitro* matured oocytes [9].

In conclusion, superovulation and IVM have the potential to affect imprint erasure and establishment in oocytes, although the results are not all in agreement.

Epigenetic effects in the embryo

The inevitable connection of subfertile patients, superovulation, *in vitro* fertilization, and culture makes it difficult to investigate the separate contribution to epigenetic deregulation in preimplantation embryos and blastocysts. Moreover, *in vivo* control embryos are lacking. Nevertheless, interesting information is obtained from the analysis of human surplus embryos of low quality (low number of blastomeres and/or low morphological grade) that were not suitable for transfer or for cryopreservation. Six out of 32 (19%) Day 3 embryos showed aberrant methylation at a single CpG within *H19* DMR; five of these showed a complete loss of methylation and one was hypomethylated. It is unlikely that this is caused by paternal transmission, since the sperm samples that were used to fertilize these embryos showed normal methylation [10]. In another study, it was shown that in some DNA strands in cells of abnormally developing morulas and blastocysts, the relaxation of methylation comprises not only a single CpG but the whole strand [11]. Again, the corresponding sperm samples showed complete methylation. This suggests a lack of imprint maintenance induced by *in vitro* manipulation as the main cause. Five cryopreserved good quality blastocysts that were donated for research all showed normal methylation. The relation between embryo quality and abnormal methylation needs further investigation but could be reassuring when considering transmission of ART-induced epigenetic effects to the offspring. Which is cause and which is effect in the relation between embryo quality and *H19* DNA hypomethylation is unknown.

From these limited number of analyzed embryos there is no evidence that one of the two fertilization methods, IVF or ICSI, differently affects vulnerability for methylation defects. Moreover, the effect of the culture medium is not investigated in the human. However, it was shown recently that the birth weight of children that as an embryo were cultured in one of two different culture media, differed 112 g after adjustment for several confounders [12]. This resembles the results in animal studies where the addition of serum to the culture medium affects the growth of the fetus and the expression of several imprinted genes

[3]. Market-Velker and colleagues compared six different culture media (Whitten's, KSOM supplemented with amino acids (KSOMaa), Global, HTF, P1MB, and G1/G2) and found that all media, albeit to a different extent, affected DNA methylation of imprinted genes (*H19*, *Mest*, and *Snprn*) in mouse blastocysts, as compared with *in vivo*-derived blastocysts. All media systems also led to loss of imprinted gene expression of *H19* [13].

Epigenetic effects in placenta and umbilical cord blood

Numerous studies compared methylation and/or expression of imprinted genes in placental tissue and/or umbilical cord blood (UCB) from IVF and naturally conceived pregnancies (see Table 12.2 and [5] for a more extensive overview of studies).

In the targeted gene studies analyzing multiple imprinted genes, mainly *H19* and *MEST* show altered methylation patterns after IVF, while other regions remain unaffected (Table 12.2). Rancourt *et al.* analyzed the DNA methylation of six DMRs (MEST, GRB10, KCNQ1, SNRPN, H19, and IGF2 DMR0) and found a hypomethylation of *MEST* and *H19* together with a hypermethylation of *SNRPN* in placental tissue of IVF singletons, as compared with non-IVF controls [14]. Interestingly, the corresponding UCB was hypomethylated at *KCNQ1* only. This inconsistency in DNA methylation effects between placental and fetal tissue is also often reported in animal studies on imprinting effects of ART. The methylation in fetal tissue is less affected compared to placental tissue. Since both paternally and maternally methylated regions are involved, and since the loss or gain in methylation concerns only a minority of the alleles (i.e. only a few percent hypo- or hypermethylation is recorded), the epigenetic deregulation is expected to occur at a time point after fertilization. It might also be caused by a superovulation primed uterine environment since the infants conceived with ovulation induction alone were also hypomethylated at *H19* and *SNRPN* (placental tissue) and *SNRPN* and *KCNQ1* (UCB). At birth, no phenotypic differences were noted between the groups.

Very similar results were seen in a comparable study analyzing placental tissue from IVF and *in vivo*-conceived pregnancies. *H19* and *MEST* were hypomethylated after IVF, whereas *IGF2, IG-DMR, MEG3, SNRPN, PEG3,* and *KCNQ1OT1* showed a

Table 12.2 DNA methylation and gene expression studies in ART-conceived human offspring at birth and during childhood. See van Montfoort et al. [5] for a more extensive overview of the studies

Studies	ART	No. (ART)	Sample	Control group	CpGs analyzed	Gene / DMR analyzed	Methylation (M) or Expression (E) analyzed	Epigenetic outcome in ART group	Clinical outcome in ART group
At birth									
Katari et al. (2009)	IVF	10	UCB, placenta	Naturally conceived children	Imprinted + non-imprinted	1536 CpG sites	M + E	23% CpG sites differed in UCB and 16% in placenta. Imprinted genes not extra vulnerable for deregulation compared to non-imprinted. 4/11 tested genes with differential methylation also showed differential expression	Lower birth weight
Tierling et al. (2010)	IVF + ICSI	112	UCB, amnion membrane	Naturally conceived children	Imprinted	KCNQ1OT1 H19 SNRPN MEST GRB10 GTL2 GNAS locus	M	Slight hypermethylation of MEST in IVF samples compared to ICSI and control	Lower birth weight and length
Nelissen et al. (2013)	IVF + ICSI	35	Placenta	Naturally conceived children	Imprinted	H19 IGF2 IG-DMR MEG3 SNRPN MEST PEG3 KCNQ1OT1	M + E	Hypomethylation at H19 and MEST in IVF accompanied by an increased expression of H19. No difference in IGF2 and MEST expression	Similar birth weight
Rancourt et al. (2012)	IVF (ICSI unknown) OI	59 27	Placenta + UCB	Naturally conceived children	Imprinted	MEST GRB10 KCNQ1 SNRPN H19 IGF2 DMR0	M + E	In placenta: Hypomethylation at H19 and MEST and hypermethylation at SNRPN in IVF. Hypomethylation at H19 and hypermethylation at SNRPN in OI. In UCB: Hypermethylation at KCNQ1 in IVF. Hypermethylation at SNRPN and KCNQ1 in OI. No differences in expression	Lower birth weight (~ 100 g, NS)

At childhood

Kanber et al. (2009)	ICSI + SGA	19	Buccal smear from children aged 4–7 years	Normal weight children after spontaneous conception	Imprinted	*KCNQ1OT1* *MEST* *PEG3* *H19* *GTL2* *PLAGL1*	M	1/19 hypermethylated at *KCNQ1OT1* and *MEST*	SGA
Oliver et al. (2012)	IVF + ICSI	66	Blood from children aged 4–10 years	Naturally conceived children	Imprinted + non-imprinted	*H19* *SNRPN* *KCNQ1OT1* *IGF2* Global DNA methylation Genome-wide promoter methylation	M	No differences	Lower birth weight taller, lower BMI, higher level of serum IGF2 and HDL and lower level of IGFBP1 and triglycerides

ART, assisted reproductive technology; AS, Angelman syndrome; BMI, body mass index; DMR, differentially methylated region; HDL, high-density lipoprotein; ICSI, intracytoplasmic sperm injection; IVF, *in vitro* fertilization; NS, not significant; OI, ovulation induction; PWS, Prader–Willi syndrome; SGA, small for gestational age.

normal methylation pattern [15]. In contrast to the single CpG methylation approach applied in many studies, this study shows that the hypomethylation is consistently observed in all CpG sites analyzed within the DMR. A higher transcript abundance of *H19* was recorded. Birth weight was similar in both groups.

Besides imprinted genes, also non-imprinted ones can be affected. An extended analysis of more than 1500 genes in placental tissue and UCB indicated that there is no increased vulnerability of imprinted genes for IVF-related methylation disturbances when compared to non-imprinted genes [16]. Around 23% of the CpG sites analyzed in UCB were hypo- or hypermethylated and 16% were in placental tissue. Four out of 11 tested genes that were differentially methylated also showed a difference in expression level. Some of these genes are involved in metabolic disorders.

Next to an affected metabolism, ART-induced epigenetic aberrations might also affect the placental functioning. A large-scale protein analysis revealed 20 differentially expressed proteins, including proteins involved in transmembrane transport, metabolism, nucleic acid processing, stress response, and cytoskeleton. Together with the observations of a thicker maternal–fetal placental barrier and a decreased number of apical microvilli at the placental barrier [17], this suggests a reduced maternal–fetal exchange in the placenta after an IVF treatment.

Epigenetic effects in IVF children

To assess potential epigenetically induced health risks for IVF offspring, DNA methylation in IVF children is assessed. The investigation of organ-specific methylation alterations (e.g. in liver where in rodents environmentally induced differences in expression and methylation of metabolically important genes have been found [3]) is not possible in human, which limits the analyses to blood or buccal cells. Kanber *et al.* (Table 12.2) analyzed the methylation of 6 loci in 19 small-for-gestational-age children born after ICSI and found a hypermethylation in one child (defined as >60% methylation) of *KCNQ1OT1* and *MEST* without further phenotypic abnormalities [18]. In a larger cohort no significant differences in DNA methylation at four imprinted DMRs, as well as global DNA methylation and genome-wide promoter methylation were observed [19]. Interestingly, these samples were collected from children that were also subjected to

anthropometric measurements and serum screening for several metabolic and growth factors. *In vitro* fertilization-conceived children were taller than the controls and also had a more favorable lipid profile [20].

Epigenetic effects transmitted by the subfertile parents

Besides the *de novo* induction of epigenetic effects by ART, the possibility of transmittance of these effects from the subfertile patient to their offspring should be taken into account. Although an extensive reprogramming of epigenetic marks during gametogenesis takes place, some elements escape this reprogramming allowing for transgenerational epigenetic inheritance (TEI). This phenomenon and examples of TEI are described in van Montfoort *et al.* [5].

Whether subfertility and epigenetic disturbances in human oocytes are correlated and whether these possible epigenetic disturbances can be transmitted to the next generation is difficult to investigate since oocyte retrieval from subfertile women is always inevitably connected to hormonal stimulation.

Effect of male subfertility on DNA methylation in spermatozoa

In the male germline, the paternal and maternal imprints are erased in the fetal prospermatogonia. The male imprints are reestablished after birth in the adult spermatogonial stage, before the spermatocytes enter meiosis I and hence are completely methylated in mature spermatozoa. A disturbance in spermatogenesis, whether it is in concentration, morphology or motility, is associated with incorrect imprinting. An overview of the numerous studies showing this is given in van Montfoort *et al.* [5]. In general, in spermatozoa from oligozoospermic men, the occurrence of hypermethylation of maternal imprints, and the hypomethylation of paternal imprints like *H19* and IG-DMR is increased, especially in semen samples with $<10 \times 10^6$/ml spermatozoa. In normozoospermia only a few CpGs within a DMR are aberrantly methylated, while in azoospermia this ranges from only a few to all CpGs. The latter occurs only in a minority of alleles and thus in a minority of the spermatozoa. Although less extensively investigated, a reduced sperm motility and morphology are also associated with aberrant methylation at imprinted regions.

Global DNA methylation of non-imprinted sequences such as long and short interspersed nucleotide elements (LINE1 and SINE) is not affected in azoospermia (see Chapter 6).

Is there evidence for transmission of methylation defects in spermatozoa to IVF offspring?

The numerous aberrations in DNA methylation in spermatozoa from the subfertile male might be worrying. However, transmission of these defects to viable offspring is not so evident. To the best of our knowledge this has never been reported. The reported reduced fertilization rate and increased embryo developmental arrest in ART after using this methylation-defective sperm suggest that spermatozoa with aberrant imprints have reduced capacity to fertilize the oocyte or to guide the embryo through the first stages of development. However, the embryos were not analyzed, and so paternal transmission is not confirmed.

In trophoblastic villi samples from ART miscarriages between six and nine weeks of gestation, *H19* methylation defects were found. For part of these samples, similar defects were found in the spermatozoa from the father [21]. This suggests transmittance, but with no viability for the offspring.

Perinatal and childhood outcome of IVF children: epigenetic influence or not?

In vitro fertilization singletons show an increased risk for very preterm birth (<32 weeks), preterm birth (<37 weeks, relative risk (RR) 1.4–3.0), very low birth weight (<1500 g, RR 2.7–3.8), low birth weight (<2500 g, RR 1.4–1.6), small for gestational age (odds ratio (OR) 1.6), and perinatal mortality (OR 2.2–2.4). Also an increased risk for congenital malformations like neural tube defects, septal heart defects, and esophageal atresia is reported, with a RR between 1.3 and 1.4 according to meta-analyses [5].

Recently, interest is directed towards physiological and metabolic outcome parameters. An extensive examination of 233 age- and gender-matched IVF and spontaneously conceived children of subfertile parents aged 8–18 years showed that weight and height gain between 3 months and 1 year, peripheral skin-fold thickness, systolic and diastolic blood pressure, fasting glucose level, and dehydroepiandrosterone sulfate (DHEAS) and luteinizing hormone (LH) level in pubertal girls are all higher in the IVF group [22]. Fasting insulin level, bone mass, pubertal maturity, follicle-stimulating hormone (FSH) level, and hip and waist circumference were similar. In another study, systemic (flow-mediated dilation and carotid intima-media thickness) and pulmonary vascular function was decreased in IVF children, whereas blood pressure was equal to the control group [23]. Vascular function in the naturally conceived siblings from the IVF children and in children conceived after hormonal stimulation only was normal, suggesting that an ART factor and not a parental factor is at stake. In a younger IVF population of around 6 years old, the IVF children were taller and had a slightly more favorable lipid profile indicated by the higher HDL and lower triglycerides level, and an increased serum IGF2 level [20].

When assuming a random distribution of genotypic variation among ART and non-ART offspring, a genetic component for these perinatal and childhood IVF outcomes is unlikely. Therefore, it is reasonable to assume that this is an effect of an epigenetic adaptive response to the preimplantation embryo environment. Further, for most of the congenital malformations (like neural tube defects and heart defects) the incidence decreases when the mother takes folic acid supplementation, which is a factor in the DNA methylation cycle, during the periconception phase. The physiological outcomes suggest a predisposition for metabolic syndrome, just as seen in offspring that were *in utero* during the Dutch Hunger Winter and in animal studies where the maternal diet was changed during conception phase (see the "Gene–environment interactions" section, above). Furthermore, *in vitro* culture of mouse embryos leads to similar outcomes like increased systolic blood pressure, changes in postnatal organ weight, and altered angiotensin converting enzyme (ACE) and PEPCK activity in serum and liver, respectively [3]. In these examples altered gene expression and methylation levels are also described. Altogether, these outcomes fit in the DOHaD paradigm with the fetal programming concept. This concept states that the fetus is programmed in order to prepare itself for life after birth. Based on the fetal environment (i.e. nutritional and endocrine status) epigenetic adaptations in organs and tissues are made, that permanently adjusts the physiology of these organs and the metabolism of the fetus. This ensures optimal health if both the prenatal and postnatal environment match. If not, an extra burden is put on the organs and tissues that might lead to chronic diseases in later life.

Discussion and conclusion

As can be derived from the studies described in this chapter, ART can cause epigenetic imprinting changes in oocytes, embryos, placental tissue, and UCB. However, as yet, the health effects for the offspring are not so clear-cut.

Ovarian hyperstimulation is a candidate for epigenetic deregulation in oocytes. However, the effects seen later in development, i.e. in embryos or placental tissue, are mosaic rather than showing a complete de- or re-methylation. This supports the idea that methylation errors are due to imprint maintenance failure in part of the embryo rather than imprint establishment in the gamete. Further, the effect of a hormone-induced changed environment of the female reproductive tract, as seen in animals, should not be neglected, but is difficult to analyze in humans.

In human blastocysts methylation defects have been reported, but mainly in the arrested embryos not suitable for transfer. This might be an *in vitro* culture effect since no defects in the spermatozoa were found. It seems as if both natural selection (developmental arrest) and laboratory selection of embryos based on morphology largely reduce the risk for major epigenetic effects in ART offspring. This is supported by the low frequency (although increased) of imprinting disorders reported after ART. Also the risk of transmitting methylation defects from azoospermic men to viable IVF offspring appears small.

Besides aberrant methylation of a DMR, indicative of an epimutation, aberrant methylation can also be a single CpG error, most likely reflecting stochastic methylation errors without phenotypic or functional consequences. The techniques used often make it impossible to distinguish between an epimutation of the whole allele or a stochastic effect of a single CpG site. Although methylation aberrations in a large part of the DMR have been reported in placental tissue [15], many studies analyzing placental tissue and UCB often analyzed only one or a very few CpGs per DMR. An ART-induced increased rate of stochastic errors will presumably not lead to an increased risk immediately, but might put ART offspring one step ahead for environment-induced stochastic DNA methylation

errors to reach the threshold that will lead to disease. This might explain the increased vulnerability of ART offspring for the physiological effects like increased blood pressure or the higher fasting glucose level that were reported, or make them more vulnerable for late-onset diseases such as cardiovascular disease or cancer.

The physiological outcomes reported in ART children suggest that the DOHaD paradigm not only refers to the fetal period but also the embryonic period. Knowledge about a direct effect of preimplantation environment on epigenetic regulation of genes important for metabolism is lacking. However, indications exist that at least part of the relation between embryo environment and postnatal physiological outcome might be regulated by an affected placenta. Since the placenta is the first organ to develop after *in vitro* exposure of preimplantation embryos, changes in the embryonic environment might affect the inner cell mass (ICM)/trophectoderm (TE) differentiation or programming. This is supported by the fact that ART-induced methylation defects of imprinted genes, which play an important role in placenta function, are mainly seen in placental tissue and hardly in fetal tissue (UCB) or blood of an IVF child. It is evident from animal and human studies that epimutations in imprinted genes can lead to alterations in the morphology and physiology of the placenta with subsequent consequences such as abnormal fetal growth and perhaps organ-specific fetal programming of genes important in metabolism [24]. (Suggestive for this is that, in an analysis of around 1500 CpG sites of which most resided in the promoter region of non-imprinted genes, ART-induced methylation differences were more abundant in the UCB as compared to the placenta. Some of the affected genes are indeed involved in metabolic disorders [16].) The increased vulnerability of the placenta or TE is substantiated by the increased risk for placental defects after ART, like placenta praevia [1], the aberrant values of first-trimester pregnancy serum markers produced by the placenta (PAPP-A), and the structural abnormalities in ART placentas [17].

In general, although the risk for creating and transmitting major epigenetic defects, i.e. epimutations, in ART seems small, the possible effect of smaller epigenetic effects should not be underestimated as long as many issues regarding epigenetically induced disease risk remain unknown. Also, the role of ART-induced aberrant epigenetic regulation in the placenta and its possible adverse effects for ART offspring deserves attention.

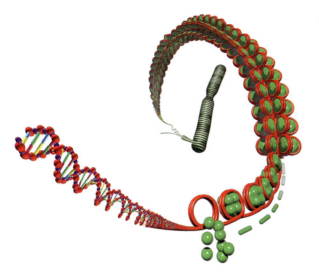

Figure 1.2 DNA is organized in chromatin. © Science Photo Library.

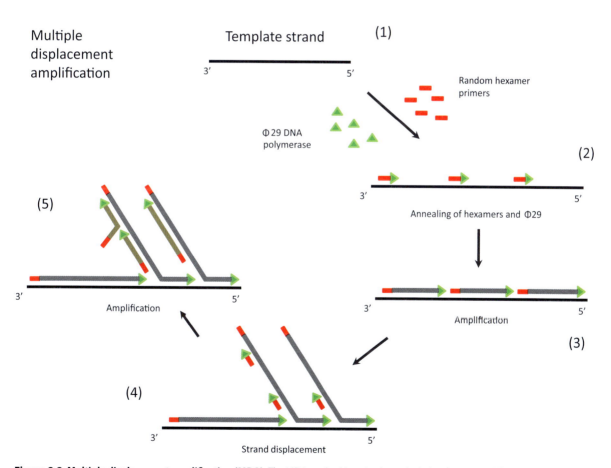

Figure 2.2 Multiple displacement amplification (MDA). The MDA method is an isothermal whole genome amplification method involving: (**1**) the annealing of random primers onto the denatured DNA template; (**2–3**) amplification of the DNA strands at constant temperature using, for example, the φ29 DNA polymerase; (**4**) strand displacement that (**5**) exposes the newly synthesized DNA strands for further amplification.

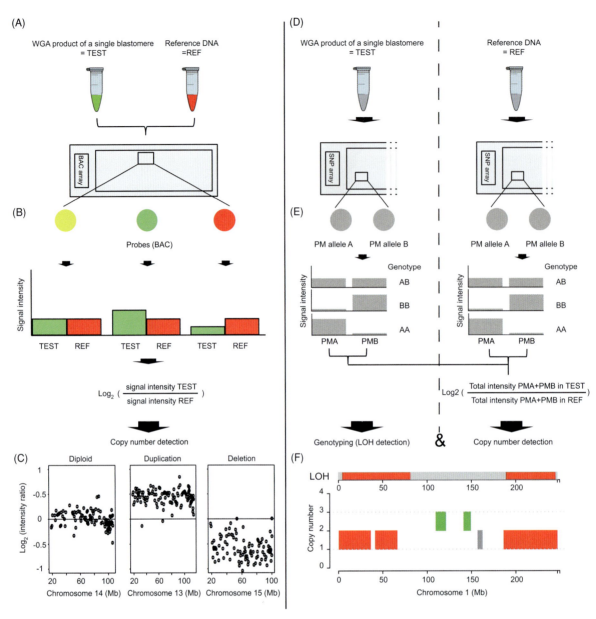

Figure 2.3 Single-cell aCGH and SNP array analysis. Analyzing the genome of a single blastomere using bacterial artificial chromosome (BAC) arrays (**A–C**) or SNP arrays (D–F). (**A**) The whole genome amplification (WGA) product of a single blastomere "TEST" sample is fluorescently labeled (green) and a reference DNA "REF" sample is marked with a different fluorophore (red). The labeled TEST and REF samples are hybridized simultaneously on a BAC array, and (**B**) the intensities of the fluorescent signals resulting from hybridized TEST and REF DNA are measured for each spot containing DNA of a specific BAC probe. The ratio of both signals is representative of the relative copy number in the TEST sample compared to the REF sample. Equal signal intensities for TEST and REF indicate a diploid region in the TEST sample (left bars) if the REF sample is diploid for the locus interrogated by the BAC probe. In this scenario, a higher or lower TEST signal versus the REF signal indicates a DNA gain (middle bars) or DNA loss (right bars) in the TEST respectively. Log$_2$ intensity ratios across all BAC probes are normalized, segmented, and used for copy number detection. (**C**) Log$_2$ intensity ratios (Y-axis) for each probe according to their genomic location (X-axis). The left panel shows a diploid chromosome 14 in a single blastomere demonstrating log$_2$ intensity ratios rippling around 0. The middle and right panel show, respectively, a duplication of chromosome 13 and a deletion of chromosome 15 in the same single blastomere. (**D,E**) The WGA product of a single blastomere is labeled and hybridized to a SNP array (left of panel **D,E**). Reference DNA sample(s) are hybridized each to a separate SNP array (right of panel **D,E**). (**E**) The labeled DNA will bind a set of single-stranded probes interrogating, respectively, the A and B allele for each SNP on the array. These are depicted as perfect-match probes (PM) for the A and B allele of a SNP (gray dots). Gray bar-plots represent different examples of signal intensities for PM-A and PM-B allele probes that can be obtained in scenarios of AB, BB, or AA genotypes for this SNP, respectively. The genotypes inferred from PM-probe signals can be used to detect stretches of loss of heterozygosity (LOH) in the genome. Log$_2$ intensity ratios per SNP can be calculated *in silico* from the PM-A and PM-B probe signals obtained for both the TEST sample and REF sample(s). The log$_2$ intensity ratios are used to detect copy number aberrations in the TEST sample as compared to the REF sample(s). (**F**) The bottom panel shows the calculated copy number (Y-axis) for chromosome 1 (X-axis) in a single blastomere as deduced from SNP array analysis. Red signifies deletions, green duplications. The top panel of (**F**) shows the detection of regions of LOH (red) using the same SNP array data. The LOH is detected in the deleted 1p- and 1q-terminal regions, confirming that these deletions are real.

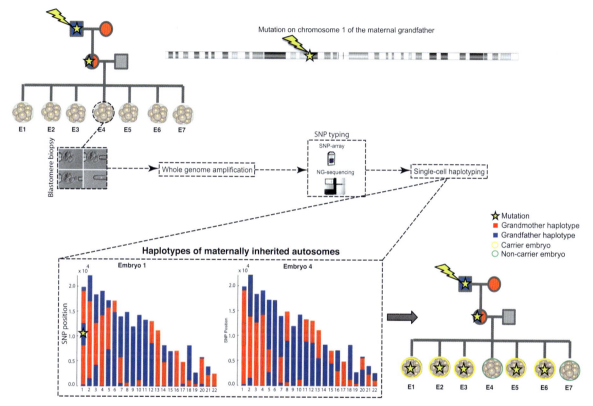

Figure 2.5 A schematic overview of the workflow for haplotyping single blastomeres of *in vitro* fertlilization embryos. In the depicted pedigree, a blue color represents the grandfather's homologous chromosomes and a red color represents the grandmother's homologous chromosomes in the maternal lineage of an embryo. After a single blastomere biopsy of the Day 3 cleavage-stage embryos and genotyping of the whole genome amplification (WGA) products, single-cell haplotypes can be deduced. Following haplotyping of the single blastomere genotypes, the homologous recombinations that occurred between the homologous chromosomes in maternal meiosis I are revealed by the transitions of red and blue haplotype blocks on the maternally inherited chromosomes. The X-axis represents the 22 autosomes and the Y-axis represents the relative SNP position along the chromosome. The transmission of the genetic risk allele (depicted as a star) can now be tracked through the pedigree, and carrier embryos (embryos 1, 2, 3, 5, and 6) as well as non-carrier embryos (embryos 4 and 7) can be identified.

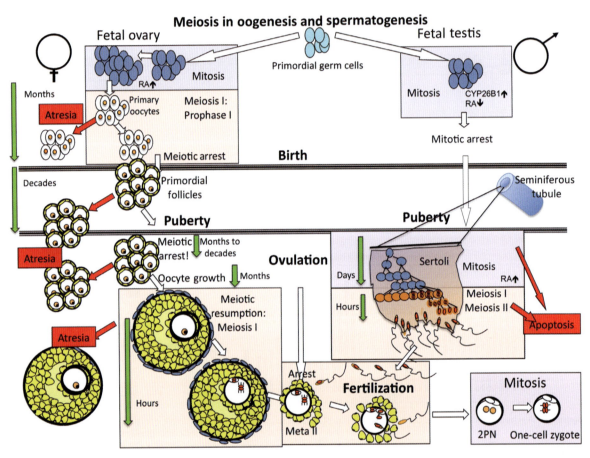

Figure 3.2 Germ-cell formation and timing of meiosis in oogenesis (left side) and spermatogenesis (right side). For further explanation, see text.

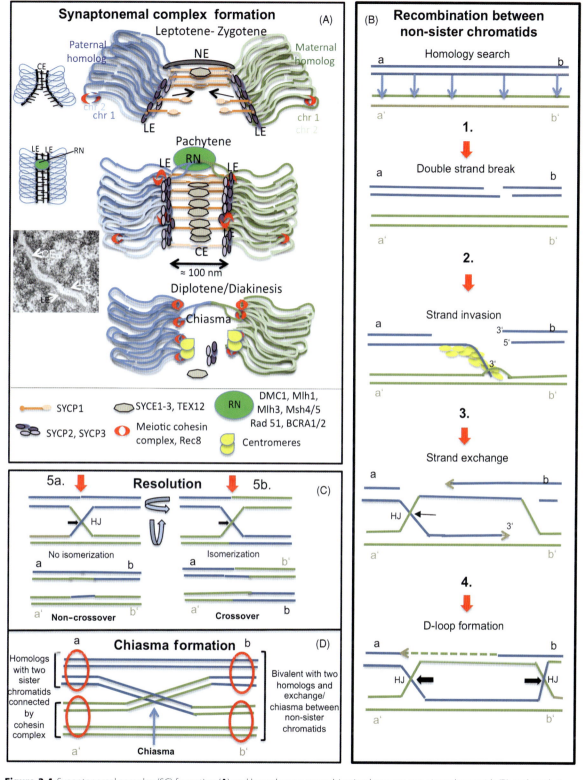

Figure 3.4 Synaptonemal complex (SC) formation (**A**) and homologous recombination between non-sister chromatids (**B**), and resolution of recombination after non-crossover or crossover (**C**), and chiasama formation (**D**). DNA strands from parental homologs are symbolized by different colors (blue and green, respectively). Proteins involved in the SC (**A**) in lateral elements (LE) with SYCP2 and 3 proteins, central element (CE) containing SYCE1–3 and TEX12 proteins, cohesion (red clips) with meiotic Rec8 cohesin that physically attach the sister chromatids to each other or to the LE, transversal fibers (orange) containing SYCP1 protein, and recombination nodules (RN) containing recombination enzymes (DMC1, Mlh1, Mlh3, Msh4/5, Rad 51, BCRA1/2) are presented. Chr 1 and Chr 2: sister chromatids in paternal and maternal homolog. Left: top view, right tangential section of SC and homologs are depicted at successive stage of prophase I (**A**). Events in recombination between non-sister chromatids (steps 1.–4. and 5a. and 5b., in **B** and **C**, respectively) leading to chiasma formation (**D**) are shown.

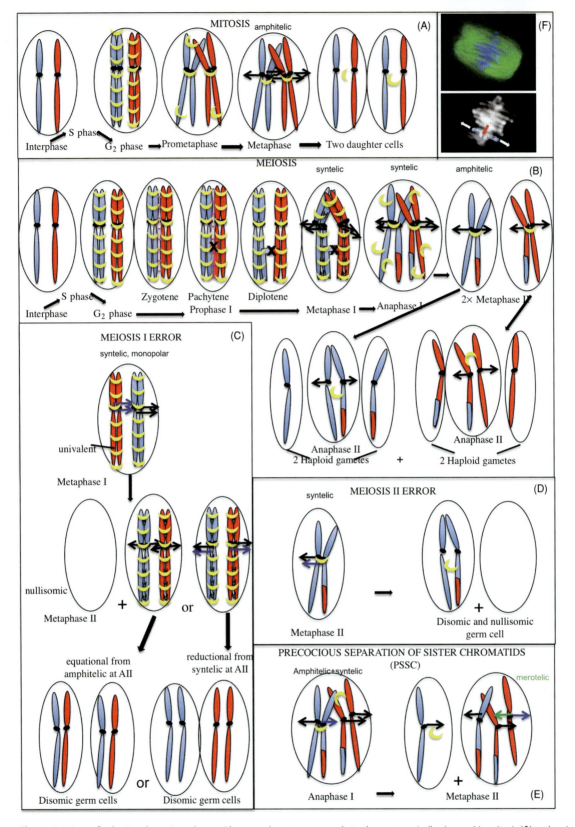

Figure 3.5 Loss of cohesion along sister chromatid arms and centromeres and attachment to spindles (arrows) in mitosis (**A**) and meiosis (**B–F**). Homologs with their two sister chromatids are colored in blue and red, respectively (**A–E**), cohesion complexes between sister chromatids in yellow and exchanges by crossover/chiasmata by black X (**B**). Aberrant chromosome attachment/orientation is indicated by blue arrows in typical meiotic errors at first meiosis (**C**), second meiosis (**D**), and precocious separation of sister chromatids (PSSC) (**E**), or by green arrow in case of merotelic attachment of one centromere to both spindle poles (**E**). Alignment of bivalents (blue and white) in the spindle (green fluorescence) in mouse meiosis I oocyte (**F**): one condensed bivalent is outlined in blue in which the centromeres of the homologs are attached to opposite spindle poles (white arrows) while the chiasma physically connecting the parental homologs lies at the spindle equator (red arrow). For further explanation, see text.

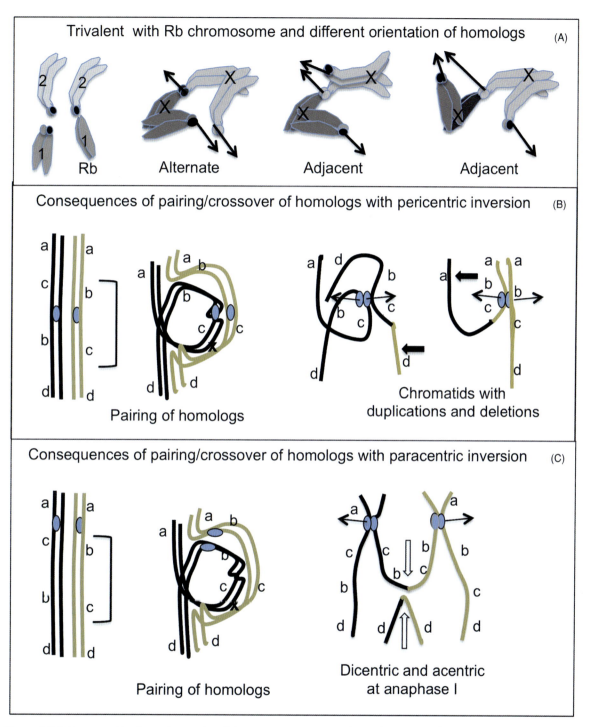

Figure 3.7 Pairing, recombination, and separation of chromosomes in meiocytes that are heterozygous for a Robertsonian translocation chromosome (Rb) (**A**), a balanced pericentric inversion (**B**), or a paracentric inversion (**C**). For further explanation, see text.

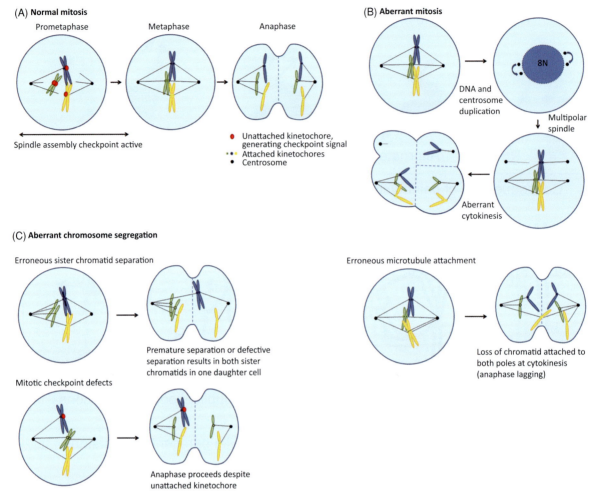

Figure 4.1 (**A**) Schematic representation of normal chromosome alignment and segregation. At prometaphase, the spindle assembly checkpoint is activated at each unattached kinetochore. Microtubule capture of both kinetochores of a chromosome results in silencing of the checkpoint and chromosome alignment at the metaphase plate. Anaphase is not initiated until all chromosomes have achieved bipolar attachment to the spindle and congression to the spindle midzone. During anaphase, the sister chromatids are pulled apart. After invagination of the cell membrane and completion of cytokinesis, the sister chromatids are equally separated to the two daughter cells. (**B**) Losses and gains of whole chromosomes during mitosis can be explained in several ways. Aberrant mitosis can cause chromosome loss. Too many centrosomes can result from errors in centrosome duplication or skipping cytokinesis, producing polyploidization (8N). Multiple centrosomes induce multipolar spindles and chromosome malsegregation. (**C**) Mitotic nondisjunction results in reciprocal loss and gain of a chromosome in the two daughter cells. This can be caused by erroneous sister chromatid separation (chromatids separate prematurely or not at all) or mitotic checkpoint defects that fail to prevent anaphase before all chromosomes are properly attached. Anaphase lagging results in loss of a sister chromatid from one daughter cell and can be the result of erroneous microtubule attachment (merotelic attachment).

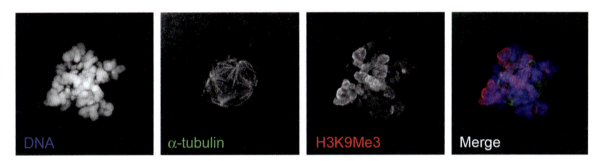

Figure 4.2 Confocal image of a human tripronuclear zygote at prometaphase, showing chromosomes (DNA) together with immunolocalization of tubulin protein in the spindle (α-tubulin) and trimethylation of histone 3 on lysine 9 (H3K9Me3). Z-stack images were merged into a single image. Maternal and paternal chromosomes are in the process of congression in a spindle that displays multiple poles. Staining for H3K9Me3 reveals a parental epigenetic asymmetry: maternal chromosomes can be observed to be enriched for H3K9me3, whereas paternal chromosomes have very low levels.

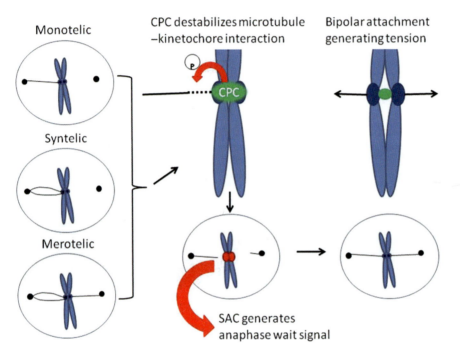

Figure 4.3 Schematic representation of erroneous, non-bipolar, attachments and how they are corrected by joint action of the chromosomal passenger complex (CPC) and the spindle assembly checkpoint (SAC). The CPC localizes to the region between the kinetochores and phosphorylates several proteins present in the kinetochore, resulting in destabilization of microtubule–kinetochore attachments. The CPC thereby generates unattached kinetochores that activate the SAC. The SAC in turn prevents anaphase, providing the chromosome the opportunity to form new attachments. As soon as bipolar attachment is achieved, tension is generated across the kinetochores, pulling them apart. The CPC can no longer reach its targets, enabling microtubule–kinetochore attachments to become stable and resulting in deactivation of the SAC.

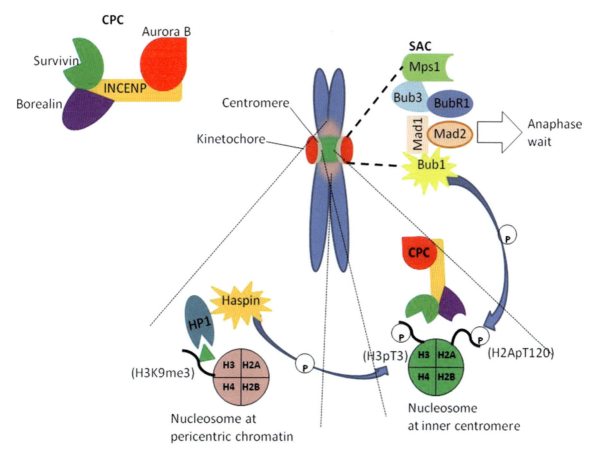

Figure 4.4 Schematic representation of the molecular mechanisms ensuring chromosomal passenger complex (CPC) recruitment to the inner centromere. Phosphorylated H3T3 is generated by haspin kinase, which is recruited to pericentric heterochromatin by HP1 bound to H3K9me3. During prometaphase, phosphorylated H2AT120 is generated by Bub1 kinase, which is recruited to the kinetochore as part of the spindle assembly checkpoint (SAC). This recruitment is promoted by Aurora B. The overlap between H3pT3 and H2ApT120 defines the inner centromere and recruits the CPC: Survivin binds H3pT3, whereas Borealin binds indirectly to H2ApT120. Aurora B is then correctly placed to phosphorylate different protein targets to destabilize chromosome-microtubule attachment errors until bipolar attachment is achieved. The SAC in the mean time generates a signal that prevents anaphase and Aurora B activity is required for maintenance of this signal.

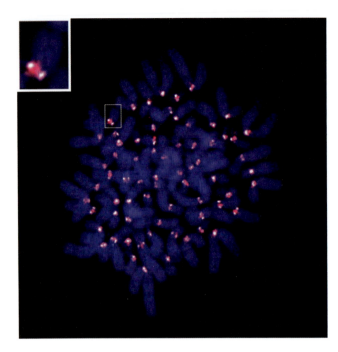

Figure 4.5 Immunolocalization of the CPC subunit INCENP and the centromere on a chromosome spread from a human tripronuclear zygote. Each chromosome (blue) displays two paired signals for the centromeres (white). INCENP (red) is located between the centromeres, on the region referred to as the inner centromere. The insert shows an enlargement of the boxed chromosome.

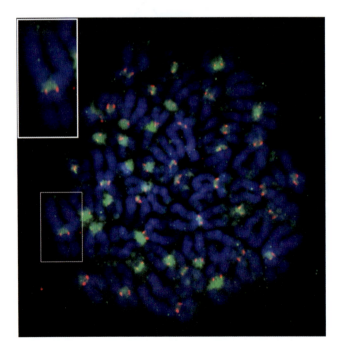

Figure 4.6 Immunolocalization of trimethylation of histone 3 on lysine 9 (H3K9Me3) and the centromere on a chromosome spread from a human fetal fibroblast cell line. Each chromosome (blue) displays two paired signals for the centromeres (red). Enrichment for H3K9Me3 can be observed on the regions surrounding the centromeres, referred to as the pericentric heterochromatin. The insert shows an enlargement of the boxed chromosome.

(A)

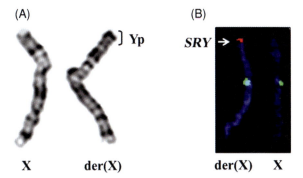

X   der(X)

(B)

SRY →

der(X)   X

Figure 7.4 Partial karyotype and fluorescence *in situ* hybridization (FISH) analysis in the XX male. (**A**) Chromosome analysis detected a derivative chromosome X containing the Yp segment at the distal short arm of X chromosome. (**B**) FISH analysis with *SRY* specific probe (red signal, arrow) shows that the *SRY* gene is present in the derivative X chromosome. The centromere of the X chromosome is colored in green.

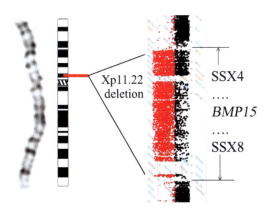

Xp11.22 deletion

SSX4
....
BMP15
....
SSX8

G-banded chromosome analysis detects imbalances > 5 Mb

Microarray analysis showing 4.5-Mb microdeletion detected in female with premature ovarian insufficiency

Figure 7.7 Array comparative genomic hybridization can detect submicroscopic Xp deletion. Partial high resolution G-banded karyotype and ideogram of the X chromosome shows a normal X chromosome in a woman with premature ovarian insufficiency. Array comparative genomic hybridization detected a 4.5 Mb deletion in the Xp11.22 region encompassing the *BMP15* gene.

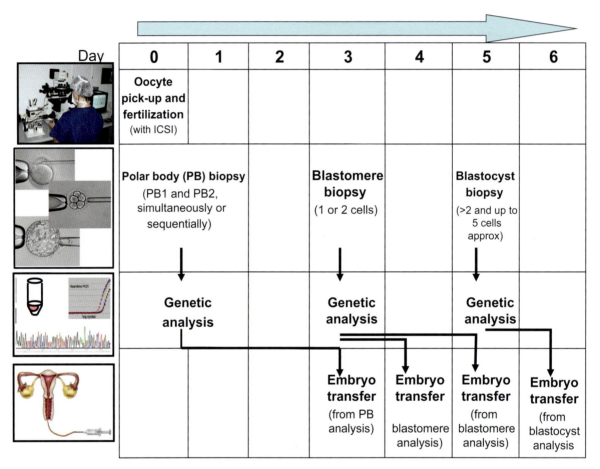

Day	0	1	2	3	4	5	6
	Oocyte pick-up and fertilization (with ICSI)						
	Polar body (PB) biopsy (PB1 and PB2, simultaneously or sequentially)			**Blastomere biopsy** (1 or 2 cells)		**Blastocyst biopsy** (>2 and up to 5 cells approx)	
	Genetic analysis			**Genetic analysis**		**Genetic analysis**	
				Embryo transfer (from PB analysis)	**Embryo transfer** (from blastomere analysis)	**Embryo transfer** (from blastomere analysis)	**Embryo transfer** (from blastocyst analysis

Figure 11.1 A representation of the procedure of preimplantation genetic diagnosis (PGD), including the option of the three developmental stages at which cells suitable for PGD analysis can be biopsied, and the timing of genetic analysis and embryo transfer.

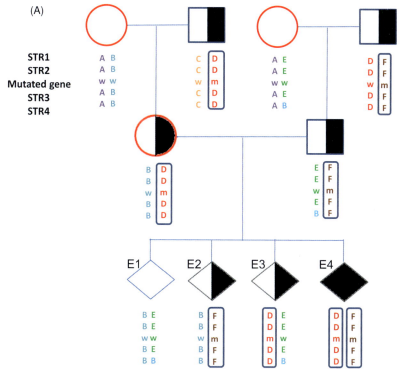

(A)

Figure 11.2 (A) The phase of informative short tandem repeats (STRs) syntenic to a disease locus in an imaginary family. (B) The sizing of the informative parental STRs following analysis on automatic sequencer.

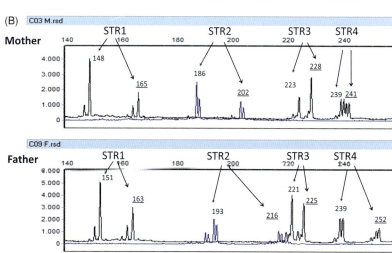

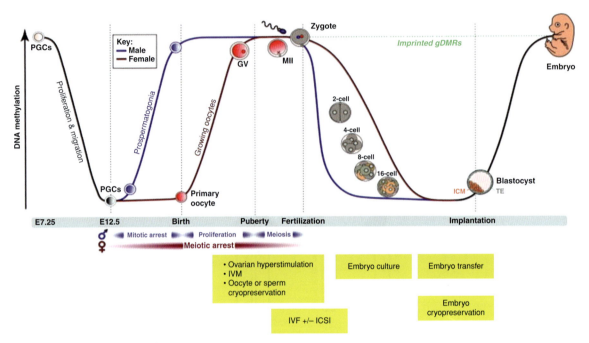

Figure 12.1 DNA methylation changes during developmental epigenetic reprogramming. The two phases of epigenetic reprogramming are schematically depicted. See text for an extensive description. The yellow boxes below indicate the timing of ART procedures in relation to reprogramming events. gDMRs, germline differentially methylated region; ICM, inner cell mass; ICSI, intracytoplasmic sperm injection; IVF, *in vitro* fertilization; IVM, *in vitro* maturation; PGCs, primordial germ cells; TE, trophectoderm. Adapted with permission from Smallwood and Kelsey [2].

References

1. Williams C, Sutcliffe A. Infant outcomes of assisted reproduction. *Early Hum Dev* 2009; 85: 673–7.

2. Smallwood SA, Kelsey G. *De novo* DNA methylation: a germ cell perspective. *Trends Genet* 2012; 28: 33–42.

3. Watkins AJ, Fleming TP. Blastocyst environment and its influence on offspring cardiovascular health: the heart of the matter. *J Anat* 2009; 215: 52–9.

4. Roseboom TJ, Painter RC, van Abeelen AF *et al.* Hungry in the womb: what are the consequences? Lessons from the Dutch famine. *Maturitas* 2011; 70: 141–5.

5. van Montfoort AP, Hanssen LL, de Sutter P *et al.* Assisted reproduction treatment and epigenetic inheritance. *Hum Reprod Update* 2012; 18: 171–97.

6. Sato A, Otsu E, Negishi H *et al.* Aberrant DNA methylation of imprinted loci in superovulated oocytes. *Hum Reprod* 2007; 22: 26–35.

7. Market-Velker BA, Zhang L, Magri LS *et al.* Dual effects of superovulation: loss of maternal and paternal imprinted methylation in a dose-dependent manner. *Hum Mol Genet* 2010; 19: 36–51.

8. Fortier AL, Lopes FL, Darricarrere N *et al.* Superovulation alters the expression of imprinted genes in the midgestation mouse placenta. *Hum Mol Genet* 2008; 17: 1653–65.

9. Al-Khtib M, Perret A, Khoueiry R *et al.* Vitrification at the germinal vesicle stage does not affect the methylation profile of H19 and KCNQ1OT1 imprinting centers in human oocytes subsequently matured *in vitro*. *Fertil Steril* 2001; 95: 1955–60.

10. Chen SL, Shi XY, Zheng HY *et al.* Aberrant DNA methylation of imprinted H19 gene in human preimplantation embryos. *Fertil Steril* 2010; 94: 2356–8.

11. Ibala-Romdhane S, Al-Khtib M, Khoueiry R *et al.* Analysis of H19 methylation in control and abnormal human embryos, sperm and oocytes. *Eur J Hum Genet* 2011; 19: 1138–43.

12. Nelissen EC, Van Montfoort AP, Coonen E *et al.* Further evidence that culture media affect perinatal outcome: findings after transfer of fresh and cryopreserved embryos. *Hum Reprod* 2012; 27: 1966–76.

13. Market-Velker BA, Fernandes AD, Mann MR. Side-by-side comparison of five commercial media systems in a mouse model: suboptimal *in vitro* culture interferes with imprint maintenance. *Biol Reprod* 2010; 83: 938–50.

14. Rancourt RC, Harris HR, Michels KB. Methylation levels at imprinting control regions are not altered with ovulation induction or *in vitro* fertilization in a birth cohort. *Hum Reprod* 2012; 27: 2208–16.

15. Melissen ECM, Dumailin JCM, Daunay A *et al.* Placentas from pregnancies conceived by IVF/ICSI have a reduced DMA methylation level at the H19 and MEST differentially methylated regions. *Hum Reprod* 2013; 27: 1117–26.

16. Katari S, Turan N, Bibikova M *et al.* DNA methylation and gene expression differences in children conceived *in vitro* or *in vivo*. *Hum Mol Genet* 2009; 18: 3769–78.

17. Zhang Y, Zhao W, Jiang Y *et al.* Ultrastructural study on human placentae from women subjected to assisted reproductive technology treatments. *Biol Reprod* 2011; 85: 635–42.

18. Kanber D, Buiting K, Zeschnigk M *et al.* Low frequency of imprinting defects in ICSI children born small for gestational age. *Eur J Hum Genet* 2009; 17: 22–9.

19. Oliver VF, Miles HL, Cutfield WS *et al.* Defects in imprinting and genome-wide DNA methylation are not common in the *in vitro* fertilization population. *Fertil Steril* 2012; 97: 147–53.

20. Miles HL, Hofman PL, Peek J *et al. In vitro* fertilization improves childhood growth and metabolism. *J Clin Endocrinol Metab* 2007; 92: 3441–5.

21. Kobayashi H, Hiura H, John RM *et al.* DNA methylation errors at imprinted loci after assisted conception originate in the parental sperm. *Eur J Hum Genet* 2009; 17: 1582–91.

22. Ceelen M, van Weissenbruch MM, Vermeiden JP *et al.* Pubertal development in children and adolescents born after IVF and spontaneous conception. *Hum Reprod* 2008; 23: 2791–8.

23. Scherrer U, Rimoldi SF, Rexhaj E *et al.* Systemic and pulmonary vascular dysfunction in children conceived by assisted reproductive technologies. *Circulation*; 125: 1890–6.

24. Nelissen EC, van Montfoort AP, Dumoulin JC *et al.* Epigenetics and the placenta. *Hum Reprod Update* 2011; 17: 397–417.

Ethical considerations in human reproductive genetics

Guido de Wert and Wybo Dondorp

Introduction

This chapter on ethical considerations focuses on current debates in three different but interlinked corners of the field of reproductive genetics: donor conception, preimplantation genetic testing, and preconception screening. Donor conception leads to the birth of children to which one of the partners is socially, but not genetically, related. Whereas for decades, the genetic link between the child and the donor was not regarded as something to be given much attention, this has considerably changed since the start of the new century, leading to a new emphasis on genetic connectedness, and to debates about what this should or should not be taken to mean for donor conception as a way of creating families. Some of these debates will be summarized in the next section, entitled "Ethics of anonymity and disclosure in donor conception". The following "Genetic screening of gamete donors" section discusses the ethics of genetic screening and testing of gamete donors. Now that new next generation sequencing (NGS) technologies are expected to make broad scope testing for many genetic conditions feasible and affordable, the ethical question becomes what we should test donors for and why. The next two sections ("Preimplantation genetic diagnosis" and "Preimplantation genetic screening") are devoted to preimplantation genetic testing: a relatively new, highly dynamic, form of reproductive genetics. Current ethical debates concentrate on preimplantation genetic diagnosis (PGD), i.e. testing of embryos on behalf of couples at risk of transmitting a specific genetic disorder (discussed in the "Preimplantation genetic diagnosis" section). As important, however, is the ethics of routine testing of *in vitro* fertilization (IVF) embryos, i.e. preimplantation genetic screening (PGS). Although it is still unclear what the

precise value of this technology may turn out to be, the possible scenario of NGS-based "comprehensive PGS" raises a number of challenging ethical issues (discussed in the "Preimplantation genetic screening" section). Moving from clinical to community genetics, the last section of this chapter, entitled "Preconception carrier screening" discusses possible uses of preconception carrier screening (PCS). Ethically, the question is whether such screening should be understood as a prevention tool in a public health context, or as a form of reproductive screening with its traditional emphasis on non-directivity and autonomous choice. And moving back to the clinic: should professionals insist on PCS for IVF-patients as part of responsible assisted reproduction?

Ethics of anonymity and disclosure in donor conception

The use of donor sperm or oocytes allows medically assisted reproduction for: (a) people in heterosexual relations who themselves do not have functional gametes; (b) for lesbian or gay couples and single women; and (c) for those who – because of a risk of transmitting a serious genetic disease to their offspring – do not wish to make use of their own gametes. Donor insemination was initially contested because the role of the donor was regarded by many as interfering with the exclusiveness of the marital bond. Several cultural and/or religious groups still reject donor conception for reasons related to adultery and honor, or because of normative views opposed to severing reproduction from sex. Of course, these arguments are not relevant for the discourse of secular medical ethics.

The moral basis of donor conception rests on the view that persons who have children with the help of a

---

Textbook of Human Reproductive Genetics, eds Karen Sermon and Stéphane Viville. Published by Cambridge University Press.
© Cambridge University Press 2014.

donor are the parents of that child and that the origin of the gametes would not in any way change this. In most (Western) jurisdictions, this is explicitly recognized by the law, at least when treatment is provided through regulated or recognized clinics. In the early days of sperm donation the corollary of this understanding was that recipients of donor sperm would do best by keeping their use of this service a secret, including for their children born as a result. This was also a means of protecting the male partner against the stigma of infertility. At the time, openness was only recommended in cases where donor conception was chosen because of a genetic risk (in order to protect the child against unnecessary anxiety about his or her own health prospects).

The past decades have seen an important change in that recipients are now encouraged to tell their children already from an early age about how they were conceived. Factors leading to this change include the use of donor conception by lesbian couples and single women (for whom openness is not much of an issue), the use of "known" oocyte donors (often a sister or friend), the more general cultural climate favoring transparency and openness, and a growing interest in genetic inheritance as testified in television programs where people try to trace their lost biological parents or siblings. As a consequence, the donor is no longer seen as just a provider of reproductive material, but as a person who had a role in the conception of the new individual and whose identity may be of interest to his or her offspring.

In several Western countries, this has led to legislation putting an end to donor-anonymity. This involves collecting and preserving identifying information about the donor (either locally or centrally) and giving donor-conceived persons the right to access this information as soon as they reach adulthood. Sweden had already issued such legislation in 1984 and a number of countries have followed since, including the UK, the Netherlands, Norway, Finland, New Zealand, and several Australian states. In Europe, those defending this change refer to jurisprudence of the European Court of Human Rights, in which it is stated that persons have "a vital interest (…) in receiving the information necessary to uncover the truth about an important aspect of their personal identity" [1]. However, it is also clear from the same jurisprudence that the protection of this interest does not lead to an absolute right, but has to be weighed against the privacy interests of others. In other countries, including

Denmark, Belgium, France, Spain, Portugal, and Greece, the law requires donor anonymity. Whereas some of those countries make an exception for donation by a "known donor" (e.g. Belgium), other countries do not, meaning that those bringing their own donor have to participate in a donor-exchange program (as in France).

From an ethical point of view, these differences between countries suggest that the force of the arguments behind the lifting of donor anonymity may not be as obvious as some think they are. To the extent that the claim of a "vital interest" of donor-conceived persons is meant to be empirical, its factual basis is weak [2]. In studies among children knowing that they were conceived through anonymous donor conception, the fact that they had no information about the identity of the donor was not found to seriously impact their well-being. The idea that many are desperately seeking their progenitors is based partly on the sometimes traumatic experiences of those who found out that they were donor conceived only later in life and partly on extrapolation from the entirely different context of adoption. Whereas adopted children have to adjust to the fact that they were for whatever reason separated from their birth parents, donor-conceived children never had other parents than those in whose family they were born. However, donor-conceived persons who do find it important to know who the donor was have an interest in being able to access this information. The ethical argument for putting an end to donor anonymity is that this would protect the interest of donor-conceived persons without unduly interfering in the reproductive freedom of would-be parents.

Internationally, there is a strong movement suggesting that the lifting of donor anonymity is not enough. According to those holding this view, the problem remains that many recipient couples decide not to tell their children about how they were conceived, thus denying them the opportunity of finding out about their genetic roots. Additional arguments are the lack of access to one's true medical family history and the risk of unknowingly marrying a half-brother or half-sister. It has also been argued that the state should not make itself complicit to deception by allowing the provision of donor conception services to recipients who have no intention to tell. Proposals for additional regulations aimed at imposing transparency upon unwilling parents include a mandatory annotation of donor-conceived status on the birth certificate as is now legally required in the Australian state of Victoria. It has also been proposed that donor conceived persons should receive an explanatory letter at their 18th birthday. The idea behind these proposals is that parents will decide to tell their children before they find out anyway. In its recent report on ethical aspects of information sharing in donor conception, the Nuffield Council on Bioethics has rejected the call for mandatory openness [2]. The Council stated that although openness is generally advisable, there is no justification for imposing this upon parents who may have sound moral reasons why in their specific situation (e.g. belonging to a cultural or religious group with negative views about donor conception) disclosure is not the best policy for all concerned.

With regard to "lacking medical history" and "risk of incest" as additional arguments for mandatory openness, these are not as strong as many seem to think. In fact the incest risk is very low (even further reduced by current limits to the number of families that may be helped with the sperm of one donor) [3] and as important health risks will be screened out (see below), additional information about family history would not in most cases have clinical consequences. However, as stated in the Nuffield Council report, "Health professionals need to be aware of the importance of not making automatic assumptions of biological connections between children and their parents" [2]. A specific situation is where the non-genetically related parent suffers from a serious genetic disease. In order to avoid unnecessary anxiety in the child, as well as unnecessary health checks, parents do have a moral duty in such cases to tell their child how it was conceived.

The call for mandatory openness and the related proposal to make the lifting of donor anonymity retrospective, flow from a view about the importance of genetic relatedness that is ill at ease with the moral basis of donor conception as referred to above. British sociologist Ilke Turkmendag has warned that, "There is a remarkable difference between disclosing to children their means of conception, and imposing on them that their genetic relatedness to the gamete donor is an indispensable component of their personal identity, and that development of their identity may depend on finding identifiable information about their 'real' biological parents" [4]. The irony is that instead of solving any problems for those children, this will make life more difficult, both for them and their parents.

Genetic screening of gamete donors

In the past decades, guidelines have been formulated in several countries giving recommendations for screening of gamete donors, including screening for infectious diseases and genetic screening. With regard to genetic screening, this mainly consists of an extensive medical history of the donor and his or her first-degree relatives taken by a qualified genetics professional. Excluding donors who either have or have had a serious hereditary condition themselves, or with a positive family history for such disorders, significantly reduces the transmission risk related to the use of donor gametes. Although donors may also be tested for specific genetic risks, present guidelines are reticent about this. In line with European legislation, British and other national European guidelines require selective testing for carrier status of autosomal recessive disorders with higher frequencies in the candidates' population of origin [5]. In the USA, where preconception carrier testing for some such disorders is universally recommended to persons of reproductive age (see "Preconception carrier screening" section, below), the American Society for Reproductive Medicine (ASRM) has advised that all gamete donors undergo this testing, and have ethnicity-based carrier testing in addition to that [6]. A further difference exists with regard to testing donors for balanced chromosome translocations. Whereas the British guidelines say that all gamete donors should be karyotyped, the ASRM recommendations state that this is not required (but "optional"), given the small risk that healthy young donors with a negative family history will have offspring with a significant chromosomal abnormality.

Occasionally and inevitably, cases are reported where despite genetic screening according to present recommendations, a serious but rare genetic condition was found either in donor offspring or in a person who is or was a gamete donor. Typically, such cases attract high level media attention and lead to societal concerns about whether the present guidelines for genetic testing are sufficient. Reports of such cases in the medical and scientific literature also often end in a call for more testing. Until now, feasibility and costs limit the extent to which donor testing can be expanded. This may change with the prospect of affordable NGS, which would allow simultaneous testing for a large number of mutations and risk factors. Inevitably, this will give a further boost to the call for expanded testing. One concern about this development is that the suggestion of a "zero risk" policy may have the unwanted effect of sending a message of false reassurance to candidate recipients. It is therefore unfortunate that instead of making clear that there is no such thing as reproduction without risk, some commercial centers advertise the wider scope of their donor testing as a competitive edge. There is a clear danger that medicolegal standards for what recipients can expect donors to be tested for, will be determined by such competition rather than by scientific evidence and professional ethics. A further concern is that in commercial settings, NGS-based testing will be used to select for what recipients regard as desirable non-health related traits, as soon as genetic determinants for those traits are identified. Together, these concerns underscore the need for a proactive debate within the field about what donors should be tested for and why [7].

Ethical reasons for donor screening are related to professional responsibilities with regard to the couple (or the woman) who requested their help, and to the future child. The couple has a rightful claim to good quality care, including the provision of donor sperm or gametes that do not carry a major risk of a serious hereditary disorder. The fact that donor gametes are part of the service provided by the center makes the situation different from cases in which assisted reproduction involves the use of the own gametes of the male and female partners. As in the latter case the aim is to help this couple to have a child; any inherent genetic risks that a well-informed couple is willing to take are part of their reproductive project and must be accepted in principle, unless doing so would amount to violating the further responsibility of professionals not to expose future children to a high risk of seriously diminished quality of life. In donor conception, things are different. Not only are donor gametes part of the service provided by the center, they are also replaceable in principle, whereas the gametes used in partner conception are not. Professionals providing this service should at least avoid using donors known to carry a risk of transmitting a serious hereditary disorder. Taking a medical history is a simple way of establishing whether this is the case. Additional testing may be a further means to avoid reproductive risks. However, whether such testing is justified depends on whether it would be proportional. This involves balancing the amount of further risk reduction that one may thus achieve on the one hand, and the inevitable drawbacks

of donor testing on the other. One of these is costs. More testing makes donor conception more expensive, entailing higher opportunity costs in societies reimbursing assisted reproduction, and putting the service out of reach of a larger group of candidate recipients in countries where it is only available on a commercial basis. As said, NGS may make expanded testing sufficiently affordable to overcome this problem. A second drawback is that more testing will lead to draining the pool of available donors, by excluding candidates with relatively small risks.

Finally, the call for expanded testing tends to ignore the possible impact that a positive test may have on the donors themselves. An example of this is testing oocyte donors for fragile X syndrome (FXS). Whereas there should be no debate about excluding women diagnosed as carriers either of a full mutation (FM) or of a premutation (PM) from being a donor, the question is whether the remaining risk connected to using undiagnosed (FM or PM) carriers should be avoided by routine testing of all oocyte donors for FXS carrier status, as is done in several US centers. The ASRM guidelines state that this is an option to be considered, even if such testing is "not required." However, this ignores the reasons behind the consensus that FXS carrier testing should not be offered to the general population [8]. There is much uncertainty and controversy about the clinical importance of findings in a "gray zone" (intermediate alleles), leading to different proposals about cut-offs. It is tempting to think that when testing oocyte donors, this would not be much of a problem as one can simply decide to also exclude candidates with these findings. But that indeed ignores that this may leave the donor in a state of great uncertainty about her own reproductive risk. Moreover, should a carrier become pregnant and want to avoid the birth of an affected child by opting for prenatal diagnosis (PND), counseling, and decision-making will be extremely difficult if the fetus turns out to be a female FM-carrier, giving a 50% chance that this will lead to an unaffected girl. Finally, FXS testing will identify carriers at risk of adult-onset disorders including premature ovarian insufficiency (PO), and untreatable adult-onset fragile X-associated tremor/ataxia syndrome (FXTAS) [8]. It has been suggested that sperm donors should also be tested for FXS carrier status [9]. Male carriers may transmit the PM, but expansion to a FM in offspring of a male PM carrier is extremely rare. However, their daughters will have a one in four risk of having an affected child. Testing sperm donors would therefore mainly serve to avoid the transmission of carrier status rather than avoiding disease in the immediate offspring. A strong reason for not considering this is that at least one-third of male carriers will develop "fragile-X-associated tremor/ataxia syndrome" (FXTAS), meaning that testing may have the adverse effect of revealing a genetic predisposition for a serious and untreatable late-onset disorder. Ignoring the implications of these outcomes for the donor amounts to treating him or her as a mere contributor of reproductive material; in fact, to reduce the donor to his or her gametes. From the point of view of medical ethics, that is clearly at odds with the principle of respect for persons.

A conceivable development that requires separate consideration is expanded testing of donors for carrier status of autosomal recessive disorders. It is expected that with NGS-technology it will become affordable to specifically test for mutations of genes involved in hundreds of such disorders simultaneously, whereas at present donors are (selectively) tested for only some. The argument in favor of considerably widening the scope of this testing is that although these disorders are individually rare, together they account for a considerable burden of disease: 1–2% of all couples are at a 25% risk of having an affected child [10]. As donors and recipients may also be carriers for the same recessive disorder(s), the question emerges whether expanded carrier testing would be a good idea. Importantly, the concern about draining the donor pool does not apply, as carriers can be matched with recipients who have tested negatively for the same disorder. In practice, since matching is also done for general donor characteristics, adding carrier status for recessive disorders can make it more difficult to find a suitable donor in concrete cases than it often already is. This may be an argument for limiting the scope of testing to those recessive mutations which clearly lead to serious health problems in affected individuals. A further reason for targeting this approach to a well-defined panel of genes is that testing for mutations of which the genophenotype relationship is insufficiently clear may lead to uncertainty for donors (and recipients) about their personal reproductive risks that cannot be properly addressed in the context of a donor conception program. Although these considerations call for careful assessment of the conditions and mutations to be included in the panel, they do not amount to reasons for thinking that expanded

carrier testing of donors (and recipients) would as such be morally problematic. Clearly, proper implications counseling would be essential, also to avoid false reassurance.

Preimplantation genetic diagnosis

Preimplantation genetic diagnosis is still somewhat controversial [11]. A first objection of (some of) the critics is that embryo selection is at odds with the "sanctity of human life." The dominant view in ethics, however, holds that the preimplantation embryo has a relatively low moral status – it is definitely not yet a human person, with a right to life. Obviously, otherwise, not only IVF as currently practiced, but also intrauterine devices (IUDs), insofar as these prevent the implantation of fertilized oocytes, would be fully unacceptable – and maybe even more so traditional prenatal screening, PND, and (selective) termination of pregnancy. A second objection is that IVF/PGD carries disproportional burdens and risks for women. But clearly, balancing the burdens and risks of the different reproductive options – including the use of donor gametes, PND, and PGD – for women/couples at high risk of having an affected child is rather personal. A significant number of women prefer PGD as it allows them to have healthy, genetically related children while avoiding a traumatic selective termination of a wanted pregnancy. For infertile couples who opt for IVF/ICSI anyway, PGD may be far more attractive than a non-selective transfer followed by PND and, possibly, a selective termination. Third, there is the slippery slope argument, which points to possible future abuses of PGD, although even these critics themselves disagree about what precisely constitutes "abuse." Furthermore, they often exaggerate the feasibility of producing "designer babies." The slippery slope argument does not seem to be a strong argument to reject and prohibit PGD altogether – it simply underscores the need to engage in an ethical and societal debate about "where to draw the line."

PGD within the "medical model"

Assuming that the "a priori" objections to PGD are not convincing and that the debate about the acceptability of PGD per se is a rearguard action, the real issue is to define acceptable indications and conditions for good clinical PGD practice. There is a strong consensus that PGD is morally justified if it is linked to the "medical model," i.e. if it aims at avoiding the conception of a child affected with a serious disease or handicap. To date, PGD has been reported for almost 200 genetic conditions, and the numbers are steadily increasing (see Chapter 11). For some, this illustrates the relevance and potential of PGD, for others, this underscores the urgency of the question: how serious does a disorder/handicap have to be in order to qualify for PGD? It is regularly proposed to impose a detailed, restrictive list of all acceptable indications. However, such a list is problematic: many disorders have a variable expression, the list would need constant updating, it could well entail a discriminatory message about the ("unworthy") lives of people affected with the conditions enlisted, and, last but not least, it disregards that the family history and personal experiences and circumstances of the applicants should be taken into account; after all, they have an expertise brought on by daily experience with the disease that medical experts often lack. Let us now have a brief look at some particular applications.

PGD for untreatable, midlife-onset disorders

In the category of PGD for untreatable midlife-onset disorders, Huntington's disease (HD) is the paradigm case. Critics object that PGD for midlife (let alone late)-onset disorders is unwarranted as the child will have (many) decades of good and unimpaired living. This view seems to disregard, however, that the prospect of HD – a progressive, lethal, highly invalidating disorder – imposes an extremely severe burden on the members of affected families. It should be no surprise, then, that HD is one of the main, and widely accepted, indications for PGD in practice.

Still, in more recent debates at least three ethical questions arise [12, 13]. First, what about the future loss of parental competence in carriers of HD? Can reproductive physicians involved in IVF accept this risk, taking into account their professional responsibility for the welfare of the future child; more particularly, their responsibility to avoid high risks of serious harm? And what if the prospective father or mother is already symptomatic? Black-and-white approaches seem to be inadequate. Although the development of HD symptoms in a parent is, no doubt, always burdensome for children, many children are able to cope reasonably well. Relevant variables include the coping skills of the partner not

affected with HD, communication about HD among family members, and the quality of the network of the family. Further discussion is needed to see how these variables would allow decisions to be made case-by-case. Second, what about exclusion-PGD? Though the procedure is "unnecessary" in 50% of the cases, the weighing of other relevant factors, including the wish not to know one's genetic status and the burdens involved in IVF/PGD, is rather personal. Apparently, applicants consider this option to be valuable. Possible unnecessary embryo loss cannot be regarded as a major moral obstacle in view of the dominant view regarding the lower status of the embryo. And third, what about applicants who carry a reduced penetrance allele (RPA) – entailing 35–39 CAG repeats – for HD? Is their risk serious enough for a PGD-indication? Preimplantation genetic diagnosis may indicate that the embryo carries an RPA or (after expansion) a full penetrance allele (FPA). It is estimated that some two-thirds of the future children carrying an RPA will have HD in (late) adulthood, before the age of 75. Furthermore, these children are at significant risk that their own children will carry a FPA (after expansion). Preimplantation genetic diagnosis aimed at the non-transfer of embryos with a FPA or an RPA is morally justified in view of this combination of risks.

PGD for preventable/treatable conditions, caused by mutations with an incomplete penetrance

A second category is PGD for preventable or treatable conditions that are caused by mutations with an incomplete penetrance. A good example of this category is hereditary breast and ovarian cancer (HBOC), testing for which hopefully will become more easily available and less expensive now that the Myriad patent on the genes has been lifted by the US Supreme Court in late Spring 2013. Preimplantation genetic diagnosis for relevant mutations of *BRCA1* or *BRCA2* is somewhat more controversial than PGD for HD, because the penetrance of these mutations is incomplete and (future) carriers have preventive and/or therapeutic options, including preventive mastectomy and ovariectomy. But obviously, although the penetrance is incomplete, it is still very high – the cumulative risk for breast and ovarian cancer may be even higher than 90%. And preventive surgery has major implications for women's welfare, whereas it is not 100% effective. A thought experiment might help here: would you tell parents of a boy at high genetic risk of future testicular cancer to not worry because they may opt for preventive castration? Preimplantation genetic diagnosis for *BRCA1* or *BRCA2* is widely – and we think rightly – considered to be morally justified. Likewise, PGD may be justified for other hereditary cancers and for some of the cardiogenic conditions. The view that the availability of treatment makes PGD obsolete is one-dimensional and too restrictive – if children's and families' quality of life is seriously (adversely) affected even though treatment is available, PGD may still be a reasonable option.

PGD for mitochondrial disorders

There seems to be a growing interest in PGD for mitochondrial DNA (mtDNA) disorders caused by a mutation in the mtDNA, such as Leigh syndrome and MELAS. Ideally, one would like to transfer embryos without a (detectable) mutant load. But sometimes, these embryos are not available after PGD, so one has to consider a transfer of the embryo with the lowest mutant load, so with the highest probability of leading to a healthy child. Obviously, the aim of PGD, then, changes from elimination of risk, to risk reduction. Possible objections include that this is at odds with the proper aim of PGD and with the doctor's responsibility to take account of the welfare of the future child thus conceived. Even though these objections do not provide compelling arguments to regard risk-reducing PGD as a priori unacceptable, in view of the responsibility to avoid a high risk that a child will be born with a seriously diminished quality of life (high risk of serious harm), a cut-off point (a threshold of mutant load) should be determined below which embryos are considered to be eligible for transfer. If only embryos above the threshold are found, options are limited to either engage in a new IVF/PGD cycle or to stop trying PGD. As it is the professional's responsibility to not only avoid a high risk of serious harm, but to also try to further reduce any risks that are not per se prohibitive, it should be considered whether it would be possible and proportional to start another cycle, possibly resulting in embryos with a lower or even zero mutant load. Looking for better embryos should not be seen as morally required if an embryo with a mutant load below the cut-off point is available. The number of cycles should be determined on a case-by-case base, also depending on, for example, the specific mutation, the wishes of couple (especially the woman involved), and the number of cycles allowed and reimbursed in

a country. Taking into account the complexities and uncertainties involved, especially in the case of PGD for unstable mtDNA mutations with an unpredictable outcome, PGD should be embedded in a scientific research protocol. As follow-up studies involving children thus conceived are at the same time valuable from a scientific point of view, but ethically controversial, this issue should be addressed in further ethical debate as well [14].

Two proportionalities (depending on whether IVF should be counted in or out)

To conclude this section on medical indications for PGD, we would like to make a more general remark. As we have suggested, the moral acceptability of PGD depends on the "proportionality" of the procedure, something that will have to be determined for specific applications. This criterion requires that (a) the efforts, burdens, and possible risks of IVF for women involved, (b) the possible risks of IVF and the (so far: theoretical) risks of PGD for future children thus conceived, (c) the inherent embryo loss, and (d) the costs of the procedure, must be in proportion to the benefit of avoiding the conception of an affected child. However, when looking at the proportionality of PGD, it seems logical and justified to make a distinction between two types of situations. In the first, most common, situation, fertile people undergo IVF/PGD just in order to avoid the birth of an affected child. In the second, a couple opts for IVF/ICSI because of subfertility, and wants to add PGD in order to avoid the transmission of a particular genetic disorder. The proportionality principle seems to imply that in the latter situation the criteria for acceptable PGD-indications may be somewhat more permissive; after all, the decision to engage in IVF/ICSI (and accept its risks, burdens, costs, and inherent embryo loss) has already been made for reasons of infertility treatment – the couple will have IVF/ICSI *anyway*. As there will mostly be more than one suitable embryo, and "not selecting" is not an option, the decision to engage in targeted PGD is relatively simple to justify. Clearly, the justification and implications of such a "double standard" need further analysis and debate.

PGD for "indirectly medical" cases

Some applications of PGD do not fit the medical model *stricto sensu*, as (at least part of) the testing is not linked with possible health problems of the future child, whereas there still is a link to the medical model in the wider sense, in that the testing may be relevant for the health of a "third party" [15]. These applications are, then, "indirectly medical" or "intermediate" between medical and non-medical.

A first example is PGD/HLA typing. The main ethical condition is that the future child (the term "donor" is a misnomer, of course) should be truly welcome – it should not be valued just as a cell bank. Regulations in Europe differ. Some countries, like the Netherlands and France, allow PGD/HLA-typing only in the context of (in addition to) PGD for a particular disease, and prohibit the procedure if aimed to treat a child affected with a non-genetic disorder. From an ethical perspective this policy is debatable, as the future child may be welcomed "for itself" in the latter context as well. The "take-home baby rate" is, unfortunately, relatively low. This should be clearly communicated to the applicants beforehand in order to avoid undue optimism. An alternative, possibly more effective, future option might be the selection of matched embryos from which embryonic stem cells (hESC) could be derived to produce hematopoietic stem cells for therapy [16].

A second example is PGD/sex selection to avoid reproductive dilemmas in (healthy) future children. Think of the case of a male patient suffering from hemophilia. Some of these males prefer to conceive male progeny only, because sons will not carry the mutation, whereas all daughters will be healthy carriers, who themselves will be at risk to have affected boys. Even though the procedure would not be done to avoid a disease or health risk in the child to be conceived, PGD in such situations may still be morally justified in view of the importance of avoiding a substantial trans-generational health risk.

PGD within the "autonomy model"

According to what may be called the "autonomy model," prospective parents are free to use PGD in order to select embryos on the basis of any characteristic they prefer, whether health-related or not. Opponents argue that selecting for non-medical characteristics violates the autonomy of the future child as the child is reduced to an object of parental ambitions and ideals. But would embryo selection on the basis of characteristics that do not limit the possible life plans of the future child or that are useful in carrying out almost any life plan ("general purpose means")

really violate the future child's autonomy? Should one not say that prospective parents undermine the ethical standard only when they deliberately try to direct the child toward a predetermined life? Anyway, the technical possibilities to use embryo selection for making "superbabies," whatever that may be, are regularly widely exaggerated in the mass media.

A paradigm case for the autonomy model in the current context is PGD/sex-selection for non-medical reasons. Sex selection for non-medical reasons is prohibited in many countries. From an ethical point of view, however, this is not evident [17]. Even though individual requests may stem from discriminatory attitudes or stereotyping views regarding the difference between boys and girls, it does not follow that sex selection for non-medical reasons is inherently sexist [18]. The fear that allowing it will result in a distortion of the sex ratio does not seem convincing either, at least not in Western countries, where a preference for boys is weak or absent. Moreover, the suggestion that sex selection for non-medical reasons will reinforce gender stereotypes to the detriment of children's development and women's position in society, are speculative at best. Since the conclusion must be that arguments against allowing sex-selection for non-medical reasons are weak, banning the practice may amount to an unjustified infringement of reproductive freedom. However, even if sex selection (limited perhaps to "family balancing") may be acceptable in itself, a further question still concerns the proportionality of the means. Clearly, the use of preconception sperm selection technologies for this purpose (if safe and effective) is more easily justified than PGD [17].

A second case is PGD for "dysgenic" reasons. The paradigm case regards a deaf couple's request of PGD in order to selectively transfer embryos affected with (non-syndromic) deafness. The couple may point to psychosocial and developmental risks of hearing children growing up with (two) deaf parents. Concerns include that (young) hearing children will have difficulties in understanding the implications of their parents' disability and related behavior, that deaf parents will have only limited access to the experiences of hearing children, and that there is a risk of role inversion. Furthermore, applicants may argue that "deafness is not a handicap, but just a variant on the spectrum of normalcy." After all, deaf people have their own rich culture and their own (non-verbal) language. One can reasonably doubt, however, whether the "just a variant" view is tenable; after all, outside the microcosmos of the deaf subculture, deafness is a disability which causes a variety of serious and lifetime challenges. Though deaf people still can (and usually do) live a reasonably happy life, selection for deafness is at odds with the professional responsibility of the reproductive doctor [11]. The couple's relational concerns should be tackled by educational support and advice, not by "dysgenic" PGD. Interestingly, ongoing technology development may contribute to solving the current moral puzzle [19]. Until now, cochlear implants are controversial, amongst other things, because their success is patchy. However, when the perfect version of the cochlear implant would become available in the future, parents will clearly harm a child they leave deaf. To select for a deaf child, then, becomes self-defeating.

Preimplantation genetic screening

Preimplantation genetic screening to check the number of pronuclei (PGS-PN) is the classical type of PGS. Zygotes with three pronuclei (tri-pronuclear (3PN) zygotes) are not transferred as these are not able to develop into a viable child. This screening is so self-evident that it is not even mentioned in debates on PGS. The non-transfer of 3PN-zygotes is, so we assume, even accepted by adherents to the "sanctity of life" doctrine; even they will consider it an absurdity to presume that there would be a moral duty to transfer an embryo lacking the potential to become a viable child.

PGS for aneuploidy

There are no valid categorical moral objections to PGS for aneuploidy (PGS-A). After all, its primary aim, i.e. to increase the success rate of IVF, is commendable, while the means, namely to exclude embryos affected with serious chromosomal aberrations, which often lack viability, from transfer is clearly morally acceptable. Some proponents of PGS-A on the basis of polar bodies (PBs) claim that this strategy has a moral advantage in comparison with PGS-A on the basis of a blastomere biopsy, as the PB approach would regard, so they argue, just oocytes, thus avoiding embryo selection (see Chapter 11). This view, is, however, not evident. After all, the PB approach would involve both the first and the second PB. As the second PB is generated only after the penetration of the oocyte by the sperm, the underlying issue regards the status of the presyngamy zygote: is this still an oocyte or already an

embryo? Views differ: in German law, the presyngamy zygote is not yet an embryo, but according to Dutch law, it is. However, we doubt as to whether it is justified to make a fundamental ethical difference between "intra-" and post-fertilization PGS.

Preimplantation genetic screening for aneuploidy is still controversial because of the lack of evidence of its efficacy. In view of this lack of evidence, both the European Society of Human Reproduction and Embryology (ESHRE) and ASRM discourage the routine use of PGS-A. It is disquieting that some proponents of PGS-A uncritically claim that its efficacy has already been proved years ago and that PGS-A is just a matter of good clinical practice. Clearly, this is at odds not only with the interests of IVF-patients, but also with professionals' responsibility to avoid futile interventions and to enable society to distribute scarce resources available for health care in a just and evidence-based way. Although some recent publications suggest that modified strategies of PGS-A may well have an added value [20], many questions remain and the outcomes of these studies should be interpreted carefully. The message that PGS-A should only be offered in the context of randomized controlled clinical trials, aimed at a systematic evaluation of its presumed advantages and possible disadvantages, is still valid [21].

Proponents' enthusiasm for PGS-A may make us forget that there may be a link between the high number of chromosomal aberrations in human IVF-embryos and the stimulation protocols used [22]. Milder stimulation may well lower the number of aneuploid and mosaic embryos (see Chapter 4). To disregard this possibility while implementing PGS-A is like filling a bucket full of holes.

The broader the scope of PGS-A, the more different chromosomal abnormalities may be found, ranging from lethal or very serious to (relatively) mild. Obviously, reasonable people may well disagree about what abnormality they consider to be relatively mild and, in their situation, acceptable. This may create conflicts between doctors who want to only transfer "normal" embryos and applicants, who may be willing to have an affected embryo transferred if no unaffected embryo is available. This situation is not unique to PGS, but one may expect this to happen more frequently here than in the context of (targeted, single-disease) PGD. Who, then, has decision-making authority concerning the transfer of chromosomally "abnormal" embryos?

As PGD is often presented as "an early type of PND," it may easily be assumed that the normative framework for PND applies to the preimplantation context as well. This, however, is not the case. In the context of PND, the principle of respect for reproductive autonomy is of paramount importance. One of the implications is, that if PND has an unfavorable ("positive") result, it is up to the woman (together with her partner) to decide about a possible termination of pregnancy – the counselor should refrain from directive counseling, and provide support, whatever she decides to do. If one would simply extrapolate this guideline to the context of PGD or PGS, the choice as to whether or not to have an affected embryo transferred must lie with the prospective parents. But clearly, a (partial) shift of the locus of decision-making seems to be inevitable. After all, in medically assisted reproduction, doctors are causally and intentionally involved in creating a child. This creates a professional responsibility to take account of the welfare of the possible future child. It seems that a strong consensus has emerged that doctors involved should avoid "high risks of serious harm" [23]. How, then, to make this operational in the current context? It is our impression that many, if not most, medical doctors consider the transfer of any affected embryo to be at odds with their professional responsibility. But we would argue that there may well be exceptions to the rule to "never transfer an affected embryo." What matters first and foremost is that professionals stick to the bottom line: they should never transfer an embryo with a defect that carries a high risk of serious harm. But what if an infertile couple would insist on transferring an embryo with, for instance, an XXY karyotype (Klinefelter syndrome) when there is no "normal" embryo available for transfer? A doctor's refusal to transfer this embryo (and other embryos with mild aberrations) cannot be justified by referring to professionals' responsibility to avoid a high risk of serious harm and would in fact be symptomatic of a disputable hypertrophy of professional responsibility. Furthermore, we wonder as to whether such a refusal would not be inconsistent in view of the widespread practice of accepting the transmission of, for example, "hereditary infertility" when treating male infertility caused by a Y-deletion by means of ICSI. Needless to say, clinics' transfer policy should be given due attention in pre-PGS counseling in order to avoid misunderstandings and facilitate timely reflection, dialogue, and well-considered, "shared," decision making.

"Comprehensive" PGS

Next generation sequencing technology may, at least in theory, allow PGS to test for chromosomal aberrations, all (more common) Mendelian disorders, many susceptibilities for complex disorders, and genetic co-determinants for non-medical traits, including personality traits, simultaneously. This approach may seem to be ideal, as one could at the same time select the most viable embryo for transfer (increasing the take-home baby rate), optimally reduce the risk of having an affected child, and select "the best embryo" for transfer, also in terms of the health prospects of the future child. However, an unmitigated enthusiasm for such "comprehensive" PGS is naïve, and at best premature, as this screening raises a series of complex ethical and ethically relevant questions and issues [24], including the following (this sketch is not meant to be exhaustive):

To begin with, what, precisely, would be the proper aim of comprehensive PGS? Basically, there seem to be at least two possibilities, at least in theory. The first would be: to exclude genetic risks for progeny. But clearly, this aim would be self-defeating and illusory, as we are all "fellow mutants"; each of us, and each embryo carries various mutations and predispositions for disorders. Most of these will relate to complex, multifactorial, disorders, some will relate to Mendelian diseases. Anyway, risk-free reproduction does not exist, either *in vivo* or *in vitro*; if one would want to eliminate any genetic risk for future children, one should refrain from any transfer – or better: from reproduction altogether. A second possible aim of comprehensive PGS would be to select, from the batch of available embryos, the embryo with the best prospects of a healthy (or maybe broader: a flourishing) life. But what criteria are most relevant in this regard (see below)?

A rather practical concern regards the quality of the information generated by whole genome sequencing and analysis on a single-cell basis. In more technical terms: what about the analytical and clinical validity of this information? Obviously, the more false positive results, the lower the number of embryos available for transfer, and the lower the take-home baby rate. Furthermore, most of the information will be related to risk factors for common complex disorders. This information is by definition probabilistic, and often has a rather low predictive value. This will easily undermine the clinical utility of the information. The *onus probandi* regarding the often claimed better quality of future screening panels and methods is, obviously, on the side of the proponents of such screening.

Next, considering the complexity of comprehensive PGS, traditional informed consent would simply be impossible. Could a so-called "generic consent" for comprehensive PGS be ethically (and legally) acceptable – and if so, on what conditions?

Another autonomy-related concern is that prospective parents would regularly, if not systematically, be confronted with rather complex, if not impossible, trade-offs. In theory, it may be simple to develop risk profiles that facilitate prospective parents' well-considered choice. But what about clinical practice, taking into account the fact that all embryos will carry many predispositions for a great number of common disorders – constituting "profiles" that may have a different meaning for different "stakeholders" in view of their own family history and experience?

A related issue regards, again, decision-making authority: who has the final say, the doctor or the prospective parents (see above)? Even if all parties agree that "the best embryo" should be transferred, there will be, so we presume, regular disagreement about what this means if confronted with complex risk profiles of, say, some 10 embryos. Obviously, before implementing comprehensive PGS, a proactive reflection about material and procedural criteria and trade-offs to be made regarding embryo-transfer is required.

Last, but not least, comprehensive PGS may provide "unexpected" (predictive) information about the genetic status of (one of) the prospective parents themselves, thereby undermining their right not to know. Likewise, it may involve an interference with the future child's right not to know, i.e. the right of the child to later decide for itself whether or not to be tested for genetic risks for future diseases. In theory, the latter could be prevented by not transferring embryos carrying such risk factors, but, again, as we are all "fellow mutants," there may well be no embryo suitable for transfer. Or would it be morally acceptable to adopt a narrower (less extensive) interpretation of future children's right not to know, and accept comprehensive embryo profiling and related transfers of embryos with known genetic risk factors for later onset preventable and/or treatable disorders?

Our conclusion is that comprehensive PGS, although attractive in theory, would be fully dispro-

portional at the moment. Is meets neither the basic "technical" criteria related to analytic and clinical validity nor the fundamental requirement of proportionality. Furthermore, some ethical issues urgently need further analysis.

Part of this analysis should be a comparative analysis of comprehensive PGS on the one hand and broad scope preconception carrier screening (PCS) of IVF-couples, followed by more targeted PGD on the other. This strategy (PCS-PGD) could have various advantages [24]. It could facilitate prospective parents' reproductive autonomy in that they would have both more time for reflection and more reproductive options if proven to be at high risk of having an affected child (see "Preconception carrier screening" section, below). Furthermore, as the PCS-PGD strategy would entail targeted testing of embryos, it can be designed to avoid invasions of the right not to know of future children. However, issues related to the feasibility of informed decision-making and the decisional authority of couples and clinicians need further scrutiny.

Preconception carrier screening

Given the potential importance of preconception testing in the context of assisted reproduction (see "Genetic screening of gamete donors" and "Preimplantation genetic screening" sections, above), the question emerges whether PCS should not also be offered as a form of population screening to all persons or couples of reproductive age. The case for PCS is especially strong with regard to testing for carrier status of autosomal recessive disorders. Carrier couples (1/100–1/50) have a 25% risk of having an affected child but, as they themselves are healthy, the great majority will not be aware of this risk [10]. As a consequence, affected children are in most cases born in families where this was not anticipated. Only after an affected child is born, can measures be taken to avoid the recurrence risk in further pregnancies and to inform relatives that they may be carriers as well. Preconception carrier screening has the potential to change this by allowing those without a positive family history for such disorders to find out about their risk and take this into account when making reproductive decisions. In order to avoid having an affected child, carrier couples may refrain from having children, may decide to have children through IVF and PGD, may decide to have children with the help of donor gametes, or may risk starting a pregnancy and have PND and a possible abortion should the fetus turn out to be affected.

In several Mediterranean and Asian countries or regions with a high frequency of beta-thalassemia and other hemoglobinopathies, carrier screening programs were already set up in the 1970s [25]. Many of these programs have led to a significant decrease in the birth prevalence of those disorders. They are often targeted at adolescents (in a high school setting), couples who wish to register for getting married (premarital), but also at pregnant women. These programs are very much driven by a public health aim: to as far as possible eradicate a disease with a high impact on the health of the population. Given the burden of disease caused by hemoglobinopathies in countries where the carrier frequency may be as high as 40%, this is perfectly imaginable. However, a concern about these programs is that most are either mandatory or that "voluntary" participation is based on anything but meaningful informed consent. Moreover, premarital programs sometimes present "cancellation of marriage" as an option to be considered if both partners turn out to be carriers. Similar concerns have been raised about carrier screening programs targeting other disorders in other communities, for instance the well-known "Dor Yeshorim" carrier screening program for Tay–Sachs disease and other disorders with a high frequency in Jewish populations [26].

In the literature about the ethics of carrier screening, two different accounts of the aim of such programs are distinguished [27]. These are related to distinct normative frameworks and traditions. One is the prevention aim that is also driving other population screening programs in the context of public health initiatives. The second approach derives from the traditions of individual reprogenetic counseling and prenatal screening for fetal anomalies (such as trisomy 21) that some (but not all) pregnant women would regard as a reason for abortion. Precisely because of a concern that reproductive decisions (more specifically: decisions about a possible termination of pregnancy) would be determined by societal interests or professional views about preferable outcomes, the emphasis in these traditions has always been on non-directive counseling aimed at serving autonomous decision-making. Whereas in the public health approach informed consent is regarded as a side-constraint to achieving a societal aim, the genetic counseling approach reverses this order. In this perspective, providing options for autonomous choice is the very aim of

reproductive screening and societal benefits in terms of a lower number of affected children are a welcome side-effect.

The practical importance of these different frameworks for evaluating carrier screening shows in debates about whether such screening should be offered pre- or post-conceptionally. When offered post-conceptionally (e.g. the hemoglobinopathy carrier screening currently offered to all pregnant women in the UK), reproductive options if both partners turn out to be carriers are much more limited than with preconception screening. During pregnancy, the only way to avoid the birth of an affected child is PND and a possible abortion. Moreover, the decision must be made under the pressure of time, in an emotionally charged period where meaningful autonomous choice may be more difficult to achieve. In a public health-driven program these concerns may be considered as not weighing up against the clear benefit that, as a target population, "pregnant women and their partners" are much easier to reach than the diffuse category of "persons or couples of reproductive age." However, in the contrasting perspective on carrier screening that emerges from the tradition of genetic counseling, the drawbacks of the prenatal approach weigh much heavier. From this perspective, post-conception carrier screening is clearly suboptimal, which is not to say that such programs cannot have a useful role as a backup.

Clearly, the case for accepting a prevention approach to carrier screening is stronger to the extent that the target disease(s) has (have) a higher impact on the health of the population or community. In such programs, it is absolutely crucial that conditions are put in place to ensure that participation is voluntary and based on relevant and balanced information and that individual choices with regard to possible post-test courses of action are fully respected. Guarantees are also needed to counteract possible stigmatizing and discriminatory effects within the community, as well as to avoid other psychosocial harm.

Where carrier screening is offered universally rather than to specific higher risk populations, the autonomy framework should determine the set up of the program. Current recommendations of American professional societies to universally offer preconception testing for certain disorders such as cystic fibrosis (CF) [28] and spinal muscular atrophy [29] are based on this perspective. In Europe, initiatives beyond specific higher risk groups have until now been limited.

A recent scientific consensus document drawn up on the initiative of the European Cystic Fibrosis Society has explored the conditions for introducing PCS for CF [30], and a report from the UK Human Genetic commission has suggested that policy makers should consider the potential benefits of PCS for would-be parents [31]. With the advent of NGS-technologies these debates are bound to enter a new phase, as it will become possible to determine individual carrier status for many more (autosomal and X-linked) recessive conditions than are included in current screening programs, without significantly increasing the costs. Whether and to what extent such expanded PCS fulfills accepted criteria for responsible screening will have to be determined by assessing the clinical validity and utility for each of the separate conditions to be included in the panel. The earlier discussion of carrier testing for FXS ("Genetic screening of gamete donors" section) underscores the importance of this. Preconception carrier screening that would lead to couples making far-reaching reproductive decisions on the basis of test results of which the clinical implications are poorly understood, is at odds with the aim of enhancing reproductive choice.

The reasoning in this last section has suggested that the best approach would be to offer PCS to all of reproductive age, as that would provide all parents to-be with the widest range of reproductive options, including but not limited to both PND and PGD. But while PCS for all is not yet introduced in most countries, separate questions can still be asked with regard to the place of PCS in the context of assisted reproduction. In the earlier "Genetic screening of gamete donors" section, we discussed the option of testing donors and recipients for carrier status of autosomal recessive disorders, in order to enable matching of carrier donors with non-carrier recipients. But given the significant risk for all couples to be a "carrier couple" (a risk that will be even much higher in case of consanguineity), it would seem that a strong case can be made for offering PCS to all IVF-couples, as a matter of good quality care. At the end of the earlier "Preimplantation genetic screening" section, we briefly discussed the option of broad-scope PCS followed by targeted PGD to avoid the transfer of homozygous (or otherwise affected) embryos, as a possible alternative for comprehensive PGS. Here again, the precise target disorders and mutations will have to be carefully selected in order to avoid far-reaching decisions on the basis of PCS-findings of which the

clinical implications are insufficiently clear. An important further question is whether the offer of PCS to IVF-couples should be as non-directive as when PCS is offered to the general population. Given the professional's responsibility to take account of the welfare of the future child, a more directive stance may well be justified.

References

1. Mikulić vs Croatia, February 7, 2002, no. 53176/99.

2. Nuffield Council on Bioethics. Donor conception: ethical aspects of information sharing: www.nuffieldbioethics.org/sites/default/files/Donor_conception_report.pdf

3. Sawyer N. Sperm donor limits that control for the "relative" risk associated with the use of open-identity donors. *Human Reprod* 2011; 25: 1089–96.

4. Turkmendag I. The donor-conceived child's "right to personal identity": the public debate on donor anonymity in the United Kingdom. *J Law Soc* 2012; 39: 58–72.

5. Association of Biomedical Andrologists; Association of Clinical Embryologists; British Andrology Society; British Fertility Society; Royal College of Obstetricians and Gynaecologists. UK guidelines for the medical and laboratory screening of sperm, egg and embryo donors. *Hum Fertil (Camb)* 2008; 11: 201–10.

6. Practice Committee of the American Society for Assisted Reproductive Technology. Recommendations for gamete and embryo donation: a committee opinion. *Fertil Steril* 2013; 99: 47–62.

7. Brown S. Genetic aspects of donor conception. In *Principles of Oocyte and Embryo donation*. Ed. M V Sauer. London, UK: Springer Verlag, 2013.

8. Musci TJ, Moyer K. Prenatal carrier testing for fragile X: counseling issues and challenges. *Obstet Gynecol Clin North Am* 2010; 37: 61–70.

9. Wirojanan J, Angkustsiri K, Tassone F *et al*. A girl with fragile X premutation from sperm donation. *Am J Med Genet A* 2008; 146: 888–92.

10. Ropers HH. On the future of genetic risk assessment. *J Community Genet* 2012; 3: 229–36.

11. De Wert G. Preimplantation genetic testing: normative reflections. In *Preimplantation Genetic Diagnosis*, 2nd edn. Ed. J Harper. Cambridge, UK: Cambridge University Press, 2009.

12. De Wert G. Ethical aspects of prenatal testing and preimplantation genetic diagnosis for late-onset neurogenetic disorders: the case of Huntington's disease. In *Prenatal Testing for Late-onset Neurogenetic Diseases*. Eds, G Evers-Kiebooms, M Zoeteweij,

P Harper. Oxford, UK: BIOS Scientific Publishers Ltd, 2002.

13. De Die-Smulders CE, de Wert GM, Liebaers I *et al.* Reproductive options for prospective parents in families with Huntington's disease: clinical, psychological and ethical reflections. *Hum Reprod Update* 2013; 19: 304–15.

14. Bredenoord AL, Dondorp W, Pennings G *et al.* PGD to reduce reproductive risk: the case of mitochondrial DNA disorders. *Hum Reprod* 2008; 23: 2392–401.

15. De Wert G. Preimplantation genetic diagnosis: the ethics of intermediate cases. *Hum Reprod* 2005; 20: 3261–6.

16. De Wert G, Liebaers I, Van de Velde H. The future (r)evolution of preimplantation genetic diagnosis/human leukocyte antigen testing: ethical reflections. *Stem Cells* 2007; 25: 2167–72.

17. Dondorp W, De Wert G, Pennings G *et al.* ESHRE Task Force on ethics and Law 20: sex selection for non-medical reasons. *Hum Reprod* 2013; 28: 1448–54.

18. Warren MA, *Gendercide: The Implications of Sex Selection*. Lanham, MD: Rowman and Littlefield Publishers, 1985.

19. Glover Y. *Choosing Children. Genes, Disability and Design*. Oxford: Clarendon Press, 2006.

20. Rubio C, Rodrigo L, Mir P *et al.* Use of array comparative genomic hybridization (array-CGH) for embryo assessment: clinical results. *Fertil Steril* 2013; 99: 1044–8.

21. Mastenbroek S. One swallow does not make a summer. *Fertil Steril* 2013; 99:1205–6.

22. Baart EB, Martini E, Eijkemans MJ *et al.* Milder ovarian stimulation for in-vitro fertilization reduces aneuploidy in the human preimplantation embryo: a randomized controlled trial. *Hum Reprod* 2007; 22: 980–8.

23. ESHRE Task Force on Ethics and Law 13. The welfare of the child in medically assisted reproduction. *Hum Reprod* 2007; 22: 2585–8.

24. Hens K, Dondorp W, Handyside AH *et al.* Dynamics and ethics of comprehensive preimplantation genetic testing: a review of the challenges. *Hum Reprod Update* 2013; 19: 366–75.

25. Cousens NE, Gaff CL, Metcalfe SA *et al.* Carrier screening for beta-thalassaemia: a review of international practice. *Eur J Hum Genet* 2010; 18: 1077–83.

26. Raz AE, Vizner Y. Carrier matching and collective socialization in community genetics: Dor Yeshorim and the reinforcement of stigma. *Soc Sci Med* 2008; 67: 1361–9.

27. De Wert GM, Dondorp WJ, Knoppers BM. Preconception care and genetic risk: ethical issues. *J Community Genet* 2012; 3: 221–8.

28. ACOG Committee. Opinion no. 486: update on carrier screening for cystic fibrosis. *Obstet Gynecol* 2011; 117: 1028–1031.

29. Prior TW. Professional Practice and Guidelines Committee: carrier screening for spinal muscular atrophy. *Genet Med* 2008; 10: 840–2.

30. Castellani C, Macek M Jr, Cassiman JJ *et al.* Benchmark for cystic fibrosis carrier screening: a European consensus document. *J Cyst Fibros* 9: 165–78.

31. Human Genetics Commission. Increasing options, informing choice: a report on preconception genetic testing and screening, April 2011: //f.hypotheses. org/wp-content/blogs.dir/257/files/2011/04/ 2011.HGC_.-Increasing-options-informing-choice-final1.pdf

Index

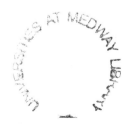

MEDICAL RADIOLOGY

Diagnostic Imaging

Editors:
A. L. Baert, Leuven
M. Knauth, Göttingen
K. Sartor, Heidelberg

V. Donoghue (Ed.)

Radiological Imaging of the Neonatal Chest

2nd Revised Edition

With Contributions by

P. G. Bjørnstad · A. Calder · V. Donoghue · G. F. Eich · B. Eidem · L. Garel · I. Gassner
T. E. Geley · H. W. Goo · C. J. Kellenberger · D. Manson · C. McMahon · A. C. Offiah
C. M. Owens · S. Ryan · L. Sena · B. Smevik · A. Twomey

Foreword by

A. L. Baert

With 303 Figures in 661 Separate Illustrations, 53 in Color and 10 Tables

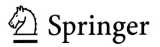 Springer

Veronica Donoghue, MD
Consultant Pediatric Radiologist
Department of Radiology
Children's University Hospital
Temple Street
Dublin 1
Ireland
and
The National Maternity Hospital
Holles Street
Dublin 2
Ireland

Medical Radiology · Diagnostic Imaging and Radiation Oncology
Series Editors:
A. L. Baert · L. W. Brady · H.-P. Heilmann · M. Knauth · M. Molls · C. Nieder · K. Sartor

Continuation of Handbuch der medizinischen Radiologie
        Encyclopedia of Medical Radiology

Library of Congress Control Number: 2007925876

ISBN 978-3-540-33748-5 Springer Berlin Heidelberg New York

Springer is part of Springer Science+Business Media

http//www.springer.com
© Springer-Verlag Berlin Heidelberg 2008
Printed in Germany

Medical Editor: Dr. Ute Heilmann, Heidelberg
Desk Editor: Ursula N. Davis, Heidelberg
Production Editor: Kurt Teichmann, Mauer
Cover-Design and Typesetting: Verlagsservice Teichmann, Mauer

Printed on acid-free paper – 21/3180xq – 5 4 3 2 1 0

Foreword

Lung and heart malformations, as well as acquired diseases, represent a major portion of the life-threatening conditions in neonates of low gestational age. Radiological imaging is one of the main tools to define the most appropriate therapeutic approach in order to improve the survival chances of these infants.

This second, completely revised and updated edition provides a comprehensive overview of the embryologic and anatomical aspects of neonatal chest conditions. It also presents very clearly our current knowledge of imaging techniques of the neonatal chest, as well as their therapeutic relevance for a correct postnatal management.

The editor, Dr. V. Donoghue, has been very successful in engaging several international experts in the field, all with outstanding qualifications, and I would like to congratulate her for the expeditious and excellent coordination of the editorial preparatory workflow of this book.

I am confident that this outstanding volume will stimulate great interest among both general and specialised pediatric radiologists, as well as among neonatologists and pediatricians and that it will meet with the same success as its first edition.

Leuven   ALBERT L. BAERT

Preface

This second edition of "Radiological Imaging of the Neonatal Chest" once again gives a detailed update on the clinical management of the various neonatal conditions, with emphasis on the impact of therapeutic interventions on the imaging findings. Antenatal and postnatal imaging of chest malformations is again discussed, together with some controversies regarding postnatal management of asymptomatic patients with these conditions. The chapters on clinical management, embryology, hyaline membrane disease, infection and chest wall abnormalities have been updated with little change in the imaging and treatment of infants with meconium aspiration syndrome.

In this edition the use of multidetector CT, which has revolutionised the imaging of vascular tracheobronchial compression syndromes and other airway disorders, is discussed and this technique now plays a central role in the modern evaluation of the newborn suspected with these abnormalities.

There are chapters devoted to all imaging modalities used to examine the heart and great vessels. In addition to high resolution ultrasonography, multidetector CT can provide exquisite extracardiac vascular detail with very short imaging times, often without sedation. In addition, there is now more widespread use of magnetic resonance imaging in the investigation of congenital cardiac abnormalities. As a result, in many institutions, both MDCT and MRI have replaced many diagnostic angiocardiography examinations in these newborns and this in turn has led to closer collaboration between paediatric radiologists and paediatric cardiologists in many centres. However, as the rate of diagnostic catheter studies is decreasing, the number of catheter-based interventional cardiac procedures is steadily increasing and this is addressed in the chapter on angiocardiography.

As many departments have installed computed or digital radiography, there is also a chapter devoted to this topic.

All of these changes prompted the preparation and publication of this second volume.

This book is intended primarily for use by paediatric radiologists, including those in training. It will also be of interest to neonatologists, paediatric cardiologists, paediatricians and paediatric surgeons.

I am most grateful to the international experts in the various fields of clinical neonatal chest medicine and diagnostic and interventional neonatal chest imaging who have written the various chapters, and I thank them for their excellent contributions. I hope this book will be accepted as a working and reference text for all those involved in caring for the neonate.

Dublin   VERONICA DONOGHUE

Contents

Embryology and Anatomy of the Neonatal Chest

1

Stephanie Ryan

CONTENTS

S. Ryan, MD
Radiology Departments, Children's University Hospital, Temple St., Dublin 1, Ireland and The Rotunda Hospital, Parnell Square, Dublin 1, Ireland

1.1
Embryology

1.1.1
Introduction

Embryology of the airway and lungs, of the heart and great vessels and of the other thoracic structures is well described in specialist texts on the subject Fitzgerald (1994), Larsen (1997). This section will summarise these with special reference to those aspects of embryology that are relevant to the radiological diagnosis of neonatal chest conditions.

1.1.2
Early Embryonic Development

At the end of the 3rd week, the embryo is a flat three-layered disc. In the 4th week a complex folding process occurs during which the flat germ disc is changed to a structure recognisable as a vertebrate. At completion of this process the early gut and the pleural and pericardial cavities are laid down.

Differential growth of the different parts of the developing embryo results in the process of embryonic folding. Whilst the embryonic disc is growing rapidly in length, the yolk sac is stagnating. The expanding disc is forced to bulge into a convex shape. The cephalic and lateral regions of the embryo begin to fold on day 22 and the caudal region on day 23. Due to this folding the edges of the germ disc from the cephalic, lateral and caudal regions are brought together in the ventral midline. A fusion of the three germ layers, the ectoderm, mesoderm and endoderm, from opposite sides of the embryo occur resulting in a three-dimensional form in which the endoderm is converted into a tubular structure termed the gut tube. This is divided into the cranial foregut, the future midgut, which remains open to the yolk sac, and the caudal hindgut.

With the midline fusion of the ectoderm along the ventral midline, the intraembryonic coelom is formed. The coelom or cavity is formed initially from the lateral plate mesoderm splitting into a somatic and splanchnic portion. The serosal membranes that line the body cavity, the somatopleure and splanchnopleure, derive from this lateral plate mesoderm. In the chest cavity these will form the parietal and visceral pleura and pericardial membranes.

The coelomic cavity extending the length of the embryo becomes divided by three partitions into the pleural, pericardial and peritoneal cavities. These will be further discussed with the development of the diaphragm.

1.1.3
Embryology of the Airway and Lungs

On day 22, a ventral protrusion develops from the foregut, called the laryngotracheal groove and later the laryngotracheal tube. The proximal part of this develops into the larynx and trachea and becomes continuous with the pharynx. The distal part enlarges and forms the lung bud, which becomes the primordium of the lungs. The epithelium of the groove becomes that of the larynx, the trachea and the bronchi and lungs. The lung bud is enclosed and retains a covering of splanchnopleuric mesoderm as it develops. This mesoderm gives origin to the muscle and cartilaginous tissue of the airways and the lung vasculature. Initially the mesoderm is a loose mesenchyme supplied by primitive systemic arteries. The pulmonary arteries arise form the sixth aortic arch and replace the systemic arteries in the mesenchyme at around 6 weeks.

By days 26–28 the lung bud enlarges and divides into a right and left bronchial bud from which the two lungs will develop (Fig. 1.1). The branching of the bronchial buds continues in the 5th week and forms three secondary bronchial buds on the right and two secondary bronchial buds on the left. There is continued growth and bifurcation in a dichotomous fashion of the bronchial buds and the associated splanchnopleure to gradually fill the pleural cavity that has developed through partition of the coelomic cavity. The terminal bronchioles are formed at the 16th generation of division, some as early as 20 weeks. These will divide to form two or more respiratory bronchioles. Respiration is possible at about 25 weeks and the process is essentially complete by week 28. These respiratory bronchioles

become invested with capillaries and are termed terminal sacs or primitive alveoli that then mature until birth. Throughout early childhood, up until the 8th year there is a continuous production of additional alveoli.

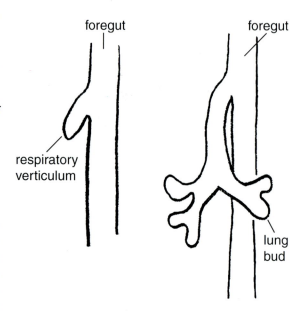

Fig. 1.1. Development of lung buds

1.1.3.1
The Maturation of the Lungs

The maturation of the lungs is described in four periods:

(1) Pseudoglandular period: from the 5th to the 17th week. By week 17 all the major lung elements have formed except those involved in gas exchange. Respiration is not possible.

(2) Cannalicular period: 16–25 weeks. This period overlaps the pseudoglandular period. Cranial parts of the developing lung mature faster than the caudal parts. The lumina enlarge, there is vascularisation of the lung tissue, and the respiratory bronchioles appear with some terminal sacs formed. Respiration is possible at the end of this period.

(3) Terminal sac period: 25–34 weeks. Many more terminal sacs are formed. The epithelium thins and capillaries bulge into the terminal sacs. Type 1 alveolar cells appear. By 23–24 weeks, type 11 pneumocytes develop that produce pulmonary surfactant. By 25–28 weeks there are sufficient terminal sacs present to permit survival of the premature infant.

Before this there is insufficient alveolar area and poor vascularisation.

(4) Alveolar period: from late foetal life to the 8th year. The epithelium of the terminal sacs becomes squamous. By late foetal life the alveolar capillary membrane is thin enough to allow gas exchange. At term, one fifth to one eighth of the adult number of alveoli is present in the newborn. Most of the remaining alveolarisation occurs within 6 months of birth at term.

Respiratory movements are present before birth with aspiration of amniotic fluid. Developed lungs at birth are half inflated with fluid, which is replaced by air in the first breaths. Lungs of a stillborn infant are firm and not aerated.

1.1.3.2
The Blood Supply of the Lungs

The blood supply of the lungs is derived from the splanchnopleuric mesoderm that covers the lung bud as it develops. It is supplied by the sixth arterial arch. The bronchial arteries arise from the thoracic aorta. A venous plexus surrounds the developing bronchial buds and drains to the left atrium.

1.1.4
Embryology of the Heart

The heart forms in the cardiogenic mesoderm in the floor of the pericardial coelom at the cranial end of the germ disc. Initially two tubes are formed that fuse to form a primitive heart tube. Between weeks 5 and 8 this tube loops and septates, forming four chambers and separating the pulmonary and systemic circulations (LAMERS 1992).

1.1.4.1
The Primitive Heart Tube

On day 19 two lateral endocardial tubes develop and soon afterwards the process of embryonic folding (described with development of the lungs) brings these tubes into the midline of the thoracic region where they fuse to form the primitive heart tube.

This tube has six inflow veins inferiorly:
- Two common cardinal veins, each formed by confluence of paired posterior cardinal veins draining the trunk and two anterior cardinal veins draining the head;

- Two vitelline veins drain the yolk sac and
- Two umbilical veins bring oxygenated blood from the placenta.

The tube has two outflow tracts superiorly, the paired dorsal aortae, which have come to form two arches due to embryonic folding.

1.1.4.2
Early Chamber Formation

On day 21 and over the next 5 weeks constrictions and expansions of the primitive heart tube result in the formation of primitive chambers (Fig. 1.2). Starting at the inferior "venous" end, these are:
- Right and left sinus horns and the sinus venosus. The right sinus horn will become the venous return and the left will become the coronary sinus draining only the myocardium.
- Primitive atrium, will become both atria.
- Primitive ventricle, early left ventricle.
- Bulbus cordis, which will form most of the right ventricle.
- Conotruncus will become the conus cordis and the truncus arteriosus.

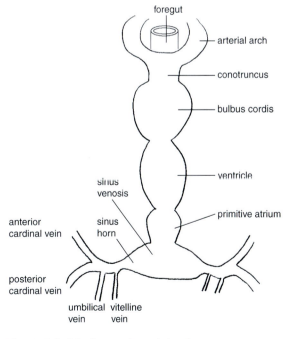

Fig. 1.2. Primitive heart tube and chambers

1.1.4.3
Development of the Heart Wall

The myocardium develops from the splanchnopleuric mesoderm that surrounds the heart tube. Initially the myocardium is separated from the endothelial heart tube by gelatinous material, cardiac jelly. Visceral pericardium and parietal pericardium also develop, but the dorsal mesocardium (the heart's mesentery) is absorbed early so that the pericardial space is continuous all around the heart. The fibrous pericardium develops later. The heart starts to beat on day 22 and blood begins to circulate throughout the embryo over the next few days.

1.1.4.4
Folding of the Heart

The primitive heart tube enlarges and elongates and on day 23 it begins to loop and fold. The bulbus cordis is displaced inferiorly, anteriorly and to the right, the ventricle to the left and the primitive atrium and the sinus venosus posteriorly and superiorly (Fig. 1.3). By day 28 the primitive chambers have assumed their relative positions as in the neonatal heart.

1.1.4.5
Development of the Atria

As the venous return from most of the body shifts in week 4 to the right side, the right sinus horn becomes the superior and inferior vena cavae, part of which, with the sinus venosus, becomes incorporated in the smooth walled part of the right atrium at 6 weeks.

Meanwhile, at the beginning of the 5th week the primitive atrium develops a pulmonary vein that bifurcates into right and left veins that grow towards the lungs where they anastomose with developing veins in the lung buds. These veins and their first order branches become incorporated into the atrial wall as two right and two left pulmonary veins.

1.1.4.6
Development of the Atrial Septum

On day 28 the conotruncus pressing on the atrial roof results in the formation of a depression and later a septum, the septum primum, which separates the right and left atrium (Fig. 1.4). The foramen below the septum primum is called the ostium primum. With further growth, the ostium primum fuses with the endocardial cushions that are separating the ventricles and the atria, thus obliterating the ostium primum. Perforations in the superior part of the septum primum become the ostium secundum before the ostium primum closes.

A second, thicker muscular septum grows from the roof of the atria to the right of the septum primum. This septum secundum has a defect inferiorly, the foramen ovale. Blood from the superior vena cava passes to the primitive right atrium. Oxygenated blood from the placenta in the inferior vena cava passes from the right atrium through the formaen ovale in the lower part of the septum secundum and through the ostium secundum in the upper part of the septum primum, to get to the left atrium. The increase in left atrial pressure after birth closes the septum primum against the septum secundum.

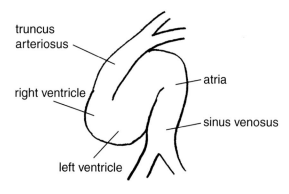
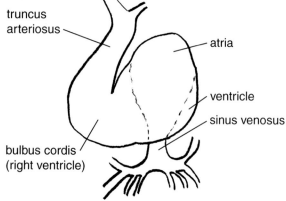

Fig. 1.3a,b. Folding of the heart tube

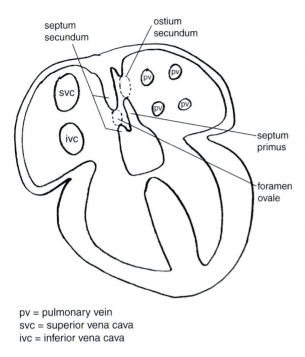

pv = pulmonary vein
svc = superior vena cava
ivc = inferior vena cava

Fig. 1.4. Development of the atrial septum

1.1.4.7

Development of the Ventricles, the Atrioventricular Canals, the Valves and the Outflow Tracts

In the primitive heart tube the atria are in line with the left ventricle and the entire outflow of the heart is from the right ventricle. At day 28 thickening of the endocardium around the atrioventricular canal, called superior and inferior and right and left endocardial cushions, develops to separate the atrium and the left ventricle. Fusion of the superior and inferior endocardial cushions forms the septum intermedium, which separates the right and left AV canals. (The interatrial septa fuse with this septum.) Extensive remodelling in the 7th week allows the right AV canal to be aligned with the right atrium and the left with the left ventricle. Simultaneously the left ventricle is brought into the line of the conus cordis. Part of the conus cordis is incorporated in the outflow tracts of both ventricles.

At the end of the 4th week a muscular septum forms that separates the ventricles and this continues to grow from below upward almost to the septum intermedium. A persisting gap allows access from the left ventricle into its outflow tract. The atrioventricular valves develop between the 5th and 8th week.

During the 7th and 8th weeks the conotruncus divides into separate pulmonary and systemic outflow vessels from the right and left ventricles, respectively. These spiral around each other as the pulmonary artery and aorta. Development of the valves at the outflow of the ventricles and closure of the final part of the interventricular septum finally results in the fully developed configuration of the four-chambered heart with separate pulmonary and systemic circulations.

1.1.5
Embryology of the Oesophagus

The oesophagus is derived from the foregut. Pharyngeal arch mesoderm gives rise to the muscle of its upper part, which is supplied by the recurrent laryngeal nerves. The muscle of its lower part arises from splanchnic mesoderm, which is supplied by autonomic nerves.

1.1.6
Embryology of the Diaphragm

Four embryonic structures contribute to the formation of the diaphragm:
  a) the septum transversum,
  b) the paraxial mesoderm of the body wall,
  c) the oesophageal mesenchyme, and
  d) the pleuroperitoneal membranes (Fig. 1.5).

The migration of myoblasts from the septum transversum into the pleuroperitoneal membranes draws the C2, 3 and 4 innervation of the phrenic nerve inferiorly as the septum transversum migrates cranio-caudally. However, the main contribution of the septum transversum is to the central tendon of the diaphragm.

The outermost rim of the diaphragm muscle is formed from the body wall paraxial mesoderm and is innervated by spinal nerves from C7-T12. The right and left crura of the diaphragm are muscular bands formed by condensation of mesenchyme associated with the foregut at the vertebral levels L1-L3. The pleuroperitoneal membranes separate the definitive pleural cavities from the peritoneal cavity. They are transverse membranes that grow ventrally from an oblique line connecting the root of the 12th rib with the tips of the ribs 12 through 7. The membranes fuse with the posterior edge of the septum transversum closing off the pleuroperitoneal canals by the 7th week. The left pleuroperitoneal canal is larger than the right and closes later, a difference that may account for the fact that congenital hernias of the abdominal viscera are more common on the left side than on the right.

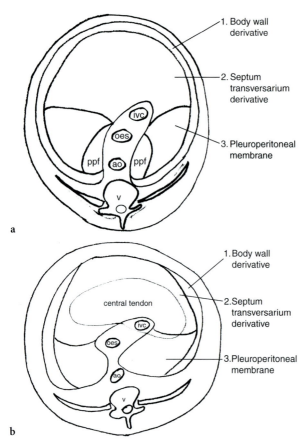

Fig. 1.5a,b. Development of the diaphragm. **a** Before 7 weeks. (ppf = pleuroperitoneal foramen). **b** neonatal diaphragm showing the origins of its components

1.1.7
Embryology of the Thoracic Wall

1.1.7.1
Vertebrae

Somites separate from the paraxial mesoderm in a craniocaudal sequence until day 30. Commencing in the cervical region the somites subdivide into three kinds of mesodermal primordium: the myotomes, the dermatomes and the sclerotomes. The sclerotomes give origin to the vertebral bodies and vertebral arches. The ventral portion of the sclerotome encloses the notochord and forms the rudi-

ment of the vertebral body. The dorsal part of the sclerotome encloses the neural tube and forms the rudiment of the vertebral arch. Vertebral bodies are formed in response to substances from the notochord (e.g., chondroitin sulphate). Vertebral arches require interaction with surface ectoderm for their formation.

Abnormalities in the induction of the somites may result from abnormal induction of the sclerotome. Defective induction of vertebral bodies on one side may result in a severe lateral scoliosis.

The sclerotomes are arranged segmentally, and whilst migrating towards the neural tube and the notochord, split into a cranial half and a caudal half. The caudal half of each sclerotome fuses with the cranial half of the succeeding sclerotome to form intersegmental vertebral rudiments.

The intervertebral discs are fibrous and form between the vertebral bodies at the segmental levels. Cells of notochordal origin initially form the core of each disc, the nucleus pulposus, probably to be later replaced by cells of sclerotomal origin, and the surrounding annulus fibrosus develops from sclerotomal cells.

1.1.7.2
Ribs

Small condensations of mesenchyme develop along the lateral aspect of the vertebral arches of the developing neck and trunk vertebrae. These are termed costal processes and on day 35 in the thoracic region the distal tips of these processes lengthen to form ribs. Ventrally, the first seven ribs connect to the sternum through the costal cartilages by day 45 and are termed true ribs. Ribs 8–12 do not articulate directly with the sternum and are termed false ribs.

Initially, the ribs are cartilaginous and later ossify through a process termed endochondral ossification. In the 6th week a primary ossification centre appears near the angle of each rib and ossification then proceeds distally. The secondary centres of ossification do not appear in the heads and tubercles of the ribs until adolescence.

1.1.7.3
Sternum

In the centrolateral body wall a pair of longitudinal mesenchymal condensations termed the sternal bars appear. In the 7th week the most cranial of the ribs makes contact with them and the bars meet along the midline and begin to fuse, progressing in a cranio-caudal sequence to terminate with the formation of the xiphoid process in the 9th week.

The cartilaginous precursors of the sternal bars ossify, like the ribs, in a craniocaudal sequence from the 5th month to shortly after birth, thus producing the definitive components of the sternum–the manubrium, the body and the xiphoid process. The xiphoid process does not ossify until after birth.

1.1.7.4
Intercostal Muscles and Dermis

After the sclerotome migrates medially to contribute to the development of the vertebrae, the portion that remains is termed a dermamyotome. This separates into a myotome and a dermatome. The dermatome contributes to the dermis of the ventral trunk (skin and connective tissue). The myogenic cells differentiate from the myotomes, which split into two components, the epimeres and the hypomeres. The dorsal epimeres give rise to the deep muscles of the back, the erector spinae and the transversospinalis groups. The ventral hypomeres form the muscles of the ventral and lateral body wall: the three layers of intercostal muscles.

1.2
Anatomy of Neonatal Chest Radiology

1.2.1
Introduction

Neonatal thoracic anatomy is similar to thoracic anatomy at any other age. Detailed accounts may be had in standard anatomy and radiological anatomy textbooks (RYAN 2004). This section will deal with the anatomy as seen on radiographs and other imaging with emphasis on the differences between neonates and older children or adults.

1.2.2
Airway and Lungs

The trachea is a fibromuscular tube supported by 16 to 20 cartilaginous rings that are deficient pos-

teriorly. It extends from the C4 level to T4 in the neonate (T5 in the older child). The trachea may be "buckled" on a chest radiograph, especially one taken in expiration. It is seen to straighten considerably with deep inspiration. It buckles anteriorly and to the right. It will buckle to the left if the aortic arch is right sided.

At the carina the trachea bifurcates. The right main bronchus is more vertical, at 32° to midline, than the left main bronchus, which lies at 51° to midline in the neonate. The carinal angle becomes smaller in the older child. The bronchi can be visible to their second or third order of branching on a neonatal chest radiograph, especially behind the heart. This is not abnormal as it would be in an adult CXR.

Lungs should be symmetrically radiolucent on a chest radiograph. Radiographs taken with some rotation result in asymmetric lung density. The left lung has two lobes, and the right has three, but the pleural fissures may be incomplete in the neonate. The horizontal fissure on the right is sometimes visible on the radiograph as a pencil-thin line equidistant from the apex and the diaphragm. The oblique fissures are not usually visible on AP chest radiographs.

The borders of the lungs are visible on a chest radiograph because of the lucency of the lung against the denser heart, mediastinum or diaphragm. Both hemidiaphragms should be entirely visible on an AP chest radiograph including the medial part of the left hemidiaphragm below the heart.

The pulmonary artery is visible below the aortic knuckle on radiographs of older children, but is masked by the normal thymus in neonates. The pulmonary arteries can be seen on a radiograph as they branch at the hilum. The right pulmonary artery divides into an upper lobar artery and interlobar artery. The latter can be clearly seen on a radiograph, and its diameter may equal that of the trachea. Large vessels should not be visible in the periphery of the lungs on a radiograph. Radiographs taken with the beam angled cranially result in accentuation of the upper lobe vascularity.

1.2.3
Heart and Great Vessels

The internal anatomy of the neonatal heart is best imaged by echocardiography. Cardiac MR may be used for the evaluation of congenital heart disease in the neonate. CT and MR are used for imaging the great vessels.

The chest radiograph shows the overall heart size and to a certain extent can show relative enlargement of certain chambers. The thymus (see below) can result in apparent heart enlargement. The cardiac diameter on the lateral view is independent of the thymus and may be easier to interpret if the AP view is confusing.

On an AP chest radiograph, the right heart border is formed by the right atrium, the left by the left ventricle. The upper part of the cardiac silhouette is covered by the thymus. On the lateral radiograph the anterior border of the heart is hidden by the thymus; the posterior border is formed by the left atrium.

The aortic arch is hidden by the thymus, but the descending aorta is usually visible lateral to the left border of the spine where its lateral border is defined by the adjacent lung (Fig. 1.6).

1.2.4
Thymus

The mediastinum in neonates appears widened due to the relatively large thymus gland. In neonates the thymus may extend superiorly as far as the thyroid gland and inferiorly to the lower border of the heart. It widens on expiration and elongates and rises on inspiration. It has two asymmetrical lobes.

On the AP chest radiograph it may blend imperceptibly with the cardiac silhouette or its inferior border may be marked by notches on either side. The protruding triangular configuration called the sail sign is less common in neonates than in older babies (Fig. 1.6). The lateral border of the thymus may be sharp or may fade gradually. It may have an undulating border reflecting its soft nature and moulding by the overlying ribs. Lung markings are usually visible through the thymic shadow.

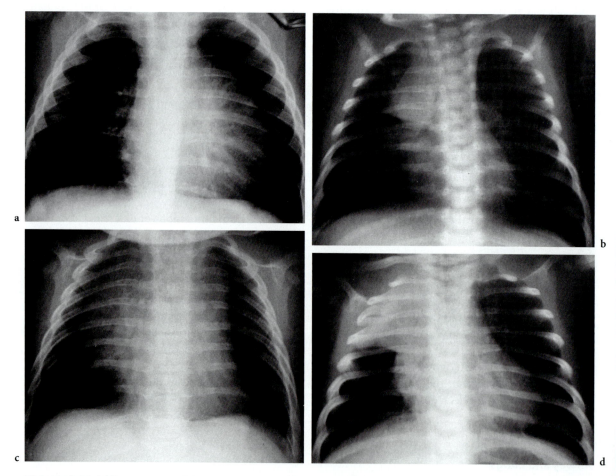

Fig. 1.6a–d. Variable appearance of thymus on neonatal AP chest radiograph. **a** Thymus blends with left heart border giving impression of cardiomegaly. **b** Thymus protrudes from right upper mediastinal border as "sail sign". **c** Large but normal thymus mimics right mediastinal mass. **d** Thymus mimics right upper lobe density

On a lateral chest radiograph the thymus is anterior and superior to the heart. It obliterates the superior mediastinal lucent space that is visible in adults. While it can extend posterior to the trachea, a posterior mediastinal mass is less likely to represent a normal thymus.

The thymus may simulate cardiac enlargement, a mediastinal mass or pulmonary disease especially right upper lobe pneumonia (Fig. 1.6). It is most important to remember that a normal thymus never deviates the trachea or other structures. Fluoroscopy may be helpful to determine the true nature of an apparent abnormality. On fluoroscopy the thymus can be seen to be soft and move with respiration. Rotation can identify a characteristic lateral border that was not clear on the radiograph.

The thymus is visible on ultrasound, CT and MR (Fig. 1.7). It has a homogenous appearance on all three imaging modalities. It has a CT density of approximately 38 Hounsfield Units and enhances uniformly. On MR it is very bright on T2-weighted sequences and brighter than muscle on T1-weighted sequences.

1.2.5
The Chest Wall and Diaphragm

The AP diameter of the neonatal chest is almost as big as the transverse diameter, giving the chest a cylindrical configuration. A small amount of rotation while taking the radiograph will result in asymmetry of the appearance of the radiograph. The degree of rotation is judged by the length of the anterior ribs on the right and left side. The method used in adults of judging the distance between the medial end of each clavicle and the spinous process of the vertebrae is not possible since the spinous processes are not ossified in neonates.

Diaphragmatic movement can be particularly well assessed by ultrasound in neonates because their small size allows visualisation of both hemidiaphragms simultaneously in the coronal plane. Paradoxical movement on one side can be seen with real time scanning.

Folds of skin over the thoracic wall may be visible on a chest radiograph as fat lines or because they are outlined by air. If these lucent lines superimpose the lateral lung border they may simulate a pneumothorax (Fig. 1.8). If the line can be seen to extend beyond the lung its true nature is clear. Otherwise a decubitus or other view may be necessary to rule out a pneumothorax.

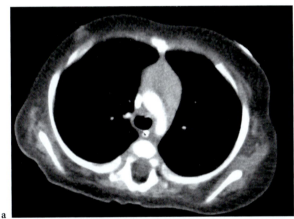

a

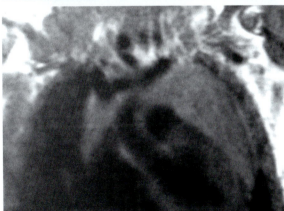

b

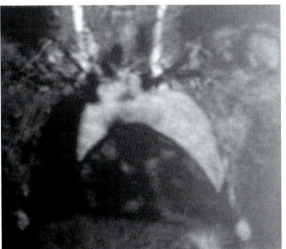

c

Fig. 1.7a–c. Neonatal thymus on cross-sectional imaging. **a** Contrast-enhanced CT. **b** Coronal T1 MRI. **c** Coronal STIR MRI

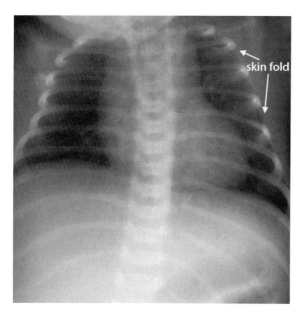

Fig. 1.8. AP chest radiograph, a skin fold simulates a pneumothorax (*long arrow*). However, the skin fold can be seen to extend beyond the lung (*short arrow*)

References

Further Reading

Fitzgerald MJT, Fitzgerald M (1994) Human embryology. Balliere Tindall, London

Lamers WH, Wessels A, Verbeek FJ et al (1992) New findings concerning ventricular septation in the human heart: implications for maldevelopment. Circulation 86:1194–1205

Larsen WJ (1997) Human embryology, 2nd edn. Churchill Livingston, New York

Ryan S, McNicholas M, Eustace S (2004) Anatomy for diagnostic imaging, 2nd edn. WB Saunders, London

Update on Clinical Management of Neonatal Chest Conditions

Anne Twomey

CONTENTS

2.1
Introduction

The past 4 decades have been marked by extraordinary advances in the treatment of critically ill neonates. With the advent of intensive care coupled with advances in modern technology, the face of neonatal medicine has changed forever. This has resulted in improved survival and decreased morbidity among term and preterm gestation infants. Nowhere is this more eloquently seen than in the fact that the limits of viability have now extended to lower gestational ages. Most of these improvements are directly related to the better management of neonatal lung conditions such as respiratory distress syndrome in preterm infants and meconium aspiration syndrome and persistent pulmonary hypertension of the newborn in term infants. In addition, a better understanding of various congenital abnormalities of the chest such as congenital diaphragmatic hernia has allowed us to manage these infants better in the immediate postnatal period as well as allowing us to consider novel new ways of treating these conditions such as with foetal intervention. This chapter will outline the recent key advances that have impacted on the management of neonatal lung conditions. Firstly, the area of mechanical ventilation will be discussed, including newer modes of ventilation such as high frequency ventilation, liquid ventilation and extracorporeal membrane oxygenation. Attention will then be turned to two new drug therapies: surfactant, which has become established as a standard part of the management of preterm infants and, more recently, nitric oxide, which is being used in the management of hypoxic respiratory failure in term infants. Lastly a mention will be made of the role of prenatal diagnosis and foetal surgery in the treatment of selected neonatal chest conditions.

2.2
Ventilatory Support

Without doubt, the ability to support and treat various respiratory disorders in the neonate has led to an increase in survival among lower gestational age infants and critically ill term infants. Continuous positive airway pressure (CPAP) and conventional mandatory ventilation (CMV) remain the mainstays, although more recently, high frequency ventilation (HFV) and liquid ventilation (LV) have been evaluated as alternative ventilatory modes.

A. Twomey
Consultant Neonatologist, The National Maternity Hospital, Holles Street, Dublin 2 and Children's University Hospital, Temple Street, Dublin 1. Ireland

2.2.1
Continuous Positive Airway Pressure

Continuous positive airway pressure (CPAP) has been an important tool in the treatment of neonates with respiratory distress syndrome (RDS). The mechanisms by which CPAP produces its beneficial effects include an increase in alveolar volumes and functional residual capacity (FRC), better alveolar recruitment and stability and redistribution of lung water. The result is an improvement in ventilation-perfusion matching. However, high CPAP levels can lead to side effects including over distension, an increased risk of air leaks, carbon dioxide retention, cardiovascular impairment, decreased lung compliance and possibly an increase in pulmonary vascular resistance.

Multiple clinical trials have evaluated the use of CPAP in neonates with respiratory disorders. Meta-analyses have generally concluded that in preterm infants with RDS, the application of a continuous distending pressure is associated with a decrease in mortality and a decrease in the need for assisted ventilation (Ho et al. 2002a). One notable side effect, however, is that the incidence of air leaks is increased (Ho et al. 2002a). The applicability of these results to current practice is difficult to determine as four of the five trials included in the above analysis were carried out in the 1970s in the presurfactant era and infants studied were quite mature ranging between 31-34 weeks gestation. CPAP is most beneficial if used early on in the treatment of neonates with established RDS as it decreases the need for subsequent positive pressure ventilation (Ho et al. 2002b). Again, most of the trials included in this analysis were conducted in the presurfactant era on more mature infants. Prophylactic CPAP commenced soon after birth (within 2 h) regardless of respiratory status in preterm infants has not been shown to decrease the need for subsequent intubation and intermittent positive pressure ventilation (Subramaniam et al. 2005). However, of the two studies included in this meta-analysis, one was done in the presurfactant era and the other reported outcomes for infants in the 28-31-week gestational age group. There was insufficient evidence in the meta-analysis to evaluate the benefits or harm of prophylactic nasal CPAP in very preterm infants, a group that warrants particular attention. CPAP is also effective in preventing failure of extubation in preterm infants after a period of endotracheal intubation and intermittent positive pressure ventilation (Davis and Henderson-Smart 2003).

One of the most controversial areas currently in neonatology is the appropriate early management of respiratory distress syndrome in extremely low birth weight (ELBW) infants. The debate centers on the use of early CPAP after delivery compared with the use of prophylactic or early surfactant. Although there is good evidence that prophylactic and early surfactant reduces mortality and respiratory morbidity, few of these studies have large numbers of the smallest babies, and none of the studies randomised infants in the placebo or control group to treatment with early CPAP (Soll 1997, Soll 1998, Soll and Morley 2001, Yost and Soll 2001). On the other hand, there is increasing concern that the use of mechanical ventilation, especially in the first few days of life, seems to considerably increase the risk of chronic lung disease (CLD) (Van Marter et al. 2000). A retrospective analysis of eight different neonatal units by Avery et al. (1987) found that the use of CPAP and the acceptance of higher PaCO2 and lower pH were associated with a reduction in the incidence of CLD. The critical question, therefore, is if it is better to avoid mechanical ventilation at all costs in the most vulnerable group of preterm infants by using early CPAP or does the benefit of intubation with the administration of early surfactant outweigh any subsequent morbidities seen with the use of mechanical ventilation.

Historically, respiratory support for very preterm babies has been intubation and mechanical ventilation and so many clinicians have questioned whether ELBW infants could, in fact, be managed successfully with CPAP alone. The neonatal intensive care unit in Columbia has consistently reported a low rate of CLD and a much greater use of CPAP compared with early intubation and mechanical ventilation. Their experience has been presented in more detail in a recent article (Ammari et al. 2005). The authors report that of 87 infants between the ages of 23–25 weeks gestation, 69% were treated with initial CPAP. Overall, 31% of these 87 infants were maintained solely on CPAP. Of the group of infants between 26–28 weeks, 95% were started on CPAP in the delivery room and 78% were successful in requiring only CPAP as their treatment. Of infants <699 g at birth, 73% were started on CPAP and the overall success of CPAP alone was 33%. They reported fewer pneumothoraces in the group of infants started on CPAP than for the infants who were CPAP failures or who were initially intubated in the delivery room. Only 51% of infants who were CPAP failures and 53% of infants ventilated from birth received surfactant.

Booth et al. (2006) have also recently reported that a high proportion of their very preterm infants (<27-week gestation) intubated at birth for prophylactic surfactant were successfully extubated and treated with nasal CPAP during the 1st week of life without requiring re-intubation during that time. Of note, no baby <660 g sustained nasal CPAP without requiring re-intubation, whereas 25% of infants born at 23 or 24 weeks of gestation were successful in doing so. This suggested that diaphragmatic and intercostal muscle bulk may be more important than the maturity of the respiratory drive in sustaining ventilation on CPAP. Based on the above, it would seem that with appropriate experience and attention to detail, it is possible to manage a percentage of extremely preterm infants on nasal CPAP soon after birth.

If early CPAP is to be advocated, should exogenous surfactant be administered in conjunction with it, and what is the appropriate timing of administration? The results of published surfactant trials in ventilated patients cannot be extrapolated to this population. The strategy of a short intubation to deliver surfactant with subsequent extubation to CPAP compared with CPAP alone was first reported by Verder et al. in 1994. This group found that in infants (25–35 weeks gestation) with moderate to severe RDS (as defined by an arterial to alveolar ratio of less than 0.22) treated with nasal CPAP, a single dose of surfactant significantly reduced the need for subsequent mechanical ventilation from 85% to 43%. There was no difference in the incidence of CLD between the groups. Tooley and Dyke (2003) compared infants who had received surfactant followed by a rapid extubation to those who had received surfactant with ongoing mechanical ventilation. Again, no differences were detected between the groups. The IFDAS trial, which is currently published in abstract form, randomized infants between 27–29 weeks of gestation into one of four treatment arms: early CPAP and prophylactic surfactant, early CPAP with or without subsequent rescue surfactant, early intubation and ventilation with prophylactic surfactant, and conventional management (Thomson 2002). CPAP was reportedly initiated within 6 h of birth (the study did not require the use of CPAP in the delivery room). It was found that infants treated with CPAP had a shorter mean duration of mechanical ventilation. No differences were detected in the rates of CLD or other complications between the groups. A recent meta-analysis addressing the effect of early surfactant administration with brief ventilation (<1 h)

versus the more conventional approach of selective surfactant administration and continued mechanical ventilation found that the former strategy was preferable in terms of preventing the need for mechanical ventilation (Stevens et al. 2004). However, there was insufficient evidence to reliably evaluate any effect on the rate of CLD. It should be noted that most of the infants enrolled in the studies quoted in the meta-analysis were greater than 28-week gestation. In summary, infants with RDS can be successfully treated with a brief intubation for surfactant administration and a rapid extubation to CPAP. Those infants treated with early surfactant replacement therapy and CPAP are less likely to need mechanical ventilation than infants who are treated with nasal CPAP and later surfactant therapy. To date, there have been no reported benefits in terms of the incidence of CLD, and there remains a paucity of data on long-term neurodevelopmental outcome. It is also not clear from the studies which infants (in terms of birth weight and/or gestational age) are most likely to benefit from this rapid extubation approach, nor is it clear at what point in time in the course of RDS disease progression should one recommend intervention with intubation for the purpose of surfactant administration.

What is clearly missing from the literature are any randomized controlled trials comparing the use of CPAP initiated in the delivery room with the use of prophylactic or early surfactant. There are currently three prospective trials underway that will hopefully address this issue. The COIN trial has enrolled infants between 25–28 weeks of gestation who showed spontaneous breathing in the delivery room after stabilisation with subsequent evidence of RDS. Infants were randomised to nasal CPAP or intubation with surfactant administration. Enrolment is now completed and results are awaited. The Vermont-Oxford Network is carrying out a three-armed trial in which infants from 26–29 weeks of gestation are randomized to either intubation with early prophylactic surfactant with subsequent stabilisation on ventilator support, intubation with early prophylactic surfactant with rapid extubation to CPAP or early stabilisation with CPAP with selective intubation and surfactant administration for clinical indications. Finally, the SUPPORT trial is enrolling infants of 24–27 weeks gestation, and these infant are randomised to either CPAP beginning in the delivery room with criteria for subsequent intubation or intubation with surfactant treatment within 1 h of birth with continuing ventilation with criteria for extubation. It is hoped that the results of these trials will be available within the next 2–3 years.

While we do not have unequivocal answers to all our questions at this time, FINER (2006), in a recent editorial, voiced a sensible and practical approach until such time as more definitive information becomes available. He is of the opinion that for more mature infants ≥26 weeks gestation, early CPAP started at delivery with intubation and surfactant administration for those infants who show a significant oxygen requirement and immediate extubation to CPAP for infants with an adequate respiratory effort appears reasonable. While he does not specifically address the point at which he would recommend intervention with intubation, he does note in his editorial that the criteria for intubating an infant assigned to CPAP in each of the three prospective trials currently in progress are remarkably similar and include a PaCO2 >60–65 mmHg (8–8.5 kPa), an FiO2 >40–60% and significant apnoea. With regards to the immediate management of infants <26 weeks of gestation, he is less definitive. The success of CPAP alone as a modality increases with increasing gestational age, and CPAP alone is unlikely to be successful for more than a minority of infants weighing <600 g or of <24-week gestation. While these percentages will likely increase as individual units gain more experience with the use of CPAP, his current preference, in the absence of the results of the current trials underway, is to err on the side of intubating infants <26 weeks' gestation and to administer surfactant within the first 30 min of life followed by aggressive attempts to extubate the infant to CPAP within the next 24–48 h.

In summary, the role of CPAP in the management of RDS in ELBW infants is still being elucidated. Results of ongoing trials are anxiously awaited. Further studies that include longer-term neurodevelopmental follow-up are required to determine the safety and effectiveness of the earlier use of CPAP without surfactant, the acceptance of higher PaCO2 and the use of higher levels of CPAP in ELBW infants with RDS.

More recently, nasal intermittent positive pressure ventilation (NIPPV) has been utilized as a method of augmenting nasal CPAP. It has the added advantage of delivering ventilator breaths via the nasal prongs. A review of randomised controlled trials comparing NIPPV to nasal CPAP has found that NIPPV is more effective in preventing failure of extubation (DAVIS et al. 2001). No studies have yet described the use of NIPPV as first line therapy for early respiratory disease. Further work is needed to determine if the use of NIPPV confers benefits in terms of the rate of CLD, etc. The impact of synchronization of NIPPV with infants' breaths in terms of safety and efficacy has also to be established.

2.2.2
Continuous Mandatory Ventilation

CMV plays a critical role in the care of neonates. With the increasing survival of premature infants, CMV is being used on smaller and sicker infants for longer durations. There is evidence to suggest that mechanical injury from ventilation plays a role in the pathogenesis of chronic lung disease. Ventilator-associated lung injury was traditionally thought to have been due to the use of high pressures, thus the name "barotrauma". However, recent laboratory-based and clinical research has raised questions about this purported mechanism. Experimentally, investigators have used high and low lung volumes and pressures in an attempt to determine if volume or pressure is the major culprit responsible for lung injury in the immature animal. By using negative pressure ventilation and chest strapping, investigators have been able to dissociate the magnitudes of volumes and pressures. These studies have consistently demonstrated that markers of lung injury (pulmonary oedema, epithelial injury and hyaline membrane) are present with the use of high volume and low pressure, but not with the use of low volume and high pressure. Thus many investigators and clinicians prefer the term "volutrauma" to the more classic term of "barotrauma" (DREYFUSS and SAUMAN 1998, HERNANDEZ et al. 1989, DREYFUSS and SAUMON 1993). Armed with this information, attempts are now being made to optomise particular ventilatory strategies in certain lung diseases in an effort to minimise barotrauma and volutrauma. This offers the theoretical advantage of improving gas exchange with the smallest amount of lung injury. These strategies have been derived by the application of basic concepts of pulmonary mechanics, gas exchange and control of breathing to the particular lung disease in question. To demonstrate a benefit in adopting particular ventilatory strategies, it is necessary to show an improvement in blood gases and/or a decrease in morbidity. Not surprisingly, the complexities of the multiple patient presentations along with the myriad of available ventilatory changes mean that definitive conclusions are hard to reach. Suffice it to say that more research is needed.

RDS is characterised by low compliance and low functional residual capacity. An optimal CMV strategy would include conservative indications for CMV, the use of the lowest PIP (positive inspiratory pressure) and tidal volume required, moderate PEEP (peak end expiratory pressure) (3–5 cm H_2O), permissive hypercapnia, judicious use of sedation and aggressive weaning (OCTAVE Study Group 1991, POHLANDT et al. 1992, MARIANI et al. 1999). Studies have shown that relatively high ventilatory rates (60 breaths/min) result in a decreased incidence of pneumothorax. Shorter inspiratory times (the time allowed for inflation to occur) also promote weaning, decrease the risk of pneumothorax and allow the use of higher ventilator rates (CARLO and AMBALAVANAN 1999). Overall, most clinicians favour a short inspiratory time, high rate, low tidal volume strategy. Unlike RDS, the lung disease in chronic lung disease of prematurity (CLD) is usually heterogenous with varying time constants among different lung areas. The time constant is the product of resistance and compliance and is a measure of the time needed for the airway pressure delivered by the ventilator to equilibrate throughout the lungs. If the time constant is prolonged (therefore, implying that the lungs are more difficult to inflate and deflate), more time is needed for inflation and deflation to occur. Infants with CLD often do better with higher PEEPs (4–6 cm H_2O). In addition, they often respond to longer inspiratory times as this allows more time for equilibration of the airway pressure to occur. The use of longer inspiratory times results in improved tidal volumes and better carbon dioxide elimination. Longer expiratory times and lower flow rates are also preferred. Hypercarbia and a compensated respiratory acidosis are often tolerated to avoid increasing lung injury with aggressive CMV (CARLO and AMBALAVANAN 1999).

Persistent pulmonary hypertension of the newborn (PPHN) may be primary or associated with meconium aspiration syndrome, prolonged intrauterine hypoxia or congenital diaphragmatic hernia (CDH). The best ventilatory strategy in this condition is also controversial with marked differences in management style being evident among different neonatal units (WALSH-SUKYS et al. 2000). In general, the inspired oxygen (FiO2) is adjusted to maintain PaO2 between 10–12 kPas (80–100 mmHg) to minimise hypoxia-mediated pulmonary vasoconstriction. Ventilatory rates are adjusted to maintain an arterial pH between 7.45–7.55. Care is taken to avoid extremely low PaCO2 (<20 torr), which can

cause cerebral vasoconstriction. The availability of inhaled nitric oxide, a selective pulmonary vasodilator, has added greatly to our ability to care for these critically ill infants and has been accompanied by a reduction in the need for extracorporeal membrane oxygenation. The widespread availability of this drug means that current ventilatory strategies will need to be reassessed as it may be neither necessary nor beneficial to maintain low-normal PaCO2.

While continuing study is needed to delineate the best ventilatory strategy in each lung condition, there is, nevertheless, a consensus that CMV, by its very nature, can and does lead to lung injury. On this basis, it is recommended that clinicians aim for more gentle ventilatory strategies in which gas trapping and alveolar overdistension are minimised while blood gas targets are modified to accept higher than normal PaCO2 and lower than normal PaO2 values. This concept of "permissive hypercapnia" or "controlled mechanical hypoventilation" suggests that respiratory acidosis and alveolar hypoventilation may be an acceptable price to pay for the prevention of pulmonary volutrauma. Two large retrospective studies designed to determine risk factors for lung injury in neonates concurred on the potential importance of this strategy, noting that higher PaCO2 values were associated with less lung injury (GARLAND et al. 1995, KRAYBILL et al. 1989). Using multiple logistic regression, these two studies independently concluded that ventilatory strategies leading to hypocapnia during the early neonatal course resulted in an increased risk of lung injury. MARIANI et al. (1999) have recently reported their experience of permissive hypercapnia in preterm infants. Surfactant-treated infants (birth weight 854±163 g, gestational age 26±1.4 weeks), receiving assisted ventilation during the first 24 h after birth, were randomised to permissive hypercapnia (PaCo2 45–55 mmHg) or to normocapnia (PaCO2 35–45 mmHg). The number of patients receiving assisted ventilation during the intervention period was lower in the permissive hypercapnia group (P<0.005). During that period, the ventilated patients in the permissive hypercapnia group HAD (rather than have) a higher pCO2 and lower PIP, MAP and ventilator rate than those in the normocapnia group. While it is clear that this ventilatory strategy is feasible and seems safe, the more important issue is whether it improves long-term outcome in these infants. A Cochrane review assessing whether a strategy of permissive hypercapnia in mechanically ventilated neonates led to improvements in short- and long-term outcomes found that there was no difference in the incidence of death, chronic lung disease, severe intraventricular haemorrhage or periventricular leucomalacia between the groups (WOODGATE and DAVIES 2001). On that basis, it was felt that this ventilation strategy could not be recommended to reduce mortality or pulmonary or neurodevelopmental morbidity. Until more evidence is available that supports the safety and benefits of this strategy, it would seem wise to avoid the exposure of ventilated newborns to either severe hypocapnia or hypercapnia.

Recent advances in respiratory technology have transformed standard mechanical ventilators. Ventilators are now highly sophisticated machines that offer the unique ability to provide rapid and precise control of gas delivery and ventilatory support in various ways, while allowing for the monitoring and alarming of virtually every aspect of the procedures involved. Most infants who require ventilation continue to breathe spontaneously. Spontaneous breathing facilitates venous return and ventilation-perfusion matching. Some infants tolerate ventilation very well, whereas others seem to "fight the ventilator" with increased agitation and decreased oxygenation and are possibly at increased risk of barotrauma and intraventricular haemorrhage (GREENOUGH et al. 1984, PERLMAN et al. 1985). Because of this, efforts were made to create ventilators that would synchronise with the infant's own respiratory effort. Currently, there are two modes of synchronised ventilation. Firstly, assist/control ventilation, also known as patient-triggered ventilation, delivers a positive pressure breath in response to the patient's inspiratory effort (assist) provided the latter exceeds preset threshold criteria. This mode also provides the safety of a guaranteed mechanical breath rate set by the operator if no patient effort is detected (control). The backup control rate ensures a minimum mandatory minute ventilation in case the patient stops making inspiratory efforts. It is suggested that this is an excellent mode of ventilation for use in premature infants in the acute phase of their illness because it requires the least amount of patient effort and produces improved oxygenation at the same mean airway pressure (DONN et al. 1994). Other authors have reported that prolonged support of low birth-weight infants (<28 weeks) might not be feasible because of patient fatigue (CHAN and GREENOUGH 1993). The overall evidence, however, is that patient-triggered ventilation reduces the duration of time from weaning to extubation in mechanically ventilated neonates and may have a beneficial effect on secondary outcome measures such as chronic lung disease and intraventricular haemorrhages (GREENOUGH et al. 1984, PERLMAN et al. 1985, SINHA and DONN 1996), but these findings require verification in larger studies. Synchronised intermittent mandatory ventilation (SIMV) refers to a ventilatory mode where the mechanically delivered breaths are delivered at a fixed rate, but are synchronised to the onset of the patient's own breath. During apnoea, ventilator breaths continue to be delivered at the pre-ordained SIMV rate. Unlike Assist/Control, in SIMV, the ventilatory support can be varied according to the rate set by the clinician from very low rates to high rates making it a very flexible mode of ventilation. However, a low set SIMV rate is undesirable when the patient's ventilatory demand is high. Similarly, reducing the SIMV rate to a very slow rate (<20 breath/min) may be unwise when discontinuation of mechanical ventilation is imminent as this may impose significant work of breathing on the intubated baby and contribute to weaning failure (DIMITRIOU et al. 1995). While SIMV has been found to be as effective as CMV, no major benefits were observed in a large randomised controlled trial (BERNSTEIN et al. 1996). A third method of ventilation is pressure support ventilation (PSV), and it is often used coupled with SIMV. This is defined as patient-initiated, pressure-targeted and patient-controlled ventilation, which is generally flow cycled (PERLMAN et al. 1985). It is designed to assist the patient's spontaneous breathing with an inspiratory pressure "boost". PSV reduces the work of breathing, created by the resistive forces of endotracheal tubes, the ventilatory circuit and demand valve systems. In PSV, once the breath is triggered by the patient's inspiratory effort, a preset system pressure is rapidly delivered and maintained throughout inspiration by adjustment of machine inspiratory flow. The inspiration ends when the inspiratory flow falls below a preset value, usually determined as a percentage of delivered volume or flow (this has been called flow synchronization). This prevents inflation extending into expiration reducing the rate of asynchrony. Although PSV closely resembles Assist/Control ventilation, it seems because of its unique design, PSV is better customised to support and synchronise with patient effort because the patient has control of both the inspiratory flow rate and inspiratory time. The main role of PSV is to assist respiratory muscle activity and so reduce workload. The use of PSV in neonates and infants has been poorly studied, although it looks promising (DONN et al.

1994). The addition of pressure support to SIMV can reduce oxygen consumption (KANAK et al. 1985) and shorten the duration of weaning (JAUNIEAUX et al. 1994). PSV may also have a role to play in infants who are chronically ventilator dependent such as those infants with chronic lung disease.

As stated earlier, while individual studies have shown synchronized ventilation to be beneficial, a meta-analysis of relevant randomized controlled trials has shown that the only positive benefit noted is a shorter duration of ventilation when compared to conventional ventilation delivered at rates of less than 60 breaths per minute (GREENOUGH et al. 2004). There is no significant effect on the incidence of chronic lung disease or death. Nevertheless, this shorter duration of ventilation would support the use of synchronized ventilation as the preferred mode of ventilation in newborn infants. Comparing PTV to SIMV, it was noted that in preterm infants in the recovery stage of respiratory distress, PTV was associated with a shorter duration of ventilation and so this method of ventilation may offer some advantage when weaning preterm neonates. Further work in this important area is still needed. While it is assumed that these modes of ventilation result in improved synchrony with the infants' breaths, none of the randomised trials report on whether synchronous ventilation was actually achieved. It also remains to be seen if certain ventilators and trigger devices perform better with specific respiratory diagnoses.

More recently, the strategy of proportional assist ventilation (PAV) has been touted. Conventional modes of patient-triggered ventilation, as outlined above, typically synchronise one or two events of the ventilator cycle to certain points in the respiratory cycle. In contrast, with PAV, the applied airway pressure is servocontrolled throughout each spontaneous breath (adaptive ventilation). Essentially, it functions by tailoring the ventilator pressure contour to the specific derangements in lung mechanics and by a near perfect synchronization with the infant's own respiratory effort (SCHULZE and BANCALARI 2001). To date, there is little published on its use in newborn infants. One study comparing PAV with assist-control and with conventional intermittent mandatory ventilation in 36 low birth weight infants with mild to moderate acute respiratory illness reported that during PAV, infants achieved equivalent respiratory gas exchange with significantly lower mean and peak transpulmonary pressures compared with the other two modes (SCHULZE et al. 1999). No unde-

sirable side effects or complications were observed. While the results are encouraging, additional studies with clinically significant long-term end points are necessary before PAV can be recommended for broader clinical use in this population.

Until recently, the mode of ventilation most frequently used in virtually all conventional mechanical ventilators was time-cycled, pressure-limited ventilation in which peak inspiratory pressure was set by the clinician and not exceeded by the ventilator. This results in consistent pressure delivery, but inconsistent tidal volume delivery, which becomes a function of the patient's own pulmonary mechanics, particularly compliance. As it appears that "volutrauma" may, in fact, contribute more to ventilator-associated lung injury, attention has once again been focused on volume-targeted ventilation (SINHA and DONN 2001). This mode of ventilation attempts to deliver a consistent tidal volume. While it has been in use in paediatric and adult practice for many years, technological limitations of the older ventilators precluded their use in the preterm infant because they were unable to accurately deliver the small tidal volumes required when ventilating these small babies. With recent advances in ventilator design, this problem has been overcome, and it is now possible to offer volume ventilation in the newborn population. The major difference between volume-targeted ventilation and pressure-limited ventilation is that the former targets a specific volume of gas to be delivered either from the ventilator or to the patient. The ventilator then makes adjustments to the peak inspiratory pressure or to the inflation times from inflation to inflation to try and deliver that volume. As with pressure-limited ventilation, there are different forms of volume-targeted ventilation. The first is "volume-controlled ventilation" also known as "volume-support ventilation". Here, the clinician sets a desired tidal volume. The duration of inflation then depends on the time it takes for that volume to be delivered (i.e., volume-cycled not time-cycled), and inflation ends as soon as that volume has been delivered. If the volume is not delivered in the preset inspiratory time, then the desired volume may not be delivered. The rate of flow, PIP and inspiratory time may all vary from breath to breath. The only constant is the tidal volume delivered into the ventilator circuit. Like pressure-limited ventilation, volume-controlled ventilation can be synchronized with an infant's own respiratory effort. Options include synchronised intermittent mandatory ventilation and Assist-Control. In addition, pressure support ventilation is often provided in combination with volume-controlled SIMV. The level of pressure support provided can be selected by the clinician. As PSV is pressure-limited, the tidal volume delivery on these breaths depends on respiratory mechanics and may be variable. To overcome this, some ventilators have combined pressure support with a guaranteed minimum tidal volume delivery. The second form of volume-targeted ventilation is known as "volume-guarantee ventilation". This is a form of time-cycled, pressure-limited ventilation (i.e., preset inspiratory time determines the duration of inflation, and the maximum pressure set by clinician limits maximum PIP), where a preset expiratory tidal volume is selected. By analysing the inspired and expired tidal volumes, the ventilator then adjusts the peak inspiratory pressure to try and maintain the set expired tidal volume for the next inflation ensuring that for each inflation the tidal volume delivered to the baby is as close as possible to that set by the operator. This method of ventilation provides a volume-targeted strategy within the limits of time-cycled, pressure-limited ventilation. It must be remembered that volume-controlled and volume-guarantee ventilations are distinct entities, despite being linked by a strategy of presetting tidal volume. The difference in flow patterns, inspiratory times and degree of limitations of PIP may interact with the spontaneously breathing infant in very different ways. Lastly, some other ventilators provide a time-cycled, pressure-limited "volume-limited" strategy where the pressure support for any inflation is aborted if the measured inspired tidal volume exceeds a preset upper limit. Of note, the inflating pressures are not automatically adjusted if the inspired tidal volume falls to less than the preselected value. Hence, this mode does not provide assurance of tidal volume delivery in the same way as the modes of ventilation mentioned above.

While there is a sound theoretical basis for the use of volume-targeted strategies in the neonates, because volume-targeting ventilation has only become available for use in neonatal practice recently, clinical trials are few. Meta-analysis of four trials comparing the use of volume-targeted ventilation strategies with time-cycled pressure-limited ventilation did not identify any adverse outcomes associated with their use, but it also failed to show any benefit in the clinically significant long-term outcomes of death and neurodevelopmental impairment (Mc-Callion et al. 2005). There was a significant reduction noted in the rates of intraventricular haemor-

rhage and pneumothorax along with the number of days of IPPV required in the volume-targeted group, but the small numbers of studies and the small numbers of infants enrolled in each trial means that caution must be exercised before widespread application of volume targeting in neonatal intensive care units occurs. Further randomised controlled trials, powered to assess effects on important outcomes such as death, CLD or neurodevelopmental disability are required to determine if this new mode of ventilation should routinely be used in preference to conventional pressure-limited modes in neonates

One final strategy that deserves mention is that of continuous tracheal gas insufflation (CTGI). The added dead space of the endotracheal tube and the ventilator adapter adds to the anatomic dead space and reduces alveolar minute ventilation. In smaller infants or in infants with increasing severity of lung disease, dead space becomes the largest proportion of the tidal volume. With tracheal gas insufflation, gas delivered to the distal part of the endotracheal tube during exhalation washes out this dead space and the accompanying carbon dioxide. Reports on the use of CTGI in neonates have found it allows the use of low-volume ventilation over a prolonged period and reduces the duration of mechanical ventilation (Dassieu et al. 2000). Its exact role in preterm infants and infants with severe lung disease has yet to be elucidated.

In summary, conventional mandatory ventilation is a mainstay in the care of critically ill neonates. In recent years, a combination of a better understanding of the pathophysiology of neonatal lung diseases, the use of disease-specific ventilatory strategies and technological advances in ventilators have all contributed to significant reductions in mortality and morbidity. Large multicentred clinical trials with long-term follow-up are now urgently required to determine the optimal mode of ventilation in critically ill neonates who are suffering from a wide variety of pathological processes.

2.2.3
High Frequency Ventilation

With the realisation that lung injury appeared to be more closely related to cyclic changes in lung volume (Dreyfuss and Sauman 1998, Hernandez et al. 1989, Dreyfuss and Saumon 1993), considerable interest has been generated over the past 15 years in the application of high frequency ventilation (HFV) to the neonatal population. This technique allows ventilation with very small tidal volumes and offers the theoretical advantage of avoiding lung injury.

Henderson and Chillingworth first noted in 1915 that smoke blown down a tube formed a long, thin spike and the quicker the puff, the thinner and sharper the spike. They concluded "there may easily be gaseous exchange sufficient to support life even when the tidal volume is considerably less that the dead space". Emerson in 1959 patented a device that, by vibrating air into the patient's lungs, had the potential for enhancing gas exchange (EMERSON 1959). Subsequently, SJOSTRAND (1980) reported his groups' modification of standard conventional ventilators to allow their use at frequencies of 60–120/min. In 1974, HEIJMAN and SJOSTRAND first reported the application of HFV to neonates with respiratory distress syndrome (RDS). The era of HFV began and its use became more widespread. The early days of HFV were characterised by device confusion leading many to believe that HFV was a technology in search of a disease. More recently, despite many studies of HFV in animal models of RDS showing promising results in the prevention of lung injury, results of clinical studies of this ventilatory technique are not as promising. Controversy continues to surround the indications for HFV in newborns and whether HFV is more effective than other modes of ventilation for neonatal respiratory failure, whether HFV reduces adverse outcomes or whether HFV is more likely to result in significant long-term complications compared to CMV.

HFV can essentially be defined as ventilation at a rapid rate (at least two to four times the natural breathing frequency) using tidal volumes that are less than the anatomic dead space. Gas transport during HFV cannot be explained by the classic concepts of ventilation and lung mechanics. Although the precise mechanisms by which gas exchange occurs during HFV remain incompletely understood, a number of different mechanisms have been suggested to explain the phenomenon and each may play a role within different segments of the lung. Similar to CMV, bulk convention may be important during HFV in ventilating the most proximal alveoli. The Pendelluft effect, which allows the exchange of gases among lung units with different time constants, is felt to be particularly important when ventilation occurs at tidal volumes less than anatomic dead space (LEHR et al. 1985, FREDBERG et al. 1985). Other mechanisms that may help to explain the gas exchange include "asymmetric velocity profiles"

(where convective gas transport is enhanced by asymmetry between inspiratory and expiratory velocity profiles that occur at branch points in the airways), Taylor dispersion (augmented diffusion due to turbulent air currents that result from interaction between axial velocity and the radial concentration gradient in the airways) and molecular diffusion. With regard to oxygen exchange, as in all forms of mechanical ventilation, it is essential to maintain adequate lung volumes and to avoid atelectasis. Despite major differences in the design and function of high frequency ventilators, the strategy of improving oxygenation during HFV and CMV is similar. In both, the aim is to maximise ventilation-perfusion matching while avoiding impairment of cardiac output. With HFV, a high mean airway pressure is used to recruit alveoli and maintains lung volumes above functional residual capacity. In contrast to CMV, HFV maintains lung volumes at a relatively constant level and uses small changes in tidal volume to accomplish ventilation. Mean airway pressure and its corollary, lung volume, are very difficult to quantify during HFV and make the comparison of different modes of HFV and CMV very difficult. Mean tracheal pressure is obviously very different from mean alveolar pressure, making the precise manipulation of HFV parameters problematic. Therefore, comparisons between CMV and HFV regarding airway pressure and adequacy of oxygenation are meaningless. However, peak airway pressures are generally lower in HFV because of the smaller delivered tidal volume and this should theoretically lead to a lower incidence of barotrauma.

There are three main types of high frequency ventilators-high frequency oscillatory ventilators (HFOV), high frequency flow interrupters (HFFI), and high frequency jet ventilators (HFJV). HFJV employs a high pressure source to deliver a volume of gas through a small-bore injector cannula. It is used in parallel with a conventional ventilator that provides positive end-expiratory pressure (PEEP) and intermittent "sigh" breaths to help prevent atelectasis. Expiration is passive (i.e., dependent of chest wall and lung recoil). HFFIs operate on a principle similar to jet ventilation. Gas from a high pressure source is delivered into a standard ventilator circuit and endotracheal tube. To produce high frequency breaths, the flow of gas is interrupted by a valve mechanism. Expiration, in this case, is also passive. HFOV employs a piston or diaphragm to oscillate a bias flow of gas resulting in both positive and negative pressure fluctuations. Because of the negative pressure deflection during the expiratory cycle of the oscillated breaths, expiration is active. This has the advantage of allowing shorter expiratory times and gas trapping may be less of a problem.

Several animal studies have examined the role of HFV in reducing ventilator-induced lung injury. Early studies examining the use of HFOV in animals that had experimental RDS showed that using low mean airway pressures during HFV resulted in progressive atelectasis and hypoxaemia. In contrast, when used with a strategy to optimise lung inflation with higher mean airway pressures, HFOV applied to baboons, monkeys, and rabbits promoted uniform lung inflation, improved gas exchange and lung mechanics and reduced the number of inflammatory mediators (McCulloch et al. 1988, deLemos et al. 1987, Jackson et al. 1991). These effects were even greater when HFOV was used in concert with surfactant treatment (Froese et al. 1993, Jackson et al. 1994). In addition, if HFOV, using a high mean airway pressure/lung volume strategy, was initiated immediately in preterm baboons with RDS, HFOV prevented the deterioration in gas exchange and lung mechanics characteristically seen in animals treated with CMV (Meredith et al. 1989). Early treatment with HFOV also prevented the morphologic changes of hyaline membrane disease seen in the conventionally treated animals (Jackson et al. 1991, Meredith et al. 1989). However, it was not as effective in reducing the pathological findings of acute lung injury when initiated later in the course of RDS, after several hours of CMV (deLemos et al. 1992). These studies and others mentioned earlier lend support to the hypothesis that volutrauma, rather than barotrauma, is the primary cause of acute lung injury secondary to assisted ventilation and that HFOV, which uses a relatively static lung volume and minimal cyclic volume changes, may protect the surfactant deficient lung from injury. Such data lead to an evolution in the clinical application of HFV.

Studies in infants using HFV are hard to interpret as many different ventilators have been used along with many different ventilatory strategies. In the early to mid-1980s, several small studies reported that infants with severe RDS who were failing on CMV could achieve adequate gas exchange with HFJV or HFOV at significantly lower mean airway pressures. These findings prompted the National Institute of Health (NIH) to conduct a multicentered randomised controlled trial in the mid 1980s on 673 preterm infants weighing between 750 g and 2 kg using HFOV. The results of the study showed that HFOV did not reduce the incidence of bronchopulmonary dysplasia or death and an association was seen between the use of HFV and other adverse outcomes including air leak and intracranial haemorrhage (HIFI Study Group 1989). On reviewing the study subsequently, it was felt that the ventilatory strategy applied was fundamentally flawed. Several large studies subsequently, using a high lung volume approach, revealed more promising results than the original NIH trial. These later trials looked at HFV as the initial mode of ventilation in preterm infants who had RDS (early intervention) and as rescue therapy in preterm and term infants who had severe lung disease and/or air leak syndrome (rescue therapy). A Cochrane review of 11 randomised trials involving 3,275 infants comparing elective HFOV in the treatment of preterm infants with RDS (early intervention) to conventional mechanical ventilation found that elective HFOV did not offer any important advantages (Henderson-Smart et al. 2003). There was possibly a small reduction in the rate of CLD with HFOV use, but the evidence was weakened by the inconsistency of this effect across trials, and it was not found to be significant overall. Adverse effects on short-term neurological outcomes were observed in some studies, but again these effects were not significant overall. There was inadequate information about effects on long-term outcome. Another meta-analysis published in the Cochrane Database looks at the use of elective HFJV compared to CMV in preterm infants with RDS (Bhuta and Henderson-Smart 1998a). The overall analysis shows a benefit in pulmonary outcomes in the group electively ventilated with HFJV. Of concern was the significant increase in periventricular white matter injury seen in one trial that used lower mean airway pressures when ventilating with HFJV (Wiswell et al. 1996). In this trial, hypocarbia was not found to be independently associated with an adverse outcome, although observational studies have suggested that marked hypocarbia is associated with an increased risk of cystic periventricular leucomalacia (PVL) (Graziani et al. 1992, Fujimoto et al. 1994). With regards to long-term outcomes, the HIFI trial has reported respiratory morbidity and neurodevelopmental outcome up to 2 years of post-term age for 77% of survivors (HIFI Study Group 1990). Growth and clinical respiratory status did not differ between the two groups, but neurodevelopmental outcome was worse in the HFOV group, in keeping with the excess of major cranial ultrasound abnormalities identified in the original report. The United Kingdom Oscillation study (UKOS) randomly assigned 797 infants born between 23 and 28 weeks gestation to receive either HFOV or CV within 1 h of birth (JOHNSON et al. 2002). No difference was found in short-term outcomes including mortality, CLD and neonatal cranial ultrasound scan appearances. This group has recently reported on the 2-year respiratory and neurodevelopmental outcome of 73% of the 585 surviving infants (MARLOW et al. 2006). No difference between the groups was identified supporting their original conclusion that HFOV and CV are equally effective for the early treatment of respiratory distress syndrome. At this stage, it would seem that the literature suggests that HFV is comparable and possibly offers some advantage over CMV in the treatment of preterm infants with uncomplicated RDS (COURTNEY et al. 2002). The caveats attached to this are many. Certain experience in the use of HFV is essential and the clinical trials using HFV with a low lung volume strategy offer a cautionary note. Despite animal data suggesting that the early application of HFV modifies the sequence of lung injury initiated by CMV, results of the clinical trials have not really shown HFV to prevent chronic lung disease. This is likely due to the complex, multifactorial aetiology of chronic lung disease in extremely premature infants and the mode of ventilation used in these infants may have less of an impact on overall outcome than other perinatal and neonatal factors that play a role in the disease. Further studies looking at long-term neurodevelopmental outcomes are still required. As conventional mechanical ventilation of neonates continues to advance with an improved ability to monitor tidal volumes, better synchronization with the infant's own respiratory effort and "auto-weaning" of inspiratory pressures as lung compliance improves and as the current trend of using non-invasive modes of ventilation in preterm infants from birth gains support, EICHENWALD (2006), in a recent editorial, argues that equivalence of HFOV with conventional ventilation may not be sufficient to recommend its routine use in this population.

HFV has also been used in the rescue treatment of premature infants with pulmonary interstitial emphysema and air leak syndromes. KESZLER et al. (1991) found HFJV to be superior to CMV in infants with pulmonary interstitial emphysema. Infants had a lower mortality rate and a more rapid improvement in radiological appearance. There was no increased incidence of adverse outcomes including chronic lung disease or intraventricular haemorrhage. Another large study looked at the role of HFOV in air leak syndrome in infants with severe RDS (HiFO Study Group 1993). While fewer children on HFOV developed air leak, no difference in the progression or resolution of air leak was observed between the groups with established air leak syndrome at the time of randomisation. Of concern, however, was that there was an increased rate of intraventricular haemorrhage of any grade in infants treated with HFO. There was also a stronger, but non-significant trend towards an increase in the more severe grades of IVH in this group. Cochrane reviews on the use of rescue HFV in preterm infants conclude that there is currently insufficient information on its use to make recommendations for practice (BHUTA and HENDERSON-SMART 1998b, JOSHI and BHUTA 2006). The small amount of data that exists suggests that harm may outweigh any benefits. As in the other clinical scenarios, more studies are needed before definite recommendations can be made regarding the use of HFV as a rescue therapy in this population.

Limited data are available on the use of HFV in term or near term infants as a rescue therapy for severe respiratory failure or persistent pulmonary hypertension. The causes of respiratory failure in this group of infants are heterogeneous and include RDS, congenital pneumonia, meconium aspiration, pulmonary hypoplasia and congenital diaphragmatic hernia. Only one prospective randomised trial of HFV in near-term and term infants with respiratory failure has been performed (CLARK et al. 1994). In this study, 81 infants >34 weeks gestation and >2 kg referred for ECMO were randomised to HFOV or CMV. In the crossover design, those who failed the initial treatment were switched to the alternative ventilator mode. The proportion of infants who failed their initial treatment was comparable between the HFOV and CMV groups. However, of those who failed conventional ventilation, 63% responded to HFOV, significantly more than the 23% that responded to CMV after failing therapy with HFOV. No significant difference in mortality or morbidity was observed. A meta-analysis carried out in 2001 looking at this issue was only able to identify one trial that was appropriate for inclusion, namely that by CLARK et al. (BHUTA et al. 2001). On that basis, the review concluded that there is inadequate data to support the routine use of rescue HFOV in term or near term infants with severe pulmonary dysfunction. Uncontrolled rescue studies in term infants indicate that HFOV might be of value in neonates with intractable respiratory failure who are candidates for ECMO (Kohlet et al. 1988, Carter et al. 1990). In the case series of Carter et al. (1990), 46% of ECMO candidates treated with HFOV recovered without the need for ECMO. The response rate, however, does appear to be disease specific with infants who have homogenous lung diseases such as RDS or pneumonia more likely to respond to HFV that those with heterogeneous lung diseases such as meconium aspiration syndrome. The question that now must be posed is whether the long-term outcome of these infants treated with HFOV is comparable to those treated with ECMO. In view of the increasing use of HFOV in practice, more randomised controlled trials are urgently needed to establish its role more accurately. The area is complicated by the diverse pathology in these infants and also by the occurrence of other interventions (such as surfactant, nitric oxide and inotropes). Any future randomisation should be stratified according to disease and it is essential that long-term outcomes be reported.

Nitric oxide (NO) is being increasingly utilised as a treatment for persistent pulmonary hypertension of the newborn (PPHN). Recent work has suggested that lung volume recruitment with HFOV may enhance the response to inhaled nitric oxide in infants with persistent pulmonary hypertension (PPHN) complicated by parenchymal lung disease. Kinsella et al. (1997) conducted a prospective randomised trial comparing CMV with inhaled nitric oxide to HFOV alone in 203 infants with severe pulmonary hypertension. Treatment failure resulted in crossover to the alternative treatment, which led to combination treatment with HFOV and inhaled nitric oxide. The response rate, defined as a sustained PaO2 >60 mmHg (8 kPas), was significantly higher for the HFOV plus nitric oxide group than for either therapy alone in infants who had RDS or meconium aspiration.

In summary, HFV is an important development in the management of preterm and term infants with respiratory failure. Clinical trials have demonstrated that HFV with a high volume strategy is a safe and comparable alternative to CMV. Its place in the therapeutic armamentarium will undoubtedly continue to evolve in the years to come particularly with the advent of advanced modes of fully synchronized and volume-targeted conventional mechanical ventilatory modes along with the trend to use smaller tidal volumes and higher levels of PEEP with conventional ventilation.

2.2.4
Extracorporeal Membrane Oxygenation

Extracorporeal membrane oxygenation (ECMO) is a complex technique for providing life support that has been in use for just a little over 25 years. It oxygenates blood outside the body, obviating the need for gas exchange in the lungs and if necessary, provides cardiovascular support. It is used in the management of neonates with respiratory failure as a result of a lung insult that is generally complicated by pulmonary hypertension and significant extra-pulmonary right-to-left shunting of blood. These infants have severe hypoxaemia that persists despite conventional ventilation and they are predicted to be at great risk of dying.

There are two types of EMCO that are employed. The first is venoarterial (VA) ECMO, which gives support to both heart and lung function. In brief, cannulas are placed to drain venous blood from the right atrium (usually via the internal jugular to superior vena cava/right atrial junction or femoral vein to right atrium). This venous blood then goes to a pump (using a roller-head device) that advances the blood to the membrane oxygenator. The latter is made of silicone rubber and is similar to the extracorporeal lungs used in cardiac bypass. As blood passes through the oxygenator, oxygen is added and carbon dioxide is removed. The oxygenated blood is then rewarmed and returned to the arterial circulation. Arterial return is directed into the arch of the aorta via cannulation of the right carotid or femoral artery. With more blood being drained into the ECMO circuit, less blood will flow through the damaged native heart/lung circulation. This will decrease the amount of ventilator support required to maintain gas exchange. Ventilator settings and concentrations of inspired oxygen can be minimised to avoid ongoing barotrauma/volutrauma and oxygen toxicity as the damaged lung attempts to heal itself. As the lung heals and native gas exchange becomes more efficient, the need for ECMO support decreases, and blood flow through the circuit is correspondingly decreased until native pulmonary function alone is sufficient to sustain the infant. The cannulas are then removed from the infant and ECMO can be discontinued. One of the major disadvantages of VA ECMO is that the carotid artery frequently requires ligation although now many centres repair the vessel during decannulation with reportedly good results and continued patency on follow-up examinations (Karl et al. 1990, Crombleholme et al. 1990). Venovenous (VV) ECMO allows supplementation of pulmonary gas exchange, but relies on adequate function of the heart to perfuse the body. The venous blood is drained from the right atrium or the inferior vena cava. It is then sent to the ECMO circuit and membrane oxygenator where it undergoes removal of carbon dioxide and addition of oxygen as in VA ECMO. The saturated blood is then rewarmed and returned to the patient's venous circulation. Recirculation at the tip of the insertion of the cannulas can be limited (although not completely eliminated) by careful placement of the venous cannulas, thereby preventing large amounts of the returning oxygenated blood from reentering the ECMO circuit before it reaches the systemic circulation. Since the proportion of cardiac output drained into the ECMO circuit (approximately 50%) with VV ECMO is less, the arterial saturation in VV ECMO is also less than that seen with VA ECMO. To maintain adequate oxygen delivery, some oxygen uptake via the lungs must be maintained. This usually requires that higher levels of inspired oxygen be maintained through the ventilator than in VA ECMO. PEEP is also used to retain lung expansion and optomise oxygenation. In patients who develop cardiac dysfunction or who do not receive enough systemic oxygen despite VV ECMO, conversion to VA ECMO is possible. The advantage of VV ECMO is that it limits the risk of embolisation to the central nervous system of air, clots or debris returning form the ECMO circuit. It also avoids potential damage to or ligation of the carotid artery. For a diagrammatic representation of the ECMO circuit, the reader is referred to Chap. 6, Figure 6.7.

The first adult patient to be offered long-term support with a membrane oxygenator for life-threatening pulmonary disease was a 24-year-old man treated by Dr. J.D. Hill for ARDS (HILL et al. 1972). The perfusion lasted a total of 75 h and had a favourable outcome. The early adult ECMO experience is best summarised in the 1979 report by Zapol et al. of the nine hospital collaborative trial conducted under the auspices of the National Institute of Health. Ninety patients were admitted to the study, of which 48 were treated with mechanical ventilation alone and 42 were treated with mechanical ventilation plus partial venovenous, venoarterial or mixed bypass support. Ultimately only three of the control patients and four of the ECMO patients survived. There were, however, many explanations for the disappointing outcomes with many of the patients who had died demonstrating

extensive pulmonary fibrosis (SHORT and PEARSON 1986). If ECMO was going to demonstrate an advantage, it was thought it would have to be used in patients with readily reversible diseases or conditions. This requirement led investigators to pursue the use of ECMO in the treatment of neonatal pulmonary disease. Bartlett was the first to use ECMO to support a neonate in 1973, and he treated the first neonatal survivor in 1975 (BARTLETT et al. 1976). The first randomised trial of ECMO in neonates was carried out by Bartlett et al., and it demonstrated the efficacy of ECMO in the management of respiratory failure when compared to conventional ventilation (BARTLETT et al. 1985). A subsequent randomised trial in Boston produced similar conclusions (O'ROURKE et al. 1989). These studies, however, had used adaptive designs and were criticised as this may have introduced bias. The UK Collaborative ECMO Trial Group subsequently carried out a randomised controlled trial and published their findings in 1996 (UK Collaborative ECMO Trial Group 1996). The eligibility criteria included infants with severe respiratory failure [defined as an oxygenation index (OI) of greater than or equal to 40 or an arterial partial pressure of carbon dioxide >12 kPa for at least 3 h], gestational age at birth 35 completed weeks or more, birth weight 2 kg or more, age less than 28 days and less than 10 days of high pressure ventilation. Once the infant had met the criteria, the infant was randomised to transfer to one of five regional centres for ECMO or to continued conventional management in the referring hospital. Use of HFV, inhaled nitric oxide and surfactant was allowed. A total of 185 children were enrolled, 93 were allocated to the ECMO arm and 92 were allocated to conventional management. At trial entry, 19% of the cases had a congenital diaphragmatic hernia. Of the 93 allocated to ECMO, 84% actually received ECMO support. The overall mortality rate differed significantly between the ECMO and the conventional management groups (32% vs. 59%, $P=0.005$), which was equivalent to one extra survivor for every three to four infants allocated to ECMO. This benefit was sustained even when severe disability at 1 year of age was taken into account ($P=0.002$). Mortality among infants with a primary diagnosis other than CDH was 21% in the ECMO group compared with 49% in the control group ($P=0.0006$). The trial results left little doubt that allocation to ECMO reduced the risk of death or severe disability. The one potential confounding factor in this study, which may have overestimated the benefit of ECMO, was that infants randomised to receive ECMO were transferred to a regional centre, which may have had greater expertise in treating critically ill infants. On the other hand, infants randomised to the conventional arm remained in the smaller referring units and they may not have received optimal conventional management. Not unexpectedly, more infants in the conventional management group were treated with HFV (33% vs. 11%), surfactant (41% vs. 33%) or both especially in the later years of the study. Whether even greater use of these treatments would have improved outcome after conventional care is uncertain. Meta-analysis of the above trials in addition to another trial carried out by Bifano et al. reported a clear benefit for the ECMO policy in terms of reducing mortality (ELBOURNE et al. 2002).

While ECMO has clearly been shown to be beneficial, an appreciation of the long-term outcome of these infants is essential if ECMO is to be regarded as a useful modality. The UK Collaborative ECMO Trial Group has reported the neurodevelopmental outcome of its cohort at both 4 years and 7 years of age (UK Collaborative ECMO Trial Group 2001, UK Collaborative ECMO Trial Group 2006). With regards to the primary outcome of death or severe disability at 4 years, 34 of 93 infants in the ECMO group (37%) compared to 54 of 92 infants in the conventionally treated group (59%) were affected, a statistically significant finding (P=0.004). The results were equivalent to one additional child surviving without severe disability for every four to five children referred for ECMO. This benefit was evident in all stratified analyses based on principal diagnosis and disease severity, although the numbers were small. Equally, there was a higher proportion of known survivors without any disability in the ECMO allocated group. A higher respiratory morbidity was documented in the children treated conventionally (UK Collaborative ECMO Trial Group 2001, BEARDSMORE et al. 2000). By 7 years of age, 76% of the children assessed (56 ECMO cases and 34 conventional treatment cases) recorded a cognitive level within the normal range with no differences recorded between the trial groups. Learning problems were similar in the two groups and there were notable difficulties with spatial and processing tasks. A higher respiratory morbidity and increased risk of behavioural problems among children treated conventionally persisted. Progressive sensorineural hearing loss was found in both groups. Hence, the beneficial influence of ECMO

was still present at 7 years. The authors go on to state that the evidence at 7 years of age strongly suggests that the underlying disease processes (and associated physiological instability) appear to be the major influence on morbidity rather than the use of ECMO itself.

Therefore, the use of ECMO appears to increase the likelihood of intact survival. However, questions that still need to be answered include whether ECMO is more useful for some category of patients than others. Certainly, patients who have been ventilated at high ventilator pressures for long periods are poor candidates as they likely have irreversible pulmonary disease. Most centres attempt to avoid this problem by reserving ECMO for those patients who have only received mechanical ventilation for less than 14 days. To date, the main indications for ECMO in neonates are meconium aspiration syndrome, congenital diaphragmatic hernia (CDH), pneumonia/sepsis, RDS and PPHN. Although the lungs are usually severely affected by the disease processes, the uniqueness of the neonate's pulmonary vasculature and the presence of functional right to left shunts can magnify the severity of the hypoxaemia. The failure of the pulmonary vascular resistance to decrease after delivery or a postnatal increase in the resistance associated with pulmonary disease, resulting in PPHN, is a situation found only in neonates. Its reversibility and the ability of the infant's lung to recover from the underlying insult allow for the use of ECMO with encouraging results currently being reported. In the UK study, the benefit of ECMO was seen in all of the above diagnostic categories with the exception of congenital diaphragmatic hernia (UK Collaborative ECMO Trial Group 1996). Unfortunately, the number of infants with CDH randomised to either arm was too small and it was not possible to draw definitive conclusions. Four out of 18 infants with CDH randomised to ECMO survived to discharge, whereas there was no survivor among the 17 infants randomised to the conventional group. However, by 4 years of age, 16 of the 18 in the ECMO arm had died or were severely disabled. There is now a strong case to further study the role of ECMO and other treatments (such as inhaled nitric oxide, HFV and surfactant) in the management of infants with CDH who require anything more than modest respiratory support (oxygenation index >20) in the first 12 h of life. The second question to be addressed is the selection of patients for ECMO. Trying to determine which patients are failing less invasive therapies and have reversible injury that may improve with lung rest provided by ECMO is still difficult. Various mortality prediction criteria have been put forth as indicators of when ECMO rescue is best applied. These criteria were developed to identify patients with a predicted mortality of 80% or greater (KIRKPATRICK et al. 1983). However, many of these criteria were derived from historical data for respiratory failure patients at single institutions or extrapolated from neonatal respiratory failure data (NADING 1989). In addition to being developed retrospectively, these criteria were only meant to be used at specific centres where the review had been conducted and were not intended to be transferable. A more obvious limitation of the criteria was their inability to be revised on the basis of changes or improvements in conventional treatment. For example, with the increasing use of HFV that uses a higher mean airway pressure than CMV, calculated oxygenation indices (which have been used as predictors of high mortality) are higher, but this may not necessarily translate to an increased risk of death. Hence, criteria that define a mortality rate of 80% during one epoch will not necessarily predict the same risk in a future epoch. In centres that use ECMO, it is impossible to redefine 80% mortality unless that centre is willing to deny patients treatment with ECMO. Because of these limitations, it is not surprising that criteria developed at an earlier time do not have the same predictive value when used in different institutions or indeed with the evolution of time (DWORTEZ et al. 1989). Currently the most widely used predictor is the oxygenation index, which considers the degree of oxygenation as well as the mean airway pressure required to achieve that level of oxygenation. One of the weaknesses of this criterion is that it is not disease specific. Its uniform application assumes that the pathophysiology and clinical course are similar for all conditions for which ECMO is used. As stated earlier, it would be particularly useful to have specific criteria for the use of ECMO in the management of CDH that would also include the timing of operative repair. The problem of higher calculated oxygenation indices in cases where HFV is employed has already been mentioned. Further data collection and analysis are essential to help develop treatment algorithms for instituting therapies such as ECMO and this should hopefully lead to better predictors of death. The final question to be asked is the correct timing of institution of ECMO. The extent to which

the respiratory and neurological morbidity among infants assigned to receive ECMO reflects the underlying condition or the treatment offered is still a major source of debate although the follow-up data at 7 years reported by the UK Collaborative ECMO trial group would suggest that the former is more important. Whether the initiation of ECMO when the oxygenation index is between 25 and 40 would result in a better outcome is as yet unanswered.

In summary, although there was appropriate concern regarding the use of ECMO in the treatment of neonatal respiratory failure during the initial stages of clinical use, there is no doubt now that ECMO can be used successfully to support neonates and the result is a reduction in the mortality rate without an apparent increase in neurodevelopmental disability. Despite this, around the world, rates of ECMO referral have fallen and the use of interventions such as nitric oxide and high frequency ventilation has increased (HINTZ et al. 2000). While use of these interventions has been shown to decrease the need for ECMO, the studies have not definitely reported improvements in survival or long-term outcomes. Nevertheless, avoidance of ECMO as an end point seems to be widely accepted as desirable. Of concern is that despite these interventions, a significant number of infants still go on to require ECMO. If long-term morbidity, as some clinical evidence suggests, is in fact due to damage that occurs before the initiation of ECMO, then one must worry about unnecessarily delaying ECMO once standard ECMO referral criteria have been reached. More recently, some authors have reported longer patient ventilator times and longer ECMO runs in those in whom ECMO initiation is delayed (HUI et al. 2002, GILL et al. 2002). ECMO, despite its invasive nature, is an established therapy with predictable mortality and morbidity rates. Should new therapies be tested before initiating ECMO only if the results of phase 1 or 2 trials are at least as promising as the ECMO alternative? Should ECMO be accepted as a standard of care against which other therapies should be tested rather than the safety net for the introduction of these new therapies into the neonatal intensive care unit for prospective trials? Whatever the answers, it is clear that more work is needed to determine those infants most suitable for ECMO and the appropriate timing in the disease process when ECMO should be utilized. Without doubt, the role of ECMO in practice is evolving. It, however, should not be forgotten that ECMO is clearly a life-saving therapy for selected patients.

2.2.5
Liquid Ventilation

The use of exogenous surfactant indicated that reducing surface tension in the alveoli resulted in improved gas exchange at lower ventilatory settings. This was accompanied by a reduction in barotrauma and an improvement in mortality. With the realisation that a reduction in surface tension could have a significant impact clinically, investigators turned their attention once again to the idea of liquid ventilation (LV).

Perflurochemical (PFC) liquids are fluorinated hydrocarbons in which the hydrogen atom has been replaced by fluorine atoms. For perflubron, a bromine atom is added as well. These fluids are stable chemicals that are clear, odourless, colourless and insoluble in water. They are denser than water and soft tissue and their surface tension and viscosity are generally low. Certain PFC liquids have higher vapour pressures than water and will evaporate much faster than water at body temperature. Of particular importance is the fact that these liquids have exceptionally high gas solubility and can dissolve as much as 20 times the amount of oxygen and more than three times as much carbon dioxide as water. Oxygen solubility is three times that of whole blood. In general, PFC fluids are non-toxic and biochemically inert. In addition, they are radiopaque (the presence of bromine atoms in PFCs confers even greater radiopacity). More than 100 different PFC liquids exist although only a few commercially available liquids meet both the physiochemical property requirements and purity specifications for respiratory applications. PFC fluids diffuse from the lung into the circulation and are distributed with blood flow to body tissues. Because PFC liquids are nearly insoluble in water, essentially all of the PFC in the blood and tissues is dissolved in lipid. Extensive studies in animals and adult humans have examined the physiology, toxicity and biodistribution of PFC when used intravascularly. The concentration of PFC in the blood after intravascular administration is several orders of magnitude greater than any blood or tissue level reported following LV. Low levels are found in the liver with the highest levels being found in the lung followed by fat tissue. PFC is not metabolised and is eliminated intact by evaporation during exhalation or transpiration through the skin (SHAFFER et al. 1999, GREENSPAN et al. 1998, WOLFSON and SHAFFER 2005).

Early work with PFC liquids as a respiratory support medium involved total immersion of the animals. If the liquid was oxygenated continuously, the animals could survive for hours by spontaneously breathing, but the increased work of breathing soon led to fatigue. In the early 1970s, mechanical ventilators capable of ventilating liquids were designed to compensate for the increased work of breathing. Early studies with these ventilators reported improved oxygenation and better removal of carbon dioxide. A system for time-cycled, pressure-limited total liquid ventilation (TLV) was developed. In TLV, the respiratory gases are transported solely in the dissolved form through tidal volume exchange of PFC to and from the lung. All gas-liquid interfacial tension is eliminated and the lung is provided with maximal protection from inflation pressures as lung volume is recruited, compliance is increased and inflation pressures and pulmonary barotrauma are reduced. Functionally, the system resembles an extracorporeal membrane oxygenation circuit. The inspiratory cycle is performed by pumping warmed and oxygenated PFC liquid from a fluid reservoir into the lung. Expiration is in large part active, accomplished by pumping liquid from the lung with passive assist of the lung recoil. During the expiratory cycle, fluid is filtered, returned to a gas exchanger for desired levels of oxygenation and carbon dioxide scrubbing, and returned to the fluid reservoir. The TLV may have a closed or open circuit. In the closed circuit, expired gas is circulated through a carbon dioxide scrubber, and PFC fluid is conserved by condensing vapour in the expired gas; the condensed vapour is pumped back into the gas exchanger. In the open circuit, condensed vapour in the expired gas is returned in a similar fashion, and non-condensed PFC loss due to evaporation is measured and returned to the system. In this way, total fluid inventory is closely monitored and the PFC lung volume is tightly controlled, thus maintaining global lung protection. Because PFC liquids have a high heat capacity, the patient's body temperature can be regulated easily and closely by the liquid temperature during ventilation. Over the years, the liquid ventilator has been refined sufficiently to allow computer operation using the same control modes as gas ventilators, that is, time-cycled, pressure or volume limited, inspiratory and expiratory times. In TLV, the ventilator rate is generally set around five breaths/min due to the longer diffusion time of gases through liquids, and tidal volume (approximately 15 ml/kg) is used to regulate minute ventilation and therefore PaCo2. Unlike gas ventilation, TLV allows unique control and measurement of functional residual capacity (FRC) by monitoring the change in weight as liquid is exchanged between the subject and the TLV system. FRC and inspired oxygen can be adjusted to optimise oxygenation.

Based on the successful recovery of animals to gas ventilation in the presence of a lung partially filled with PFC liquid following TLV, research then focused on interfacing PFC liquid with gas ventilation. An alternative method of supporting pulmonary gas exchange with PFC liquid is to deliver a volume of PFC to the lung, less than or equal to the FRC, and then continue with gas ventilation. The PFC liquid in the lungs can function similarly to an artificial surfactant for RDS or a lavage medium for other types of pulmonary dysfunction. It is reinstilled periodically to maintain the desired amount of liquid in the lung and replace evaporative losses. This technique is known as partial liquid ventilation (PLV). PLV is similar to TLV as it utilizes the alveolar recruitment capabilities of a low surface tension fluid to establish an adequate FRC in a surfactant-deficient or impaired lung. The PFC liquid is oxygenated and CO_2 is exchanged in the lung through various forms of mechanical gas ventilation. During PLV, the air liquid interface in the lung is not eliminated completely so some of the major mechanical advantages of a liquid-liquid interface may not be appreciated (such as removal of debris and homogeneous ventilation). However, PLV requires only minimal technical devices, a syringe to administer the fluid and a standard mechanical gas ventilator to move tidal volumes of gas. This technique offers specific advantages over gas ventilation for many pulmonary disorders particularly where surfactant therapy is not an option.

Since then, many different strategies and techniques have been tried. Continuous TLV, brief periods of TLV for 3–5 min, rapid instillation of a bolus of oxygenated PFC (30 mlg/kg) with the ventilator disconnected or slow infusions of oxygenated or unoxygenated PFC in doses of up to 30ml/kg over 15 min during continuous gas ventilation. Intrapulmonary delivery of PFC in droplet or vapour form has also been explored in various animal models. The latter can be achieved by aerosolisation, vapourisation or by bubbling the inspiratory gas flow through a heated PFC liquid reservoir to create a PFC saturated inspired gas. The optimum PFC filling strategy and the effect of

any subsequent gas ventilation scheme including high frequency, assist control, synchronised and spontaneously breathing strategies are still under extensive investigation.

In the neonatal population, there are a number of situations where the infant might benefit from liquid ventilation. In RDS, preterm infants have homogenous surfactant deficiency and immature parenchyma leading to atelectasis. While surfactant and antenatal steroids have substantially improved the clinical outcome of these infants, they would appear to have the most to gain from LV, particularly if the technique is applied early. Surface tension forces are reduced or eliminated, atelectasis can be prevented or remedied and the liquid environment of the developing foetal lung can be reproduced. The need for excessive ventilator pressures and inspired oxygen concentrations are also diminished. Term infants who present with consolidated collapsed lungs with an aggressive inflammatory process and extremely poor compliance can also potentially benefit by lung recruitment and improved compliance in addition to the benefit of having gas exchange maintained while lavaging the lungs. Infants with congenital diaphragmatic hernias face the dilemma of pulmonary hypoplasia, pulmonary hypertension and surfactant deficiency. PFC liquids have the potential to maximise recruitment of the hypoplastic lung while minimising the surface tension forces allowing more efficient ventilation and reduction of barotrauma (SHAFFER et al. 1999, WOLFSON and SHAFFER 2005).

The first human trials of PFC liquid breathing were conducted in Philadelphia in 1989 and were initiated in near death infants with severe respiratory failure. TLV was administered in two 3–5-min cycles separated by 15 min of gas ventilation (GREENSPAN et al. 1990, GREENSPAN et al. 1989). A gravity-assisted approach was used and tidal volumes of liquid were given to a liquid-filled lung for two sequential 5-min cycles. The infants tolerated the procedure well and showed improvement in several physiological parameters including lung compliance and gas exchange. Improvement was sustained after LV was discontinued. All of the infants ultimately died from their underlying respiratory disease, but TLV was shown to support gas exchange and allow residual improvement in pulmonary function following return to CMV. Further clinical trials were then limited by the need for a medically approved liquid ventilator and a medical grade breathing fluid. Subsequent human protocols have used a PLV approach to LV. Leach and collaborators reported 13 preterm infants who had severe RDS in whom CMV has failed. The infants were treated with PLV for up to 76 h. Their lungs were filled with perflubron to approximately 20ml/kg and supplemental doses were generally administered hourly. The study was not randomised or blinded. The arterial tension of oxygen increased by 138%, the dynamic compliance by 61% and the oxygenation index reduced from a mean of 49 to 17 within 1 h of initiation. It was concluded that clinical improvement and survival occurred in some infants who were not predicted to survive (LEACH et al. 1996). PRANIKOFF et al. (1996) reported the results of four patients with CDH who were being managed on extracorporeal life support for up to 5 days. PLV was performed in a phase 1/11 trial for up to 6 days with daily dosing. The technique appeared to be safe and possibly associated with improvement in gas exchange and pulmonary compliance. In a similar study, GREENSPAN and coworkers (1997) treated six term infants who had respiratory failure and were failing to improve while receiving ECMO. They administered PLV with hourly dosing for up to 96 h. They concluded the technique appeared to be safe, improved lung function and recruited lung volumes in these infants. These initial studies of PLV in neonates were encouraging and suggested the feasibility of this technique in the neonate with severe RDS or ARDS. However, to date, there has been no reported randomised controlled trial of this technique in the neonatal population. Research in this area has been hampered by a lack of investment. This appears to stem from the time when the preliminary results of a phase 2–3 clinical trial in adults with ARDS were reported in 2001. While the study demonstrated that PLV was safe and well tolerated, it failed to show that PLV offered any incremental benefit over conventional treatment (WOLFSON and SHAFFER 2005). The results of the trial, unfortunately, have not been published in full and only limited data have been reported in abstract form (FUHRMAN et al. 1998). A recent Cochrane review looking at the role of PLV in paediatric ARDS concluded that there currently was no evidence from randomised controlled trials to support or refute the use of PLV in children with acute lung injury or acute respiratory distress syndrome, and it called for more adequately powered, high quality randomised controlled trials to assess its efficacy (DAVIES and SARGENT 2004). It is clear that further studies are needed in this area. It must also be said that a lack of efficacy of PLV in adult

trials should not necessarily preclude its study in the neonatal population. Until more information is available, it is currently not possible to define the role of this promising technique more clearly in the neonatal population.

In addition to its respiratory applications, PFC liquids may possess other qualities that are potentially beneficial. Firstly, PFC liquids are radiopaque, resulting in a whitened lung on standard radiograph. This means that they can be used as a diagnostic imaging adjunct in addition to supporting gas exchange. Radiographic studies of the perflubron-filled lungs of animals and humans with CDH may provide information on the degree of pulmonary hypoplasia, which in turn may allow a better determination of the prognosis. Secondly, there is growing evidence from several laboratories to suggest that intratracheal administration of PFC liquids may reduce pulmonary inflammation and injury. The mechanism of action has been speculated as a direct modification of cell function and chemotaxis. Thirdly, PFC liquids may help promote lung growth. Neonatal lambs were studied for 21 days following isolation and PFC distension of the right upper lobe to maintain up to 10 mmHg of intrabronchial pressure. The results demonstrated accelerated growth based on increased right upper lobe volume to body weight ratio, total alveolar number, total alveolar surface area, normal histological appearance, normal airway space fraction and normal alveolar numerical density compared with controls. Lastly, the physiochemical properties and physiological responses associated with PFC liquid ventilation suggest that PFC liquid may provide the means to deliver therapeutic agents directly to the lung including anaesthetic agents, antibiotics, steroids and gene therapy products (SHAFFER et al. 1999, GREENSPAN et al. 1998, WOLFSON and SHAFFER 2005).

The use of PFC liquids as an alternative respiratory medium is a rapidly evolving field. They have the potential to facilitate gas exchange with less risk of barotrauma and they may complement existing forms of respiratory management such as surfactant therapy, ECMO, HFOV and NO. With continued research towards establishing the efficacy and safety of the biological interaction of PFC fluids, LV should hopefully assume an integral role in clinical medicine in the not too distant future. We await further definition of the application and limitations of this alternative therapeutic approach to neonatal respiratory management.

2.3

New Drug Therapies

Respiratory distress syndrome in premature infants is a disease characterised by surfactant deficiency and its management has been revolutionised by the introduction of exogenous surfactant therapy. Nitric oxide is a potent vasodilator that acts specifically on the pulmonary vasculature when given as an inhalation. Its ability to selectively lower the pulmonary vascular resistance has provided clinicians with the first drug to treat the newborns with persistent pulmonary hypertension of the newborn.

2.3.1

Surfactant

The development of exogenous surfactant therapy was a significant and historical advance in neonatal intensive care. Pulmonary surfactant is a complex mixture of phospholipids, neutral lipids and specific proteins. It spreads as a monoloayer at the air liquid interfaces of the lung and lowers surface tension. By so doing, it prevents atelectasis at end expiration, thus preventing alveolar collapse. Phosphatidylcholine is the major component, constituting about 60% of total phospholipids, and dipalmitoylphosphatidylcholine (DPPC) is the primary surface-tension lowering phospholipid. The physical effects of surfactant depend on the interaction between phospholipids and surfactant-associated proteins, of which at least four have been identified (SP –A –B –C –D). These apoproteins are synthesised and secreted by type 2 alveolar cells. The hydrophilic protein SP-A improves surface properties and regulates secretion and recycling of surfactant constituents by alveolar cell. The hydrophobic proteins SP-B and SP-C facilitate the adsorption and spreading of lipids. In addition, SP-A and SP-D seem to play a role in the host defence mechanisms of the lung (JOBE and IKEGAMI 2000).

AVERY and MEAD first described the association of surfactant deficiency with respiratory distress syndrome (RDS) (AVERY and MEAD 1959). In healthy neonates, the pool size of endogenous alveolar surfactant is at least 100 mg/kg. In preterm infants, it is usually less than 10 mg/kg. Surfactant deficiency causes alveolar collapse, increased work of breathing and progressive respiratory failure. As a consequence of lung injury during the course of the disease or its treatment, serum proteins leak into the air spaces and further inhibit surfactant function. The recognition that these infants were deficient in surfactant offered an exciting opportunity for treatment. FUJIWARA and coworkers (1980) were the first group to use natural surfactant extract to treat premature infants with RDS. They treated a series of ten premature infants with severe RDS with surfactant-TA (Surfacten), a modified bovine surfactant extract. Shortly after this, a number of different natural and synthetic surfactant preparations came on the market. Natural surfactant extracts are obtained from animal (mainly bovine or porcine sources) or in some cases human sources and many are modified subsequently by the addition of phospholipids or other surface active materials to optomise their surface-tension-lowering properties. These natural surfactants contain variable amounts of the surfactant proteins, but the hydrophilic proteins SP-A and SP-D are removed during the extraction process. The preparations vary in composition, concentration and volume as well as in recommended dose. In addition, different retreatment doses, dosing intervals and criteria for retreatment exist for the various preparations. Synthetic or "artificial" surfactants are composed of DPPC and spreading agents such as unsaturated phosphatidylglycerol or tyloxapol and hexadecanol, which are added to replace the function of the surfactant proteins. As a result, synthetic surfactants do not adsorb and spread as quickly as natural surfactants. Following Fujiwara's first uncontrolled trial of surfactant replacement, more than 30 randomised controlled clinical trials of surfactant replacement have been conducted to assess different aspects of surfactant therapy. In general, these trials have used two approaches: prophylactic administration of surfactant to high risk premature infants in the delivery room concurrently with the initiation of breathing and resuscitation (prevention trials) or administration of surfactant to premature infants with moderate to severe RDS at 2–24 h of age once the diagnosis has been made (rescue or treatment trials). Prevention trials offer the theoretical advantage of replacing surfactant before the onset of RDS thereby avoiding the secondary barotrauma that may result from short periods of assisted ventilation. It is also argued that surfactant may distribute more homogeneously when administered immediately at birth. Rescue trials offer the advantage of treating only those infants who have the clinical signs of RDS, thus eliminating the potential risks associated with treating surfactant-sufficient infants who would receive no benefit from the treatment, not to mention the unnecessary cost. The findings of these trials have been systematically reviewed and reported in the Cochrane Database.

Overall, the administration of prophylactic natural or synthetic surfactants to infants judged to be at risk of RDS (intubated infants <30 weeks gestation) results in a pronounced reduction in neonatal mortality by about 40% and in the incidence of pneumothorax by 30–70% (SOLL 1997, SOLL 1998). The introduction of surfactant into general clinical use in 1989 coincided with a decline in the general infant mortality in the US from 8.5% in 1989 to 6.3% in 1990 and this was attributed primarily to fewer deaths from respiratory causes among preterm infants. The incidence of chronic lung disease (CLD) is not consistently lower in surfactant-treated infants irrespective of the type of surfactant used. There is, however, an increased survival without BPD after treatment with natural surfactants. A similar trend is also seen in the group treated with synthetic surfactants, but the finding was not statistically significant. The incidence of IVH is essentially unaffected. Although no individual study reported an increase in the incidence of haemodynamically significant PDA, the meta-analysis suggests an increased risk of PDA in infants treated with synthetic surfactants. This risk is of marginal statistical significance. Several of the trials using Exosurf (one of the synthetic surfactants) reported an increased incidence of pulmonary haemorrhage and this was borne out in the meta-analysis. Although many of the randomised controlled trials of other surfactant products did not report on pulmonary haemorrhage, this outcome was addressed retrospectively in analyses by RAJU et al. (1993). Pulmonary haemorrhage remains a small but consistent complication (2% in treated infants, 1% in control infants) and appears to occur with both synthetic and natural surfactants. It occurs mainly in small infants and it can occur many hours after successful treatment. Although, pulmonary haemorrhage has been associated with a PDA, its cause is not known and it does not appear to be preventable. Despite this complication, it should be noted that it does not overshadow the impact on overall survival.

The rational for prophylactic administration of surfactant is provided by the observation that in animal studies a more uniform and homogeneous distribution of surfactant is achieved when it is administered into a fluid-filled lung. In addition, there is a belief that administration of surfactant into a previously unventilated or minimally ventilated lung results in diminished lung injury. Even brief (15–30 min) periods of mechanical ventilation before surfactant administration in animal models have been shown to cause acute lung injury resulting in alveolar-capillary damage, leakage of proteinaceous fluid into the alveolar space and release of inflammatory mediators (JOBE and IKEGAMI 1998). Once again, the Cochrane Database of systematic reviews has looked at this area. Eight randomised controlled trials, each using natural surfactant preparations, compared the effects of administering surfactant prophylactically to infants (within 15 min) or selectively to infants with established RDS (from 1.5–7.4 h) (SOLL and MORLEY 2001). To date, there are no trials comparing the use of prophylactic surfactant administration with very early selective administration, for example, at 30–60 min of life. The results suggest that prophylactic surfactant administration to infants judged to be at risk of developing respiratory distress syndrome (infants <30–32 weeks gestation) compared to selective use of surfactant in infants with established RDS results in a decreased risk of pneumothorax, a decreased risk of pulmonary interstitial emphysema and a reduction in neonatal mortality. In a secondary analysis of infants less than 30 weeks gestation, similar clinical improvements were noted. This is not surprising as the benefits of prophylactic surfactant administration over selective administration would most likely be seen in the group of infants at highest risk of RDS and neonatal mortality. Importantly, there was no significant difference in the incidence of IVH, PVL, PDA, necrotising enterocolitis (NEC) or retinopthy of prematurity (ROP). What is not clear from this review is exactly what criteria should be chosen to judge "risk" in these infants. At what point do the benefits of prophylactic surfactant outweigh the risks of intubation and exposure to mechanical ventilation? Based on the above information, the threshold would appear to be around 30 weeks gestation, but from our earlier discussion on the use of early CPAP in the extremely low-birth weight population (see Sect. 2.2.1), it may be that this cut off should be as low as 26 weeks (SURESH and SOLL 2001, FINER 2006). This is a point that is currently hotly debated and will hopefully be answered in the not too distant future as the results of ongoing clinical trials become available.

In the initial trials using prophylactic surfactant, the drug was administered as a bolus immediately after intubating the infants after birth, with a goal of giving the drug before the infant took its first breath.

This approach delays the initiation of neonatal resuscitation, including positive pressure ventilation, and is associated with a risk for surfactant delivery into the right main stem bronchus or oesophagus. It has been shown in a randomised trial that prophylaxis may be administered with equivalent or greater efficacy in small aliquots given soon after resuscitation and confirmation of endotracheal tube placement (KENDIG et al. 1998). This would suggest that early administration before the first breath may be unnecessary.

In preterm infants who do not receive prophylaxis, many of the arguments in support of prophylactic surfactant administration are also supportive of early surfactant treatment in established RDS. A comparison of early selective versus delayed selective surfactant therapy for newborns intubated for respiratory distress within the first 2 h of life has also been the subject of a meta-analysis (YOST and SOLL 1999). For the purpose of the analysis, early administration was defined as surfactant administration to infants intubated for respiratory distress within the first 2 h of life and it excluded those infants who were intubated specifically for surfactant dosage. Four randomised controlled trials have been evaluated. Early administration of surfactant in these trials consisted of the administration of the first dose of surfactant with the 1st 30 min (1 study), 1st h (1 study) or 1st 2 h of life (two studies). Two of the studies used natural surfactant and two used synthetic surfactant. The selective treatment group received surfactant anywhere between 1.5 and 8 h of age. The findings concluded that early selective surfactant administration led to a decreased risk of acute pulmonary injury (pneumothorax and pulmonary interstitial emphysema) and a decreased risk of neonatal mortality and chronic lung disease compared to delaying the treatment of such infants until they develop established RDS. Therefore it would seem prudent, in preterm infants who have not received prophylactic surfactant, that the first dose of surfactant be administered as early as possible should they develop severe enough RDS (i.e., as soon as they are intubated). It is hard to judge the relative value of early surfactant treatment compared to true prophylactic use of surfactant in the absence of any randomised trials that have directly compared these policies. Nevertheless, it would appear that the earlier surfactant is given to infants with RDS, the better the outcome. The difficulty still remains in judging which infants are at risk of surfactant deficiency. Improved

identification of these infants would improve the selection criteria for prophylactic or early selective surfactant treatment. This is an important area for future research.

Although both synthetic and natural surfactants are effective, their composition differs. A meta-analysis incorporating 11 randomised trials studied the effects of natural versus synthetic surfactant for the treatment of RDS. Trials were included if using either a prophylactic or selective treatment strategy. Greater earlier improvement in the requirement for ventilator support, fewer pneumothoraces and fewer deaths were associated with natural surfactant extract treatment. A trend towards improved survival without bronchopulmonary dysplasia was noted. The meta-analysis did comment that natural surfactants may be associated with an increase in intraventricular haemorrhages, though the more serious haemorrhages (grade 3-4) were not increased. Despite these concerns, the overall conclusion was that natural surfactant extract would seem to be the more desirable choice to currently available synthetic surfactants (SOLL and BLANCO 2001).

Many of the initial trials of surfactant therapy tested a single dose of surfactant. Surfactant may become rapidly metabolised or functionally inactivated by soluble proteins and other factors in the small airways and alveoli. Multiple doses of surfactant are believed to be useful because they can overcome such inactivation. Two randomised controlled trials have looked at this question. In the first trial, second and third doses were given 12 and 24 h after the initial treatment at about 6 h of age if the infant remained on assisted ventilation. There was a reduced frequency of pneumothoraces from 18% with a single dose to 9% with three doses and the death rate at 28 days was also reduced (21% compared to 13%, $P<0.05$) (SPEER et al. 1992). In the second study of 75 infants with RDS, those who received multiple doses had better oxygenation during the first several days of life (DUNN et al. 1990). A meta-analysis of these studies concluded that multiple doses of surfactant in infants with established respiratory distress syndrome was associated with greater improvements in oxygenation and ventilatory requirements, a decreased risk of pneumothorax and a trend towards improved survival (SOLL 1999). There were no differences in other outcome measures or in the rates of complications. Approximately 70% of the infants randomised to the multiple dose regimen actually received multiple doses. In a third study in which a synthetic surfactant was used in a prophylactic manner (826 infants weighing 700–1,100 g at risk of developing RDS were given either one or three doses of Exosurf), the use of two doses of surfactant in addition to a prophylactic dose led to a decrease in mortality, respiratory support, necrotising enterocolitis and other outcomes when compared to a single prophylactic dose (Corbet et al. 1995). In the OSIRIS trial, in which synthetic surfactant was used, a two-dose treatment schedule was found to be equivalent to a treatment schedule permitting up to four doses of surfactant (the OSIRIS Collaborative Group 1992). In summary, therefore, the ability to give multiple doses of surfactant to infants with ongoing respiratory insufficiency leads to an improved outcome and appears to be the most effective policy. The definition of "ongoing respiratory insufficiency" has also been the subject of debate. The question of what criteria to use for administration of repeat doses of surfactant has been addressed by two studies, both of which used natural surfactant. In one study, the retreatment criteria compared were an increase in the fraction of inspired oxygen by 0.1 over the lowest baseline value (standard retreatment) versus a sustained increase of just 0.01 (liberal retreatment) (Dunn et al. 1991). There was no difference in complications of prematurity or duration of respiratory support. Short-term benefits in oxygen requirement and ventilatory support were noted, however, in the liberal retreatment group. In another study, retreatment at a low threshold (FiO2 >30%, still requiring endotracheal intubation) was compared with retreatment at a higher threshold (FiO2 >40%, mean airway pressure >7 cm H_2O) (Kattwinkel et al. 2000). Again, there were minor short-term benefits to using a low threshold with no difference in major clinical outcomes. In a subgroup of infants with RDS complicated by perinatal compromise or infection, however, infants in the high threshold group had a trend towards higher mortality than the low threshold group. Based on current evidence, it seems appropriate to use persistent or worsening signs of RDS as criteria for retreatment with surfactant. It is uncertain whether a low threshold strategy should be used in certain subgroups of infants or with certain preparations of surfactant. Further clinical studies should help address some of these questions.

As stated earlier, the synthetic surfactants used in the aforementioned studies are composed of phospholipids, some of which have additional dispersion agents and polymers. They do not contain the highly lipophilic proteins that are found in native surfactant in situ. More recently, newer synthetic surfactant preparations have been developed that include peptides or whole proteins that, when added to an aqueous dispersion of phosphoplipids, function in a fashion similar to endogenous pulmonary surfactant protein. Lucinactant (Surfaxin) is a combination of phospholipids with a new peptide called sinapultide. The peptide (developmental name KL4 peptide) mimics domains of surfactant protein B (SP-B). Lusupultide (Venticute) is another new synthetic surfactant that contains recombinant SP-C and phospholipids. The rationale for the development of these protein-containing synthetic surfactants includes both practical and theoretical considerations. Synthetic surfactants would have highly reproducible composition with potentially less batch-to-batch surfactant protein variability, would be more readily available with no dependence on an animal source and could theoretically be produced in large quantities. Furthermore, synthetic surfactants may lessen the risk of inflammation and immunogenicity associated with animal-derived surfactants as well as the theoretical risk of infection (Pfister et al. 2006). A recent study compared the use lucinactant administered prophylactically with the natural surfactant, beractant (Survanta), and the synthetic surfactant, colfosceril palmitate (Exosurf) (Moya et al. 2005). Lucinactant significantly reduced the incidence of RDS at 24 h when compared with colfosceril. In addition, the incidence of BPD at 36 weeks post-gestational age was also significantly less common in the lucinactant group when compare to the colfosceril group. The RDS-related mortality rates at 14 days of life were lower in the lucinactant group compared to either the beractant or colfoseril palmitate groups. The authors concluded that lucinactant was a more effective surfactant preparation than colfosceril palmitate and that it was an effective therapeutic option for preterm infants at risk of RDS. A second study by Sinha et al. (2005) compared lucinactant used prophylactically in infants at risk of RDS with the natural surfactant, poractant (Curosurf). Lucinactant and poractant were found to be similar in terms of efficacy and safety when used for the prevention and treatment of RDS among preterm infants. As more clinical trials are undertaken, it is likely that the role of these newer synthetic surfactants in the treatment of RDS will be further elucidated.

There are few therapies for which the cumulative evidence of benefit is as much as that for surfactant therapy for RDS in premature infants. However, it is now becoming clear that exogenous surfactant may have a role to play in other non-RDS lung conditions with secondary surfactant deficiency such as meconium aspiration syndrome, pulmonary haemorrhage, congenital diaphragmatic hernia, etc. These disorders generally either have dysfunction and inactivation of endogenous surfactant or deficits in the composition of available endogenous surfactant. Surfactant production can be altered by damage to the type 2 alveolar cells by inciting agents. Proteins from plasma, red blood cells or meconium may inhibit surfactant properties and production. The products of inflammation, such as cytokines, other mediators, proteases and reactive oxygen species may interfere with surfactant function and processing of the substances in the alveoli.

Uncontrolled studies of surfactant treatment in infants with meconium aspiration syndrome suggest that surfactant may be of benefit in MAS. In a pilot study of seven infants with MAS treated with surfactant, all seven infants demonstrated an improvement in respiratory failure (AUTEN 1991). KHAMMASH et al. (1993) treated 20 infants with severe MAS. Improvement in the oxygenation index and arterial-to-alveolar ratio was noted in 75% of the treated infants in the 6 h following surfactant instillation. None of the treated infants required further experimental therapy, including ECMO. In infants who were already on ECMO, surfactant therapy was noted to improve lung function and decrease the time on ECMO (LOTZE 1998). A meta-analysis of the use of surfactant in term infants with MAS found that it reduced the need for ECMO, but no difference was noted in the overall mortality (SOLL and DARGAVILLE 2000). The relative efficacy of surfactant therapy compared to or in conjunction with other approaches to treatment including inhaled nitric oxide, liquid ventilation and high frequency ventilation remains to be tested. Other approaches to surfactant therapy, including the use of surfactant lavage, may prove to be of benefit in this condition in the future. With regards to the use of surfactant in pulmonary haemorrhage, PANDIT et al. (1995) carried out a retrospective study of 15 infants. There was an improvement in the oxygenation index 3 to 6 h following surfactant treatment particularly in the near-term infants. No infants deteriorated following surfactant treatment. In another study, AMIZUKA et al. (2003) treated 27 infants with haemorrhagic pulmonary oedema. A good response, defined as a ventilatory index <0.047 at 1 h after treatment was found in 82% of cases. Both authors suggest that

further investigations including randomized controlled trials are now required to evaluate the effectiveness of surfactant in this condition. Many studies in animal models of congenital diaphragmatic hernias and from infants with this abnormality suggest that a deficiency of surfactant plays a role in the pathophysiology of the disease. There is limited experience to date on treating infants with this disorder. Bos et al. (1991) reported improved oxygenation in four infants treated, whereas GLICK et al. (1992) treated seven infants and believed that surfactant improved survival. In contrast, LOTZE et al. found no benefit of administration of a natural surfactant to infants with CDH who were already on ECMO. While there have been several additional reports on the use of surfactant in this condition (NAKAYAMA 1991, KARAMANOUKIAN 1994, FINER 1998), it is impossible to determine from these studies whether surfactant administration is beneficial since multiple other interventions such as high frequency ventilation, inhaled nitric oxide and ECMO were also utilized. It is clear that a lot more research in this area is required. Use of surfactant therapy for any disorder other than RDS must be considered experimental at this stage. Much work remains to be done to address the optimum type of surfactant to use, the appropriate dose, the method of delivery and the duration of treatment in each of the specified disorders.

In conclusion, surfactants are a new class of drugs specifically designed for the neonatal population. Prophylaxis or treatment of neonatal RDS with either natural or synthetic surfactant is now a clinical reality. With either, the incidence of pneumothorax and mortality is reduced and more infants survive without BPD. The earlier the treatment, the better the outcome is. There is some benefit in using multiple dose regimens. New surfactants combining peptides or proteins based on human surfactant-protein sequences with synthetic lipids are being developed and need to be further evaluated along with possible new techniques such as aerosolisation. The primary goal should be to reduce BPD and mortality from RDS even further. Surfactant is not a substitute for attempts to increase foetal maturation and thus prevent RDS, by delaying preterm delivery and by using maternal corticosteroid therapy. It is nevertheless a rational treatment strategy that is based on sound physiological principles and extensive experimental and clinical therapy. Use of surfactant for conditions other than RDS must still be regarded as experimental.

2.3.2
Nitric Oxide

Successful adaptation of the newborn to postnatal conditions requires a dramatic transition of the pulmonary circulation from a high resistance state in utero to a low resistance state within minutes after birth. This fall in pulmonary vascular resistance (PVR) allows for a nearly ten-fold rise in pulmonary blood flow and ensures that the lung can assume its postnatal role in gas exchange. Some infants fail to achieve or sustain the normal decrease in PVR at birth, which in turn leads to severe respiratory distress and hypoxaemia, a condition referred to as persistent pulmonary hypertension of the newborn (PPHN). PPHN is a syndrome that can occur in association with diverse neonatal cardiorespiratory disorders such as meconium aspiration, sepsis, pneumonia, ARDS, asphyxia, CDH and lung hypoplasia. Although striking differences exist among these conditions, they all share common pathophysiological features, including high PVR leading to extrapulmonary right to left shunting of blood flow across the ductus arteriosus or foramen ovale. PPHN remains a major clinical problem, contributing significantly to morbidity and mortality in both term and preterm infants.

Initial attempts at treating PPHN were aimed at reducing PVR with a combination of hyperventilation and hyperoxia, both of which resulted in worsening lung injury and contributed further to the morbidity and mortality of the disease. Pulmonary vasodilator drug therapy was often unsuccessful due to the concomitant systemic hypotension and the inability to achieve or sustain pulmonary vasodilation. In many centres, the only treatment available for those that failed conventional therapy was ECMO. Effective treatment of PPHN suffered because of a lack of an agent that could cause selective and sustained pulmonary vasodilation. This all changed with the identification of a potent short-acting substance called nitric oxide. Nitric oxide (NO) is a major regulator of vascular smooth muscle tone. Generated enzymatically by one of several NO synthases from L-arginine in the vascular endothelium, NO rapidly diffuses to underlying smooth muscle. Here, it activates guanyl cyclase by binding to its haem component leading to the production of cyclic GMP. This, in turn, relaxes vascular and bronchial smooth muscle. NO has a high affinity for the iron of haem proteins, including reduced haemoglobin, forming nitrosyl haemoglobin (NOHb), which is then oxidised

to methaemoglobin with the production of nitrate. As a result, when given as an inhalation, NO relaxes pulmonary smooth muscle and is inactivated before it can affect the systemic vascular bed.

Early reports of the use of this inhaled substance in term infants with PPHN showed both acute and sustained improvements in oxygenation (ROBERTS et al. 1992, KINSELLA et al. 1992). Since then, there have been a number of large randomised controlled trials confirming that NO improves oxygenation and reduces the need for extracorporeal membrane oxygenation (ECMO). The Neonatal Inhaled Nitric Oxide Group (1997) reported on 235 infants less than 4 days old born >34 weeks gestation and with an oxygenation index of >25. Cases of congenital cardiac disease and congenital diaphragmatic hernias were excluded. The infants were randomised to receive inhaled NO or a control gas. Infants failing to respond to either treatment were eligible to receive ECMO. Use of other therapies such as HFV or surfactant was allowed. Sixty-four percent of the control group compared to 46% of the inhaled NO (iNO) group died within 120 days or were treated with ECMO ($P=0.006$). The difference in mortality between the two groups was not significantly different (iNO Group – 14%, control group – 17%), but significantly fewer infants in the iNO group required EMCO (39% vs. 54%). The iNO group had significantly greater increases in PaO2 and in oxygenation index. There was no difference in the length of hospitalisation, duration of mechanical ventilation or incidence of air leak or chronic lung disease between the two groups. Of interest, this group did not require evidence of PPHN on echocardiography for inclusion in the trial. This is based on studies that have shown that iNO improves the matching of ventilation with perfusion and may reduce intrapulmonary shunting in the absence of a direct intracardiac shunt such as is seen in PPHN. In a similar analysis of 58 infants with persistent pulmonary hypertension (although in this group, prior treatment with HFV was an exclusion criterion), 53% of infants experienced a doubling of systemic oxygenation with iNO compared to only 7% with the control gas ($P=0.002$). The use of ECMO was significantly reduced (iNO group 40% vs. control group 71%, $P=0.02$). The number of deaths was similar in both groups (ROBERTS et al. 1997). Both studies confirmed that NO improved oxygenation and reduced the need for ECMO. The I-NO/PPHN Study Group reported their findings in 1998. A total of 155 patients were randomised to receive either a control gas or nitric oxide at 5, 20 or 80 ppm. The patients had not received surfactant and there was no concomitant use of HFV. The aim had been to randomise 320 patients, but the trial was halted in June 1996 because of slow recruitment. It is likely that the study's limitations on surfactant and HFV impacted on this as these modalities were increasingly being used. The study calculated a major sequelae index comprising the incidence of death, neurological injury and BPD as well as the use of ECMO. The MSI rate was not significantly different between the iNO and control groups (50% and 59%, respectively). The use of ECMO was 22% in the iNO group versus 34% in control patients. With the exception of elevated levels of NO2 and methemoglobin levels in the group receiving 80 ppm, no adverse effects were noted. While there was not a statistically significant reduced MSI in the iNO group, there was a 35% decline in the need for ECMO in the pooled iNO group even without the concomitant use of surfactant and HFV therapies, a finding that compares with earlier studies (The Neonatal Inhaled Nitric Oxide Study Group 1997, ROBERTS et al. 1992). Of equal importance was the finding that survival with ECMO was the same in both groups, despite the fact that the time to ECMO was greater in the iNO group (42±22 vs. 22±15 h). This allayed a fear at the time that iNO may merely delay the use of ECMO, an accepted and proven therapy. Another group published information on 248 infants >34 weeks gestation with an OI index of 25 or greater. This group included cases of CDH (The Clinical Inhaled Nitric Oxide Research Group 2000). Each infant was assigned to one of five diagnostic groups–meconium aspiration syndrome, sepsis, RDS, lung hypoplasia (including CDH) and idiopathic. Neonates were randomised to receive iNO 20 ppm for a maximum of 24 h followed by 5 ppm for no more than 96 h or a control gas. The findings of the study were that the use of ECMO was less common in the iNO group (38%) than in the control group (64%) (P=0.001). This was true for all pulmonary diagnostic groups except neonates with CDH (89% vs. 92%). In those treated with ECMO, the median time to treatment was the same in both groups (5 h on the control group (range 1–86 h) and 9 h in the NO group (range 2–150 h). There was no difference in the overall mortality between the two groups. The incidence of chronic lung disease was lower in the neonates treated with iNO (7% vs. 20%, P=0.02) and the incidence of neurological problems was the same in each group. These results concurred with the findings of the Neonatal Inhaled Nitric Oxide Study (1997),

demonstrating that NO was effective across a broad range of diagnoses, the only exception being neonates with CDH in whom iNO did not reduced the use of ECMO or improve the outcome. One other important finding born out by earlier studies was that low dose iNO was effective and that there was no apparent need for higher does. This study also limited the time for administering iNO, in an effort to avoid delaying ECMO, a proven therapy in PPHN, beyond the point in which its efficacy might be reduced. The use of nitric oxide for respiratory failure in infants born at or near term has been the subject of a recent Cochrane review (FINER and BARRINGTON 2006). Fourteen studies were included. Inhaled nitric oxide was found to improve the outcome in hypoxic term and near term infants by reducing the incidence of the combined endpoint of death or need for ECMO. The reduction seemed to be entirely a reduction in the need for ECMO; mortality was not reduced. Oxygenation improved in approximately 50% of infants receiving nitric oxide. The oxygenation index decreased by a mean of 15.1 within 30–60 min after commencing therapy and PaO2 increased by a mean of 53 mmHg. Whether infants had clear echocardiographic evidence of PPHN or not did not appear to affect the outcome. The outcome of infants with CDH was not improved and, in fact, there was a suggestion that outcome was slightly worsened. The incidence of disability, deafness and infant development scores were all similar between tested survivors who received iNO or not. On the evidence currently available, the meta-analysis concluded that it appeared reasonable to use inhaled nitric oxide in an initial concentration of 20 ppm for term or near term infants (>34 weeks gestation) with hypoxic respiratory failure who did not have a congenital diaphragmatic hernia. The therapy was found to be very potent in reducing the need for ECMO with an NNT of 5.3. It can still be questioned whether a decreased need for ECMO, a therapy of proven benefit, is, in fact, a real benefit (see Sect. 2.2.4). However, as ECMO is invasive, expensive and associated with clinically important complications, a reduction in ECMO requirement using a less invasive and safer treatment does promise to be a therapeutic advance. The meta-analysis was not able to comment on whether the use of iNO resulted in a delay in the initiation of ECMO and consequently a poorer outcome as this issue was not adequately tested in the trials included. This is an important area for future research. It appeared appropriate to reserve therapy for those who were severely ill. Commencing therapy earlier did not appear to further reduce ECMO requirements or mortality. Thus starting therapy when the OI exceeds 25 or when the PaO2 while receiving 100% O2 is less than 100 mmHg is consistent with the published evidence. While the meta-analysis found that the use of iNO at lesser OIs appeared to decrease progression to severe disease, this was not accompanied by an increase in survival, a decrease in ECMO requirements or an improvement in any other reported clinical outcome when compared to waiting to see whether the patient deteriorates. It may be, however, that long-term outcomes are improved by preventing more severe disease. This question has yet to be answered. Further unresolved issues include whether pretreatment with surfactant improves the response to iNO in humans, whether iNO is more effective during high frequency ventilation rather than conventional ventilation or whether improved or earlier treatment with more conventional modalities including surfactant and HFV are as effective as iNO. Long-term outcome information on patients treated with iNO is also required. The follow-up study of the Neonatal Inhaled Nitric Oxide Study Group (2000), which noted no differences in neurodevelopmental, behavioural or medical abnormalities between the two groups at 2 years of age, provides us with some reassuring information.

Another area of current investigation is the role of iNO in preterm newborns with hypoxemic respiratory failure. The role of endogenous NO production in vasoregulation of the preterm pulmonary circulation and the effects of iNO in the preterm newborn have received less attention than in the term infant. Preterm infants with respiratory failure do have an increase in pulmonary artery pressure, but it is rarely sufficient to cause reversal of ductal flow and, therefore, the haemodynamic profile of preterm infants differs from that of term infants. ECMO is not used for preterm infants and so its requirement cannot be used as an outcome criterion. Equally, entry criteria used for studies in term infants may not be applicable to preterm infants as measurements such as the oxygenation index may not predict mortality to the same extent at the same levels. Because of the above, results of trials in term infants cannot be applied to the preterm population. A meta-analysis of the information published to date on this group of infants has recently been carried out (BARRINGTON and FINER 2006). Currently, there is no evidence from eight randomised trials to support the use of inhaled nitric oxide in preterm infants with respiratory failure. Rescue therapy of very sick preterm

infants who met criteria for poor oxygenation did not improve their survival, survival without BPD or brain injury. Oxygenation did appear to be improved in the short-term. While the meta-analysis did not recommend the routine use of iNO as a rescue therapy, it did emphasise that further studies were warranted because of the intriguing results of one study by SCHREIBER et al. (2003). In this study, infants <34 weeks gestation and <2 kg and <72 h of age were randomised to receive nitric oxide as part of routine therapy while intubated. There was a significant reduction in the combined outcome of death or BPD and a significant reduction in the rate of grade 3 or 4 IVH or PVL in those treated with iNO. In addition, cognitive outcome at 2 years of age was improved in the treated group (MESTAN et al. 2005). The infants studied were less ill at the time of enrolment and confirmation of the efficacy of such an approach would be important. It may be that infants who are already sick enough to fulfil the entry criteria of rescue studies may already have suffered brain and pulmonary injury that is too severe to be improved by nitric oxide while routine "prophylactic" use may be able to reduce the incidence of some such injuries. Again, more work in this area is needed.

While iNO therapy improves oxygenation in over 50% of neonates with PPHN, some infants do not show a response and others deteriorate subsequently while on iNO. This has led to the investigation of alternate and complementary approaches to iNO. These include the use of vasodilators such as prostacyclin or PGE2, NO precursors such as L-arginine, phosphodiesterase inhibitors such as sildenafil and free radical scavengers such as superoxide dismutase. All of these therapies remain investigational at this point in time with limited or no data in neonates with PPHN. It may be possible in the future to decrease morbidity and mortality in PPHN further as specific strategies aimed at correcting alterations in NO and prostacyclin biology are discovered.

In summary, available evidence supports the use of iNO beginning at initial doses of 20 ppm in term or near-term infants who have hypoxic respiratory failure and who do not have a congenital diaphragmatic hernia. Although brief exposures to higher doses (40–80 ppm) appear to be safe, sustained treatment with 80 ppm increases the risk of methaemoglobinaemia. The lowest effective initial does for iNO in term newborns has not yet been determined. While iNO has reduced the need for ECMO by about 40%, not all patients will experience a sustained improvement in oxygenation and some will still require ECMO. This has raised concerns about the use of iNO in centres that do not have access to ECMO facilities as it has been well demonstrated that infants rapidly become tolerant to iNO and withdrawal of iNO during transport may lead to an acute deterioration (KINSELLA et al. 1995). In addition, there is currently much debate in the literature about the possible adverse effects on infants if there is a delay in the initiation of ECMO. More work in this area is urgently needed. Another important question to be addressed is if the use of iNO earlier in the course of the disease when the oxygenation index is less than 25 will result in improved outcomes. The use of inhaled NO in the preterm population as a rescue therapy is not currently recommended.

2.4
Prenatal Medicine

Prenatal ultrasonography has permitted not only the detailed assessment of foetal anatomy and the recognition of structural defects, but it has also allowed the characterisation of their natural history. Advances in prenatal diagnosis over the past decade have provided new insights into the pathophysiology of thoracic malformations such as congenital diaphragmatic hernia (CDH), congenital cystic adenomatoid malformation of the lung (CCAM), pulmonary sequestration (PS) and foetal hydrothorax (FHT). In many respects, the natural history of each of these malformations has proven entirely different from our understanding of their postnatal history. For each of these thoracic lesions, there is a so-called "hidden mortality". Many foetuses with CDH, CCAM, PS or FHT die in utero from the consequences of a large space-occupying thoracic mass that causes mediastinal shift and hydrops. In addition, many infants may die shortly after birth from pulmonary hypoplasia before transfer to a tertiary referral centre can be made. Therefore, the observed mortality of these conditions is artificially lowered in a tertiary referral centre. Consequently, the prenatal diagnosis of any of these malformations engenders a worse prognosis than the same condition diagnosed after birth. Along with a greater understanding of the natural history and pathophysiology of these malformations has come the development of prognostic indicators and the opportunity to treat conditions in utero that would otherwise be fatal.

Foetal therapy has advanced from simple thoracentesis to the placement of thoracoamniotic shunts in FHT, pulmonary resection in CCAM and complete repair of CDH in utero.

The detection of CDH prenatally allows time both in which to prepare the family, but also to plan delivery in a tertiary referral site. It allows determination of the size and position of the hernia, the presence of the liver in the thoracic cage and the presence of other associated congenital anomalies that may impact on survival. The presence of pulmonary hypoplasia is an important determinant of survival in CDH, but is extremely difficult to predict. Harrison et al. have proposed that foetuses with a good prognosis can be identified by the absence of liver herniation into the thorax, a high lung-to-head ratio (LHR) and late (>25 weeks gestation) herniation of the abdominal viscera into the thorax (HARRISON et al. 1998, LIPSHUTZ et al. 1997, ALBANESE et al. 1998). Conversely, foetuses with liver herniation into the hemithorax and a low lung-to-head ratio have a poor prognosis with conventional postnatal management. The lung-to-head ratio is a sonographic measurement that compares the right lung size with head circumference (corrected for gestational age) and is calculated between 24 and 26 weeks gestation. Specifically, overall survival was 47% with a LHR range of 0.62–1.86, and an LHR less than 1 was associated with no survivors despite ECMO, whereas all patients with a LHR ratio more than 1.4 survived. LHR values between 1 to 1.4 were associated with a 38% survival although 75% required ECMO (LIPSHUTZ et al. 1997). While these initial results are encouraging, this measurement still needs to be validated further. The availability of a reliable predictive marker for CDH would be invaluable and it would allow us to determine those infants who would benefit from surgery as well as from other interventions such as HFV and ECMO. With the recognition that some infants had a very poor prognosis, attention then focused on attempting to repair the CDH in utero in an effort to prevent or minimise pulmonary hypoplasia. Complete surgical repair in utero for foetuses without liver herniation did not improve survival over standard care (75% vs. 86%) (HARRISON et al. 1997). As the outcome for these infants was so good irrespective of in utero intervention, foetal surgery with all its associated risks was not felt to be warranted. However, infants with liver herniation and hence an overall poor prognosis did very poorly when undergoing complete repair in utero. The repair was technically impossible secondary to kinking of the umbilical vein when the liver was reduced causing cardiovascular collapse (HARRISON et al. 1993). To combat this, a strategy of temporary tracheal occlusion or PLUG (Plug the Lung Until it Grows) was devised (HARRISON et al. 1998). Obstruction of the flow of foetal lung fluid was found to accelerate foetal lung growth, reduce herniated viscera and ameliorate pulmonary hypoplasia (DiFIORE et al. 1994). Initially, an external clip was applied to the trachea at open surgery via a hysterotomy. Subsequently, the introduction of video-fetoscopic techniques (Fetendo) allowed dissection of the foetal trachea and placement of the occluding clip without hysterotomy. Harrison's group reported their experience of foetal surgery on infants in the poor prognosis category (diagnosis before 25 weeks, left-sided hernias only, LHR <1.4 and no other major anomalies) (HARRISON et al. 1998). Infants who received standard care had a survival rate of 38%. Infants in the open tracheal occlusion group had a survival rate of 15%, whereas infants treated with the Fetendo procedure had a survival rate of 75%. Initial fetoscopic treatment of CDH utilized radially expanding uterine trocars to surgically manipulate the foetal trachea in place, perform a neck dissection and place temporary occlusive titanium clips. These clips, however, required removal prior to birth, and as a result, an additional operative procedure was developed – the ex utero intrapartum treatment strategy (EXIT). EXIT allowed clip removal and neonatal intubation prior to cord transection (essentially on placental support) by way of caesarean incision. Although beneficial in terms of pulmonary growth, this technique was flawed due to associated tracheal complications that occurred because of the fetoscopic neck dissection. Modification led to the current technique of endoscopic placement of a detachable balloon directly into the foetal trachea (SKARSGARD et al. 1996). A randomised controlled trial funded by the NIH of foetal endoscopic tracheal occlusion for severe CDH was reported by HARRISON et al. (2003). Women carrying foetuses that were between 22 and 27 weeks gestation and that had severe left-sided CDH (defined as liver herniation, LHR <1.4) with no other detectable abnormalities were randomly assigned to foetal endoscopic tracheal occlusion or standard care. The primary outcome was survival at the age of 90 days. Secondary outcomes were measures of maternal and neonatal morbidity. Of the infants randomized to the intervention, two of the infants underwent a tracheal clip procedure and the remaining nine infants were treated with the balloon-occlusion technique. Enrolment was stopped after 24 patients because of the unexpectedly high survival rate with standard care and the conclusion of the data safety monitoring board that further recruitment would not result in significant differences between the two groups (survival rates were 73% in the tracheal occlusion group and 77% in the standard care group with no difference detected between the two groups). Premature rupture of membranes and preterm delivery occurred in 100% of those receiving antenatal surgical treatment with a mean age at delivery of 30.8 weeks. The conclusion of the trial was that tracheal occlusion did not improve survival or morbidity in this cohort of foetuses with CDH. The rate of survival at 90 days of age among foetuses assigned to standard care was unexpectedly high at 77% given the 38% survival quoted in a similar group of historical controls, and the authors felt that this may be due to the "trial effect". The study design required that infants in both treatment groups be delivered, resuscitated and intensively treated in a unit experienced in caring for critically ill newborns with pulmonary hypoplasia. Therefore, "standard care" in the study was really optimal care and the authors cautioned about the general applicability of the results of the trial. The 16 survivors of this trial were prospectively followed and remarkably, despite the fact that the infants in the tracheal occlusion group were significantly more premature, follow-up at 1 and 2 years noted no differences in the neurodevelopmental outcome between the two groups (CORTES et al. 2005). DEPREST et al. (2006) felt that the NIH trial lacked the power to document the potential advantage of prenatal therapy in the more severe cases of CDH. His group carried out percutaneous foetal endoluminal tracheal occlusion with a balloon between 26–28 weeks gestation. In severe cases (liver herniation and LHR <1.0), tracheal occlusion increased lung size as well as survival with an early 7-day survival, late neonatal 28-day survival and survival to discharge of 75%, 58% and 50%, respectively, compared to 9% in contemporary controls. It was also possible to restore the airway prior to birth. This was done either by foetal tracheobronchoscopy at 34 weeks with retrieval of the balloon or by ultrasound-guided puncture of the balloon. In-utero removal avoided the burden of an EXIT procedure and neonatal survival improved (83% compared to 33%). His group feels that foetal endoluminal tracheal occlusion can be considered a minimally invasive foetal therapy improving outcome in highly selected cases. The jury on foetal intervention in this condition is still out. As future refinements in tocolytic and surgical methods develop and as the incidence and associated risks of prematurity decline, tracheal occlusion may have a larger role to play in the management of the more severe cases of CDH given its documented benefit in inducing pulmonary growth. Again, it remains to be seen exactly which infants will benefit most from this intervention.

Congenital cystic adenomatoid malformations (CCAM) are characterised by an overgrowth of terminal respiratory bronchioles that form cysts of various sizes. Prenatally, they can be divided into two categories based on their gross anatomy and ultrasonographic findings. Macrocystic lesions contain single or multiple cysts that are 5 mm in diameter or larger on prenatal ultrasound, whereas microcystic lesions appear echogenic on ultrasound. Bronchopulmonary sequestrations are masses of non-functioning lung tissue that are supplied by an anomalous systemic artery and do not have a bronchial connection to the native tracheobronchial tree. On prenatal ultrasound, they appear as well-defined, echo-dense, homogeneous masses. They may be mistaken for microcystic CCAMs unless colour flow Doppler detects a systemic artery from the aorta to the lung mass. Huge foetal lung lesions have reproducible pathophysiological effects on the developing foetus. Oesophageal compression by the thoracic mass can interfere with foetal swallowing and lead to polyhydramnios. Foetal hydrops may also develop secondary to vena caval obstruction and cardiac compression from the large masses causing extreme mediastinal shift. In some cases, the CCAM or BPS may secrete fluid or lymph and cause foetal hydrops from a tension hydrothorax. Although a large pulmonary lesion diagnosed in utero is an ominous finding, the natural history of these conditions is very variable. Adzick et al. (1998) reported that 15% of their CCAMs decreased in size during the pregnancy and most (68%) extralobar pulmonary sequestration lesions shrank dramatically before birth. Although regression of a lung lesion and associated hydrops has been reported, this is a rare occurrence (daSilva et al. 1996). The management of these lesions during pregnancy will depend on the size of the lesion, the gestational age of the foetus and the development of foetal hydrops, a harbinger of foetal or neonatal death. If the foetus is at 32–34 weeks gestation, consideration should be given to antenatal steroids and early delivery. However, if the foetus develops hydrops before 32 weeks gestation, in utero therapy has been considered. Options tried include foetal thoracentesis, but this has often been found to be ineffective because of rapid reaccumulation of fluid (Adzick et al. 1998). At best, it may serve as a temporising manoeuvre before shunt replacement or resection. Thoracoamniotic shunting of a large predominant cyst in a CCAM may be beneficial provided that there is not a large associated solid component. Successful decompression of a CCAM in a 20-week-gestation foetus was reported by Clark et al. (1987), and since then, there have been many more reports of successful shunt placement in unilocular CCAM lesions (Bernaschek et al. 1994). Adzick's group has managed nine hydropic CCAM pregnancies using thoracoamniotic shunting (Adzick 2003). There was a 61% mean reduction in mass volume following shunt placement. Hydrops resolved following shunting in all cases. The average shunt to delivery time was 13 weeks and 2 days and foetal or neonatal loss was one of nine (11%). They have also treated three foetuses with bronchopulmonary sequestration and hydrops (Adzick et al. 1998). The hydrops appeared to be a consequence of a tension hydrothorax from fluid or lymph secreted by the mass. The hydrops resolved after weekly foetal thoracocentesis in one case and thoracoamniotic shunt placement in the two other cases. All three foetuses survived after delivery at 33–35 weeks gestation, required ventilatory support and subsequently underwent BPS resection. One problem commonly reported with these shunts, however, is that many of them become dislodged or clog even after relatively short periods of time. Furthermore, not all cases will lend themselves to catheter decompression, i.e., large multicystic CCAMs and surgical resection have been attempted in these cases. Adzick et al. (2003) have performed foetal pulmonary lobectomies in 22 cases of CCAM associated with foetal hydrops at 21 to 31 weeks gestation with 11 healthy survivors aged 1–12 years on follow-up. Resections involved a single lobectomy in 16 patients, right middle and lower lobectomies in four patients, extralobar BPS resection in one patient and one left pneumonectomy for CCAM. In one multicystic case, a thoracoamniotic shunt had failed to decompress the mass effect adequately before open foetal surgery. In the 11 foetuses that survived, foetal CCAM resection led to hydrops resolution in 1–2 weeks, return of the mediastinum to the midline within 3 weeks and impressive in utero lung growth. Follow-up developmental testing has been normal in all 11 survivors. However, 11 foetuses did not survive and 6 of these died intraoperatively, usually after developing profound bradycardia after delivery of the mass from the foetal chest. These results demonstrate that surgical resection is reasonably safe, technically feasible, can reverse hydrops over 1–2 weeks and can allow sufficient lung growth to permit survival and normal postnatal development (ADZICK 2003). The clinical focus is now shifting from the technical details of the foetal surgical procedure to the crucial need for better postoperative maternal-foetal monitoring, reliable intraoperative foetal intravascular access and intraoperative foetal echocardiographic haemodynamic assessment in an effort to further reduce the significant morbidity and mortality still associated with this intervention. The role of laser therapy or techniques such as radiofrequency thermal ablation to decrease the size of the foetal lung lesion has still to be elucidated.

Lastly, foetal hydrothoraces, either unilateral or bilateral, are pleural effusions in the foetus that may be primary, due to a chylous leak, or secondary, where the effusions are part of a generalised fluid retention associated with immune or non-immune hydrops. The management of pleural effusions in the foetus is complicated by the difficulty in distinguishing primary from secondary FHT. Chylothorax is the most common cause of primary pleural effusion in the newborn. They are usually unilateral and associated with a good prognosis. In contrast to the neonate, secondary FHT is much more common in the foetus and may be due to a wide variety of maternal and foetal disorders including chromosomal anomalies, cardiovascular anomalies, haematological and gastrointestinal anomalies. Large foetal pleural effusions can lead to hydrops and can cause pulmonary hypoplasia secondary to pulmonary compression. Once again, intervention would depend on the gestational age, the presence of hydrops and the presence of other associated anomalies. Intervention in utero is possible in selected cases. Treatment options usually include single or repeated thoracocenteses and/or thoracoamniotic shunting (MORIN et al. 1994).

There have been significant strides made during the last decade in understanding the natural history and pathophysiology of foetal thoracic lesions. Largely as a result of advances in prenatal ultrasonography, it is now possible to diagnose these lesions in utero and to advise parents on prognosis. It is also feasible to offer the possibility of foetal intervention for the most severely affected cases. However, large gaps still remain in our knowledge. We are unable to accurately predict

pulmonary hypoplasia, the most devastating consequence of foetal thoracic lesions. Selection criteria for foetal intervention are not well defined. The efficacy and superiority of foetal surgery over standard care are still under scrutiny. Most cases of foetal surgery are reserved for those cases with foetal hydrops and a uniformly dismal outcome. Whether foetal surgery is beneficial in the absence of hydrops is difficult to say and made more difficult by the knowledge that some of these lesions undergo spontaneous resolution over time. Equally, until we can better detect and treat preterm labour, the "Achilles heel" of foetal surgery, foetal intervention cannot be undertaken lightly. The diagnosis and treatment of foetal thoracic lesions remain a formidable challenge, but one that can be met with cautious optimism due to the option of foetal intervention, something that was not considered a possibility before.

2.5
Conclusion

The opening decade of the twenty-first century is an exciting time for neonatology because of technical and therapeutic breakthroughs in many areas. Translational research on basic pulmonary biology has rapidly moved from the bench to the bedside, yielding dramatic results. The challenge now is to conduct the clinical research that will establish the evidence on which new therapies are based. Many of the questions will need to be addressed in large, well-designed randomised controlled clinical trials that will hopefully be carried out in the not too distant future.

Reference

Adzick NS, Harrison MR, Crombleholme TM et al (1998) Fetal lung lesions: management and outcome. Am J Obstet Gynecol 179:884–889

Adzick NS (2003) Management of fetal lung lesions. Clin Perinatol 30:481–492

Albanese CT, Lopoo J, Goldstein RB et al (1998) Fetal liver position and perinatal outcome for congenital diaphragmatic hernia. Prenat Diagn 18:1138–1142

Amizuka T, Shimizu H, Niida Y, Ogawa Y (2003) Surfactant therapy in neonates with respiratory failure due to haemorrhagic pulmonary oedema. Eur J Pediatr 182:697–702

Ammari A, Suri M, Milisavljevic V et al (2005) Variables associated with the early failure of nasal CPAP in very low birth weight infants. J Pediatr 147:341–347

Auten RL, Notter RH, Kendig JW et al (1991) Surfactant treatment of full-term newborns with respiratory failure. Pediatrics 87:101–107

Avery ME, Mead J (1959) Surface properties in relation to atelectasis and hyaline membrane disease. Am J Dis Child 97:517–523

Avery ME, Tooley WH, Keller JB et al (1987) Is chronic lung disease preventable? A survey of eight centers. Pediatrics 79:26–30

Barrington KJ, Finer NN (2006) Inhaled nitric oxide for respiratory failure in preterm infants (Review). Cochrane Database of Systematic Reviews 2006, Issue 1

Bartlett RH, Gazzaniga AB, Jefferies R et al (1976) Extracorporeal membrane oxygenation (ECMO) cardiopulmonary support in infancy. Trans Am Soc Artif Intern Organs 22:80

Bartlett RH, Roloff DW, Cornell RG et al (1985) Extracorporeal circulation in neonatal respiratory failure: a prospective randomized study. Pediatrics 76:479–487

Beardsmore C, Dundas I, Poole K et al (2000) Respiratory function in survivors of the United Kingdom Extracorporeal Membrane Oxygenation Trial. Am J Respir Crit Care Med 161:1129–1135

Bernaschek G, Deutinger J, Hansmann M et al (1994) Fetoamniotic shunting: report of the experience of four European centers. Prenat Diagn 14:821–833

Bernstein G, Mannino FL, Heldt GP et al (1996) Randomized multicenter trial comparing synchronized and conventional intermittent mandatory ventilation in neonates. J Pediatr 128:453–463

Bhuta T, Henderson-Smart DJ (1998a) Elective high frequency jet ventilation versus conventional ventilation for respiratory distress syndrome in preterm infants (Review). Cochrane Database of Systematic Reviews 1998, Issue 2

Bhuta T, Henderson-Smart DJ (1998b) Rescue high frequency oscillatory ventilation versus conventional ventilation for pulmonary dysfunction in preterm infants (Review). Cochrane Database of Systematic Reviews 1998, Issue 2

Bhuta T, Clark RH, Henderson-Smart DJ (2001) Rescue high frequency oscillatory ventilation versus conventional ventilation for infants with severe pulmonary dysfunction born at or near term (Review). Cochrane Database of Systematic Reviews 2001, Issue 1

Booth C, Premkumar MH, Yannoulis A et al (2006) Sustainable use of continuous positive airway pressure in extremely preterm infants during the first week after delivery. Arch Dis Child 91:F398–F402

Bos AP, Tibboel D, Hazebroek FWJ et al (1991) Surfactant replacement therapy in high-risk congenital diaphragmatic hernia. Lancet 338:1279

Carlo WA, Ambalavanan N (1999) Conventional mechanical ventilation: traditional and new strategies. NeoReviews e117–e126

Carter JM, Gerstmann DR, Clark RH et al (1990) High-frequency oscillatory ventilation and extracorporeal membrane oxygenation for the treatment of acute neonatal respiratory failure. Pediatrics 85:159–164

Chan V, Greenough A (1993) Randomised controlled trial of weaning by patient triggered ventilation or conventional ventilation. Eur J Pediatr 152:51–54

Clark RH, Yoder BA, Sell MS (1994) Prospective randomised comparision of high frequency oscillation and conventional ventilation in candidates for extracorporeal membrane oxygenation. J Pediatr 124:447–454

Clark SL, Vitale DJ, Mintom SD et al (1987) Successful fetal therapy for cystic adenomatoid malformation associated with second trimester hydrops. Am J Obstet Gynecol 157:294–297

Corbet A, Gerdes J, Long W et al (1995) Double-blind randomized trial of one versus three prophylactic doses of synthetic surfactant in 826 neonates weighing 700 to 1,100 g: effects on mortality rate. J Pediatr 126:969–978

Cortes RA, Keller RL, Townsend T et al (2005) Survival of severe congenital diaphragmatic hernia has morbid consequences. J Pediatr Surg 40:36–45

Courtney SE, Durand DJ, Asselin JM et al (2002) High frequency oscillatory ventilation versus conventional mechanical ventilation for very low birthweight infants. N Eng J Med 347:643–652

Crombleholme TM, Adzick NS, deLorimier AA et al (1990) Carotid artery reconstruction following extracorporeal membrane oxygenation. Am J Dis Child 144:872–874

daSilva OP, Ramamam R, Romano W et al (1996) Nonimmune hydrops fetalis, pulmonary sequestration and favorable neonatal outcome. Obstet Gynecol 88:681–683

Dassieu G, Brochard L, Benani M, Avenel S, Danan C (2000) Continuous tracheal gas insufflation in preterm infants with hyaline membrane disease. Am J Respir Crit Care Med 162:826–831

Davies MW, Sargent PH (2004) Partial liquid ventilation for the prevention of mortality and morbidity in paediatric acute lung injury and acute respiratory distress syndrome (Review). Cochrane Database of Systematic Reviews, Issue 4

Davis PG, Lemyre B, De Paoli AG (2001) Nasal intermittent positive pressure ventilation (NIPPV) versus nasal continuous positive airway pressure (NCPAP) for preterm infants after extubation (Review). Cochrane Database of Systematic Reviews, Issue 3

Davis PG, Henderson-Smart DJ (2003) Nasal continuous positive airway pressure immediately after extubation for preventing morbidity in preterm infants (Review). Cochrane Database of Systematic Reviews, Issue 2

deLemos RA, Coalson JJ, deLemos JA et al (1992) Rescue ventilation with high frequency oscillation in premature baboons with hyaline membrane disease. Pediatr Pulmonol 12:29–36

deLemos RA, Coalson JJ, Gerstmann DR (1987) Ventilatory management of infant baboons with hyaline membrane disease. Pediatr Res 21:594–602

Deprest J, Jani J, Cannie M et al (2006) Prenatal intervention for isolated congenital diaphragmatic hernia. Curr Opin Obstet Gynecol 18:355–367

DiFiore JW, Fauza DO, Slavin R et al (1994) Experimental fetal tracheal ligation reverses the structural and physiological effects of pulmonary hypoplasia in congenital diaphragmatic hernia. J Pediatr Surg 29:248–256

Dimitriou G, Greenough A, Griffin F, Chan V (1995) Synchronous intermittent mandatory ventilation modes compared with patient triggered ventilation during weaning. Arch Dis Child 72:F188–190

Donn SM, Nicks JJ, Becker MA (1994) Flow synchronised ventilation of preterm infants with respiratory distress syndrome. J Perinatol 14:90–94

Dreyfus D, Saumon G (1993) Role of tidal volume FRC and end-inspiratory volumes in development of pulmonary edema following mechanical ventilation Am Rev Respir Dis 148:1194–1203

Dreyfuss D, Saumon G (1998) Ventilator-induced lung injury. Lessons from experimental studies. Am J Respir Crit Care Med 157:294–323

Dunn MS, Shennan AT, Possmayer F (1990) Single- versus multiple- dose surfactant replacement therapy in neonates of 30–36 weeks gestation with respiratory distress syndrome. Pediatrics 86:564–571

Dunn MS, Shennan AT, Zayack D et al (1991) Bovine surfactant replacement therapy: A comparison of two retreatment strategies in premature infants with RDS. Pediatr Res 29:212A

Dwortez AR, Moya FR, Sabo B et al (1989) Survival of infants with persistent pulmonary hypertension without extracorporeal membrane oxygenation. Pediatrics 84:1–6

Eichenwald EC (2006) High frequency oscillatory ventilation: is equivalence with conventional mechanical ventilation enough. Arch Dis Child 91:F315–F317

Elbourne D, Field D, Mugford M (2002) Extracorporeal membrane oxygenation for severe respiratory failure in newborn infants (Review). Cochrane Database of Systematic Reviews 2002, Issue 1

Emerson JM (1959) Apparatus for vibrating portions of a patient's airway. US Patent 2:918–919

Finer NN, Tierney A, Etches PC et al (1998) Congenital diaphragmatic hernia: developing a protocolized approach. J Pediatr Surg 33:1331–1337

Finer N (2006) To intubate or not–that is the question: continuous positive airway pressure versus surfactant and extremely low birthweight infants. Arch Dis Child 91: F392–F394

Finer NN, Barrington KJ (2006) Nitric oxide for respiratory failure in infants born at or near term (Review). Cochrane Database of Systematic Reviews 2006, Issue 4

Fredberg JJ, Keefe DH, Glass GM et al (1985) Alveolar pressure inhomogeneity during small amplitude high frequency oscillation. J Appl Physiol 57:788

Froese AB, McCulloch PR, Suguira M et al (1993) Optimizing alveolar expansion prolongs the effectiveness of exogenous surfactant therapy in the adult rabbit. Am Rev Respir Dis 148:569–577

Fuhrman B, Blumer J, Togo-Figueroa L et al (1998) Multicenter, randomized, controlled trial (RCT) of LiquiVent® partial liquid ventilation in paediatric ARDS. Proceedings of the Eleventh Annual Pediatric Critical Care Colloquium, Chicago, IL, A17

Fujimoto S, Togari H, Yamaguchi N et al (1994) Hypocarbia and cystic periventricular leucomalacia in premature infants. Arch Dis Child 71:F107–110

Fujiwara T, Maeta H, Chida S et al (1980) Artificial surfactant therapy in hyaline membrane disease. Lancet 1(8159):55–59

Garland JS, Buck RK, Allred EN, Leviton A (1995) Hypocarbia before surfactant therapy appears to increase bronchopulmonary dysplasia risk in infants with respiratory distress syndrome. Arch Pediatr Adolesc Med 149:617–622

Gill BS, Neville HL, Khan AM et al (2002) Delayed institution of extracorporeal membrane oxygenation is associated with increased mortality rate and prolonged hospital stay. J Pediatr Surg 37:7–10

Glick PL, Leach CL, Besner GE et al (1992) Pathophysiology of congenital diaphragmatic hernia III: Exogenous surfactant therapy for the high risk neonate with CDH. J Pediatr Surg 27:866–869

Graziani LJ, Spitzer AR, Mitchell DG et al (1992) Mechanical ventilation in preterm infants: neurosonographic and developmental studies. Pediatrics 90:515–522

Greenough A, Wood S, Morley CJ et al (1984) Pancuronium prevents pneumothoraces in ventilated premature babies who actively expire against positive pressure ventilation. Lancet 1:1–14

Greenough A, Milner AD, Dimitriou G (2004) Synchronized mechanical ventilation for respiratory support in newborn infants (Review). Cochrane Database of Systematic Reviews 2004, Issue 3

Greenspan JS, Cleary GM, Wolfson MR (1998) Is liquid ventilation a reasonable alternative? Clin Perinatol 25:137–157

Greenspan JS, Fox WW, Rubenstein SD et al (1997) Partial liquid ventilation in critically ill infants receiving extracorporeal life support. Pediatrics 99:e2

Greenspan JS, Wolfson MR, Rubenstein SD et al (1989) Liquid ventilation in preterm babies. Lancet 2: 1095

Greenspan JS, Wolfson MR, Rubenstein SD, Shaffer TH (1990) Liquid ventilation of human preterm infants. J Pediatr 117:106–111

Harrison MR, Adzick NS, Bullard KM et al (1997) Correction of congenital diaphragmatic hernia in utero VII: A prospective trial. J Pediatr Surg 32:1637–1642

Harrison MR, Adzick NS, Flake AW et al (1993) Correction of congenital diaphragmatic hernia in utero VI: Hard-earned lessons. J Pediatr Surg 28:1411–1417

Harrison MR, Mychaliska GB, Albanese CT et al (1998) Correction of congenital diaphragmatic hernias in utero IX: Fetuses with poor prognosis (liver herniation and low lung-to-head ratio) can be saved by fetoscopic temporary tracheal occlusion. J Pediatr Surg 33:1017–1023

Harrison MR, Keller RL, Hawgood SB et al (2003) A randomized trial of fetal endoscopic tracheal occlusion for severe fetal congenital diaphragmatic hernia. N Eng J Med 349:1916–1924

Heijman K, Sjostrand U (1974) Treatment of the respiratory distress syndrome–preliminary report. Opusc Med 19:235

Henderson-Smart DJ, Bhuta T, Cools F, Offringa M (2003) Elective high frequency oscillatory ventilation versus conventional ventilation for acute pulmonary dysfunction in preterm infants (Review). Cochrane Database of Systematic Reviews, 2003, Issue 4

Hernandez LA, Peevy KJ, Moise RA, Parker JC (1989) Chest wall restriction limits high airway pressure-induced lung injury in young rabbits. J Appl Physiol 66:2364–2368

HIFI Study Group (1989) High-frequency oscillatory ventilation compared with conventional mechanical ventilation in the treatment of respiratory failure in preterm infants. N Eng J Med 320:88–93

HIFI Study Group (1990) High-frequency oscillatory ventilation compared with conventional intermittent mechanical ventilation in the treatment of respiratory failure in preterm infants: neurodevelopmental status at 16 to 24 months of post term age. J Pediatr 17:939–946

HiFO Study Group (1993) Randomised study of high frequency ventilation in infants with severe respiratory distress. J Pediatr 122:609–619

Hill JD, O'Brien TG, Murray JJ et al (1972) Prolonged extracorporeal oxygenation for acute post-traumatic respiratory failure (shock lung syndrome). Use of the Bramson membrane lung. N Eng J Med 286:629–34

Hintz SR, Suttner DM, Sheehan AM et al (2000) Decreased use of neonatal extracorporeal membrane oxygenation (ECMO): How new treatment modalities have affected ECMO utilization. Pediatrics 106:1339–1343

Ho JJ, Subramaniam P, Henderson-Smart DJ, Davis PG (2002a) Continuous distending pressure for respiratory distress syndrome in preterm infants (Review). Cochrane Database of Systematic Reviews 2002, Issue 2

Ho JJ, Henderson-Smart DJ, Davis PG (2002b) Early versus delayed initiation of continuous distending pressure for respiratory distress syndrome in preterm infants (Review). Cochrane Database of Systematic Reviews 2002, Issue 2

Hui TT, Danielson PD, Anderson KD et al (2002) The impact of changing neonatal respiratory management in extracorporeal membrane oxygenation utilization. J Pediatr Surg 37:703–705

Jackson JC, Troug WE, Standaert TA et al (1991) Effect of high frequency ventilation on the development of alveolar edema on premature monkeys at risk of hyaline membrane disease. Am Rev Respir Dis 143:865–871

Jackson JC, Truog WE, Standaert TA et al (1994) Reduction in lung injury after combined surfactant and high frequency ventilation. Am J Respir Crit Care Med 150:534–539

Jaunieaux V, Duran A, Levi-Valensi P (1994) Synchronized intermittent mandatory ventilation with and without pressure support ventilation in weaning patients with COPD from mechanical ventilation. Chest 105:1204–1210

Jobe AH, Ikegami M (1998) Mechanisms initiating lung injury in the preterm. Early Hum Dev 53:81–94

Jobe AH, Ikegami M (2001) Biology of surfactant. Clin Perinatol 28:655–669

Johnson AH, Peacock JL, Greenough A et al (2002) High-frequency oscillatory ventilation for the prevention of chronic lung disease of prematurity. N Eng J Med 347:633–642

Joshi VH, Bhuta T (2006) Rescue high frequency jet ventilation versus conventional ventilation for severe pulmonary dysfunction in preterm infants (Review). Cochrane Database of Systematic Reviews 2006, Issue 1

Kanak R, Fahey PJ, Vanderwarf C (1985) Oxygen cost of breathing changes dependent upon mode of mechanical ventilation. Chest 87:126–127

Karamanoukian HL, Glick PL, Zayek M et al (1994) Inhaled nitric oxide in congenital hypoplasia of the lungs due to diaphragmatic hernia or oligohydramnios. Pediatrics 94:715–718

Karl TR, Iyer KS, Sano et al (1990) Infant ECMO cannulation technique allowing preservation of carotid and jugular veins. Ann Thorac Surg 50:488–489

Kattwinkel J, Bloom BT, Delmore P et al (2000) High-versus low-threshold surfactant retreatment for neonatal respiratory distress syndrome. Pediatrics 106:282–288

Kendig JW, Ryan RM, Sinkin RA et al (1998) Comparison of two strategies for surfactant prophylaxis in very premature infants: a multicenter randomized trial. Pediatrics 101:1006–1012

Keszler M, Donna SM, Bucciarelli RL et al (1991) Multicenter controlled trial comparing high frequency jet ventilation and conventional mechanical ventilation in newborn infants with pulmonary interstitial emphysema. J Pediatr 119:85–93

Khammash H, Perlman M, Wojtulewicz J et al (1993) Surfactant therapy in full-term neonates with severe respiratory failure. Pediatrics 92:135–139

Kinsella JP, Neish SR, Shaffer E, Abman AH (1992) Low dose inhalational nitric oxide in persistent pulmonary hypertension of the newborn. Lancet 340:819–820

Kinsella JP, Schmidt JM, Griebel J et al (1995) Inhaled nitric oxide treatment for stabilisation and emergency medical transport of critically ill newborns and infants. Pediatrics 95:773–776

Kinsella JP, Truog WE, Walsh WF et al (1997) Randomised, multicenter trial of inhaled nitric oxide and high frequency oscillatory ventilaton in severe, persistent pulmonary hypertension of the newborn. J Pediatr 131:55–62

Kirkpatrick BV, Krummel TM, Mueller DG et al (1983) Use of extracorporeal membrane oxygenation for respiratory failure in term infants. Pediatrics 72:872–876

Kohlet D, Perlman M, Kirpalani H (1988) High frequency oscillation in the rescue of infants with persistent pulmonary hypertension. Crit Care Med 16:510–516

Kraybill EN, Runyan DK, Bose CL, Khan JH (1989) Risk factors for chronic lung disease in infants with birth weights 751 to 1,000 grams. J Pediatr 115:115–120

Leach CL, Greenspan JS, Rubenstein SD et al (1996) Partial liquid ventilation with perflubron in premature infants with severe respiratory distress syndrome. N Eng J Med 335:761–767

Lehr JL, Butler JP, Westerman PA et al (1985) Photographic measurement of pleural surface motion during lung oscillation. J Appl Physiol 59:623

Lipshutz GS, Albanese CT, Feldstein et al (1997) Prospective analysis of lung-to-head ratio predicts survival with patients with prenatally diagnosed congenital diaphragmatic hernia. J Pediatr Surg 32:1634–1636

Lotze A, Mitchell BR, Bulas DI et al (1998) Multicentered study of surfactant (beractant) use in the treatment of term infants with severe respiratory failure. J Pediatr 132:40–47

Mariani G, Cifuentes J, Carlo WA (1999) Randomized controlled trial of permissive hypercapnia in preterm infants. Pediatrics 104:1082–1088

Marlow N, Greenough A, Peacock JL et al (2006) Randomised trial of high frequency oscillatory ventilation or conventional ventilation in babies of gestational age 28 weeks or less: respiratory and neurological outcomes at 2 years. Arch Dis Child 91:F320–326

McCallion N, Davis PG, Morley CJ (2005) Volume-targeted versus pressure-limited ventilation in the neonate (Review). Cochrane Database of Systematic Reviews 2005, Issue 3

McCulloch PR, Forkert PG, Froese AB (1988) Lung volume maintenance prevents lung injury during high frequency oscillatory ventilation in surfactant deficient lungs. Am Rev Respir Dis 137:1185–1192

Meredith KS, deLemos RA, Coalson JJ et al (1989) Role of lung injury in the pathogenesis of hyaline membrane disease in premature baboons. J Appl Physiol 66:2150–2158

Mestan KK, Marks JD, Hecox K et al (2005) Neurodevelopmental outcomes of premature infants treated with inhaled nitric oxide. N Eng J Med 353:23–32

Morin L, Crombleholme TM, D'Alton ME (1994) Prenatal diagnosis and management of fetal thoracic lesions. Sem Perinatol 18:228–253

Moya FR, Gadzinowski J, Bancalari E at al (2005) A multicenter, randomized, masked comparison trial of lucinactant, colfoseril palmitate and beractant for the prevention of respiratory distress syndrome among very preterm infants. Pediatrics 115:1018–1029

Nading JH (1989) Historical controls for extracorporeal membrane oxygenation in neonates. Crit Care Med 17:423–425

Nakayama DK, Motoyama EK, Tagge EM (1991) Effect of preoperative stabilization on respiratory system compliance and outcome in newborn infants with congenital diaphragmatic hernia. J Pediatr 118:793–799

O'Rourke PP, Crone R, Vacanti J et al (1989) Extracorporeal membrane oxygenation and conventional medical therapy in neonates with persistent pulmonary hypertension of the newborn: a prospective randomized study. Pediatrics 84:957–963

Oxford Region Controlled Trial of Artificial Ventilation (OCTAVE) Study Group (1991) Multicentre randomized controlled trial of high against low frequency positive pressure ventilation. Arch Dis Child 66:770–775

Pandit PB, Dunn MS, Colucci EA (1995) Surfactnat therapy in neonates with respiratory deterioration due to pulmonary haemorrhage. Pediatrics 95:32–36

Perlman LM, Goodman S, Kreusser KL et al (1985) Reduction in intraventricular haemorrhage by elimination of fluctuating cerebral blood flow velocity in preterm infants with respiratory distress syndrome. N Eng J Med 312:1353–1357

Pfister RH, Soll RF, Wiswell T (2006) Protein-containing synthetic surfactant versus protein-free synthetic surfactant for the prevention and treatment of respiratory distress syndrome (Protocol). Cochrane Database of Systematic Reviews 2006, Issue 4

Pohlandt F, Suale H, Schroder H et al (1992) Decreased incidence of extra-alveolar air leakage or death prior to air leakage in high versus low rate positive pressure ventilation: results of a randomized seven center trial in preterm infants. E J Pediatr 151:904–909

Pranikoff T, Gauger PG, Hirschl RB (1996) Partial liquid ventilation in newborn infants with congenital diaphragmatic hernia. J Pediatr Surg 31:613–618

Raju TN, Langenberg P (1993) Pulmonary haemorrhage and exogenous surfactant. J Pediatr 123:603–610

Roberts JD, Fineman JR, Morin FC et al (1997) Inhaled nitric oxide and persistent pulmonary hypertension of the newborn. N Eng J Med 336:605–610

Roberts JD, Polander DM, Lang P, Zapol WM (1992) Inhaled nitric oxide in persistent pulmonary hypertension of the newborn. Lancet 340:818–819

Schreiber MD, Gin-Mestan K, Marks JD et al (2003) Inhaled nitric oxide in premature infants with the respiratory distress syndrome. N Eng J Med 349:2099–2107

Schulze A, Bancalari E (2001) Proportional assist ventilation in infants. Clin Perinatol 28(3):561–578

Schulze A, Gerhardt T, Musante G et al (1999) Proportional assist ventilation in low birth weight infants with acute respiratory disease: A comparison to assist/control and conventional mehanical ventilation. J Pediatr 135:339–344

Shaffer TH, Wolfson MR, Greenspan JA (1999) Liquid ventilation: current status. NeoReviews e134–e142

Short BL, Pearson GD (1986) Neonatal extracorporeal membrane oxygenation: a review. J Intensive Care Med 1:47–54

Sinha SK, Donn SM (1996) Advances in neonatal conventional ventilation. Arch Dis Child 75:F135–140

Sinha SK, Donn SM (2001) Volume-controlled ventilation, variations on a theme. Clin Perinatol 28(3):547–560

Sinha SK, Lacaze-Masmonteil T, Valls i Soler A et al (2005) A multicenter, randomized, controlled trial of lucinactant versus poractant alfa among very premature infants at high risk for respiratory distress syndrome. Pediatrics 115:1030–1038

Sjostrand U (1980) High-frequency positive pressure ventilation (HPPPV): a review. Crit Care Med 8:345–364

Skarsgard ED, Meuli M, VanderWall KJ et al (1996) Fetal endoscopic tracheal occlusion ("Fentendo-PLUG") for congenital diaphragmatic hernia. J Pediatr Surg 31:1335–1338

Soll RF (1997) Prophylactic natural surfactant extract for preventing morbidity and mortality in preterm infants (Review). Cochrane Database of Systematic Reviews 1997, Issue 4

Soll RF (1998) Prophylactic synthetic surfactant for preventing morbidity and mortality in preterm infants (Review). Cochrane Database of Systematic Reviews 1998, Issue 2

Soll RF (1999) Multiple versus single dose natural surfactant extract for severe neonatal respiratory distress syndrome (Review). Cochrane Database of Systematic Reviews 1999, Issue 2

Soll RF, Blanco F (2001) Natural surfactant extract versus synthetic surfactant for neonatal respiratory distress syndrome (Review). Cochrane Database of Systematic Reviews 2001, Issue 2

Soll RF, Dargaville P (2000) Surfactant for meconium aspiration syndrome in full term infants (Review). Cochrane Database of Systematic Reviews 2000, Issue 2

Soll RF, Morley CJ (2001) Prophylactic versus selective use of surfactant in preventing morbidity and mortality in preterm infants (Cochrane Review). In: The Cochrane Library, Issue 4, 2001 Oxford: Update Software

Speer CP, Robertson B, Curstedt T et al (1992) Randomised European multicenter trial of surfactant replacement therapy for severe neonatal respiratory distress syndrome single versus multiple doses of Curosurf. Pediatrics 89:13–20

Stevens TP, Blennow M, Soll RF (2004) Early surfactant administration with brief ventilation vs selective surfactant and continued mechanical ventilation for preterm infants with or at risk for respiratory distress syndrome (Review). Cochrane Database of Systematic Reviews 2004, Issue 3

Subramaniam P, Henderson-Smart DJ, Davis PG (2005) Prophylactic nasal continuous positive airway pressure for preventing morbidity and mortality in very preterm infants (Review). Cochrane Database of Systematic Reviews 2005, Issue 3

Suresh GK, Soll RF (2001) Current surfactant use in premature infants. Clin Perinatol 28:671–694

The Clinical Inhaled Nitric Oxide Research Group (2000) Low dose nitric oxide therapy for persistent pulmonary hypertension of the newborn. N Eng J Med 342:469–474

The I-NO/PPHN Study Group (1998) Inhaled nitric oxide for the early treatment of persistent pulmonary hypertension

of the term newborn: a randomized, double-masked, placebo-controlled, dose-response, multi-center study. Pediatrics 101:325–334

The Neonatal Inhaled Nitric Oxide Study Group (1997) Inhaled nitric oxide in full-term and nearly full-term infants with hypoxic respiratory failure. N Eng J Med 336:597–604

The Neonatal Inhaled Nitric Oxide Study Group (2000) Inhaled nitric oxide in term and near-term infants: neurodevelopmental follow-up of the neonatal inhaled nitric oxide study group. J Pediatr 136:611–617

The OSIRIS Collaborative Group (1992) Early versus delayed neonatal administration of a synthetic surfactant–the judgement of OSIRIS. Lancet 340:1363–1369

Thomson M, on behalf of the IFDAS investigators (2002) Early nasal continuous positive airway pressure with surfactant for neonates at risk of RDS. Pediatr Res 45:321A

Tooley J, Dyke M (2003) Randomized study of nasal continuous positive airway pressure in the preterm infant with respiratory distress syndrome. Acta Paediatrica 92:1170–1174

UK Collaborative ECMO Trial Group (1996) UK Collaborative randomised trial of neonatal extracorporeal membrane oxygenation. Lancet 348:75–82

UK Collaborative ECMO Trial Group (2001) UK Collaborative randomised trial of neonatal extracorporeal membrane oxygenation: follow-up to age 4 years. Lancet 357:1094–1096

UK Collaborative ECMO Trial Group (2006) UK Collaborative randomised trial of neonatal extracorporeal membrane oxygenation: follow-up to age 7 years. Pediatrics 117:e845–e854

Van Marter LJ, Allred EN, Pagano M et al (2000) Do clinical markers of barotraumas and oxygen toxicity explain interhospital variation in rates of chronic lung disease? Pediatrics 105:1194–1201

Verder H, Robertson B, Greisen G et al (1994) Surfactant therapy and nasal continuous positive airway pressure for newborns with respiratory distress syndrome. N Eng J Med 331:1051–1055

Walsh-Sukys MC, Tyson JE, Wright LL et al (2000) Persistent pulmonary hypertension of the newborn in the era before nitric oxide: Practice variations and outcomes. Pediatrics 105:14–20

Wiswell TE, Graziani LJ, Kornhauser MS et al (1996) High-frequency jet ventilation in the early management of respiratory distress syndrome is associated with a greater risk for adverse outcomes. Pediatrics 98:1035–1043

Wolfson MR, Shaffer TH (2005) Pulmonary applications of perfluorochemical liquids: ventilation and beyond. Paed Respir Reviews 6:117–127

Woodgate PG, Davies MW (2001) Permisssive hypercapnia for the prevention of morbidity and mortality in mechanically ventilated newborn infants (Review). Cochrane Database of Systematic Reviews 2001, Issue 2

Yost CC, Soll RF (1999) Early versus delayed selective surfactant treatment for neonatal respiratory distress syndrome (Review). Cochrane Database of Systematic Reviews 1999, Issue 4

Zapol WM, Snider MT, Hill DJ et al (1979) Extracorporeal membrane oxygenation in severe acute respiratory failure: A randomized prospective study. JAMA 242:2193–2196

Computed and Digital Radiography in Neonatal Chest Examination

Amaka C. Offiah

CONTENTS

A. C. Offiah, BSc, MBBS, MRCP, FRCR, PhD
Consultant, Academic Paediatric Radiology, Great Ormond Street Hospital for Children, Great Ormond Street, London, WC1N 3JH, UK

3.1 General Considerations

3.1.1 Indications

In the neonate (as well as other paediatric and older age groups), chest radiography (be it digital or analogue) remains the most requested imaging modality for investigation of respiratory and cardiac pathology. This is particularly true for preterm infants and neonates on intensive care, for whom daily portable chest radiographs are not uncommon. While other imaging modalities [such as ultrasound, fluoroscopy, computed tomography (CT), nuclear medicine, bronchoscopy, angiography and magnetic resonance imaging] may subsequently be employed, radiography is the most valuable initial investigation for neonatal respiratory disorders (Arthur 2001). Some of the major indications for chest radiography in the neonate are listed below.

1. Abnormalities of aeration
   a. Congenital
      i. Developmental
         1. Tracheobronchomalacia
         2. Congenital diaphragmatic hernia
         3. Pulmonary hypoplasia
         4. Congenital lobar emphysema
         5. Congenital cystic adenomatoid malformation/pulmonary sequestration spectrum
         6. Bronchial atresia
      ii. Infection
   b. Arising from premature birth/perinatal complications
      i. Hyaline membrane disease
      ii. Transient tachypnoea of the newborn

iii. Meconium aspiration

iv. Infection

c. Acquired/iatrogenic

 i. Bronchopulmonary dysplasia

 ii. Pulmonary interstitial emphysema

 iii. Pneumothorax/air leaks

 iv. Pulmonary haemorrhage

 v. Infection

2. Abnormalities of circulation

 a. Cyanosis without congestive heart failure or respiratory distress (e.g., TGA, tetralogy of Fallot)

 b. Cyanosis with congestive heart failure or respiratory distress (e.g., Ebstein's anomaly)

 c. Congestive cardiac failure, without cyanosis (e.g., coarctation of the aorta)

 d. Collapse/shock (e.g., hypoplastic left heart syndrome)

3. Abnormalities of the thorax

 a. Neuromuscular

 b. Skeletal dysplasia

 i. Asphyxiating thoracic dystrophy

4. Lines, tubes and wires (iatrogenic)

 a. Umbilical arterial/venous catheter

 b. Percutaneous (PICC) long line

 c. Extra corporeal membrane oxygenation (ECMO) catheters

 d. Chest/mediastinal drains

 e. Endotracheal tubes (ETT)

 f. Nasogastric tubes (NGT)

5. Other

 a. As part of a skeletal survey for suspected dysplasia

 b. As part of a skeletal survey for suspected abuse (relatively uncommon in this age group)

3.1.2
Radiographic Technique

The radiographic technique remains the same whether performing analogue (film/screen) or digital radiography of the neonatal chest. The emphasis is on high quality and low exposure in keeping with the ALARA principle (see also Sect. 3.2.4). In a bid to standardise image quality, the Community of European Commissions (CEC) has developed imaging guidelines/criteria for paediatric and adult radiographic techniques (CEC 1996; EUR 1996). The assumption is that radiographs of sufficient quality to allow the depiction of important anatomical structures are therefore of sufficient quality to al-

low the detection of pathology. The CEC criteria for the paediatric chest radiograph are summarised in Table 3.1.

Table 3.1. The Commission of European Communities Quality Criteria for Chest Radiographs in Children (EUR 1996)*

Number	Criterion
1.1	Performed at peak of inspiration, except for suspected foreign body aspiration
1.2	Reproduction** of the thorax without rotation and tilting
1.3	Reproduction of the chest must extend from just above the apices of the lungs to T12/L1
1.4	Reproduction of the vascular pattern in central 2/3 of the lungs
1.5	Reproduction of the trachea and the proximal bronchi
1.6	Visually sharp reproduction of the diaphragm and costo-phrenic angles
1.7	Reproduction of the spine and paraspinal structures and visualisation of the retrocardiac lung and the mediastinum

* The CEC also recommend a standard entrance surface dose of 100 Gy (for a 5-year-old child), 60–80 kV and an exposure time of <10 ms (please note that these parameters refer to film/screen systems). However the criteria listed in the Table are applicable to all chest radiographs regardless of the imaging system used to produce them

** Visualisation = characteristic features are detectable but details are not fully reproduced; features just visible
Reproduction = details of anatomical structures are visible, but not necessarily clearly defined; details emerging
Visually sharp reproduction = anatomical details are clearly defined; details clear

It should be emphasised that these guidelines were developed for film/screen systems. However, although imaging parameters will vary, the CEC (semi-objective) criteria are applicable to all chest radiographs regardless of the imaging system used to produce them.

When obtaining the radiograph, careful positioning of the neonate should be aimed for, to avoid artefact produced by rotation; to avoid the erroneous diagnosis of cardiomegaly and/or mediastinal shift; to avoid the misdiagnosis of a pathological cause for differences in radiolucency of the hemithoraces; and to allow precise interpretation of the position of lines, catheters, etc. Neonatal chest radiographs are taken in the supine (AP) position. If possible,

the arms should be extended to prevent the scapulae from obscuring lung pathology. The beam should be centred at the nipple line and collimated to the outer chest margins (BONTRAGER 1993). With digital systems the radiographer/radiologist is able to apply electrical "shutters" as a post processing capability of the system. This practise conceals poor collimation technique, which will almost certainly have led to increased radiation exposure to the patient. In this regard, the BIR recommends that all four collimation marks be visible on any radiograph, regardless of the system from which it was produced (BIR 2001).

A good quality radiograph should not be rotated, and should extend from lung apices to the T12/L1 level (EUR 1996). If the position of umbilical venous/arterial catheters is to be assessed, then an additional abdominal radiograph (or single chest radiograph including the upper two thirds of the abdomen) is indicated.

Excessive handling of sick neonates will lead to episodes of hypoxia and bradycardia. Indeed up to 75% of hypoxemic episodes in neonates are associated with handling (LONG 1980). The radiographer obtaining a chest radiograph on a neonate on intensive care will usually have to place the cassette/imaging plate under the neonate. Careful handling is mandatory. SLADE et al. (2005) advocate the use of specially designed incubators with a facility for placing the imaging plate/cassette in a tray beneath the mattress ("under-tray" technique), thereby avoiding the need to handle the neonate altogether. These authors have shown that radiographs obtained with the under-tray technique have at least the same image quality as those obtained with the standard direct contact method.

It should be noted that although portable radiographs can be obtained with direct digital radiographic imaging (DR), cost implications are prohibitive; see Section 3.2.1.4 below.

3.1.3
Expected Findings, Normal Variants and Artefacts

3.1.3.1
The Normal Neonatal Chest Radiograph

The following refers to straight AP supine chest radiographs (Fig. 3.1). Both lungs should be symmetrically aerated, and therefore have uniform radiolucency within minutes of birth. Neonates lack the normal lordosis seen in older children; therefore the clavicles may be projected above the first ribs. The diaphragms should be dome-shaped and lie at the level of the sixth rib anteriorly or eighth rib posteriorly. However care should be taken in assessing lung volumes in the neonate by this method (BRAMSON 2005).

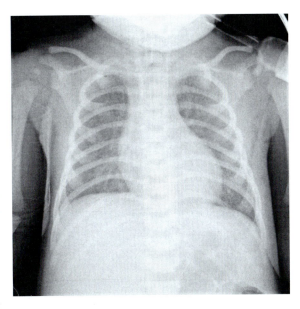

Fig. 3.1. Normal appearance of neonatal chest radiograph

The transverse cardiothoracic ratio should be <60%. The shape and size of the thymic shadow is variable; however the thymus should normally be clearly visible. Classical appearances include a wavy outer border and the "sail sign". It may occupy the entire upper chest or simulate lobar consolidation (Fig. 3.2).

Stress causes the normal neonatal thymus to involute; therefore the diagnosis of thymic aplasia (Di George syndrome) should be made with caution in a sick neonate (an ultrasound scan may be indicated). Vascular markings are well seen centrally, but are not visualised in the periphery (outer one third). An "air bronchogram" appearance may be seen in the left lower lobe behind the cardiac silhouette, and a diagnosis of pneumonia should be avoided.

The thoracic vertebrae are clearly visualised. The spinal arches may not be fused in the early neonatal period. Therefore it is normal for the vertebral bodies to have a central defect that should not be mistaken for sagittal clefts or hemivertebrae.

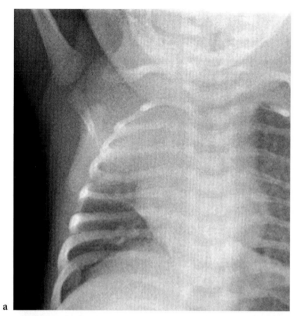

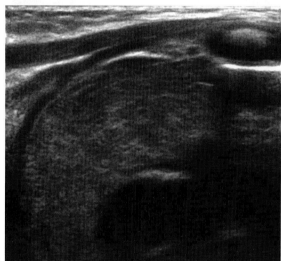

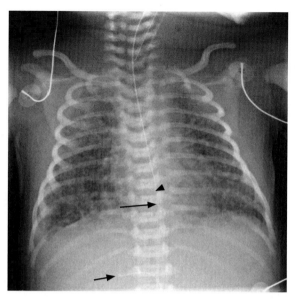

Fig. 3.3. The tip of the nasogastric tube lies at the level of T9 (*arrowhead*) and should be advanced. Note the satisfactory position of the umbilical arterial catheter (*long arrow*). The tip of the umbilical venous catheter (*short arrow*) lies within the right hepatic vein and should be withdrawn

a

b

Fig. 3.2. a This neonate had persistent "consolidation" of the right upper lobe that did not respond to treatment. **b** An ultrasound confirmed the "consolidation" to be a normal thymus

3.1.3.2
Nasogastric, Replogle and Endotracheal Tubes

Nasogastric tubes are recognisable by the continuous radio-opaque line in their walls. In the chest they should run distally in the midline to loop within the stomach. The tip should lie well below the left hemidiaphragm and if at or above the level of the gastro-oesophageal junction (Fig. 3.3) should be advanced.

Replogle tubes are double-lumen sump tubes first introduced in 1963 (Replogle 1963). They are recognised (and distinguished from nasogastric tubes) by the discontinuous radio-opaque line in their walls (Fig. 3.4).

They enable continuous suction of the upper pouch of neonates and infants with oesophageal atresia. The precise position of their tips is therefore variable; they should not be mistaken for high-lying nasogastric tubes.

The endotracheal tube also has an opaque marker in its wall. It should lie in the midline, and its tip should lie at a level between C7 and T4 (ideally between T1 and T3 as the tip moves with flexion and extension of the cervical spine; Figure 3.5). If positioned too low, the tip may enter one or other main bronchus (usually the right main bronchus or bronchus intermedius) causing collapse/partial collapse of the contralateral lung, as that lung is no longer ventilated. Note that in these situations collapse is not inevitable (Fig. 3.6).

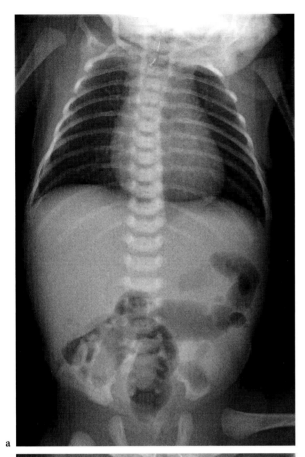

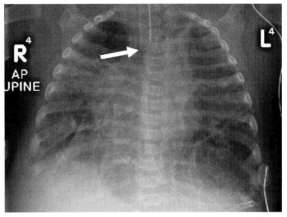

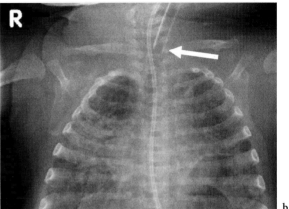

Fig. 3.5. a The tip of the ETT is in a satisfactory position on this AP supine radiograph. b A subsequent radiograph with the neonate in a prone position shows the ETT to be in a high position

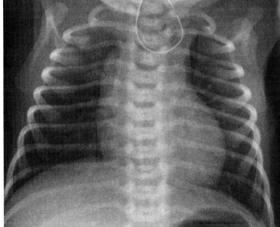

Fig. 3.4. a Neonate with oesophageal atresia. A Replogle tube lies within the upper pouch. Air within bowel loops indicates the presence of a tracheo-oesophageal fistula. b Another neonate with oesophageal atresia and a tracheo-oesophageal fistula (note the gastric air bubble). A nasogastric tube is seen to be coiled within the upper pouch. It is distinguished from the Replogle tube in (a) because of the continuous radio-opaque line in its wall

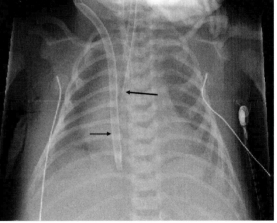

Fig. 3.6. The tip of the ETT lies in the right main bronchus (*long arrow*). There is no associated collapse. Note the VV ECMO cannula (*short arrow*)

3.1.3.3
Umbilical Arterial/Venous Catheters

An umbilical artery catheter can be distinguished from an umbilical vein catheter by the downward loop formed as the arterial catheter reaches the abdominal aorta via the internal and common iliac arteries.

It is important that the tip of the arterial catheter lies either in a low position (below L3 vertebral body) or in a high position (above T10) in order to avoid the origins of the renal arteries and celiac axis respectively. The tip of the umbilical venous catheter should be at the level of T8/T9. Occasionally the tip may enter one or the other hepatic vein (Figs. 3.3, 3.7).

The tip of percutaneous long (PICC) lines should lie within the distal IVC or SVC. If the tip lies within the right atrium, then there is a risk of cardiac arrythmias. If inserted via a femoral vein, then like an umbilical venous catheter, the tip may be misplaced and lie within a hepatic vein (Fig. 3.7).

3.1.3.4
Extracorporeal Membrane Oxygenation Catheters (ECMO)

ECMO provides support to neonates with conditions such as meconium aspiration, congenital diaphragmatic hernia and primary pulmonary hypertension. Venous blood is bypassed to an extracorporeal membrane for oxygenation before return either to the arterial circulation (providing both pulmonary and cardiac support) or to the venous circulation (providing pulmonary support alone). In either case the lungs are allowed to rest/recover, and there is a reduction in the incidence of barotrauma. Two main circuits exist; the standard venous-to-arterial circulation (VA ECMO), which requires venous and arterial cannulae (Fig. 3.8), and the increasingly popular venous-to-venous circulation (VV ECMO), for which a single double lumen venous cannula is employed (Figs. 3.6, 3.9).

The tip of the arterial catheter should lie within the innominate artery at the origin of the common carotid artery. The tip of the venous catheter should lie within the right atrium (at about the 8th /9th posterior ribs), and (in the case of VV ECMO) with the smaller arterial lumen facing the tricuspid valve. It may be difficult to confirm the position of the cannulae, and echocardiography is particularly useful in this regard. Furthermore, there is wide variation in the types of existing cannulae. Familiarity with the precise type of cannula employed locally is advised. Almost complete opacification of the lungs of a neonate on ECMO is common, and in these instances no impression can be made as to the condition of the underlying lungs (Fig. 3.9). Barnacle et al. (2006) provide a detailed review of the role played by radiography in the management of neonates on ECMO.

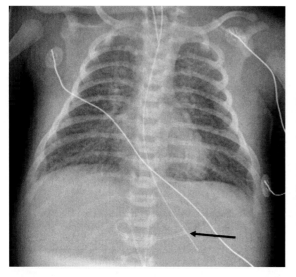

Fig. 3.7. The tip of the UVC lies within the left hepatic vein (*arrow*)

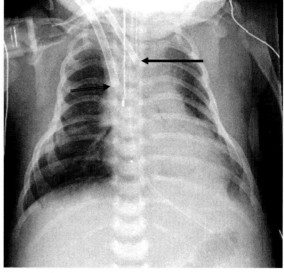

Fig. 3.8. VA ECMO with the arterial (*solid arrow*) and venous (*open arrow*) cannulae in satisfactory positions. See Figure 3.6 for VV ECMO cannula

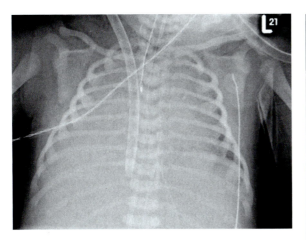

Fig. 3.9. Opacification of the lungs is an expected finding in neonates on ECMO

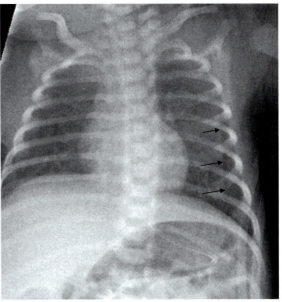

Fig. 3.10. Notice the skin fold in this neonate which mimics a left pneumothorax

3.1.3.5
Chest/Mediastinal Drains

Radiographs are performed to confirm adequate (and effective) positioning of chest and mediastinal drains, to monitor resolution of pleural fluid (although ultrasound is also useful) and to exclude complications such as subcutaneous emphysema. The role played by routine chest radiography following the removal of chest drains has been questioned. Some authors suggest that because of its low yield, chest radiography in this situation should be replaced by careful clinical monitoring as this is more effective at determining those neonates with recurrent pneumothorax or reaccumulation of pleural fluid (van den Boom and Battin 2007).

3.1.3.6
Normal Variants and Artefacts

Normal variants relating to the thymus and spine have been referred to in Section 3.1.3.1 (the normal neonatal chest radiograph). It is also important to beware of skin folds, which may mimic a pneumothorax (Fig. 3.10), and artefact related to holes in the incubator, which may mimic bullae. Other normal variants such as the azygous lobe are common to all age groups.

3.2
Digital Radiographic Systems

3.2.1
Acquisition Techniques

3.2.1.1
Introduction

There has been a rapid advance in the use of digital radiographic technology over the past decade or so. This is particularly related to the perceived benefits of picture archiving and communication (PACS) systems, which are ergonomical when compared to traditional film/screen radiography. With the "filmless" environment that is possible with digital radiography, there is no longer the need to find storage for the large number of patient packets; radiographs are no longer lost and are available (within a short space of time) to radiologists and clinicians throughout the hospital as long as there is access to an appropriate computer.

The term "digital radiography" applies to any system that at some point involves data in digital format in the acquisition, processing, display, management or storage of X-ray images. The difference between digital and traditional film/screen (analogue) imaging lies in the fact that with analogue systems the radiographic film is used for image capture, display, storage and transmission. With digital imaging these stages are separated from each other, and each may be optimised independently of the others. Of particular importance is the ability to post process digital images, which is not possible with conventional radiography. This ability is largely responsible for the reduction in the number of rejected radiographs and repeated patient exposure.

Current digital systems may be subdivided into five main categories (JAMES et al. 2001):
- Digitisation of analogue radiographs
- Fluorography (image intensifiers)
- Photostimulable phosphor plate technology (CR)
- Amorphous selenium-based systems
- Flat panel direct digital radiography (DR)

Although fluorography has a role in neonatal imaging (e.g., to monitor diaphragmatic excursion) and selenium-based technology is applicable to chest imaging, the following sections discuss in more detail only the digitisation of analogue radiographs, CR and DR as these are the most relevant to imaging of the neonatal chest. Several authors (JAMES et al. 2001; MACMAHON 2003; MCADAMS et al. 2006; PARKS and WILLIAMSON 2002; SHAEFER-PROKOP et al. 2003) have provided detailed reviews of all systems.

3.2.1.2
Digitising Analogue Images

The ability to digitise analogue images is important for several reasons. Firstly, the introduction of digital systems across and within NHS Trusts is occurring in a stepwise fashion. While it is not possible to digitise all analogue images that were obtained prior to going "digital", it may be necessary for departments to have the radiographs of certain patients archived. Secondly, referral centres receiving hard copy radiographs for a second opinion may wish to have a permanent record of the radiographs on their PACS system, particularly if the child is to receive treatment there. In addition to the PACS benefits of digitised images, the technology is also useful for teleradiology purposes, when images can be transferred to more experienced centres for expert opinion or made available to consultants who are then able to meet some of their on-call commitments from home.

There are two main systems; laser digitisers and charge couple devices (CCD). In general, laser digitisers are to be preferred as they have a wider dynamic range and superior signal-to-noise ratio (HANGIANDREOU et al. 1998). However CCD systems have a cost advantage and digitise at a rate of approximately 130 radiographs per hour compared to 100 radiographs per hour for laser digitisers (BIR 1999).

The quality of the digitised images depends on the quality of the original radiographs as well as on the quality of the digitiser. The Royal College of Radiologists teleradiology and PACS guidelines stipulate an optical density of at least 4.0 and a spatial resolution of at least 3 to 5 line pairs per mm (RCR 1999).

As far as creating teaching files is concerned, RUESS et al. (2001) performed a study that included chest radiographs of 15 neonates with pathology including (but not limited to) pneumothoraces, pneumomediastinum, RDS and tetralogy of Fallot. They showed that a low-cost flatbed scanner yields images of the paediatric chest that are significantly superior to those obtained with a digital camera-indeed demonstration of pathology was comparable to that achieved on the original radiographs.

3.2.1.3
Computed Radiography (CR)

The concept of storing an X-ray image in a phosphor screen was the first step in the development of CR, and is credited to LUCKEY (1975) working for Kodak. KOTERA et al. 1980 (working for Fuji) produced the first medical images. CR was the first, and remains the most widely used digital method for imaging the chest.

In conventional radiography, the useful optical signal is derived from light emitted as an immediate response to incident radiation exiting from the patient. However with CR, the X-ray exposure produces a latent image stored on an imaging plate containing a special photostimulable phosphor. The phosphors are usually from the barium fluorohalide family activated with europium, with BaFBR:Eu2+ being the first to be used (ROWLANDS 2002). The latent image that is produced on exposure to X-rays consists of trapped charge stored within the barium fluorohalide crystals. In essence some electrons are held at high energy levels, leaving vacancies (holes) where the electrons used to be. In conventional radiography the electrons very rapidly reoccupy the holes, releasing light and producing the definitive image as they do so. In CR, the energy is trapped (latent image) until stimulated optically. The imaging plate (IP) is held in a light-tight cassette, reducing decay of the latent image before read out. Although fading of the image is said to commence within the first 10 min following exposure, it takes more than 6 h to detect clinically significant differences when compared to an image that was read out immediately (SHAEFER-PROKOP and PROKOP 1997).

After exposure the IP is inserted into the CR reader, which consists of a laser scanner and transport system. Either a helium-neon or a semiconductor laser is used, with a spot size of 50–200 μm. Exposure to the laser scanner triggers a process known as photostimulated luminescence in which shorter wavelength (blue) light is emitted in an amount proportional to the original X-ray irradiation. This emitted light is collected with a light guide and detected with a photomultiplier tube (PMT). The electrical signals produced by the PMT are digitised to form the image on a point-by-point basis. Digital processing is introduced to adapt the image to the specific diagnostic need. Finally, by exposing the IP to strong light, any residual data can be erased, and the plate becomes reusable. The resulting images may be printed onto film allowing traditional "hard copy" interpretation with the aid of a light box. More conveniently, it is possible to view the digital images from a monitor of sufficiently high resolution ("soft copy" interpretation).

Furthermore, to obtain portable chest radiographs of sick neonates, all that is required is the exchange of a traditional film screen cassette with a CR imaging plate.

Imaging plates may be single or dual read out. In the latter, signal is collected from both sides of the imaging plate thereby increasing the signal-to-noise ratio by approximately 30% (SHAW et al. 1997); however this is associated with an increase in radiation dose.

3.2.1.4
Direct Digital Radiography (DR)

Direct digital radiography (DR) is also known as thin film transistor (TFT) or flat panel detector radiography. There are two types of DR system–direct and indirect. In contrast to CR systems where there is a need for a separate reader, with DR systems the image is sent directly to a computer for processing.

In direct DR systems, the X-ray-sensitive medium is amorphous selenium. X-rays interacting with the detector cause the excitation of electrons leaving "holes" in a manner similar to the excitation of photostimulable phosphors described above. A charged electric field guides the excited electrons to the photoconductor thus producing a latent image via the TFTs. The signal is amplified and digitised. The difference between CR and direct flat panel systems is that with the latter the absorbed X-ray energy is directly converted to a charge, by-passing the need for a scintillator.

Like CR plates, indirect flat panel detectors contain a scintillating detector (usually caesium iodide with thallium-CsI:lh or gadolinium oxysulphide–GOS). However, they also contain a light-sensitive amorphous silicon photodiode. The X-ray energy causes the scintillator to emit light, which is converted to electrical charge by the photodiode. These indirect flat panel DR systems are said to be the most amenable to real-time display (DUCOURANT et al. 2000). All DR systems are therefore self-scanning and give instant readout.

The advantage of DR is related firstly to the direct acquisition of a digital image, thereby leading to a rapid display time, and secondly to the production of images of higher quality than either CR or analogue systems (CHOTAS and RAVIN 2001; FLOYD et al. 2001). Image quality of CR and DR systems has been shown to be equivalent for portable neonatal chest radiographs even when radiation exposure for the latter was reduced to 25% (SAMEI et al. 2003). The disadvantage, however, is that the cost of DR systems coupled with the fragility of their detector hardware inhibits their use for portable imaging. Figure 3.11 illustrates the working of film/screen, CR and DR imaging systems.

3.3
Digital Image Optimisation

3.3.1
Image Display

3.3.1.1
Hard Copy Versus Soft Copy

Hard copy refers to the interpretation of printed film with the aid of a light box in a similar way to the interpretation of traditional film/screen radiographs. Printing is achieved by using the digital data to modulate the intensity of a laser beam that exposes an analogue film. Many radiology departments with newly installed CR systems continue to print radiographs until their PACS systems are well established.

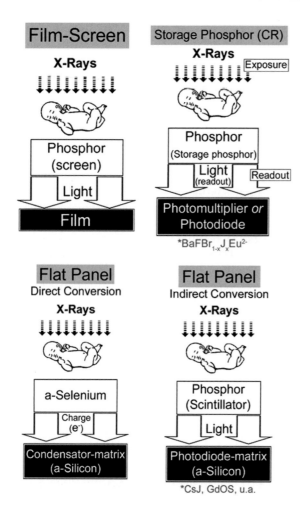

Fig. 3.11. Pictorial illustrations comparing the processes involved in analogue and digital imaging

Soft copy refers to the interpretation of images from a monitor and therefore with no need to produce a printed film. In this case the digital data are converted to an analogue video signal and projected on a cathode ray tube monitor. Soft copy images may also be obtained by digitising film as described above (Sect. 3.2.1.2). Clearly, when interpreting digital images, the resolution of the monitor will affect the degree to which structures are visualised–this is discussed further in Section 3.3.1.3.

Soft copy interpretation allows the use of post processing functions such as adjustment of contrast and brightness, image magnification, etc. All of these will help to optimise the visualisation of specific structures, e.g., lines, lung edge in suspected pneumothorax, bones, etc., from the same radiograph.

Clearly there are ergonomical and economical advantages of PACS, with an estimated saving of US$

128,009 per year or US$ 6.20 per patient for soft over hard copy interpretation (ABE et al. 2004). However it is also important to consider image quality and diagnostic accuracy of each method. In the study by ABE et al. mentioned above, there was similar diagnostic accuracy for the detection of subtle lesions from adult chest radiographs when interpreted as soft compared to hard copy. Other studies have been performed for neonatal and paediatric chest radiographs (RAZAVI et al. 1992; BRILL et al. 1996). RAZAVI et al. (1992) showed no significant difference between the two displays for demonstration of pneumothoraces and air bronchograms on chest radiographs of children; however soft copy showed a slight advantage for demonstration of interstitial disease and linear atelectasis. BRILL et al. (1996) performed a large study in which soft and hard copy display of 1,104 chest radiographs of neonatal and paediatric intensive care patients were reviewed for nine specific tubes (nasogastric, nasoduodenal, endotracheal, central venous catheter, PICC line, chest drain, pacemaker wires, umbilical areterial catheter and umbilical venous catheter) and nine specific diagnoses (lung parenchymal abnormality, pneumothorax, pneumomediastinum, pleural effusion, normal lungs, normal abdomen, pneumatosis intesitnalis, other abnormal bowel gas pattern and pneumoperitoneum). Their results showed that soft copy had similar, or slightly improved diagnostic accuracy compared to hard copy interpretation.

In summary, therefore, soft copy interpretation of neonatal chest radiographs has economical and ergonomical advantages over hard copy film interpretation, with similar (if not better) diagnostic accuracy. At the author's institution hard copy radiographs are no longer produced. Indeed the neonatal, paediatric and cardiac intensive care units all have PACS monitors, which allow the review of images by radiologists and clinicians (independently or at regular combined ward rounds).

It must be emphasised that the monitor used for initial radiological diagnosis should be of sufficient resolution for this purpose (see Sect. 3.3.1.3) and that the observer makes full use of the post processing facilities of the workstation.

3.3.1.2
DICOM

This acronym stands for Digital Imaging and Communication in Medicine. The DICOM standard is regularly reviewed, and the latest is DICOM 2007 (DICOM 2007). The standard was created as a result of problems that arose from the various digital systems available. In short, different manufacturers developed their own software packages, which meant that digital images obtained from one system could not necessarily be interpreted by the system of another manufacturer. As (for example) NHS Trusts purchased different digital systems, it was found that digital images could not be interpreted across Trusts. DICOM overcomes this problem. A DICOM-compliant system uses universally recognised standardised file formats so that images can be transferred between distant locations.

3.3.1.3
Matrix Size of Digital Systems and Monitors

Spatial resolution of standard-resolution CR plates is 2 line pairs/mm (lp/mm) – matrix size 2K × 2K; 5 lp/mm for high-resolution CR plates (matrix size 4K × 4K), and for DR systems maximum spatial resolution is 3.3 to 2.5 lp/mm.

Of further interest are the spatial resolution requirements of monitors used for soft copy interpretation. It has been shown that for chest radiography, the detection of anatomical structures and subtle abnormality is similar for 2K × 2K and 4K × 4K matrix sizes (SCHAEFER-PROKOP C et al. 1997; MIRÓ et al. 2001; UEGUCHI et al. 2005). This has significant positive implications for financial outlay and image processing and archiving solutions.

STERLING et al. (2003) showed that with the exception of diffuse pulmonary disease, Web-based bedside personal computers (linked to their hospital's PACS system) allowed a similar diagnostic accuracy as their diagnostic workstation (possible findings were normal; pleural effusion; pulmonary oedema; pneumothorax; subcutaneous and mediastinal emphysema; atelectasis; position of endotracheal tube; position of central venous line). Observers were critical care physicians and not radiologists. If such protocols are instituted, it is strongly advised that a radiologist reports all radiographs from a diagnostic workstation as soon as possible.

Most diagnostic monitors use cathode ray tube (CRT) technology. The system involves moving an electron beam to and fro across the back of the screen. As it passes the screen, the beam lights up phosphor dots on the inside of the glass tube. This process allows the illumination of active portions of the screen, gradually building up an image. Liquid crystal display monitors (LCDs) are also available. The most common LCDs depend on picture elements (pixels) formed by liquid-crystal (LC) cells.

These cells change the polarization direction of light passing through them in response to an electrical voltage. Changes in the polarization direction allow more or less light to pass through a polarizing layer on the face of the display. A change in voltage changes the amount of light. When compared to CRTs, LCDs are less bulky, lighter and require less power to run. They produce a perfectly sharp image with no geometric distortion. However the image contrast may vary with the viewing angle, and they are more costly than CRTs. Furthermore, whether LCD monitors have a diagnostic benefit is still being investigated (SCHARITZER et al. 2005).

3.3.2
Image Processing

3.3.2.1
Introduction

The ultimate goal when obtaining a radiograph of a neonate is to enable the radiologist to reach a precise and accurate diagnosis. There are factors related both to the observer and the image acquisition/display system that will affect this. Techniques to optimise the diagnostic process fall into two main categories, those aimed at improving soft copy display and those aimed at improving diagnostic accuracy by providing automated (computer-aided) diagnosis. Techniques to improve image display can be broadly subdivided into pre- and post-processing techniques.

3.3.2.2
Pre-processing

Image pre-processing includes scaling and correction techniques. Correction techniques are required because of the intrinsic non-uniformity of digital detectors. Image scaling is necessary because of the wide dynamic range (latitude) of digital systems beyond the visual perception of the human eye. Full data presentation would lead to considerable reduction in contrast resolution.

When imaging the neonatal chest, it is important that the radiographer collimates adequately, and that the neonatal chest algorithm is selected for imaging plate readout. Both collimation and algorithm selection affect the histogram analysis that is required for image scaling. Readers needing more detailed discussion of digital image pre-processing are referred to SIEBERT (2003).

3.3.2.3
Post-processing

The ability to post-process images is a significant advantage of digital over conventional radiography. When used optimally post-processing improves visualisation of pathology and allows the display of the full object irradiated range while improving local contrast (FRIJA et al. 1998). In other words bony, mediastinal and lung parenchymal detail (for example) may be clearly visualised on the same radiograph. Techniques include non-linear grey-scale enhancement, non-linear unsharp masking (edge-enhancement) and more advanced applications such as single or double exposure dual-energy subtraction (KANTOR 1997). Optimisation of parameters by departments for different examinations is advised (SCHAEFER-PROKOP and PROKOP 1997). The CEC quality criteria for chest radiography in the paediatric age group (Table 3.1) have been found useful in this regard (MOONEY and THOMAS 1998).

3.3.2.3.1
Non-Linear Grey-Scale Enhancement

In order to obtain an interpretable image, digital values must be converted to a grey-scale value. Typically this is performed with the aid of a look-up table analogous to the characteristic curve of film/screen imaging. As long as each digital input value has a unique (grey-scale) output value, then an image can be obtained (FREEDMAN and STELLAR 1997).

Table 3.2 (adapted from FREEDMAN and STELLAR 1997) summarises some of the G and R factors used in digital radiography, their interpretation and the values used at the author's institution (Fuji 5000R CR system).

3.3.2.3.2
Edge Enhancement

Edge enhancement emphasises the edges and contrast of a lesion, compensating for the lower

Table 3.2. The "G" and "R" factors in digital imaging

Abbreviation	Interpretation	Effect	Parameters for Figure 3.1
GA	Gradient angle Slope of steepest portion of LUT*	Steep slope = high contrast Gentle slope = low contrast	1.4
GC	Gradient centre Optical density point around which the GA rotates the LUT	High GC = low optical density	1.6
GS	Gradient shift (Grey scale) Affects the overall density of the image	High GS = high optical density	0.4
GT	Gradient type Basic shape of the graph Allows black/white inversion	N = upward curve M = downward curve	E
RN	Frequency number Also known as kernel size Ranges from 1 (large) to 9 (small)	Large RN emphasises larger structures Small RN emphasises smaller structures and noise	3
RT	Frequency type Blurs image in light exposure areas Options include R, T and F		R
RE	Edge enhancement	Larger number enhances edges	0.5

spatial resolution of CR systems. It may improve image quality and enhance the visualisation of pathology; however it may also suppress pathological lesions, or produce artefacts simulating pathology.

In one study, the application of a strong edge-enhancement algorithm (2K × 2K, 21-inch Barco, Kortirijk, Belgium PACS monitor) to soft copy neonatal chest radiographs improved the visualisation of small pneumothoraces, vascular catheters and other subtle findings on neonatal chest radiographs (Goo et al. 2001). The effect of altering various G and R factors on the visibility of structures is illustrated in Figures 3.12 and 3.13.

To summarise, increased edge-enhancement algorithms may be useful in certain situations, e.g., identification of lines and small pneumothoraces, particularly if alteration of contrast, brightness and magnification have not helped. However (as illustrated) high levels may lead to the production of artefact. An optimal level of edge enhancement for neonatal chest radiographs has not been established, and is likely to vary depending on clinical indication. Routine display of a single radiograph at varying levels of edge-enhancement is possible, but is not employed at the author's institution-rather all chest radiographs are displayed with a standard edge-enhancement factor of 0.5.

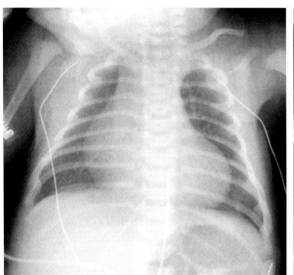
a

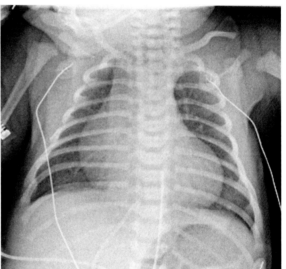
b

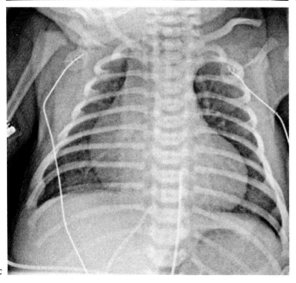
c

Fig. 3.12a–c. Effects of altering edge enhancement (RE). Notice how increasing edge enhancement exaggerates the appearance of interstitial lung markings and hardens the edges of lines, cardiac contour, rib margins, etc. **a** kV=62, mAs=2.2, grey scale (GS)=0.4, edge enhancement (RE)=0. **b** kV=62, mAs=2.2, grey scale (GS)=0.4,edge enhancement (RE)=1. **c** kV=62, mAs=2.2, grey scale (GS)=0.4,edge enhancement (RE)=2

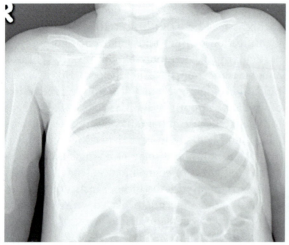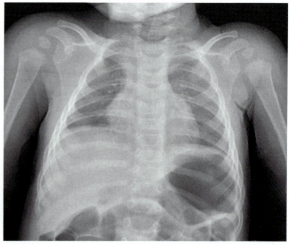

a b

Fig. 3.13a,b. Effects of altering GS. Reducing grey scale reduces the apparent contrast of the image. **a** kV=66, mAs=1.8, edge enhancement (RE)=0.5, grey scale (GS)=-0.1. **b** kV =66, mAs =1.8 edge enhancement (RE)=0.5, grey scale (GS)=0.4

3.4
Digital Image Quality

3.4.1
Introduction

In determining the quality of a radiograph, we are determining what degree of excellence that radiograph has attained. In this regard there are two main questions to be answered, namely:

How well does the imaging system perform? Answers to this question concern measures of the objective physical performance of an imaging system and are usually sought under standardised experimental conditions. They assess the technical efficacy of an imaging system. Quality in this case might be expressed, for example, in terms of spatial resolution, modulation transfer function (MTF), detector quantum efficiency (DQE), grey-scale bit resolution, dynamic range or signal-to-noise ratio (THORNBURY and EUGENE 1994, JAMES et al. 2001).

How excellent is the radiograph that is produced? This is dependent on the answers to the first question. However in the clinical setting it is also dependent on radiographic technique. Radiation exposure, patient positioning, collimation and presence of artefact all contribute to clinical image quality. In the paediatric population patient movement also contributes significantly to image quality. In the neonate this will usually be related to motion artefact secondary to ventilatory support.

In general, increased radiation dose produces an improvement in image quality. Children are at an increased lifetime risk of developing complications secondary to radiation; therefore image quality (i.e., radiation dose) cannot be increased indefinitely. A radiograph is deemed to be of sufficient quality if it is "… adequate for the clinical purpose with the minimum radiation dose to the patient…" (MARTIN et al. 1999).

Radiology departments must optimise their imaging and display parameters if the ALARA principle is to be adhered to (HUDA 2004).

A glossary of some terms used in the definition of digital image quality is found below, with the equivalent analogue terminology in brackets.

Background electronic noise: Small electronic current with no useful clinical information. It contributes to a reduction in image quality by obscuring some of the useful electronic signal. DR systems produce less noise than CR systems (mottle/noise).

Brightness: A measure of the degree of darkness of the radiograph (density).

Contrast resolution: The degree to which a digital system is able to detect differences in density between areas on the radiograph (contrast).

Dynamic range: The number of shades of grey that the system is able to depict (latitude).

Exposure index: An objective indication of the X-ray exposure to the imaging plate, the precise index varies between manufacturers (objective = density/ subjective = over or under exposure).

Linearity*: Direct relationship between exposure and density (film speed/sensitivity**).

Modulation transfer function: A function of spatial frequency, this is the ratio of information recorded to information available. An MTF of 1 implies that all available information (contrast) has been recorded (resolution).

Signal-to-noise ratio: Ratio of clinically useful electronic current to background current (sharpness).

Spatial resolution: Ability of the system to record as separate images two or more small objects placed very close together. Measured in line pairs (lp)/mm (resolution).

*Typically for digital paediatric imaging (both CR and DR) the equivalent film/screen speed should now be 400.

** Sensitivity of film/screen systems should not be confused with the Sensitivity (S) developed by Fuji as a measure of exposure (exposure index) for their systems (see Sect. 3.4.2).

3.4.2
Image Quality and Radiation Dose Considerations

Currently the best estimation of radiation risk is the linear, no-threshold model (i.e., no level of radiation is risk free). Neonates are at greatest lifetime risk of developing medical radiation induced malignancy, moreover while on intensive care, many of them will have a significant number of serial radiographs performed to monitor their disease progress.

In one study, the average number of radiographs was 10.6 and cumulative effective dose for chest radiographs for patients on a neonatal intensive care unit ranged from 0 to 1450 µSv (Donadieu et al. 2005). Factors influencing cumulative dose included gestational age, birth weight, management procedures and complications.

The CEC reference level for entrance surface dose (ESD) for mobile chest radiography in children is 80 µGy (EUR 1996), while the National Radiation Protection Board (NRPB) reference level for paediatric chest radiographs is 50 µGy (Hart et al. 2000). The range of published ESD for analogue neonatal chest radiographs is 27.8 µGy to 60 µGy (Armpilia et al. 2002; Duggan et al. 2003; Makri et al. 2006).

Due to the improved contrast resolution and post-processing tools of digital radiography, there is potential for significant dose reductions. Numerous clinical and phantom studies have been performed comparing radiation dose, image quality and diagnostic accuracy of film screen and hard/soft copy digital chest radiography (Aldrich et al. 2006; Bacher et al. 2003; Compagnone et al. 2006; Ono et al. 2005). Specific to paediatric departments, using the CEC quality criteria as a semi-objective means of assessing image quality, Hufton et al. (1998) were able to demonstrate a dose benefit for CR compared to analogue chest radiography (film speed of 400) of 33%. Other studies have also shown a dose benefit for digital radiography of the neonatal chest particularly for DR systems (Rapp-Bernahardt et al. 2005a; Rapp-Bernahardt et al. 2005b).

At the author's institution (Fuji 5000R, CR system and standard resolution imaging plates) imaging parameters for neonatal (and infant) chest radiographs are 60 kV–65 kV and 2.2–2.5 mAs.

In general, digital imaging has allowed a reduction in radiation dose while improving image quality and diagnostic accuracy, but only after careful monitoring of departmental parameters. Dose efficiency is better for dual readout than for single readout CR and for DR than either of the CR techniques even with a 50% reduction in exposure (Gruber et al. 2006).

Careful attention to other technical parameters is also important. As an example, Soboleski et al. (2006) demonstrated that their current collimation parameters (Sect. 3.1.2) caused exposure of anatomical areas outside the thorax with only a 3% yield of additional diagnostic information. Radiation exposure can be further reduced by improved collimation.

How do changes in exposure affect image quality? Unlike traditional analogue systems, digital systems are able to maintain relatively constant image density regardless of radiation exposure. Dose however cannot be reduced indefinitely as increased quantum mottle (electronic noise) reduces image quality. On the other hand, as mentioned earlier, as dose is increased, image quality increases with no significant discernable increase in density, and indeed with no improvement in diagnostic accuracy (Elsenhuber et al. 2003). Because image quality is improved with no effect on density, there is a tendency for radiation exposure to increase, "exposure factor creep." It has been shown that with analogue imaging, exposure to very low birth weight babies is extremely low (mean effective dose 0.04 mSv) (Sutton et al. 1998). It is possible that with digital systems, current exposure to these very low birth weight infants while being within recommended limits is, nevertheless, excessive. The effect of dose on image quality is illustrated in Figure 3.14.

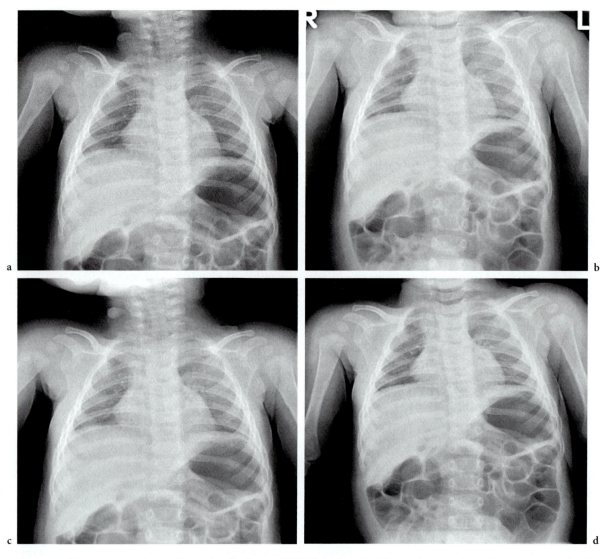

Fig. 3.14a–d. Post mortem chest radiographs all taken at 66 kV. Note the insignificant change in image density as a result of downward adjustment of S values with increasing dose. Lower exposures are associated with increased noise (mottle) best appreciated in the soft tissues of the neck and shoulders (same patient as Fig. 3.13). **a** mAs = 0.8, S=836. **b** mAs = 3.2, S = 179. **c** mAs = 6.4, S = 86. **d** mAs = 13, S = 39

It behoves radiology departments to optimise their exposure parameters particularly when a new digital system is installed, and regularly thereafter to maintain quality assurance. One of the simplest methods is to monitor the exposure index of a digital system.

The exposure index is an objective indicator of radiation dose exposure incident on the imaging plate. Different manufacturers have developed different indices:

- Agfa-Logarithm median of histogram, IgM (directly related to exposure).
- Fuji-Sensitivity, S (inversely related to exposure).

- Kodak–Exposure index, EI (directly related to exposure).

Interpretation of these indices is summarised in Table 3.3.

By correlating ESD with the exposure index, departments can optimise a range of acceptable values for specific clinical indications. In Figure 3.13, notice how there is no perceptible change in image density despite the increasing levels of exposure. The corresponding decrease in S values is the main indication of excessive radiation. Unfortunately, although the exposure index will appear on the image processing workstation and on hard copy radiographs, with

Table 3.3. Exposure indices for three major manufacturers of digital systems

Manufacturer	Exposure index	Unit	Mean receptor exposure*		
			5 µGy	10 µGy	20 µGy
			0.5 mR	1 mR	2 mR
Agfa	IgM	bels	1.9	2.2	2.5
Fuji	S	No units	400	200	100
Kodak	EI	mbels	1,700	2,000	2,300

* Note than an exposure of 1 mR is equivalent to an air dose/kerma of 10 µGy

many systems (including that at the author's institute), it is not transferred across to the archive with the digital images.

Regular audit will help to ensure that standards are maintained. At the author's institute, the mean S value for 45 neonatal portable chest radiographs was 1,020 (115–2,466). Fuji recommends S values of 100–400 for portable chest radiographs in children–although they have not specifically stated a range for neonates (MacCutcheon 2004). As S is inversely related to exposure, the recommendation by Fuji, if followed, would lead to excessive exposures. New standards need to be set for various paediatric age ranges.

3.4.3
Strategies for Dose Reduction and Image Optimisation

1. Of utmost importance is a multidisciplinary team approach. The team should consist of a (paediatric) radiologist, medical physicist, radiographer, biomedical engineer, manufacturer service engineer, manufacturer applications engineer and manufacturer-imaging scientist (WILLIS and SLOVIS 2004).
2. Obtain the best patient positioning that is practicable and collimate adequately.
3. Consider the indication. Lines, catheters, pacing wires, etc., are inherently of high contrast; their visualisation is MTF rather than noise or exposure limited. Therefore there is significant scope for dose reduction when for example the clinical indication is solely to confirm their position. The detection of low contrast structures (e.g., lung parenchymal disease) is noise/exposure limited. Nevertheless dose reductions of up to 20% have been achieved with no apparent effect on diagnostic accuracy (DON 2004).

4. With the indication in mind, set parameters that will lead to lower exposure. Improve the quality of the beam by using additional filtration (e.g., 2–3 mm aluminium).
5. DR has a higher DQE (detective quantum efficiency) than CR, i.e., DR systems are more effective at converting the same degree of radiation exposure into useful signal. If cost allows, then DR systems are to be preferred.
6. Use appropriate paediatric image processing software.
7. Purchase monitors of at least 1K × 1K resolution, and ideally 2K × 2K. Whether higher resolution monitors improve diagnostic accuracy continues to be debated.
8. Select appropriate post-processing parameters. Observers should make use of the tools of the workstation.
9. Optimise exposure parameters, taking note of the value of the exposure index, particularly when a new digital system is installed, and regularly thereafter to maintain quality assurance.
10. Keep abreast with the literature. Newer imaging plates are being developed with a view to improving DQE without affecting resolution, e.g., double-sided CR imaging plates, or CR plates that incorporate CsBr:Eu2+ needle crystals (LEBLANS et al. 2000). Close teamwork as mentioned in Point 1 above is essential.

3.5
Computer-Aided Diagnosis

Advanced techniques include single exposure and double exposure dual energy subtraction, temporal subtraction and automated identification of nodules

(MacMahon 2000; Kuhlman et al. 2006). While these techniques are entering into routine clinical use to assist the interpretation of adult chest radiographs, they have a limited role in paediatric, and even less so in neonatal chest radiography. They are mentioned here for the sake of completion.

Single and double exposure dual energy subtraction works on the principle that different tissues attenuate low and high-energy photons to different degrees. In the former a single exposure is made onto two imaging plates, which are separated by a copper filter. In the latter, two exposures (of 60 Kv and 120 Kv) with a delay of approximately 200 ms are made. This time interval is occasionally a source of misregistration artefact due to patient motion between the two exposures.

The technique allows the simultaneous display of chest radiographs on standard, soft tissue-selected and bone-selected settings. It improves the visualisation of calcified nodules, pleural disease, vascular and mediastinal masses and tracheal stenosis. Dual energy subtraction is associated with an increased radiation dose, and is not generally performed in the paediatric age group (Kuhlman et al. 2006).

Temporal subtraction involves automated registration, warping and subsequent subtraction of one chest radiograph from another, thus displaying interval change between the two (MacMahon 2003). A number of studies have demonstrated the benefits of this technique for the detection of lung nodules, heart failure and pneumonia (Jokoh et al. 2002; Tsubamoto et al. 2002; Okazaki et al. 2004). It has also been shown that in addition to improving diagnostic accuracy, temporal subtraction reduces reviewing time (Kakeda et al. 2006). Like double exposure dual energy subtraction, misregistration artefact is a possibility. However temporal subtraction has the benefit of not increasing radiation dose (as the patient will in any case have had the follow-up radiograph). Despite this advantage, the effect of temporal subtraction on diagnostic accuracy and reporting times in neonatal chest radiography has not been studied, and might be complicated by the interval growth that is seen in children, but not in adults.

Automated lung nodule detection in adults has a sensitivity of 70% to 80%, with an average of one to two false-positives per radiograph. While the technique improves observer identification of new lesions, clearly the sensitivity does not approach that of high resolution CT, and currently has no role in the interpretation of neonatal chest radiographs.

References

Abe K, Kosuda S, Iwasaki Y et al (2004) Soft copy using image processing in place of hard copy for detection of subtle pulmonary lesions: Is it actually cost-effective? Radiation Med 22:379–383

Aldrich JE, Duran E, Dunlop P, Mayo JR (2006) Optimization of dose and image quality for computed radiography and digital radiography. J Digital Imaging 19:126–131

Armpilia CI, Fife IAJ, Croasdale PL (2002) Radiation dose quantities and risk in a special care baby unit. Br J Radiol 75:590–595

Arthur R (2001) The neonatal chest X-ray. Paediatr Resp Rev 2:311–323

Bacher K, Smeets P, Bonnarens K, Hauwere AD, Verstraete K, Thierens H (2003) Dose reduction in patients undergoing chest imaging: Digital amorphous silicon flat panel detector radiography versus conventional film screen radiography and phosphor based computed radiography. AJR Am J Roentgenol 181:923–929

Barnacle AM, Smith LC, Hiorns MP (2006) The role of imaging during extracorporeal membrane oxygenation in pediatric respiratory failure. AJR Am J Roentgenol 186:58–66

BIR, British Institute of Radiology Teleradiology Working Party (1999) Teleradiology: an introduction and definition. British Institute of Radiology, London

BIR, British Institute of Radiology (2001) Assurance of quality in the diagnostic imaging department (2nd edn). BIR, London

Bontrager KL (1993) Textbook of radiographic positioning and related anatomy, 3rd edn. Mosby, New York

Bramson RT, Griscom NT, Cleveland RH (2005) Interpretation of chest radiographs in infants with cough and fever. Radiology 236:22–29

Brill PW, Winchester P, Cahill P, Lesser M, Durfee SM, Giess CS (1996) Computed radiography in neonatal and pediatric intensive care units: a comparison of 2.5×2K softcopy images vs digital hard-copy film. Pediatr Radiol 26:333–336

CEC (1996) Commission of the European Communities. European guidelines on quality criteria for diagnostic radiographic images EUR 16260 EN. Brussels: CEC, 1996

Chotas H, Ravin C (2001) Digital chest radiography with a solid-state flat-panel X-ray detector: contrast-detail evaluation with processed images processed on film hard copy. Radiology 218:679–682

DICOM (2007) http://www.dclunie.com/dicom-status/status.html#BaseStandard2007

Compagnone G, Baleni MC, Pagan L, Calzolaio FL, Barozzi L, Bergamini C (2006) Comparison of radiation doses to patients undergoing standard radiographic examinations with conventional screen-film radiography, computed radiography and direct digital radiography. Br J Radiol 79:899–904

Don S (2004) Radiosensitivity of children: potential for overexposures in CR and DR and magnitude of doses in ordinary radiographic examinations. Pediatr Radiol 34 (Suppl 3):S167–S172

Donadieu J, Zeghnoun A, Roudier C et al (2005) Cumulated effective doses delivered by radiographs to preterm infants in a neonatal intensive care unit. Pediatrics 117:882–888

Ducourant T, Michel M, Päppler T et al (2000) Optimisation of key building blocks for a large area radiographic and fluoroscopic dynamic digital X-ray detector based on a a-Si H:CsI:Tl flat panel technology. Proc SPIE 3977:14–25

Duggan L, Warren-Forward H, Smith T, Kron T (2003) Investigation of dose reduction in neonatal radiography using specially designed phantoms and LiF:Mg, Cu, P TLDs. Br J Radiol 76:232–237

Elsenhuber E, Stadler A, Prokop M, Fuchsjäger M, Weber M, Schaefer-Prokop C (2003) Detection of monitoring materials on bedside radiographs with the most recent generation of storage phosphor plates: Dose increase does not improve detection performance. Radiology 227:216–221

EUR (1996) European guidelines on quality criteria for diagnostic radiographic images in paediatrics EUR 16261 Luxembourg: European Commission 1996

Floyd C, Warp R, Dobbins J III et al (2001) Imaging characteristics of an amorphous silicon flat-panel detector for digital chest radiography. Radiology 218:683–688

Freedman MT, Stellar D (1997) Image processing in digital radiography. Sem Roentgenol 32:25–37

Frija J, de Kerviler E, de Gery S, Zagdanski A-M (1998) Computed radiography. Biomed Pharmacother 52:59–63

Goo WH, Kim HJ, Song K-S, Kim EA-R, Kim KS, Yoon CH, Pi SY (2001) Using edge enhancement to identify subtle findings on soft-copy neonatal chest radiographs. AJR Am J Roentgenol 177:437–440

Gruber M, Uffman M, Weber M, Prokop M, Balassey C, Schaefer-Prokop C (2006) Direct detector radiography versus dual reading computed radiography: feasibility of dose reduction in chest radiography. Eur Radiol 16:1544–1550

Hangiandreou NJ, O'Connor TJ, Felmlee JP (1998) An evaluation of the signal and noise characteristics of four CCD-based digitisers. Med Phys 25:2020

Hart D, Wall BF, Schrimpton PC, Bungay DR, Dance DR (2000) Reference doses and patient size in paediatric radiology. NRPB R 318. Chilton: HMSO

Huda W (2004) Assessment of the problem: pediatric doses in screen-film and digital radiography. Pediatr Radiol 34 (Suppl 3):S173–S182

Hufton AP, Doyle SM, Carty HM (1998) Digital radiography in paediatrics: radiation dose considerations and magnitude of possible dose reduction. Br J Radiol 71:186–199

James JJ, Davies AG, Cowen AR, O'Connor PJ (2001) Developments in digital radiography: an equipment update. Eur Radiol 11:2616–2626

Johkoh T, Kozuka T, Tomiyama N et al (2002) Temporal subtraction for detection of solitary pulmonary nodules on chest radiographs: evaluation of a commercially available computer-aided diagnosis system. Radiology 223:806–811

Kakeda S, Kamaka K, Hatakeyama Y, Aoki T, Korogi Y, Katsuragawa S, Doi K (2006) Effect of temporal subtraction technique on interpretation time and diagnostic accuracy of chest radiography. AJR Am J Roentgenol 187:1253–1259

Kantor C (1997) Computed radiography. Biomed Instrum Technol 31:73–75

Kotera N, Eguchi S, Miyahara J, Matsumoto S, Kato H (1980) Method and apparatus for recording and reproducing a radiation image. US patent no 4236078

Kuhlman JE, Collins J, Brooks GN, Yandow DR, Broderick LS (2006) Dual-energy subtraction chest radiography: What to look for beyond calcified nodules. Radiographics 26:79–92

Leblans P, Struye L, Willems P (2000) A new needle-crystalline computed radiography detector. J Digit Imaging 13 (Suppl 1):117–120

Long JG, Philip AG, Lucey JF (1980) Excessive handling as a cause of hypoxaemia. Pediatrics 65:203–207

Luckey GW (1975) Apparatus and method for producing images corresponding to patterns of high-energy radiation. US patent no 3859527

MacCutcheon DW (2004) Management of pediatric radiation dose using Fuji computed radiography. Pediatr Radiol 34 (Suppl 3):S201–S206

MacMahon H (2000) Improvement in detection of pulmonary nodules: Digital image processing and computer-aided diagnosis. Radiographics 20:1169–1177

MacMahon H (2003) Digital chest radiography; practical issues. J Thoracic Imaging 18:138–147

Makri T, Yakoumakis E, Papadopoulou D, Gialousis G, Theodoropoulous V, Sandilos P, Georgiou E (2006) Radiation risk assessment in neonatal radiographic examinations of the chest and abdomen: A clinical and Monte Carlo dosimetry study. Phys Med Biol 51:5023–5033

Martin CJ, Sharp PF, Sutton DG (1999) Measurement of image quality in diagnostic radiology. Appl Radiat Isot 50:21–38

McAdams HP, Samei E, Dobbins III J, Tourassi GD, Ravin CE (2006) Recent advances in chest radiography. Radiology 241:663–683

Miró SPM, Leung AN, Rubin GD et al (2001) Digital storage phosphor chest radiography: An ROC study of the effect of 2K versus 4K matrix size on observer performance. Radiology 218:527–532

Mooney R, Thomas PS (1998) Dose reduction in a paediatric x-ray department following optimization of radiographic technique. Br J Radiol 71:852–860

Okazaki H, Nakamura K, Watanabe H et al (2004) Improved detection of lung cancer arising in diffuse lung diseases on chest radiographs using temporal subtraction. Acad Radiol 11:498–505

Ono K, Yoshitake Y, Akahane K, Yamada Y, Maeda T, Kai M, Kusama T (2005) Comparison of a digital flat-panel versus screen-film, photofluorography and storage-phosphor systems by detection of simulated lung adenocarcinoma lesions using hard copy images. Br J Radiol 78:922–927

Parks ET, Williamson G (2002) Digital radiography: An overview. J Contemp Dent Pract 4:023–039

Rapp-Bernhardt U, Bernhardt TM, Lenzen H et al (2005a) Experimental evaluation of a portable indirect flat panel detector for the pediatric chest: comparison with storage phosphor radiography at different exposures by using a chest phantom. Radiology 237:485–491

Rapp-Bernhardt U, Roehl F-W, Esseling R et al (2005b) Portable flat-panel detector for low-dose imaging in a pediatric intensive care unit. Invest Radiol 40:736–741

Razavi M, Sayre JW, Taira RK et al (1992) Receiver-operating-characteristic study of chest radiographs in children: digital hard-copy film vs 2K×2K soft-copy images. AJR Am J Roentgenol 158:443–448

RCR Board of the Faculty of Clinical Radiology, The Royal College of Radiologists (1999) Guide to information technology in radiology: teleradiology and PACS. Royal College of Radiologists, London

Replogle RL (1963) Esophageal atresia: Plastic sump catheter for drainage of the proximal pouch. Surgery 54:296–297

Rowlands JA (2002) The physics of computed radiography. Phys Med Biol R123–R166

Ruess L, Uychara CFT, Shiels KC, Cho KH, O'Connor SC, Whitton RK, Person DA (2001) Digitizing pediatric chest radiographs: comparison of low-cost, commercial off-the-shelf technologies. Pediatr Radiol 31:841–847

Samei E, Hill JG, Frey GD et al (2003) Evaluation of a flat panel digital radiographic system for low-dose portable imaging of neonates. Med Phys 30:601–607

Schaefer-Prokop CM, Prokop M (1997) Storage phosphor radiography. Eur Radiol 7 (Suppl 3):S58–S65

Schaefer-Prokop C, Prokop M, Nagal S et al (1997) Impact of matrix size and exposure dose in storage phosphor chest radiography: results of an anthropomorphic phantom study. Radiology 25(P):436

Schaefer-Prokop C, Uffmann M, Eisenhuber E, Prokop M (2003) Digital radiography of the chest: Detector techniques and performance parameters. J Thoracic Imaging 18:124–137

Scharitzer M, Prokop M, Weber M, Fuchsjäger M, Oschatz E, Schaefer-Prokop C (2005) Detectability of catheters on bedside chest radiographs: comparison between liquid crystal display and high-resolution cathode-ray tube monitors. Radiology 234:611–616

Shaw CC, Wang TP, Breintenstein DS, Gur D (1997) Improvement in signal-to-noise and contrast-to-noise ratios in dual-screen computed radiography. Med Phys 24:1293–1302

Siebert JA (2003) Digital radiographic image presentation: Preprocessing methods. In: Samei E, Flynn MJ (eds) 2003 Syllabus: Categorical course in diagnostic radiology physics–advances in digital radiography. Oak Brook III: Radiological Society of North America:53–70

Slade D, Harrison S, Morris S, Alfaham M, Davis P, Guildea Z, Tuthill D (2005) Neonates do not need to be handled for radiographs. Pediatr Radiol 35:608–611

Soboleski D, Theriault C, Acker A, Dagnone V, Manson D (2006) Unnecessary irradiation to non-thoracic structures during pediatric chest radiography. Pediatr Radiol 36:22–25

Sterling L, Tait GA, Edmonds JF (2003) Interpretation of digital radiographs by pediatric critical care physicians using web based bedside personal computers versus diagnostic workstations. Pediatr Crit Care Med 4:26–32

Sutton PM, Arthur RJ, Taylor C et al (1998) Ionising radiation from diagnostic X-rays in very low birth weight babies. Arch Dis Child 78:227–229

Sutton PM, Arthur RJ, Taylor C, Stringer MD (1998) Ionizing radiation from diagnostic X-rays in very low birth weight babies. Arch Dis Child Fetal Neonatal Ed 78:F227–F229

Thornbury JR Eugene W (1994) Caldwell Lecture: Clinical efficacy of diagnostic imaging: love it or leave it. AJR Am J Roentgenol 162:1–8

Tsubamoto M, Jokoh T, Kozuka T et al (2002) Temporal subtraction for the detection of hazy pulmonary opacities on chest radiography. AJR Am J Roentgenol 179:467–471

Ueguchi T, Johkoh T, Tomiyama N et al (2005) Full-size digital storage phosphor chest radiography: Effect of 4K versus 2K matrix size on observer performance in detection of subtle interstitial abnormalities. Radiat Med 23:170–174

Van den Boom J, Battin M (2007) Chest radiographs after removal of chest drains in neonates: clinical benefit or common practice? Arch Dis Child Fetal Neonatal Ed 92: F46–F48 doi: 10.1136/dc.2005.091322

Willis CE, Slovis TL (2004) The ALARA concept in pediatric CR and DR: dose reduction in pediatric radiographic exams–A white paper conference. Executive summary. Pediatr Radiol 34 (Suppl 3):S162–S164

Hyaline Membrane Disease and Complications of Its Treatment

Veronica Donoghue

CONTENTS

4.1
Introduction

Hyaline membrane disease (HMD) or idiopathic respiratory distress syndrome (IRDS) affects premature infants, most of those concerned being born at less than 36 weeks of gestational age and weighing less than 2.5 kg. Infants of diabetic mothers are also more prone to develop the condition (ROBERT et al. 1976) because foetal hyperinsulinism interferes with the glucocorticoid axis that governs surfactant synthesis (AGRONS et al. 2005). It is a leading cause of death in live born infants. Males are affected more commonly than females, and the condition is more common in whites than blacks (CLEVELAND 1995).

V. DONOGHUE, MD
Consultant Paediatric Radiologist, Radiology Department, Children's University Hospital, Temple Street, Dublin 1, Ireland and Radiology Department, The National Maternity Hospital, Holles Street, Dublin 2, Ireland

4.2
Pathophysiology

The basic problem in this condition is a deficiency of the lipoprotein pulmonary surfactant superimposed on structural immaturity of the lungs. This lipoprotein is believed to be produced in the endoplasmic reticulum of the type II pneumocytes and is then transported through the Golgi apparatus and then concentrated into intracellular lamellar bodies. Lamellar bodies then migrate to the cell surface, where their contents are expressed onto the alveolar luminal surface by exocytosis. The surfactant phospholipids combine with four surface active apoproteins (surfactant proteins A, B, C and D), which are also produced by the type II pneumocytes, to form a complex lattice called tubular myelin (AGRONS et al. 2005; NEWMAN et al 2001). Without it alveolar surface tension is elevated, alveolar distensibility is reduced and there is collapse of the alveoli. Massive atelectasis has been identified following previous radiographic-pathological correlation in infants of 30 weeks or greater gestational age (TUDOR et al. 1976; EDWARDS et al. 1980). As a result, there is poor gas exchange, hypoxia, hypercarbia and acidosis. In HMD the alveoli are collapsed, but the alveolar ducts and terminal bronchioles are distended and lined with hyaline membranes containing fibrin, cellular debris and fluid. They are a constant finding in airspaces in infants surviving at least 8 h with lung disease and are thought to result from a combination of ischaemia, barotrauma and the increased oxygen concentrations delivered by assisted ventilation (WOOD et al. 1989). Hyaline membrane formation also occurs in other neonatal lung diseases requiring artificial ventilation and is not specific to HMD.

In a study of extremely premature infants (WOOD et al. 1989), pulmonary haemorrhage, interstitial oedema, airspace oedema and occasionally underexpansion with severe immaturity contributed to the pattern of coarse linear density or patchy consolidation. Profound oedema with associated haemorrhage was the underlying abnormality in most of the babies examined. This accounted for deterioration of the infants' condition and produced the major radiographic changes. It is suggested that there are several factors responsible for the presence of oedema (WOOD et al. 1989; BRASCH et al. 1993). Immature arterioles have a highly permeable basement membrane, a defect that is enhanced by anoxia and acidosis. With large intravascular volumes and increased pulmonary blood flow intravascular fluid loss increases. Immature vessels may lack sufficient smooth muscle to compensate for haemodynamic and osmotic changes. Interstitial pericapillary pressures lower than alveolar pressures produce transmural pressure gradients which cause capillaries to leak. When intercellular junctions leak at the type 1 pneumocyte lining layer, protein molecules in the alveolar lining fluid exert a colloid osmotic pressure, drawing water into the alveolus. At low lung volumes the less negative interstitial tissue pressure hampers fluid movement into the lymphatics. Pulmonary haemorrhage occurs because of immature sequence of clotting factors, platelet sequestration or vitamin K and enzymatic deficiency. In addition, immature capillaries have poorer wall integrity.

4.3
Radiographic Findings and New Treatments

Clinically these infants are usually symptomatic within minutes of birth, with grunting, nasal flaring, retractions, tachypnoea and cyanosis. Although the initial radiographic findings may be noted shortly after birth, occasionally the maximum radiographic findings are not present until 6–24 h of life.

Prior to the commencement of treatment, typically the radiographic findings are those of underaeration of the lungs with fine granular opacities and air bronchograms which are diffuse and symmetrical (Fig. 4.1). This appearance is due to a combination of collapsed alveoli interspersed with dilated terminal bronchioles and alveolar ducts. When the distension is less, the granularity disappears and is replaced by a more generalised opacification or a frank whiteout of the lungs (Fig. 4.2). Atelectasis is the main cause of this opacification (TUDOR et al. 1976; EDWARDS et al. 1980), but in very premature infants in particular, oedema, haemorrhage and very occasionally pneumonia are contributors (WOOD et al. 1989). Very small infants less than 26 weeks of gestation may initially have clear lungs or mild pulmonary haziness (Fig. 4.3) (NEWMAN 1999). The lungs in these profoundly premature infants are both biochemically and structurally immature and require prolonged ventilatory support.

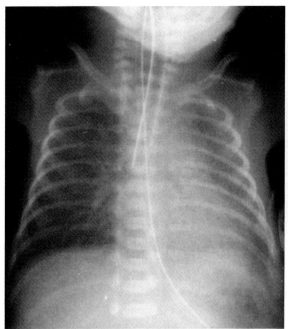
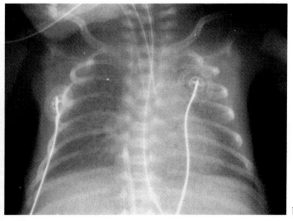

Fig. 4.1. a Mild hyaline membrane disease (HMD) with very fine granular appearance in both lungs. Note position of endotracheal tube in proximal right main bronchus. **b** Moderate HMD: the lungs have a fine granular appearance with air bronchograms. The abnormality is diffuse and symmetrical

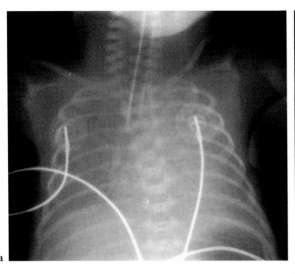
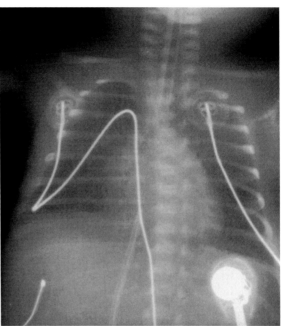

Fig. 4.2. **a** Severe hyaline membrane disease with almost complete "whiteout" of both lungs. Some air bronchogram visible in right lung. **b** Dramatic improvement after surfactant therapy

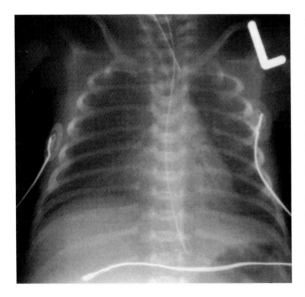

Fig. 4.3. Infant born at 25 weeks of gestation. There is a good inspiratory effort and mild perihilar haziness

Several technologies have significantly altered the clinical and radiographic evolution of HMD. Prenatal steroid administration to mothers during the 2 days prior to delivery is safe and significantly reduces the incidence of HMD in premature infants (CROWLEY et al. 1990). Though the trial results have not confirmed a definite benefit in infants born at 24–28 weeks gestation, the National Institutes of Health recommend that all pregnant women due to deliver prematurely during 24–34 weeks gestation should be considered eligible for a single course of corticosteroids (ACOG Practice Bulletin 2002). It promotes endogenous surfactant production and lung maturation in addition to inducing antioxidant enzymes (NORTHWAY 1992). A similar response can occur when maternal steroid production is increased because of the stress that is caused by prepartum maternal infection, toxaemia and other forms of prepartum stress (Thibeault and Emmanouilides 1977), but these stressful situations usually need to exist for 24 h or more before delivery (SWISCHUK 2003).

The clinical use of artificial surfactant, both animal derived and synthetically produced, has been a very important recent therapeutic advance. It is given at birth, with up to three or four additional doses in the first 48 h in selected patients. As a result, there is less need for long-term high-pressure ventilation and high oxygen concentrations. It acts rapidly, with the synthetic agents being somewhat slower in onset of action. Radiographic improvement can also occur quickly (Fig. 4.2). The surfactant is given as a liquid bolus through the endotracheal tube. It is often not evenly distributed throughout the lungs, and on the chest radiograph it is common to see areas of lung which may improve in aeration alternate with areas of unchanged HMD (Fig. 4.4) (SLAMA et al. 1999). This may produce a radiograph simulating other entities, such as neonatal pneumonia. In addition, the surfactant may reach the level of the acini, causing sudden distension, which produces a radiographic picture similar to that of pulmonary interstitial emphysema (Figs. 4.5, 4.6). It is therefore essential, when interpreting the radiographs, to correlate the picture closely with the clinical findings. In general, older and larger babies with HMD respond best to surfactant therapy (SWISCHUK et al. 1996). Smaller infants, generally under 27 weeks of gestation and weighing less than 1,000 g, do not respond so well. In these infants the biochemical abnormality manifested as surfactant deficiency can now be treated. However, the structural immaturity of the lungs is not affected by the surfactant therapy. The lungs of these infants, although becoming clear after surfactant, are still hypoplastic with fewer alveoli than normal. This leads to inadequate gas exchange and the need for prolonged ventilator-assisted treatment, which in turn leads to chronic lung problems, the most common being the development of a hazy to opaque appearance on the chest radiograph (SWISCHUK et al. 1996; ODITA 2001). This reflects the presence of pulmonary oedema and haemorrhage (WOOD et al. 1989). Several factors cause oedema. Immature arterioles have a highly permeable basement membrane, which is damaged further by hypoxia and

acidosis and oxygen toxicity. The result is seepage of fluid into the pulmonary interstitium, or "leaky lung" syndrome (SWISCHUK et al. 1996; BRASCH et al. 1993) (Fig. 4.7). Rather less commonly a radiographic pattern may evolve into a much coarser, irregular appearance similar to that seen in stage-3 bronchopulmonary dysplasia, a situation originally described as occurring at several weeks of age (NORTHWAY 1992).

A patent ductus arteriosus is normal in most premature infants and is thought to contribute to the lung disease. In the early stages of HMD the rigid noncompliant lungs and the resultant hypoxia and hypercarbia result in persistent pulmonary vasoconstriction. This may lead to right-to-left shunting through the ductus. With improved oxygenation as a result of surfactant treatment pulmonary resistance decreases, and this may lead to left-to-right shunting and consequent pulmonary oedema. This may be recognised radiographically before any clinical symptoms of a murmur develop. In addition to the pulmonary oedema, the chest radiograph may demonstrate sudden cardiac enlargement together with left atrial enlargement causing elevation or distortion of the left main bronchus (Fig. 4.8). Treatment with indomethacin may produce ductal closure, but surgery may occasionally be required.

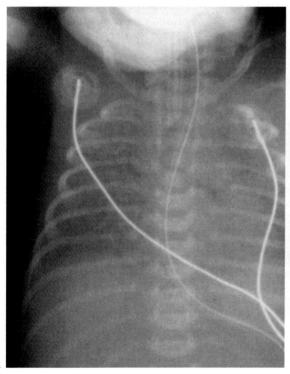

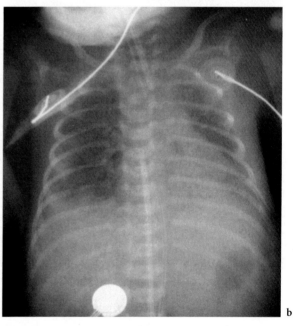

Fig. 4.4. a Severe hyaline membrane disease in a premature infant. **b** After surfactant therapy. There is better aeration of the upper lobes and the right middle lobe than of the lower lobes

High-frequency ventilation has also recently been employed to reduce the incidence of barotrauma. This is a method of mechanical ventilation that employs supra-physiological breathing rates and tidal volumes frequently less than dead space. This allows the primary goals of ventilation, oxygenation and carbon dioxide removal to be achieved without the penalty of pressure-induced injury. The aim is to achieve maximum alveolar recruitment without causing overdistension of the lungs.

As overinflated lungs compromise the systemic circulation, this is to be avoided. The radiographs of babies receiving high-frequency ventilation are not significantly different from those of babies receiving conventional ventilator therapy. However, the chest radiograph is the best diagnostic tool for assessing overinflation of the lungs. Ideally the dome of the diaphragm should project over the 8th to the 10th posterior ribs if the main airway pressure is appropriately adjusted (Fig. 4.9).

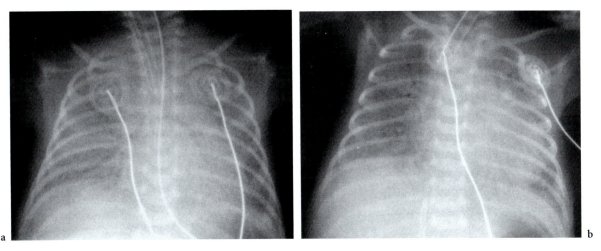

Fig. 4.5. a Severe hyaline membrane disease in a premature infant. **b** After surfactant therapy: small air bubbles in both upper lobes as a result of focal acinar distension

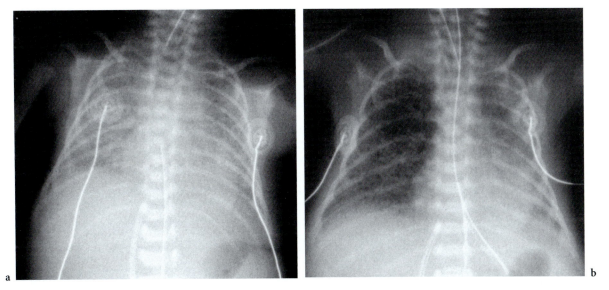

Fig. 4.6. a Severe hyaline membrane disease in an infant. **b** Significant sudden acinar distension of the right lung, similar in appearance to pulmonary interstitial emphysema. There was an improvement in the infant's clinical condition

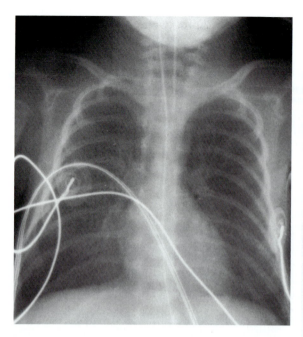

Fig. 4.7. Chest X-ray of an infant born at 25 weeks of gestation. There is bilateral perihilar hazy opacification or "leaky lung" syndrome

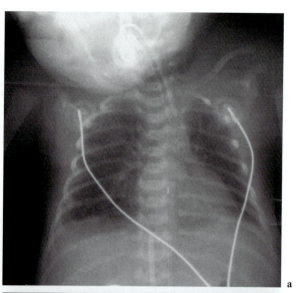

a

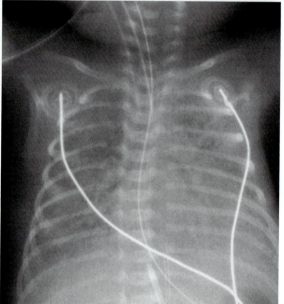

b

Fig. 4.8. a Premature infant 24 h after surfactant therapy. There is almost complete clearing of the lungs. **b** At day 3 the infant developed a patent ductus arteriosus. The heart size has increased. There is distortion of the left main bronchus. The marked bilateral pulmonary opacification is due to pulmonary oedema

Fig. 4.9. Premature infant on high-frequency ventilation. The dome of the diaphragm lies between the posterior aspects of the 9th and 10th ribs

4.4
Air Leaks

Spontaneous pneumothorax and pneumomediastinum are a cause of respiratory distress in some newborn infants. They are usually transient and do not need intervention. However, positive pressure ventilation in newborns is the most common cause of pneumothorax, pneumomediastinum, pulmonary interstitial emphysema and pneumopericardium. These have become much less common with the more routine use of artificial surfactant and high-frequency ventilation. In all instances when a terminal airway ruptures, most often as a result of air being forced into the collapsed alveoli of HMD, air leaks into the pulmonary interstitial tissues and lymphatics and results in pulmonary interstitial emphysema. This is a serious problem, as it causes stiff, poorly compliant lungs which do not empty with expiration (SWISCHUK 2003). As a result, gas exchange is poor, which in turn leads to increased ventilatory requirements (NEWMAN 1999). It may also compromise pulmonary blood flow. The abnormality may be unilateral, bilateral or confined to part of a lung. It may cause mass effect and mediastinal shift (WILLIAMS et al. 1988). Radiographically, pulmonary interstitial emphysema is seen as bubbles often radiating outwards from the hilum towards the periphery along the perivascular bundles (Fig. 4.10). Treatment includes lowering ventilatory pressures and decubitus positioning with the affected side down. Other measures, such as selective intubation of the unaffected side, have also been reported (NEWMAN 1999; SWISCHUK 2003).

When interstitial air reaches the pleural surface of the lung, if these blebs burst a pneumothorax develops (Fig. 4.10). In addition, air dissecting centrally can leak into the mediastinal or pericardial space or downwards into the peritoneal cavity. These air collections, particularly pneumothoraces, may be under tension in a ventilated infant and require rapid decompression. Occasionally air may reach the pulmonary venous system causing air embolus, which is usually fatal. Access to the systemic venous system is thought to be via the lymphatic ducts (BOOTH et al. 1995). Large pneumothoraces are usually easy to identify. A pneumothorax may be radiographically subtle because sick ventilated infants are usually placed in a supine position and free air may accumulate over the anterior surface of the lung, producing a large hyperlucent lung and increased sharpness of its mediastinal edge. When anterior pneumothoraces are bilateral the entire chest is hyperlucent with a sharp mediastinum. The thymus may also be compressed, giving the appearance of a superior mediastinal mass. As the lungs are non-compliant in HMD, they do not easily collapse and air collects anteromedially, inferiorly or in pockets (Fig. 4.10). Medial collections may be difficult to differentiate from a pneumomediastinum. If a pneumomediastinum is anteriorly located it usually outlines a thymus (Fig. 4.11), and if posteriorly located it may dissect into the subcutaneous tissues of the neck and chest wall or inferiorly into the retroperitoneum and pericardial cavity (SWISCHUK 2003; QUATTROMANI et al. 1981). These mediastinal collections are usually asymptomatic and rarely require intervention. Pneumopericardium is recognised by the presence of air completely surrounding the heart, and the pericardial sac may be visible as a white line (BURT and LESTER 1982) (Fig. 4.12). In these infants pericardial tamponade may require rapid decompression. If one is in doubt as to the location of the free air, cross-table lateral or decubitus views may help.

Skin folds should not be mistaken for pneumothoraces. These lines can often be seen to continue beyond the lung edge, and their course is usually opposite to that of the line produced by the edge of the lung in a pneumothorax.

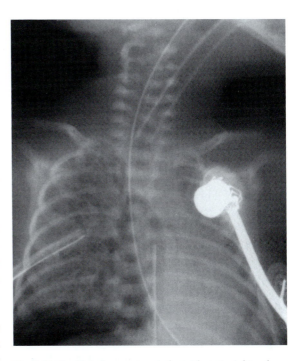

Fig. 4.10. Ventilated premature infant. There is right pulmonary interstitial emphysema and a right inferior and medial pneumothorax causing mediastinal displacement to the left side. A right chest drain is in position

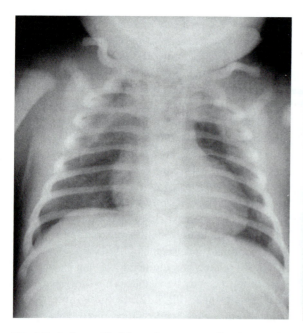

Fig. 4.11. Infant with bilateral pneumomediastinum. The thymus is clearly outlined

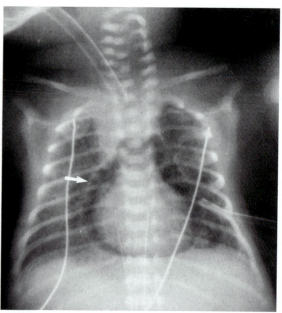

Fig. 4.12. Ventilated premature infant. There is a pneumo-pericardium. The heart is completely surrounded by air, and the pericardial sac is visible as a thin white line (*arrow*). There is also some bilateral pulmonary interstitial emphysema. A left chest drain is in position

4.5
Atelectasis

All forms of surfactant deficiency are associated with alveolar atelectasis, and its occurrence is not infrequent. The atelectasis can be segmental (Fig. 4.13), lobar or even total. There is usually intrinsic obstruction of a bronchus.

A significant cause of focal atelectasis, particularly that of the right upper lobe, is endotracheal tube malpositioning (Fig. 4.14). Atelectasis can also occur in other lobes and is frequently due to poor clearance of secretions and plugging of the endotracheal tube with mucus (Newman 1999). Additionally, atelectasis, especially of the right upper lobe, is common following extubation (Finer et al. 1979) (Fig. 4.15). The condition is usually easy to identify radiographically. There is pulmonary opacification with corresponding volume loss or ipsilateral mediastinal shift which is proportional to the degree of atelectasis.

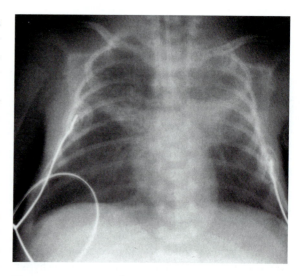

Fig. 4.13. Premature infant with segmental atelectasis both upper lobes

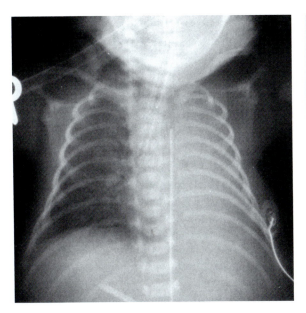

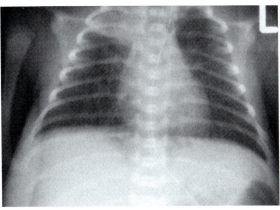

Fig. 4.15. Infant after extubation. There is right upper lobe atelectasis. In addition, there is underlying bronchopulmonary dysplasia of a moderate degree, with mild overinflation and diffuse interstitial shadowing

Fig. 4.14. The endotracheal tube tip is in the right main bronchus. There is left lung collapse as a result

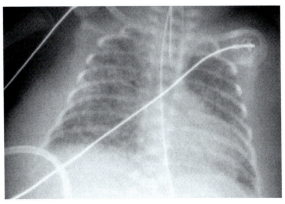

Fig. 4.16. Chest radiograph (day 12) of a premature infant born at 25 weeks gestation. There is coarse bilateral pulmonary opacification in keeping with pulmonary infection. Multiple sterile abscesses were found at post-mortem examination 2 days later

4.6
Pneumonia

Premature infants, including those with HMD, are at increased risk of pneumonia, and the two conditions frequently co-exist (CLEVELAND 1995). Viral infections are also common in hospitalised infants, and agents such as *Ureaplasma* are emerging as of importance in infants with bronchopulmonary dysplasia and prolonged ventilatory requirements (NEWMAN 1999).

It may be difficult both clinically and radiographically to determine the presence of infection in infants in the various stages of treatment for HMD. The radiographic appearance may be identical to the picture of HMD. The lungs may be compliant, with lower levels of ventilatory support required relative to the degree of pulmonary opacification seen on the chest radiograph.

The development of patchy pulmonary opacification is commonly seen on comparison of current and previous radiographs (Fig. 4.16). Radiographic alterations may be very subtle, however, especially when superimposed on chronic lung changes. Viral infections often produce diffuse peribronchial inflammation, which results in diffuse air trapping and patchy atelectasis (SWISCHUK 2003).

4.7
Pulmonary Haemorrhage

Pulmonary haemorrhage is also a superimposed problem in infants with HMD. It usually represents intrapulmonary bleeding secondary to severe hypoxia and capillary damage. In mild cases the radiographic findings are usually those of the various stages of HMD and infiltrations resulting from focal areas of superimposed microscopic haemorrhage are difficult to detect. When haemorrhage is massive it is not difficult to identify. Clinically respiratory distress develops suddenly, and blood may ooze from the nose, mouth or endotracheal tube.

- Radiographically the lungs may show homogeneous opacification and appear airless (Swischuk 2003) (Fig. 4.17). Occasionally a dramatic increase in left-to-right shunting following surfactant administration also leads to pulmonary haemorrhage (Wood 1993).

4.8
Neonatal Chronic Lung Disease

Chronic lung disease or bronchopulmonary dysplasia (BPD) is a significant long-term consequence of neonatal lung disease. The condition most commonly occurs after treatment for HMD with mechanical ventilation, but many other neonatal lung diseases which require positive pressure ventilation and oxygen therapy can result in chronic lung changes. The cumulative effects of prolonged oxygen exposure and the pressure-induced lung injury of positive pressure ventilation on the immature lungs are thought to be the primary cause of the chronic lung disease. This type of disease is characterised by terms such as necrotizing bronchiolitis, alveolar cell hyperplasia, bronchiolar squamous metaplasia and focal alveolar septal fibrosis (Agrons et al. 2005). An inflammatory response and fibrotic reaction seem to be important in its development (Northway 1992; Newman 1999; Groneck et al. 1994). Struc-

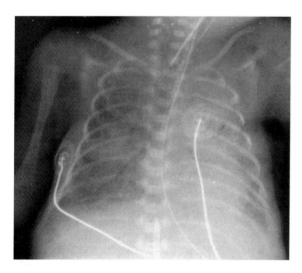

Fig. 4.17. Premature infant with HMD. Marked bilateral pulmonary opacification of a rather coarse nature in keeping with pulmonary haemorrhage. Blood oozed from the endotracheal tube

tural changes in the pulmonary arteries are similar to those seen in hypertensive vascular disease and include intimal proliferation, medial hyperplasia and adventitial thickening (Agrons et al. 2005). In long-standing chronic lung disease alveolar septal fibrosis is a predominant feature and it may vary from acinus to acinus in the same infant (Stoker 1986; Agrons et al. 2005).

Air leaks, patent ductus arteriosus and infection, which prolong the ventilatory requirements, are contributory factors. Genital ureaplasma urealyticum infection, the most common contaminant of amniotic fluid, has also been associated with the development of chronic lung disease (Theilen et al. 2004; Kotecha et al. 2004)

In 1989 the American Bureau of Maternal and Child Health and Resources Development put forward the following diagnostic criteria for BPD:
- Positive pressure ventilation during the first 2 weeks of life for a minimum of 3 days
- Clinical signs of respiratory compromise persisting beyond 28 days of age
- Requirement for supplemental oxygen beyond 28 days of age to maintain a PaO2 above 500 mmHg
- Chest radiograph with findings characteristic of BPD

A new definition of chronic lung disease has been developed for infants less than 32 weeks gestational age and greater than 32 weeks. In infants less than 32 weeks, chronic lung disease is considered of moderate severity if they require less than 30% oxygen at 36 weeks chronological age or at discharge if this occurs first. If the oxygen requirements are greater than 30% with or without ventilation or nasal CPAP the condition is considered severe. In infants greater than 32 weeks gestational age the time of clinical assessment is 56 days of postnatal age or at discharge (Jobe and Bancalari 2001). Such infants often have associated abnormalities such as pneumonia, atelectasis, aspiration, pulmonary oedema and pulmonary hypertension. Nutritional requirements are difficult to maintain and there may be poor growth and osteopenia.

Northway et al. described the condition in 1967. Their work described the course of the disease through four stages beginning at 2–3 days of life and reaching the final chronic phase at more than 1 month of age. Stage 1 at 2–3 days represents a generalised granular pattern and air bronchogram similar to that of severe HMD. Stage 2 is seen at age 4–10 days, when the chest radiograph shows almost complete opacification of both lungs. In stage 3 opacification is replaced by hyperlucent cystic areas and hyperinflation. Stage 4 represents enlargement of the cystic areas with linear strands due to fibrosis and atelectasis. Occasionally there may be cardiomegaly as the result of pulmonary hypertension. However, the radiological appearance has changed considerably since this original description of an ordered progression. Currently the severe cystic form is less common and is most frequently seen in very tiny premature infants (Fig. 4.18). Nowadays the most common radiographic appearance of chronic lung disease is that of diffuse interstitial shadowing with mild to moderate hyperinflation of the lungs of gradual onset and with little change over time (NORTHWAY 1992) (Fig. 4.15). This is thought to be due to mild diffuse alveolar septal fibrosis (HUSAIN et al 1998). It can be seen as early as the 10th to the 14th day of life. A normal chest radiograph (FITZGERALD et al. 1990) or leaky lung syndrome possibly related to increased capillary permeability and pulmonary oedema is not uncommon preceding or accompanying bronchopulmonary dysplasia in infants of extreme prematurity (Fig. 4.19). Radiographically this produces a diffuse hazy pattern (SWISCHUK et al. 1996). Ultrasonography of the chest has been used to predict the development of chronic lung disease in patients with hyaline membrane disease, but this practice is not widespread. The persistence of abnormal retrodiaphragmatic hyperechogenicity on day 9 or later has been observed in patients who were diagnosed with chronic lung dis-

ease at day 28 (PIEPER et al. 2004). Complications of bronchopulmonary dysplasia include tracheomalacia, tracheal and bronchial stenosis, atelectasis and lobar obstructive emphysema. Associated recurrent respiratory infections are also common. The entity described as Wilson-Mikity syndrome seems inseparable from BPD. It is described as seen in small infants whose first few days of life are rather uneventful. These infants develop respiratory distress later and most become oxygen dependent. Radiographically, as in BPD, the pattern is that of uneven aeration and cystic changes (WILSON and MIKITY 1960).

Most deaths from BPD occur early in infancy. In the majority of those who survive, lung recovery occurs over the first few years of life. Hyperinflation and linear shadowing representing fibrosis and deep pleural fissuring are not uncommonly seen in older children and adolescents. Survivors often have abnormal pulmonary function tests.

Though the incidence of BPD has not changed significantly despite the many technological advances, there has been a significant decrease in its severity, particularly in infants greater than 28 weeks of gestation. This unchanged incidence is largely due to the increased survival of very low birth weight premature infants. An advance in its treatment has been the use of short-term corticosteroids. These decrease inflammatory cell activity while also reducing inflammatory mediators (DURAND et al. 1995). They may also stabilise capillary permeability and prevent leaking of fluid.

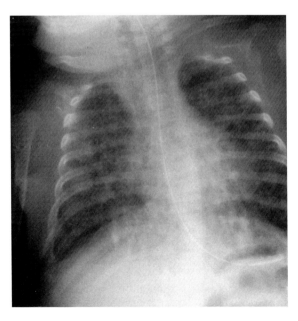

Fig. 4.18. Infant with severe bronchopulmonary dysplasia. There are hyperinflation, cystic changes and diffuse linear strands

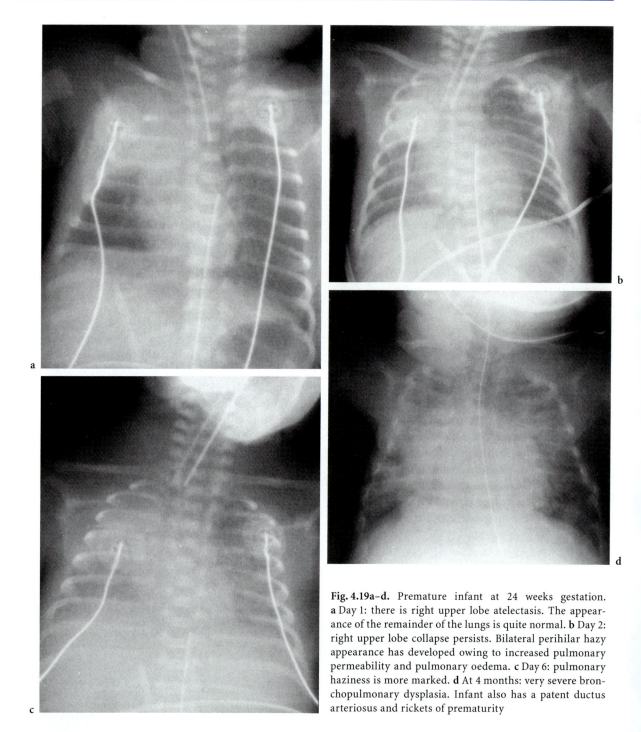

Fig. 4.19a–d. Premature infant at 24 weeks gestation. **a** Day 1: there is right upper lobe atelectasis. The appearance of the remainder of the lungs is quite normal. **b** Day 2: right upper lobe collapse persists. Bilateral perihilar hazy appearance has developed owing to increased pulmonary permeability and pulmonary oedema. **c** Day 6: pulmonary haziness is more marked. **d** At 4 months: very severe bronchopulmonary dysplasia. Infant also has a patent ductus arteriosus and rickets of prematurity

4.9
Conclusion

HMD is the most serious pulmonary abnormality in the premature infant. Exogenous surfactant and corticosteroid administration prior to delivery has had a major impact on both the clinical and the radiographic course. Chronic lung disease is still common, but is less severe than previously, especially in larger infants.

References

ACOG Practice Bulletin: Clinical Management Guidelines for Obstetrician-Gynaecologists: no. 38, September 2002. Perinatal care at the threshold of viability. Obstet Gynecol 100:617–624

Agrons GA, Courtney SE, Stocker JT, Markowitz RI (2005) Lung disease in premature neonates: radiologic-pathologic correlation. Radiographics 25:1047–1073

Booth TN, Allen BA, Royal SA (1995) Lymphatic air embolism: a new hypothesis regarding the pathogenesis of neonatal systemic air embolism. Pediatr Radiol 25 [Suppl 1]:220–227

Brasch RC, Berthezene Y, Vexler V, Rosenau W, Clement O, Muhler A, Kuwatsuru R, Shames DM (1993) Pulmonary oxygen toxicity: demonstration of abnormal capillary permeability using contrast enhanced MRI. Pediatr Radiol 23:495–500

Bureau of Maternal and Child Health and Resources Development (1989) Bronchopulmonary dysplasia (BPD) In: Guidelines for the care of children with chronic lung disease. Pediatr Pulmonol 6 [Suppl 3]:3–13

Burt TB, Lester PD (1982) Neonatal pneumopericardium. Radiology 142:81–84

Cleveland RH (1995) A radiologic update on medical disease of the newborn chest. Pediatr Radiol 25:631–637

Crowley P, Chalmers I, Keirse MJ (1990) The effects of corticosteroid administration before preterm delivery: an overview of the evidence from controlled trials. Br J Obstet Gynaecol 97:11–25

Durand M, Sardesai S, McEvoy C (1995) Effects of early dexamethasone therapy on pulmonary mechanics and chronic lung disease in very low birth weight infants: a randomized, controlled trial. Pediatrics 95:584–590

Edwards DK, Jacob J, Gluck L (1980) The immature lung: radiographic appearance, course and complications. AJR Am J Roentgenol 135:659–666

Finer NN, Moriarty RR, Boyd J, Phillips JH, Stewart AR, Vlan O (1979) Post-extubation atelectasis: a retrospective review and a prospective controlled study. J Pediatr 94:110–113

Fitzgerald P, Donoghue V, Gorman W (1990) Bronchopulmonary dysplasia: a radiographic and clinical review of 20 patients. Br J Radiol 63:444–447

Groneck P, Gotze-Speer B, Oppermann M, Giffert H, Speer CP (1994) Association of pulmonary inflammation and increased microvascular permeability during the development of bronchopulmonary dysplasia: a sequential analysis of inflammatory mediators in respiratory fluids of high risk premature neonates. Pediatrics 93:712–718

Husain AN, Siddiqui NH, Stocker JT (1998) Pathology of arrested acinar development in postsurfactant bronchopulmonary dysplasia. Hum Path 29 710–717

Jobe AH, Bancalari E (2001) Bronchopulmonary dysplasia. Am J Respir Crit Care Med 163:1723–1729

Kotecha S, Hodge R, Schaber JA, Miralles R, Silverman M, Grant WD (2004) Pulmonary ureaplasma urealyticum is associated with the development of acute lung inflammation and chronic lung disease in preterm infants. Pediatr Res 55:61–68

Newman B (1999) Imaging of medical disease in the newborn lung. Radiol Clin North Am 37:1049–1065

Newman B, Kuhn JP, Kramer SS, Carcillo JA (2001) Congenital surfactant protein B deficiency: emphasis on imaging. Pediatr Radiol 31:327–331

Northway WH (1992) Bronchopulmonary dysplasia: 25 years later. Pediatrics 89:969–973

Northway WH Jr, Rosan RC, Porter D (1967) Pulmonary disease following respirator therapy of hyaline membrane disease: bronchopulmonary dysplasia. N Engl J Med 276:357–368

Odita JC (2001) The significance of recurrent lung opacities in neonates on surfactant treatment for respiratory distress syndrome. Pediatr Radiol 31:87–91

Pieper CH, Smith J, Brand EJ (2004) The value of ultrasound examination of the lungs in predicting bronchopulmonary dysplasia. Pediatr Radiol 34:227–231

Quattromani FL, Foley LC, Bowen A (1981) Fascial relationship of the thymus: radiologic-pathologic correlation in neonatal pneumomediastinum. AJR Am J Roentgenol 137:1209–1211

Robert MF, Neff RK, Hubbell JP, Taeusch HW, Avery ME (1976) Association between maternal diabetes and the respiratory distress syndrome in the newborn. N Engl J Med 294:357–360

Slama M, Andre C, Huon C, Antoun H, Adamsbaum C (1999) Radiological analysis of hyaline membrane disease after exogenous surfactant treatment. Pediatr Radiol 29:508–511

Stoker JT (1986) Pathologic features of long-standing "healed" bronchopulmonary dysplasia: a study of 28 3- to 40-month-old infants. Hum Pathol 17:943–961

Swischuk LE (2003) Respiratory system. In: Swischuk LE (ed) Imaging of the newborn, infant and young child, 5th edn. Lippincott Williams and Wilkins, Baltimore

Swischuk LE, Shetty BP, John SD (1996) The lungs in immature infants: how important is surfactant therapy in preventing chronic lung problems? Pediatr Radiol 26:508–511

Theilen U, Lyon AJ, Fitzgerald T, Hendry GM, Keeling JW (2004) Infection with Ureaplasma urealyticum: is there a specific clinical and radiological course in the preterm infant? Arch Dis Child Fetal Neonatal Ed 89(2):F163–F167

Thibeault DW, Emmanouilides GC (1977) Prolonged rupture of fetal membranes and decreased frequency of respiratory distress syndrome and patent ductus arteriosus in preterm infants. Am J Obstet Gynecol 129:43–46

Tudor J, Young L, Wigglesworth JS, Steiner RE (1976) The value of radiology in the idiopathic respiratory distress syndrome: a radiological and pathological correlation study. Clin Radiol 27:65–75

Williams DW, Merten DF, Effmann EL (1988) Ventilator induced pulmonary pseudocysts in premature neonates. AJR Am J Roentgenol 150:885–887

Wilson MG, Mikity VG (1960) A new form of respiratory disease in premature infants. Am J Dis Child 99:489–449

Wood BP (1993) The newborn chest. Radiol Clin North Am 31:667–676

Wood BP, Davitt MA, Metlay LA (1989) Lung disease in the very immature neonate: radiographic and microscopic correlation. Pediatr Radiol 20:33–40

Transient Tachypnoea of the Newborn

5

Veronica Donoghue

CONTENTS

5.1
Introduction

Transient tachypnoea of the newborn is also referred to as retained foetal lung fluid. Normally this fluid is cleared from the lungs at, during or shortly after birth via the tracheo-bronchial system (30%), the interstitial lymphatics (30%) and the capillaries (40%) (CLEVELAND 1995). In transient tachypnoea of the newborn the normal physiological clearance of fluid is prolonged.

V. DONOGHUE
Radiology Department, Children's Univesity Hospital,
Temple Street, Dublin 1, Ireland
and
Radiology Department, The National Maternity Hospital,
Holles Street, Dublin 2, Ireland

5.2
Pathophysiology and Clinical Course

During foetal life the lungs are expanded with fluid, an ultrafiltrate of foetal serum which contributes to amniotic fluid volume (NEWMAN 1999). During and after birth the fluid is removed by the pulmonary lymphatics and capillaries (CLEVELAND 1995). Transient tachypnoea of the newborn occurs when there is slow or complete removal of the lung fluid. There is an increased incidence of this condition in infants delivered by caesarean section (MILNER et al. 1978; SWISCHUK 1970). It is postulated that the absence of squeezing of the thorax, which occurs during passage through the vaginal canal, leads to retention of lung fluid. Delayed clearance of fluid has also been reported to occur with hypoproteinaemia (STEELE and COPELAND 1972) and hyponatraemia and maternal fluid overload (SINGH and CHOOKANG 1984). There is also an increased incidence of the condition in very small, hypotonic or sedated infants and in infants who have experienced a precipitous delivery (SWISCHUK 1997). A cardiac aetiology for this condition has been suggested (HALLIDAY et al. 1981). The last authors reported mild left ventricular myocardial dysfunction in a small number of infants with transient tachypnoea of the newborn. However, transient tachypnoea is so common in the newborn period, and there are so many causes of myocardial dysfunction in the immediate neonatal period which can cause lung congestion of varying degrees, that it is difficult on the basis of this report to incriminate ventricular myocardial disease as a cause.

Mild to moderate respiratory disease without cyanosis is typically present at birth or in the first couple of hours. However, the condition does not always lead to overt respiratory distress. Clinically resolution usually occurs within 48 h, and often in 24 h or less. Treatment usually consists of supportive oxygen therapy and body temperature maintenance.

5.3
Radiographic Findings

The radiographic findings are rather characteristic (SWISCHUK 1997; WESENBERG et al. 1971). The most common appearance is mild overaeration of the lungs, perihilar interstitial shadowing, prominent blood vessels and fluid in the transverse fissure. Occasionally there are small pleural effusions (Fig. 5.1). There may be mild cardiomegaly. The radiographic appearances may be asymmetrical, and occasionally they are most marked on the right side. This right-sided predominance remains unexplained (SWISCHUK 1997; NEWMAN 1999). The radiographic changes may simulate the irregular pattern of opacification of meconium aspiration or of congenital neonatal pneumonia. Close clinical correlation may be necessary in the early stages of the disease to distinguish these. Though the findings may appear very marked in the early stages, their rapid clearance, usually within 24–48 h (Fig. 5.2), attests to the benign transient nature of the condition. In the severe cases where clearance may take up to 3 days, there should be rapid improvement on each successive image.

Focal retention of foetal lung fluid within congenital lobar emphysema has been recognised. It has been suggested that this focal retention occurs only, or mainly, within polyalveolar lobes, which is a point of difference from the classic congenital lobar emphysema (CLEVELAND and WEBER 1993). Infants with transient tachypnoea of the newborn are reported to have a significantly higher incidence of asthma in later childhood (SHOHAT 1989, SMITH et al. 2004).

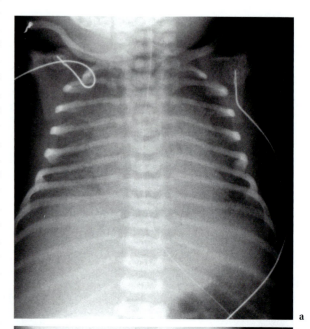

a

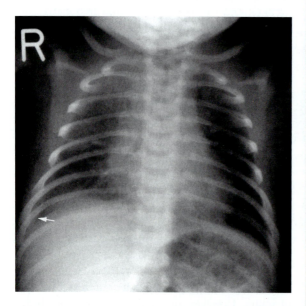

Fig. 5.1. Transient tachypnoea of the newborn. Lungs are well inflated. There is prominence of the blood vessels, perihilar interstitial shadowing most marked on the right side. There is fluid in the transverse fissure and a small right basal effusion (*white arrow*)

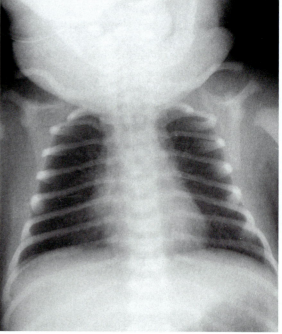

b

Fig. 5.2. a Transient tachypnoea of the newborn. Typical pattern of retained fluid. b Significant clearing of the lungs at 24 h

5.4
Conclusion

Transient tachypnoea of the newborn is a benign condition causing mild clinical symptoms that are transient. Though the radiographic features may be quite marked, resolution is usually complete by 24–48 h of age.

References

Cleveland RH (1995) A radiological update on medical diseases of the newborn chest. Pediatr Radiol 25:631–637

Cleveland RH, Weber B (1993) Retained fetal lung liquid in congenital lobar emphysema: a possible predictor of polyalveolar lobe. Pediatr Radiol 23:291–395

Halliday HL, McClure G, Reid MM (1981) Transient tachypnoea of the newborn: two distinct clinical entities? Arch Dis Child 56:322–325

Milner AD, Saunders RA, Hopkin IE (1978) Effects of delivery by caesarean section on lung mechanics and lung volume in the human neonate. Arch Dis Child 53:545–548

Newman B (1999) Imaging of medical disease of the newborn lung. Radiol Clin North Am 37:1049–1065

Shohat M, Levy G, Levy I, Schonfield T, Merlob P (1989) Transient tachypnoea of the newborn and asthma. Arch Dis Child 64(2):277–279

Singh SC, Chookang E (1984) Maternal fluid overload during labour; transplacental hyponatraemia and risk of transient neonatal tachypnoea in infants. Arch Dis Child 59:1155–1158

Smith GC, Wood AM, White IR, Pell JP, Cameron AD, Dobbie R (2004) Neonatal respiratory morbidity at term and the risk of childhood asthma. Arch Dis Child 89(10):956–960

Steele RW, Copeland GA (1972) Delayed resorption of pulmonary alveolar fluid in the neonate. Radiology 103:637–639

Swischuk LE (1970) Transient respiratory distress of the newborn-TRDN; a temporary disturbance of a normal phenomenon. AJR Am J Roentgenol 108:557–563

Swischuk LE (1997) Respiratory system in imaging of the newborn infant and young child, 4th edn. Williams and Wilkins, Baltimore

Wesenberg RL, Graven SN, McCabe EB (1971) Radiological findings in wet-lung disease. Radiology 98:69–74

Meconium Aspiration

6

CATHERINE M. OWENS

CONTENTS

6.1 Introduction

Aristotle originally coined the term 'meconium'. He used the Greek word meconium-arion to mean 'opium like' (WISWELL and BENT 1993), as he believed that meconium precipitated fetal sleep. It is probable that he recognised the association between the presence of the meconium in the amniotic fluid and subsequent fetal death or neonatal depression. Depending on the population studied, the frequency of meconium-stained amniotic fluid (MSAF) at de-

C. M. OWENS, MD
Radiology Department, Great Ormond Street Hospital for Sick Children NHS Trust, London, WC1N 3JH, UK

livery varies between approximately 8% and 19% of all term deliveries (GREGORY et al. 1974; WISWELL et al. 1990; SURESH and SARKAR 1994; FALCIGLIA et al. 1992; NATHAN et al. 1994; YODER 1994; PENG et al. 1996). Other factors, such as maternal ethnicity, result in a higher prevalence of meconium aspiration syndrome (MAS): the prevalence of MSAF in black is 1.5-fold that in white women (ALEXANDER et al. 1994), and the likelihood of MSAF increases with advancing gestational age in all ethnic groups.

Regardless of the aetiology of meconium passage, its presence is causally associated with adverse fetal and neonatal outcomes, including death, acute respiratory complications and long-term pulmonary and neurological abnormalities. Depending upon the population studied and the criteria used for making the diagnosis of MAS, approximately 2–33% of infants born through MSAF will develop MAS. Approximately a third of infants with MAS will then require mechanical ventilation (WISWELL et al. 1990; FLEISCHER et al. 1992). The complication of persistent pulmonary hypertension of the newborn (PPHN) exists in approximately one third of these infants (FLEISCHER et al. 1992). Sadly, the mortality associated with MAS is high, ranging from 4% to 19% (WISWELL et al. 1990; COLTART et al. 1989), and in a large majority of these patients mortality is due to complicating PPHN.

Subsequent neurological complications, such as early-onset neonatal seizures due to hypoxia, have also been reported in these infants born with thick MSAF (LIEN et al. 1995). Indeed, the increased likelihood of hypotonia in infants born through moderate to thick, as opposed to thin, amniotic fluid, whether meconium-stained or clear, is quite different. An article by BERKUS et al. (1994) showed a seven-fold risk of neonatal seizures, and a five-fold risk of floppy (hypotonic) infants born through moderate to thick, compared with thin, MSAF. Also of relevance is the presence of the long-term pulmonary sequelae of MAS.

A study by YUKSAL et al. (1993) showed abnormal obstructive pulmonary function tests, with increased functional residual capacity (FRC) and airway hyper-reactivity in infants at 6 months of age with a history of MAS. Those infants who required greater respiratory support in the neonatal period were significantly more symptomatic and required bronchodilator therapy more frequently. Late childhood sequelae include persistent airway hyper-reactivity and abnormal pulmonary function data later in childhood (MACFARLANE and HEAF 1988; SWAMINATHAN et al. 1989).

et al. 1994; MILLER and READ 1981). A study by ALEXANDER et al. (1994) shows that in the presence of fetal distress the odds of MSAF are twice as common as in its absence. The hypothesis that fetal hypoxia causes an increase in intestinal peristalsis, with anal sphincter relaxation resulting in meconium passage, is widely accepted. As a result of distress, fetal gasping results in meconium aspiration.

It is also thought that oligohydramnios may result in compression of the fetal head and the fetal umbilical cord, which may precipitate a vagal response and meconium passage.

6.2
Pathophysiology of Meconium Passage

Meconium is a green, viscous substance composed mainly of water (between 70% and 80%). Other components include mucus, gastrointestinal secretions, bile acids, bile, pancreatic juice, serous debris and swallowed amniotic fluid, lanugo, vernix caseosa and blood (WISWELL and BENT 1993; HOLTZMAN et al. 1989). The presence of meconium in the fetal gastrointestinal tract can be seen as early as at 10–16 weeks of gestation, and indeed at birth between 60 g and 200 g of meconium can be present in the intestinal tract of the term infant. It is uncommon for the fetus to pass meconium in utero, as there is no strong peristalsis, and this combined with the presence of a tonically contracted anal sphincter and the relative seal of a terminal cap of thick meconium, further decreases the likelihood of meconium passage. The passage of meconium is probably a physiological maturational event in many term and post-term infants, with meconium passage being rare before 37 weeks of gestation (MATTHEWS and WARSHAW 1979), but it may occur in over a third of cases of postmature pregnancy lasting longer than 42 weeks (USHER et al. 1988; MILLER and READ 1981). This may relate to higher levels of the hormone motilin, which is known to be responsible for GI motility in adults (and shown to be higher in term and post-term than preterm infants) (LUCAS et al. 1980). This further supports the hypothesis that maturation of the GI tract has a large role in the passage of meconium.

Also of great importance is the observation that the passage of meconium in utero is associated with ante- or intrapartum fetal acidaemia (NATHAN

6.3
Pathophysiology of Meconium Aspiration Syndrome

The definition of MAS is: respiratory distress in an infant born through MSAF where symptoms cannot be otherwise explained (CLEARY et al. 1992)

Many neonatal clinicians find the wide variety of chest X-ray findings amongst infants with MAS diverse enough to make specific radiographic features unnecessary as part of their diagnostic pathway, reflecting the extraordinarily complex pathophysiology of MAS. A prospective reason linking the passage of meconium and respiratory symptoms can either be secondary to aspiration of meconium in utero or at birth, or follow alterations in the pulmonary vascular system which occur as a result of asphyxia, or indeed the presence of meconium itself (Fig. 6.1) (FULORIA and WISWELL 1999). It is believed by various investigators that the presence of thick, as against moderately viscous or thin, meconium increases the likelihood of MAS (SURESH and SARKAR 1994; TING and BRADY 1975; NARANG et al. 1993). A paper by WISWELL and BENT (1993) describes a large, multicentre trial, which demonstrated a direct relationship between meconium thickness and degree of severity of subsequent respiratory disease within the neonate. It appears that the degree of symptomatology is directly related to the viscosity of meconium, and large amounts of thick meconium can potentially completely obstruct large airways. However, it is more common for the substance to migrate distally to the peripheral airways, where it causes either complete or partial obstructions (see Fig. 6.2). Complete obstruction leads to atelectasis and ventilation–perfusion (V/Q) mismatch. Par-

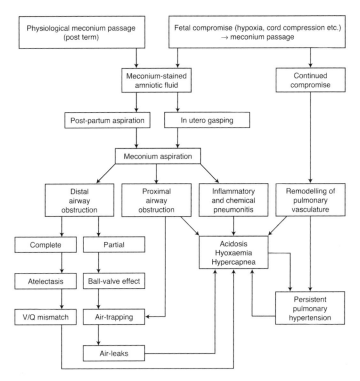

Fig. 6.1. Diagram to show the pathophysiological effects of meconium passage and meconium aspiration

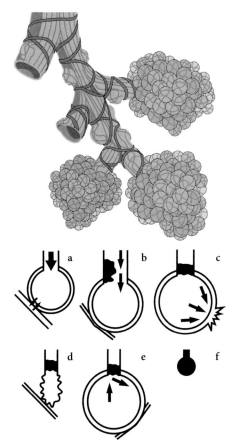

Fig. 6.2a–f. Diagrammatic representation of the dynamic effects of meconium aspiration on lung function. **a** Normal alveolar function with normal gaseous exchange across the alveolar membrane. **b** Complete obstruction of the alveolar unit with subsequent atelectasis and consequent intrapulmonary shunting. **c, d.** The 'ball-valve effect' with either (**c**) partial or (**d**) complete occlusion of the airway, and hence impossibility of air escape from the alveolar unit. **e** Overdistension and rupture of the alveolar unit with consequent air leak. **f** Atelectasis as a result of inadequate surfactant coating of the lungs due to meconium plugging

tial obstruction results in a "ball-valve" effect: gas flows into the airways on inspiration, but due to the smaller diameter on exhalation gas becomes trapped distally, and these obstructive properties result in the chest X-ray and histological findings classically seen in MAS, i.e., areas of atelectasis and consolidation adjacent to a distended hyper-expanded region (Stocker 1992; Tyler et al. 1978; Wiswell et al. 1992).

After several hours, the intense, inflammatory response to the presence of the toxic antigen (meconium) results in margination of polymorphonuclear leucocytes diffusely throughout the lungs (Stocker 1992; Tyler et al. 1978; Wiswell et al. 1992). The presence of these cells releases chemical mediators which adversely affect the tissues, and more specifically the presence of bile salts contained within meconium causes specific cytotoxicity in type II pneumocytes. This further contributes to the picture of the "chemical" pneumonitis (Oelberg et al. 1990). All of the aforementioned mechanisms lead to hypoxia, acidosis and hypercapnoea. These factors then in turn produce pulmonary vasoconstriction,

resulting in persistent pulmonary hypertension of the newborn (PPHN). Approximately two thirds of cases of PPHN are associated with MAS (Abu-Osa 1991).

Many infants respond to fetal hypoxia by remodelling pulmonary vasculature, resulting in thick muscularisation of the pulmonary vessels which aberrantly extends more distally than is appropriate along the intra-acinal vessels (Goetzman 1992;

MURPHY et al. 1984). Although there is some dispute regarding PPHN concomitant with MAS, the vicious cycle of shunting, hypoxaemia and acidosis may lead to further pulmonary hypertension, which may be either difficult or impossible to treat successfully.

Correlation of radiological appearances with outcome was studied by YEH et al. (1979), who noted that the presence of consolidation or atelectasis on the chest radiograph appeared to be more predictive of poor clinical outcome. However, Valencia and his colleagues (STOCKER 1992) were unable to predict the severity of the illness in infants with meconium aspiration accurately from the admission chest radiograph alone.

Using rabbit models of MAS, TYLER et al. (1978) showed an early onset of airway obstruction (as defined by alveolar collapse) correlated with ventilation–perfusion mismatch and an increase in functional residual capacity (FRC). In a similar model it has also been shown that chemical dysfunction in lungs is most prevalent during the early phase of MAS, with diminished dynamic and specific lung compliance, but unchanged static lung compliance suggestive of partial random obstruction of large airways (TRAN et al. 1980; WISWELL et al. 1998). Unfortunately this study is of limited duration, only considering the effects of meconium on the neonate within the first 2 hours of life; any effects occurring more than 2 hours after meconium aspiration were not, then, evaluated. Similar findings were observed by YEH et al. (1982; OELBERG et al. 1990), who evaluated pulmonary function tests in the first 3 days of life in neonates with mild MAS which did not result in the need for mechanical ventilation. It was demonstrated that dynamic and specific lung compliance were lower and airway resistance higher in these infants than in controls. It is important to note that poor correlation between the chest radiograph and clinical status may ensue, and children with substantial chest X-ray abnormalities and only minimal respiratory symptoms are observed as well as mild radiographic changes in severely ill neonates, a picture that is noted particularly in association with PPHN (CLEARY et al. 1992).

6.4
Inflammation

The presence of meconium in the airways induces an inflammatory response (see Fig. 6.3). A retrospective review of autopsied cases with histological evidence of meconium exposure showed that 60% of all cases with pulmonary inflammation were noted to be secondary to meconium aspiration.

Within an hour of exposure to meconium there is a profound pulmonary inflammatory response. Abundant neutrophils and macrophages are found in the alveoli, large airways and lung parenchyma.

Using rabbit models, in the latter stages of MAS there is characteristic microvascular endothelial damage with development of intrapulmonary shunts, alveolar collapse and cellular necrosis consistent with chemical pneumonitis (TYLER et al. 1978).

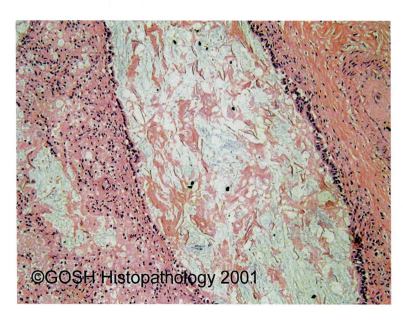

Fig. 6.3. Lung specimen from post mortem of child who died with meconium aspiration syndrome (MAS), demonstrating plugging of the airway with keratin and proteinaceous debris. (Haematoxylin-eosin)

Meconium has also been shown in vitro to inhibit the action of pulmonary surfactant function (Moses et al. 1991; Clark et al. 1987; Sun et al. 1993). In isolated rat alveolar cells, at low concentrations of meconium Higgins et al. (1996) demonstrated absence of toxicity to type II pneumocytes. However at higher concentrations of meconium (greater than 1%) he demonstrated dose-dependent cytotoxicity that was inhibited in the presence of heat-treated meconium, suggesting that a protein moiety may be partly responsible for this action (Sun et al. 1993). A cytotoxic effect of meconium has also been inferred by other investigators, who have demonstrated decreased production of surfactant protein B (SP-B) in the presence of high concentrations of meconium (Antunes et al. 1997).

As many as a third of infants with MAS develop PPHN (Fleischer et al. 1992), and approximately two thirds of infants with PPHN had associated meconium aspiration. The development of PPHN maybe a result of acidosis, hypoxia, or hypercapnoea associated with aspiration of meconium, or due to acute or chronic hypoxia in utero. The neonatal pulmonary vasculature is known to exhibit a greater vasoconstrictive response than do adult pulmonary arteries (Akopov et al. 1998). Additionally, the vessels possess a unique capability to undergo rapid changes in architecture, particularly thickening of the media and adventitia, distal extension of smooth muscle (Murphy et al. 1981) and increased tortuosity and muscularisation of the alveolar septal arterioles (Thureen et al. 1997).

6.5
Signs and Symptoms

Clinically, the infant with meconium aspiration syndrome can be quite depressed at birth, demonstrating pallor, cyanosis, apnoea, grunting and intercostal muscle retraction. As a consequence of air trapping and alveolar over-distension the chest can adopt a barrel configuration, and clinically rales and rhonchi are auscultated on physical examination.

Depending on the severity of meconium aspiration, both respiratory and metabolic acidosis may develop due to hypoxaemia and hypercarbia. The hypoxaemia and hypercarbia are secondary to ventilation–perfusion (V/Q) mismatch. Acidosis from any origin increases the risk of or potentiates PPHN.

Aspiration of meconium produces a chest radiographic picture characterised by (Tsu et al. 1979):
- Diffuse patchy nodular infiltrates, focal or general, asymmetric or symmetric
- Hyperinflation
- Air leaks
- Pleural effusion
- Cardiomegaly

Infiltrates. Complete airway occlusion results in atelectasis. This can be bilateral, diffuse, patchy or more nodular.

The lining of the alveolar sacs are more susceptible to injury and predispose to cellular necrosis which causes fluid accumulation in the airway, resulting in alveolar oedema. Cellular damage to capillary walls also results in inflammation leading to pulmonary oedema and pleural effusion secondary to leakage from capillary vascular beds (see Fig. 6.4)

Hyperinflation and Air Leaks. Partial occlusion of the airway and air sacs by meconium debris causes air trapping. (Fig. 6.5) Partial occlusion results in hyperinflation of the lungs shown by hypertransradiency of the lungs with depression of the hemidiaphragm. Overdistension of airway and terminal saccules may lead to alveolar rupture with free air dissecting into the interstitial lymphatics (Fig. 6.6a), pleural spaces (Fig. 6.6b, c) and mediastinum (Fig. 6.6d).

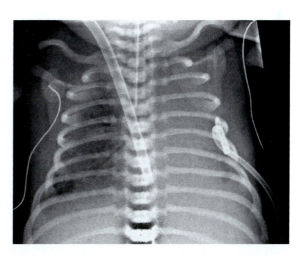

Fig. 6.4. Frontal radiograph of a child on veno-venous (VV) extracorporeal membrane oxygenation (ECMO) with coarse consolidation throughout the lungs and some overaeration of the anterior segment of the right lower lobe. There is a left basal intercostal drain draining a left pleural effusion, and a small right lamellar pleural effusion is also present

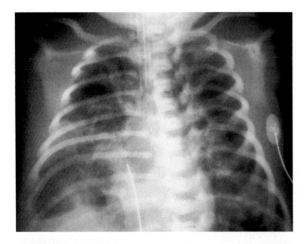

Fig. 6.5. Frontal chest radiograph showing areas of air trapping alternating with areas of atelectasis – classic features of neonatal MAS

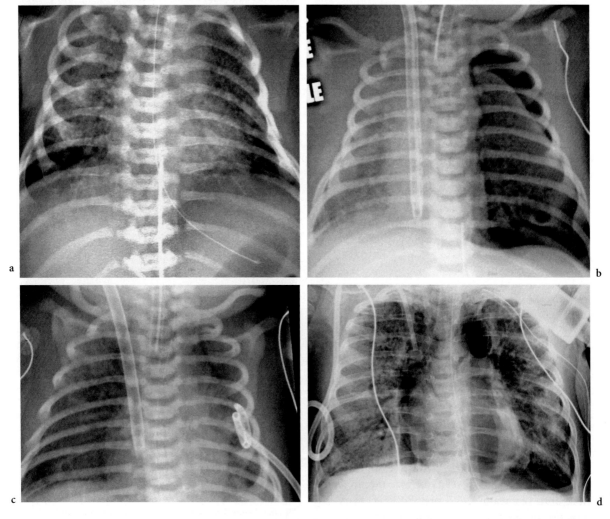

Fig. 6.6. a Frontal chest X-ray of child with MAS and early left upper lobe pulmonary interstitial emphysema (PIE). b Frontal radiograph of a child receiving VV ECMO with left-sided PIE and a large left pneumothorax causing mediastinal shift to the right. c Following suction on the intercostal drain the left pneumothorax has been almost completely drained, leaving a tiny anterior pneumothorax. d Child with MAS treated with conventional ventilation, showing extensive barotrauma-related complications with a large loculated pneumomediastinum and a left basal pneumothorax

Pleural Effusions. These are the result of inflammatory processes causing cellular necrosis and atelectasis which prevent the airway and air sacs from clearing pulmonary fluid effectively (Fig. 6.4).

Cardiomegaly. Cardiomegaly may occur as a result of direct intrauterine asphyxia associated with meconium aspiration and PPHN or the delayed effects of persistent pulmonary hypertension of the newborn.

In an interesting radiological study, Tsu et al. (1979) recorded the radiographic features present in the radiographs of 80 children with clinical and X-ray features of aspiration syndrome. The radiographic features present in the chest radiographs were divided into five separate categories, including consolidation or atelectasis, infiltration, hyperinflation, air leak and cardiomegaly. The incidence of respiratory failure was assessed in each category. The study showed that infants with consolidation or atelectasis had a higher incidence of respiratory failure and an increased mortality compared with those who did not have findings of consolidation or atelectasis (*P* 0.001) . Similarly, infants who had air leaks had a higher incidence of respiratory failure than those who did not show air leaks. The presence of air leak in infants with consolidation or atelectasis did not seem to be a significant contributing factor in causing either respiratory failure (10/17) or death (5/17), when their findings were compared with those of infants with consolidation or atelectasis but without air leak (13/27 and 18/27, respectively). Interestingly, infants who had consolidation or atelectasis as the sole radiographic feature also had a significantly higher (*P*<0.05) incidence of respiratory failure and death than those infants who had no consolidation. The authors suggest that consolidation or atelectasis appears to be the most significant determinant of respiratory failure and mortality.

This study leads to the conclusion that aspiration of meconium may produce two different radiographic patterns with different prognostic implications, i.e., one with consolidation or atelectasis, which has a poorer prognosis, and one without consolidation or atelectasis, which has a good outcome (due to aspiration of thin meconium or amniotic fluid). It appears that the initial chest X-ray with consolidation or atelectasis may be produced by aspiration of thick or sticky meconium in these infants and more severe clinical course and poorer outcome can be expected. On the other hand radiographic features of infiltration may be produced by aspiration of thin dilute meconium leading to a more benign course (similar to that of wet lung syndrome/TTN or amniotic fluid aspiration).

The authors also state that prevention is better than cure, i.e. reducing the potential of developing consolidation or atelectasis by deep oropharyngeal suctioning before delivery of the shoulder or prompt endotracheal suction of thick meconium is mandatory in cases of MASF.

6.6
Management of the Infant with Meconium Aspiration Syndrome

6.6.1
Conventional Mechanical Ventilation

One third of infants with MAS will require mechanical ventilation (Wiswell et al. 1990). The best method of ventilation management is controversial. Air leaks are a common complication of MAS (Fig 6.6a–d), especially amongst infants requiring positive pressure ventilation, and it has been shown by investigators (Yeh et al. 1982) that air trapping and increased functional residual capacity (FRC) may be exacerbated in patients on positive end expiratory pressure (PEEP) or CPAP (continuous positive airway ventilation), which are paradoxically believed to improve oxygenation in babies with MAS. The best strategy for ventilator settings once a child requires intermittent mandatory ventilation is controversial. There are advocates of using low inspiratory pressures and short inspiratory times with rapid ventilator rates to maintain arterial blood gases within normal limits, but there are no published data to substantiate their opinion that this arrangement is superior to the more commonly used ventilator settings. Additionally, one of the commoner treatments of infants with PPHN is hyperventilation (Fox and Duara 1983), with a principal goal of achieving respiratory alkalosis in an attempt to achieve vasodilatation within the pulmonary vascular bed. As two thirds of neonates with PPHN have associated MAC, hyperventilation is a common approach to the management of MAS. To date, however, there have been no prospective randomised trials comparing various mechanical ventilation strategies in the management of MAS.

6.6.2
High-frequency Ventilation

High-frequency ventilation (HFV) is a global description with several techniques, which provide effective gaseous exchange at low tidal volumes. Potential benefits of HFV may include less barotrauma, increased mobilisation of airway secretions, better attainment of respiratory alkalosis and fewer adverse histopathological changes.

6.6.3
Surfactant Therapy

Pulmonary immaturity due to surfactant deficiency is widely accepted as a primary cause of respiratory distress syndrome (RDS) in premature neonates. By contrast, however, the term infant who is more likely to suffer from MAS has a mature respiratory system with a normal alveolar surfactant pool. The surfactant deficiency seen in MAS is not the result of an insufficient quantity of surfactant, but is probably caused by inhibited surfactant function or alterations in surfactant composition. There is, however, limited information on the specific adverse effects of meconium on surfactant. In high concentrations, meconium has a direct cytotoxic effect on type II pneumocytes.

To date there has only be one randomised control trial specifically assessing the use of exogenous surfactant therapy for MAS (Findlay et al. 1996). In this study 20 affected infants were treated with 1.5+ standard dose of bovine lung surfactant administered as an infusion over 20 minutes. Significant improvements in oxygenation occurred 6–12 hours later, typically following additional surfactant doses. Six (30%) of the infants still required oxygen therapy at discharge. The authors therefore suggested further clinical trials before the widespread use of this therapy for MAS. Cleary and Wiswell (1998) conclude that surfactant therapy for MAS in humans still needs rigorous investigation.

6.6.4
Inhaled Nitric Oxide

Substantial effort has been invested in the assessment of the use of inhaled nitric oxide (INO) as a pulmonary vascular relaxing agent in the treatment of pulmonary artery hypertension.

In neonatal piglet models of MAS, Holopainen et al. (1999) found that prophylactic INO resulted in better oxygenation but did not affect the development of pulmonary hypertension. Further studies comparing the use of INO with conventional ventilation in patients diagnosed with MAS showed that INO led to better oxygenation and a lesser need for extracorporeal membrane oxygenation (ECMO) than was observed in control infants. There was no difference between the two groups in mortality, duration of mechanical ventilation or length of hospitalisation, however (The Neonatal Inhaled Nitric Oxide Study Group 1997). Roberts et al. (1997). It seems that although INO leads to better oxygenation in infants with MAS, this is not followed by any significant difference in the primary outcome (death or the need for ECMO).

6.6.5
Extracorporeal Membrane Oxygenation

The use of ECMO in the treatment of MAS was first described by Bartlett et al. (1977), who used ECMO to treat eight moribund neonates with MAS. Three of the infants survived, as compared with 90% mortality in conventionally treated groups. The use of veno-arterial (VA) ECMO became increasingly popular throughout the United States during the 1980s, with consistently encouraging results in neonates with severe MAS (Lillehei et al. 1989). Criteria for the institution of ECMO support were also refined over this time, and an oxygenation index greater than 40 was suggested as the referral criterion. The oxygenation index is calculated as follows.

$$\text{Oxygenation index} = P_{aw} + FIO_2/P_aO_2$$

where P_{aw} is the mean airway pressure, FIO_2 is the inspired oxygen fraction + 100 and P_aO_2 is the arterial oxygen tension in millimetres of mercury (mmHg). The recent publication of the UK Collaborative ECMO Trial Group (1996) has resulted in ECMO becoming a relatively well-accepted method of support for neonates with MAS in the UK. The results of the trial suggest that for every four infants receiving ECMO for MAS there was one extra survivor. Furthermore, although infants with MAS tend to be relatively less well than other term neonates with respiratory failure when treated conventionally, the converse is true when ECMO support is used. The survival figures for neonates with MAS who receive ECMO are extremely encouraging, and UK ECMO centres currently quote survival figures of around 90% for neonates in whom the primary indication is pulmonary hypertension without associated severe lung injury.

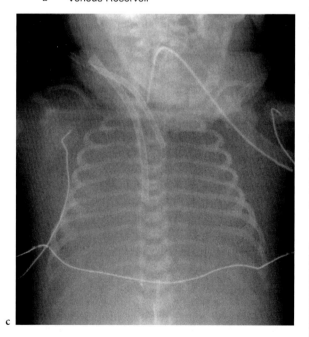

Circuit

- Arterio-venous (AV) ECMO – large bore cannulae in R common carotid artery / aortic arch and right atrium
- Circuit
  – blood out of RA → membrane → oxygenator → pump → oxygenated blood returned to aortic arch

b

Venous Drainage   Arterial

Water in
Water out
Heater

Oxygen in
Blood out
Oxygenator
Blood in
Oxygen out

a   **Venous Reservoir**   Roller Pump

c

Fig. 6.7. a Diagram and **b** summary of AV ECMO circuit **c** Chest X-ray of a child on AV ECMO. The (venous) catheter to the *right* lies in the right atrium and the more medially placed (arterial) catheter (midline) is within the right common carotid artery. An ET tube is noted, and a umbilical venous line is present with its tip at the level of the distal right atrium. The lungs are almost entirely collapsed

6.6.5.1
ECMO Technique

There are two methods of ECMO, both of which can be used to support neonates with MAS. Most ECMO centres initially used VA support, in which the right common carotid artery and internal jugular veins were cannulated, thus providing cardiac and respiratory support (Fig. 6.7a–c). More recently, however, veno-venous (VV) ECMO has emerged as the method of choice for neonates with hypoxic respiratory failure without significant haemodynamic instability (DE-LIUS et al. 1993) (Fig. 6.8).

In VV ECMO a double-lumen venous catheter is inserted into the right internal jugular vein with its tip in the right atrium. One lumen carries venous blood from the patient to the oxygenator, and the arterial lumen returns oxygenated blood to the heart (ANDREWS et al. 1983; KLEIN et al. 1985; PEEK et al. 1996) - (Figs. 6.7, 6.9). Most patients with MAS now receive VV ECMO.

Potential advantages of VV ECMO over VA ECMO are the reduced risk of intracranial haemorrhage and the theoretical advantage of preserving the intact carotid circulation. Cannulation of the arteries, as well as predisposing to arterial intracranial bleeds during ECMO (Fig. 6.10), are believed to cause haemodynamic disruption of flow after decannulation, either as a result of ligation of the vessel or because of the presence of a substrate causing turbulence or aneurysm formation if the vessel is repaired (DESAI et al. 1999; JACOBS et al. 1997).

6.6.5.2
Duration of ECMO Support

ECMO support is usually required for between 100 and 120 hours (DESAI et al. 1999) in MAS, the shortest

Arterio-venous (A-V) ECMO	Veno-venous (V-V) ECMO
Venous catheter • RA • tip = radiodense dot beyond apparent end of catheter • SVC or IVC placement → venous obstruction	• blood diverted from and returned to RA • one double lumen large bore catheter in RA • circuit provides no additional cardiac support ie. used for 'respiratory' neonates with good cardiac function • may be converted to V-A ECMO
Arterial catheter • aortic arch / origin R common carotid artery • directed down descending aorta (up overloads heart) • 'coiled' structure • small radiolucent portion beyond apparent tip	

Fig. 6.8. Table detailing AV and VV ECMO techniques

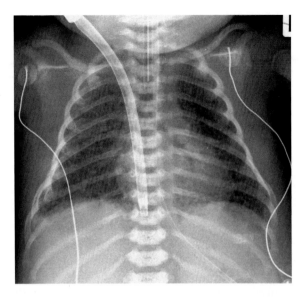

Fig. 6.9. Chest X-ray of a child with MAS treated with VV ECMO. The large VV ECMO catheter is noted with its tip in the right atrium. MAS has caused asymmetrical coarse reticulonodular change in the lungs

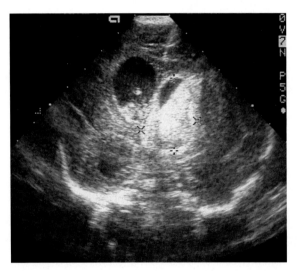

Fig. 6.10. Cranial ultrasound showing bilateral ventricular dilatation with large left intraventricular haemorrhage (IVH) in a child on ECMO

duration for any neonatal diagnosis (Fig. 6.11). This duration will inevitably be significantly increased if pressure/volume ventilation has led to air leaks before cannulation. Whilst undergoing ECMO, the infant receives resting ventilation with slow background ventilation at a moderate level of PEEP to maintain lung expansion (rate 10 per minute, pressures 20/10). Serial radiographs will show a complete

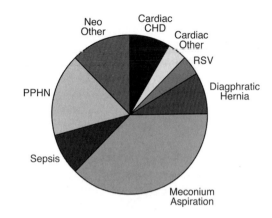

Fig. 6.11. Pie chart showing relative breakdown of indications for neonatal (*Neo*) ECMO (*CHD* chronic heart disease, *PPHN* persisting pulmonary hypertension of the newborn, *RSV* respiratory syncytial virus)

white-out during the first 2 or 3 days (Fig. 6.12a), with subsequent appearance of air bronchograms and resolution of the change as the lungs recover (Fig. 6.12b). Lung compliance can be estimated both manually and mechanically whilst the patient is on ECMO. Unless precipitous decannulation is required for other reasons, e.g. a large intracranial bleed, the infant is weaned from support when only minimal ventilatory support is needed to provide adequate lung expansion, oxygenation and gas exchange. At this stage there is usually radiological evidence of significant lung recovery.

In terms of long-term morbidity, survivors of ECMO do not appear to have a higher rate of disability or neurological damage than do conventionally treated severely hypoxic neonates with MAS, despite the greater proportion surviving.

6.7
Long-term Pulmonary Sequelae of MAS

MacFarlane and Heaf (1988) found a high prevalence of asthmatic symptoms (39%) and abnormal bronchial hyper-reactivity to exercise (33%) amongst survivors of neonatal MAS. This was much higher than the estimated prevalence of 10–12% in this age group in the general population. These children were not atopic or from atopic families and had not suffered other respiratory insults known to be associated with bronchial hyper-reactivity in later childhood. These findings of abnormal bronchial reactivity to

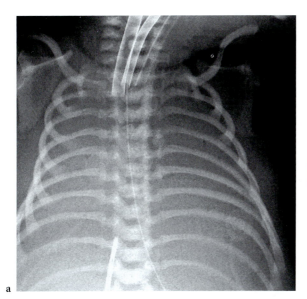

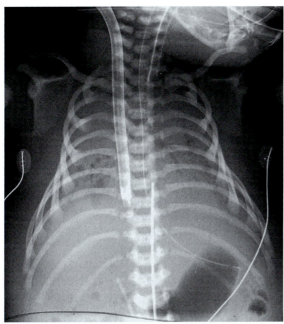

Fig. 6.12. a Chest X-ray showing complete 'white-outs' of both lungs due to low pressure maintenance ventilation (at 10 respirations per minute) for child on AV ECMO. **b** Chest X-ray of child on VV ECMO, with bilateral atelectasis and bibasal air bronchograms

abnormal bronchial reactivity, long after symptoms have resolved. It seems likely, therefore, that the developing respiratory tract is vulnerable to damage by many insults, and the nonspecific response is abnormal bronchial hyper-reactivity and limitation of airflow (MOK and SIMPSON 1984)

6.8
Conclusion

Meconium aspiration syndrome is a common neonatal problem with significant morbidity and mortality. It frequently leads to respiratory failure and even death. One third of the infants affected require ventilatory support, and a significant portion will die. MAS is the primary cause of lung disease in infants requiring ECMO oxygenation, and this despite significant advances in management. Initially emphasis should be placed on prevention and all MSAF-complicated pregnancies should be carefully monitored: in each case the obstetrician should perform thorough oropharyngeal suctioning as soon as the infant's head is in the perineum, when the paediatrician should perform thorough pharyngeal suctioning.

Endotracheal intubation and endotracheal suction should be restricted to those depressed infants who require positive pressure ventilation. Although there are no prospective randomised control trials assessing the effects of various mechanisms of mechanical ventilator strategies in the management of MAS, the use of surfactant and of inhaled NO appears to have significantly reduced the need for ECMO in the management of MAS.

Radiology has a crucial role in the management of these complex patients, and it is important to be acquainted with all forms of clinical management and their potential radiological complications.

exercise and mild expiratory air flow limitation make neonatal MAS another factor in the wide range of insults in the developing respiratory tract that can cause abnormalities of pulmonary function in later life. Aspiration of other foreign material (such as hydrocarbons or fresh water) is also associated with later abnormalities in pulmonary function, especially

References

Abu-Osa YK (1991) Treatment of persistent pulmonary hypertension of the newborn: update. Arch Dis Child 66:74–77

Akopov SE, Zhang L, Pearce WJ (1998) Maturation alters the contractile role of calcium in ovine basilar arteries. Pediatr Res 44:154–60

Alexander GR, Hulsey TC, Robillard P-Y et al (1994) Determinants of meconium-stained amniotic fluid in tern pregnancies. J Perinatol 14:259–263

Andrews AF, Klein MD, Tomasian JM, Roloff DW, Bartlett RH (1983) Venovenous extracorporeal membrane oxygenation in neonates with respiratory failure. J Pediatr Surg 18:339–346

Antunes MJ, Friedman M, Greenspan JS et al (1997) Meconium decreases surfactant protein B levels in rat fetal lung explants. Pediatr Res 41:137 (abstract)

Bartlett RH, Gazzinga AZ, Huxtable RF et al (1977) Extracorporeal circulation (ECMO) in neonatal respiratory failure. J Thorac Cardiovasc Surg 74:826–833

Berkus MD, Langer O, Samueloff A et al (1994) Meconium-stained amniotic fluid: increased risk for adverse neonatal outcomes. Obstet Gynecol 84:115

Clark DA, Nieman GF, Thompson JE et al (1987) Surfactant displacement by meconium free fatty acids: an alternative explanation for atelectasis in meconium aspiration syndrome. J Pediatr 110:765–170

Cleary GM, Wiswell TE (1999) Meconium-stained amniotic fluid and the meconium aspiration syndrome. An update (review). Pediatr Clin North Am 45:511–529

Collaborative ECMO trial group (1996) UK collaborative randomised trial of neonatal extracorporeal membrane oxygenation. Lancet 341:75–82

Coltart TM, Byrne DL, Bates SA (1989) Meconium aspiration syndrome: a 6 year retrospective study. Br J Obstet Gynaecol 96:411–414

Delius R, Anderson H, Schumacher R et al (1993) Venovenous compares favourably with venoarterial access for extracorporeal membrane oxygenation in neonatal respiratory failure. J Thorac Cardiovasc Surg 106:329–338

Desai SA, Stanley C, Gringlas M et al (1999) Five year follow-up of neonates with reconstructed right common carotid arteries after extracorporeal membrane oxygenation. J Pediatr 134:428–433

Falciglia HS, Henderschott C, Potter P et al (1992) Does DeLee suction at the perineum prevent meconium aspiration syndrome? Am J Obstet Gynecol 167:1243–1249

Findlay RD, Taeusch HW, Walther FJ (1996) Surfactant replacement therapy for meconium aspiration syndrome. Pediatrics 97:48

Fleischer A, Anyaegbunam A, Guidette D et al (1992) A persistent clinical problem: profile of the term infant with significant respiratory complications. Obstet Gynecol 79:185–190

Fox WW, Duara S, (1983) Persistent pulmonary hypertension in the neonate. J Pediatr 103:505–514

Fuloria M, Wiswell TE (1999) Resuscitation of the meconium-stained infant and prevention of meconium aspiration syndrome. J Perinatol 19:234–241

Goetzman BW (1992) Meconium aspiration. Am J Dis Child 146:1282

Gregory GA, Gooding CA, Phibbs RH et al (1974) Meconium aspiration in infants: a prospective study. J Pediatr 85:848–852

Higgins ST, Wu A-M, Sen N et al (1996) Meconium increases surfactant secretion in isolated rat alveolar type II cell. Pediatr Res 39:443–447

Holopainen R, Aho H, Laine J, Halkola L, Kaapa P (1999) Nitric oxide inhalation inhibits pulmonary apoptosis but not inflammatory injury in porcine meconium aspiration. Acta Paediatr 88:1147–1455

Holtzman RB, Banzhaf WC, Silver RK et al (1989) Perinatal management of meconium staining of the amniotic fluid. Clin Perinatol 16:825–838

Jacobs JP, Goldman AP, Cullen S et al (1997) Carotid artery pseudonaeurysm as a complication of ECMO. Ann Vasc Surg 11:630–633

Klein MD Andrews AF Wesley JR et al (1985) Venovenous perfusion in ECMO for newborn respiratory insufficiency. Ann Surg 210:520–526

Lien HM, Towers CV, Quilligan EJ et al (1995) Term early-onset neonatal seizures: obstetric characteristics, etiologic classifications, and perinatal care. Obstet Gynecol 85:163–169

Lillehei CW, O'Rourke PP, Vacanti JP, Crone RK (1989) Role of extracorporeal membrane oxygenation in selected pediatric respiratory problems. J Thorac Cardiovasc Surg 98:968–970

Lucas A, Adrian TE, Christofides N et al (1980) Plasma motilin, gastrin, and enteroglucagon and feeding in the human newborn. Arch Dis Child 55:673–677

Macfarlane PI, Heaf DP (1988) Pulmonary function in children after neonatal meconium aspiration syndrome. Arch Dis Child 63:368–372

Matthews TG, Warshaw JB (1979) Relevance of the gestational age distribution of meconium passage in utero. Pediatrics 64:30–31

MillerFC, Read JA (1981) Intrapartum assessment of the postdate fetus. Am J Obstet Gynecol 141:516–520

Moses D, Holm BA, Spitale P et al (1991) Inhibition of pulmonary surfactant function by meconium. Am J Obstet Gynecol 164:477–481

Mok JYQ Simpson H (1984) Outcome of acute bronchitis, bronchiolitis and pneumonia in infancy. Arch Dis Child 59:306–309

Murphy JD, Rabinovitch M, Goldstein JD et al (1981) The structural basis of persistent pulmonary hypertension of the newborn. J Pediatr 98:962–967

Murphy JD, Vawter GF, Reid LM (1984) Pulmonary vascular disease in fatal meconium aspiration. J Pediatr 104:758

Narang A, Nair PMC, Bhakoo O et al (1993) Management of meconium stained amniotic fluid: a team approach. Indian Pediatr 30:9–13

Nathan L, Leveno KJ, Carmody TJ et al (1994) Meconium: a 1990s perspective on an old obstetric hazard. Obstet Gynecol 83:329–332

Oelberg DG, Downey SA, Flynn MM (1990) Bile salt-induced intracellular Ca+ + accumulation in type II pneumocytes. Lung 168:297

Peek GJ, Firmin RK, Moore HM, Sosnowski AW (1996) Cannulation for neonates for venovenous extracorporeal life support. Ann Thorac Surg 61:1851–1852

Peng TCC, Gutcher GR, Van Dorsten JP (1996) A selective aggressive approach to the neonate exposed to meconium-stained amniotic fluid. Am J Obstet Gynecol 175:296–303

Roberts JD, Fineman JR, Morin FC et al (1997) Inhaled nitric oxide and persistent pulmonary hypertension of the newborn. N Engl J Med 336:605

Stocker JT (1992) The respiratory tract. In: Stocker JT, Dehner LP (eds) Pediatric pathology. Lippincott, Philadelphia, p 505

Sun B, Curstedt T, Robertson B (1993) Surfactant inhibition in experimental meconium aspiration. Acta Paediatr 82:182–189

Suresh GK, Sarkar S (1994) Delivery room management of infants born through thin meconium stained liquor. Indian Pediatr 31:1177–1181

Swaminathan S, Quinn J, Stabile MW et al (1989) Long-term pulmonary sequelae of meconium aspiration syndrome. J Pediatr 114:356–361

The Neonatal Inhaled Nitric Oxide Study Group (1997) Inhaled nitric oxide in full-term and nearly full term infants with hypoxic respiratory failure. N Engl J Med 336:597

Thureen PJ, Halliday HL, Hoffenberg A et al (1997) Fatal meconium aspiration in spite of appropriate perinatal airway management: pulmonary and placental evidence of prenatal disease. Am J Obstet Gynecol 176:967–975

Ting P, Brady JP (1975) Tracheal suction in meconium aspiration. Am J Obstet Gynecol 122:767–771

Tran N, Lowe C, Sivieri EM et al (1980) Sequential effects of acute meconium aspiration on pulmonary function. Pediatr Res 14:34–38

Tsu F, Yeh MD, Harris V et al (1979) Roentgenographic findings in infants with MAS. JAMA 242:60–62

Tyler DC, Murphy J, Cheney FW (1978) Mechanical and chemical damage to lung tissue caused by meconium aspiration. Pediatrics 62:454–459

Usher RH, Boyd ME, McLean FH et al (1988) Assessment of fetal risk in postdate pregnancies. Am J Obstet Gynecol 158:259–264

Wiswell TE, Bent RC (1993) Meconium staining and the meconium aspiration syndrome. Pediatr Clin North Am 40:955–981

Wiswell TE, Tuggle JM, Turner BS (1990) Meconium aspiration syndrome: have we made a difference? Pediatrics 85:715–721

Wiswell TE, Foster NH, Slayter MV et al (1992) Management of piglet model of he meconium aspiration syndrome with high frequency or conventional ventilation. Am J Dis Child 146:1287

Wiswell TE, Meconium in the Delivery Room Trial Group (1998) Delivery room management of the apparently vigorous meconium-stained neonate: results of the multicentre collaborative trial. Pediatr Res 43:23 (abstract)

Yeh TF, Harris V, Srinivasan G et al (1979) Roentgenographic findings in infants with meconium aspiration syndrome. JAMA 242:60–63

Yeh TF, Lilien LD, Barathi A et al (1982) Lung volume, dynamic lung compliance, and blood gases during the first 3 days of postnatal life in infants with meconium aspiration syndrome. Crit Care Med 10:588–592

Yoder BA (1994) Meconium-stained amniotic fluid and respiratory complications: impact of selective tracheal suction. Obstet Gynecol 83:77–84

Yuksel B, Greenough A, Gamsu HR (1993) Neonatal meconium aspiration syndrome and respiratory morbidity during infancy. Pediatr Pulmonol 16:358–361

Diagnostic Imaging of Neonatal Pneumonia

David Manson

CONTENTS

D. Manson, MD, FRCP
Department of Diagnostic Imaging, Hospital for Sick Children and Assistant Professor and Division Head, Pediatric Radiology, Department of Medical Imaging, University of Toronto, 555 University Avenue, Toronto, Ontario, M5G 1X8, Canada

7.1 Introduction

Respiratory infections remain a significant and formidable threat to the health and well being of the neonate despite potent antibiotics, increasingly sophisticated laboratory detection methods and technologically advanced neonatal intensive care nurseries. Although the clinical and radiological definitions of pneumonia are variable throughout medical and governmental literature, quoted incidence rates for neonatal pneumonia range between 1.5–5.0 per 1,000 live births (Keyserling 1997; Webber et el 1990).

Mortality rates from pneumonia are even more difficult to obtain and to interpret. The medical literature quotes neonatal pneumonia mortality rates between 5% and 20% (Whitsett et al. 1999). Recent reports from the Centers for Disease Control quote mortality rates from neonatal pneumonia of 3.2/1,000 live births in the United States, corresponding to 1.1% of all neonatal deaths (Document LWCK 7 2003), http://www.cdc.gov/nhcs/data/dvs/lwck7_2003pdf. The incidence and mortality in developing countries are, not surprisingly, higher, with stated mortality rates estimated at between 0.75–1.2 million neonatal deaths from pneumonia annually, accounting for 10% of all global neonatal mortality (Duke 2005).

Approximately 10% of all neonatal intensive care unit (NICU) patients will have at least one episode of pneumonia (Whitsett et al. 1999). It is estimated that 17% of very low birth weight infants will have at least one episode of a nosocomial infection (Thompson et al. 1992) of which 30% will present as a respiratory tract infection (Hemming et al. 1976). Ironically, it would seem that the increasing sophistication of neonatal care and highly specialised nursery units may actually contribute to the incidence of neonatal pneumonia and sepsis by permitting the care of increasingly premature and sick neonates who may have previously succumbed. The use of highly invasive monitoring and therapeutic equipment has life saving potential, yet they can introduce a significant iatrogenic infection potential.

7.2 Clinical Considerations

The above-quoted incidence and mortality rates demonstrate that pulmonary infection is a significant risk to the neonate, and especially to the premature infant. The reasons for this are multi-factorial. The full term neonate is considered immunologically "competent", in that most can respond appropriately to antigenic stimulation. The absolute number of T-cells is similar in the neonate to the adult as long as thymic function is normal during foetal life (ROBERTON 1996). However, there are other considerations which render the neonate relatively more susceptible to infection. Studies have documented reduced leukocyte adherence and chemotaxis, as well as complement deficiencies that result in reduced phagocytosis and intracellular killing (ROBERTON 1996; SPECK et al. 1979). Surface IgA is absent, and serum IgG can be deficient in early preterm infants for whom sufficient time for normal maternal IgG transplacental transfer has not occurred. Even if sufficient transplacental IgG transfer has occurred, this supply of IgG has a limited life span of only several weeks resulting in a physiologically normal, transient hypogammaglobulinemia in the first few months of life. Furthermore, while the neonate can initially respond to antigenic stimulation with an endogenous IgM response, conversion of this response to a more mature IgG response is delayed. These deficiencies frequently result in a neonate with a limited capability to control and/or limit the spread of invasive organisms.

As well, the physical environment of both the foetus and the neonate play significant roles in exposing them to potential pathogens. The environment of the foetus inside intact maternal amniotic membranes is generally considered partially protective from external sources of infection. Therefore, one of the most common causes of neonatal sepsis is premature rupture of maternal membranes. Nevertheless, neonatal sepsis can occur even in the presence of intact maternal membranes (KIRKPATRICK and MUELLER 1998; SPECK et al. 1979). Congenital infections can occur through transplacental spread of a variety of organisms. During and after birth, the neonate is physically exposed to potentially pathogenic organisms which may colonise the maternal vaginal canal, or may be actively infecting the mother. The neonatal nursery provides a large source of invasive monitoring and therapeutic instruments, all of which can iatrogenically introduce organisms into the infant. Nursery personnel and family members inadvertently spread nosocomial infections even if strict antiseptic technique is maintained. It is not surprising, therefore, that, since the lungs provide a "front line" exposure between the neonate and its environment, neonatal pneumonia remains a significant problem in the NICU.

Unfortunately, the clinical signs and symptoms of infection that the neonate may manifest are frequently protean and non-specific. The infant may simply demonstrate listlessness and/or decreased physical activity. Feeding intolerance or pallor may be the only initial clinical manifestations. Either apnoea or tachypnea may be present and either tachycardia or bradycardia may occur. The child may be febrile or even hypothermic. Laboratory tests may be equally non-specific, demonstrating either an increased or a decreased total white cell count. It is, therefore, common for the clinician to perform a chest radiograph to help determine if pulmonary infection is the potential cause of some of these clinically observed changes. The chest radiograph, in this situation, can become useful to localise the problem to a pulmonary aetiology, even if the radiographic changes are not sufficiently specific to diagnose pulmonary infection as the cause of the infant's symptoms. Given the fulminant potential for some etiologic pathogens which cause neonatal pneumonia, any abnormality on the chest radiograph which may suggest a pulmonary infection warrants the initiation of broad spectrum antibiotic coverage (DENNEHY 1987; KIRKPATRICK and MUELLER 1998; SPECK et al. 1979).

7.3
Radiological Considerations

When taken in isolation, the study of the radiological manifestations of neonatal pneumonia is disappointing. There are few definitive correlative studies in the literature analysing the various radiological findings of pulmonary infection and comparing them with other causes of respiratory compromise, let alone comparing them to potential etiologic microbial agents. Most studies concur that the radiological findings alone are non-specific, such that it is almost impossible to determine a causative organism by their radiographic manifestations (BURKO 1962; CURRARINO and SILVERMAN 1957; HARRIS 1963; ROBERTON 1996; WIESENBERG 1973). Furthermore, many of these neonates do not suffer from pneumonia in isolation, but may also have complicating features such as hyaline membrane disease, meconium or amniotic fluid aspiration, persistent pulmonary hypertension, transient tachypnea of the newborn, secondary ARDS, patency of the ductus arteriosus, or a variety of other causes of neonatal respiratory distress. In one of the few studies looking specifically at radiological patterns in neonatal pneumonia, HANEY et al. (1984) reviewed autopsy records of all neonates who died over a 6-year period and in whom an autopsy documented pathological changes of pneumonia as the only significant abnormality. A review of their immediate pre-mortem chest radiographs revealed that the majority of cases demonstrated bilateral air space disease. Unfortunately, a pattern indistinguishable from hyaline membrane disease was seen in 13%, and a pattern indistinguishable from transient tachypnea of the newborn was seen in 17%. A few features have been described which may be helpful in identifying pulmonary infection as the source of respiratory distress. Some authors have postulated that one finding that may help to differentiate pneumonia from hyaline membrane disease is the presence of increased lung volumes combined with air-space disease in the non-intubated neonate (HARRIS 1963; WIESENBERG 1973). Hyaline membrane disease tends to cause diffusely small lungs from surfactant deficiency, while infection may result in over-inflation of recruited airspaces. Unfortunately, only 17% of the population described by Haney et al. demonstrated increased lung volumes, and most of these children were intubated on their pre-mortem examination. Others have suggested that air-space disease in the presence of a pleural effusion is more suggestive of bacterial pneumonia than of other causes of neonatal respiratory distress, especially when group B streptococcus is the etiologic agent (HANEY et al. 1984; LEONIDAS et al. 1977; PAYNE et al. 1988). The presence of pneumatoceles may also suggest a bacterial aetiology, a finding which is not exclusive to staphylococcal pneumonia (PAPAGEORGIOU et al. 1973; WIESENBERG 1973). As well, a diffuse, bilateral, alveolar pattern that develops in the first 4–6 h of life is characteristic, although not specific, for early neonatal sepsis and pneumonia, again classically seen when group B streptococcus is the etiologic agent. Ancillary non-pulmonary chest radiographic findings may be helpful in suggesting a diagnosis. Air-space disease in conjunction with periostitis or osteomyelitic lesions may suggest congenital syphilis, while a diffusely interstitial reticulonodular pattern in conjunction with characteristic metaphyseal lucencies suggests a congenital viral aetiology. A diffuse interstitial pattern alone is nonspecific, but if associated hepatosplenomegaly and intracerebral calcifications are present, CMV pneumonitis becomes a likely aetiology. Although the initial chest radiograph may be non-specific, serial chest radiographs can be extremely useful, especially in differentiating the rapidly resolving pattern of transient tachypnea of the newborn from the more persistent pattern of neonatal pneumonia. As well, serial examinations are frequently used to follow the response to therapeutic interventions such as antibiotic administration.

7.4
Aetiologic Agents

It is best to review the major aetiologic organisms and their respective radiographic patterns according to the initial source of neonatal infection. These are commonly divided into those agents causing transplacental infection, agents acquired perinatally and those acquired postnatally or nosocomially.

7.4.1
Transplacental Infection

Transplacentally transmitted infections, conforming to the traditionally taught pneumonic of "TORCH" (or "CROTSH") are, fortunately, quite rare. The pulmonary manifestations of these particular infections are even less common. While many perinatally acquired infections gain route to the foetus/neonate via aspiration or inhalation, transplacental infections enter the foetus hematogenously, via the umbilical cord. Most infants, therefore, tend to manifest systemic and multi-organ disease rather than a primary pneumonitis. It is, therefore, not surprising that the medical literature is generally deficient in reviews of the radiological manifestations of pneumonia in infants with transplacentally acquired infections.

The most common of these disorders appears to be the fairly ubiquitous cytomegalovirus (CMV), whose presence is well documented in all ages, races and socio-economic levels throughout both the developed as well as developing countries. Fortunately, estimates of foetal infection rates are very low. Approximately 1% of all newborns demonstrate a serologic response to transplacentally acquired CMV. However, 90% of these infants are asymptomatic and demonstrate no sequelae of the infection. When clinically evident infection does occur, the primary manifestations are usually systemic, including intrauterine growth retardation, hepatosplenomegaly and thrombocytopenia. The most significant primary organ of involvement is the central nervous system, producing microcephaly, intracranial calcifications and/or sensori-neural hearing loss. Congenital CMV pneumonitis is a rare manifestation, occurring only in 1–2% of CMV infected newborns (Dworsky 1982; Stagno 1980). It is significantly more common in infants who acquire the infection from other sources such as transvaginal exposure, maternal breast milk, or neonatal blood transfusions (Dworsky 1982; Stagno 1981; Stagno et al 1980; Whitsett et al. 1999). Although the radiographic manifestations of congenital CMV pneumonitis have not undergone statistical scrutiny, it is commonly accepted that this infection manifests as a diffuse reticulonodular, non-specific, viral interstitial pattern (Dennehy 1987; Whitsett et al. 1999; Wiesenberg 1973), similar to many viral pneumonitides (Fig. 7.1).

Other, less common, transplacentally acquired pneumonitides include rubella, syphilis, Listeria monocytogenes and tuberculosis. In general, maternal infection rates with tuberculosis and syphilis are increasing in both developing and industrialised countries. This can be partially explained by the widespread increase in migration rates into industrialised countries from countries in which infections rates are relatively high. As well, the HIV world-wide epidemic has permitted many of these organisms to propagate through immunosuppressed hosts. Congenital infection rates from syphilis were increasing in the 1980s and 1990s in predominantly urban geographic foci. This trend appeared to peak in the early 1990s with over 4,000 reported cases to the Center for Disease Control in the United States, decreasing to approximately 2,000 cases in 1996 (Sanchez and Wendel 1997). Congenital syphilitic pneumonia is an uncommon manifestation of congenital syphilis, seen in only approximately 5–25% of cases of congenital syphilis (Sanchez and Wendel 1997). It is commonly referred to as "pneumonia alba", due to the pathologic whitish plaque-like appearance of the areas of consolidation. Radiologically, it usually appears as a diffuse process (Fig. 7.2), but may manifest larger patches of air-space disease corresponding to mononuclear organizing infiltrates (Roberton 1996). One helpful sign on a chest radiograph is the presence of osseous lesions such as diffuse long bone periostitis, a radiographic sign which is more commonly seen in congenital syphilis than pulmonary consolidation.

Listeria monocytogenes is a gram-positive organism which can be acquired transplacentally or perinatally and frequently presents as a pneumonitis. Maternal infection is usually within 2–3 weeks of delivery with a non-specific flu-like illness. The illness in the neonate is clinically similar to group B streptococcus, demonstrating an "early" onset variety which presents in the first 72 h of life, and a "late" onset form that becomes manifest after 7 days of life. At least 50% of those with the "early" onset form demonstrate respiratory tract involvement (Bortolussi and Schlech 2001). The predominant radiographic pattern described is fairly non-

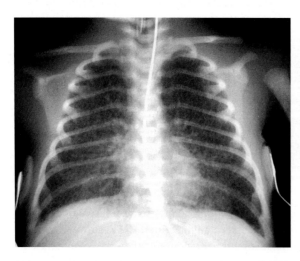

Fig. 7.1. Newborn with documented CMV pneumonia. There is a non-specific diffuse interstitial and predominantly reticular pattern, which is typical of viral pneumonitides

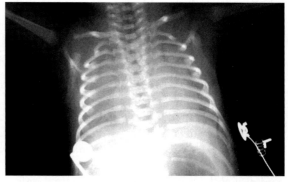

Fig. 7.2. Newborn infant born at 35 weeks of gestation to a mother treated during a previous pregnancy for congenital syphilis. The radiograph demonstrates a diffuse and bilateral pneumonitis, and the child had clinical findings of pneumonia. Associated bone changes are barely visible in the humeri, but are more apparent on other bone films. The infant responded well to appropriate antibiotics

specific. In a comprehensive review of 55 cases of neonatal listeriosis, 39 of which underwent chest radiographic examination, two equally common patterns were described (WILLICH 1967). The first is of a "bronchopneumonic" pattern of streaky and confluent opacities, and the second is a diffuse, fine interstitial pattern. It is postulated that some of the coarser interstitial densities correlate with multi-focal granulomas in medium and smaller airways. These radiographic manifestations are remarkably similar to group B streptococcal pneumonia acquired perinatally as described below (WHITSETT et al. 1999; WIESENBERG 1973).

Congenital tuberculous infection is a rare disorder, having been reported in less than 300 cases in the medical literature (STARKE 1997). It occurs secondary to disseminated maternal infection, which produces placental caseating granulomas. Pulmonary manifestations are uncommon as the usual primary site of infection is the liver from umbilical cord seeding. However, the patency of the ductus venosus and foramen ovale can result in disseminated infection relatively easily. Neonatal tuberculosis may also occur from aspiration of infected amniotic fluid, from ingestion of infected breast milk, or from inspiration of maternal respiratory droplets. Respiratory distress is a fairly common manifestation of neonatal tuberculosis, seen in approximately 72% of cases (STARKE and SMITH 2001). Parenchymal consolidation and adenopathy are common radiographic manifestations, although up to 50% of neonatal cases with radiographic findings demonstrate a miliary pattern (STARKE and SMITH 2001).

Although the pneumonic "TORCH" includes toxoplasmosis and herpes, the former uncommonly causes pneumonitis, and the latter is more appropriately considered under perinatally acquired infections. Cases reports of placental infections with influenza A (ARVIN and MALDONADO 2001), varicella (KEYSERLING 1997), adenovirus (ABZUG and LEVIN 1991) and echovirus (CHEESEMAN et al. 1977) are described, but are exceedingly rare.

7.4.2
Perinatal Infections

7.4.2.1
Clinical Considerations

Perinatally acquired infections can be clinically categorised into those which are acquired via ascending infection from the vaginal tract, those acquired transvaginally during the birth process and those acquired nosocomially in the neonatal period.

Ascending infections from the maternal vaginal tract are the usual cause of chorioamnionitis. It is estimated that maternal chorioamnionitis complicates an approximate 1–10% of all pregnancies in industrialised countries (BELADY et al. 1997), and is probably much more common in underdeveloped countries due to substandard maternal health care. Predisposing factors to chorioamnionitis include premature rupture of membranes of greater than 24 h, foetal instrumentation, increased number of vaginal examinations before birth, and prolonged labour. Although the organisms causing foetal sepsis are polymicrobial, nearly half of all infections are attributable to either group B streptococcus or E. coli (BELADY et al. 1997).

It is postulated (WIESENBERG 1973) that most organisms causing neonatal pneumonia gain entry to the infant during the birth process as the foetus takes its first gasping efforts at breathing. This may occur earlier during the course of labour in the asphyxiated infant who may swallow and/or aspirate in response to non-specific stressful events. It is for this reason that clinical signs or symptoms of maternal chorioamnionitis warrant the use of maternal perinatal intravenous antibiotics, which have been shown to significantly decrease the risk of sepsis and pneumonia in the neonate (BELADY et al. 1997).

There appear to be two separate clinical syndromes for neonatal sepsis and/or pneumonia which are significantly different with respect to symptomatology and outcome. Those infants with pneumonia or sepsis presenting within the first 48 h of life tend to have a more acute and severe clinical picture of hypotension, shock, disseminated intravascular coagulation and multi-organ failure. Mortality rates in this "early" onset form vary between 30%–50% (BOHIN and FIELD 1994; KIRKPATRICK and MUELLER 1998; SPECK et al. 1979; WHITSETT et al. 1999), especially when the offending organism is group B streptococcus. Those infants presenting after 48 h tend to have a less fulminant course with mortality rates of less than 5% (BOHIN and FIELD 1994). As well, the clinical symptoms tend to be less drastic, presenting with more isolated respiratory difficulty or less severe systemic manifestations.

7.4.2.2
Radiological Considerations

Unfortunately, the radiographic manifestations of the various etiologic agents carry very poor specificities. As noted previously, multiple studies have documented the non-specificity of the radiographic patterns of neonatal pneumonia (ABLOW et al. 1976; BURKO 1962; CURRARINO and SILVERMAN 1957; HANEY et al. 1984; HARRIS 1963; LEONIDAS et al. 1977; LILIEN et al. 1977). This holds true both in regards to differentiating between the various etiologic microbial agents, as well as to differentiating pneumonia itself from other cause of respiratory distress such as transient tachypnea of the newborn (TTN), hyaline membrane disease (HMD), and meconium aspiration. The findings which have been postulated as helpful in differentiating infection from other causes of respiratory distress include the presence of a pleural effusion (LEONIDAS et al. 1977), cardiomegaly (HUBBELL et al. 1988), and pulmonary over-inflation, the latter of which is postulated to help only in differentiating group B streptococcal pneumonia from HMD (ABLOW et al. 1976). The most common radiographic manifestation of neonatal pneumonia is a bilateral coarse pattern of perihilar reticular densities which may also involve scattered areas of air space disease (WIESENBERG 1973) (Fig. 7.3). Isolated lobar pneumonia is uncommon in this age group (ABLOW et al. 1976; CURRARINO and SILVERMAN 1957; HANEY et al. 1984; HARRIS 1963; WIESENBERG 1973), likely related both to the aspirated route of entry as well as to the inability of the neonate to control infection locally.

The radiographic differentiation of pneumonia from other processes becomes even more difficult in the preterm infant. LILIEN et al. (1977) reviewed the radiographic pattern of early onset group B streptococcal pneumonia in 73 infants, of which 86% were premature. A significantly larger portion of those preterm infants with a radiographic pattern of hyaline membrane disease (HMD) actually had both HMD and group B streptococcal pneumonia than those who had HMD alone. Nevertheless, ABLOW et al. (1976) reviewed the radiographic patterns of a smaller number of preterm infants and found that half of those who died of fulminant early onset group B streptococcal sepsis demonstrated a radiographic pattern that could not be differentiated from hyaline membrane disease. They note however that the "overall volume of the lungs is usually increased" in neonatal pneumonia. LEONIDAS et al. (1977) in their review of 67 infants of all gestational ages hospitalised for respiratory distress, found that the pattern of parenchymal lung disease was just as likely to be "typical" for pneumonia as it was to be "typical" for hyaline membrane disease. In their study, the presence of cardiomegaly or pleural effusions was more likely to represent neonatal sepsis.

7.4.2.3
Specific Agents

7.4.2.3.1
Bacterial

Group B streptococcal sepsis is one of the most common causes of neonatal sepsis. As such, there is more literature published regarding this particular agent than regarding most others. The radiographic manifestations initially described by ABLOW et al. (1976) were essentially those of hyaline membrane disease. They described a "fine, diffuse granular pattern" in 50% of infants who died of "early" onset, fatal group B streptococcal infection (Fig. 7.4), with the remainder of fatal cases demonstrating either similar findings or more focal, lower lobe opacification. Non-fatal cases tended to have a more heterogeneous pattern of mixed interstitial and air space changes.

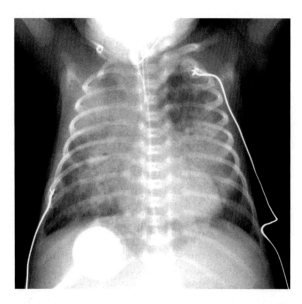

Fig. 7.3. Chest radiograph of a 1-week-old premature infant born at 26 weeks of gestational age, with documented Pseudomonas pneumonia. Bilateral air-space changes are noted on a background of diffuse interstitial changes

A subsequent study suggested that cardiomegaly and/or pleural effusions may help to differentiate group B streptococcal infection from hyaline membrane disease (LEONIDAS 1977), while admitting that there are many other causes for the presence of these findings.

There is a curious association between group B streptococcal pneumonia and the presence of an ipsilateral diaphragmatic hernia, especially when the hernia is right sided. Suggested mechanisms for the presence of this association have included a primary abnormality of lung compliance, secondary effects of mechanical ventilation on the infected lung, or direct local effects of the organism itself (POTTER et al. 1995). Whatever the mechanism, persistent ventilatory requirements or radiographic abnormalities in neonates after the treatment of group B streptococcal pneumonia should alert the radiologist to the possibility of an associated diaphragmatic hernia.

Other perinatal bacterial infections such as Pseudomonas, E. coli, Klebsiella and other streptococci have received little attention in the literature with respect to specific radiographic patterns.

7.4.2.3.2
Viral

Perinatal viral infections such as herpes, varicella, RSV and adenovirus tend to be significantly less common than the previously described bacterial causes of neonatal sepsis.

Neonatal herpes infection can be acquired transplacentally, during birth, or even postnatally. The majority of neonates acquire the virus transvaginally from a mother who is actively shedding the virus. Only a small minority of infected women are actually shedding the virus during labour (KOHL 1997). As well, only a minority of infants exposed will become clinically infected. As a result, neonatal herpetic pneumonia is an uncommon disorder, affecting approximately 1 in 7,000 live births in the United States (KOHL 1997). This rate, however, is increasing with some studies reporting a ten-fold increase over the past 20 years (KOHL 1997). Although pulmonary infection occurs in only 5–25% of infected newborns, it tends to produce a fulminant and progressive course (DOMINGUEZ et al 1984; HUBBELL et al 1988; KOHL 1997). The described radiographic findings are similar to most viral pulmonary infections, starting as bilateral interstitial perihilar reticular densities (Fig. 7.5) that can be initially quite subtle. Confluent alveolar changes occur as the infection spreads, progressing to diffuse pulmonary opacitification that may have accompanying pleural effusions (DOMINGUEZ et al. 1984; HUBBELL et al. 1988).

Varicella in the neonatal period is a rare disease. It is estimated that approximately 3,000 cases of maternal varicella occur in the United States annually (KEYSERLING 1997). Transplacental infection is extremely rare, but can result in a congenital varicella syndrome, characterised primarily by limb and

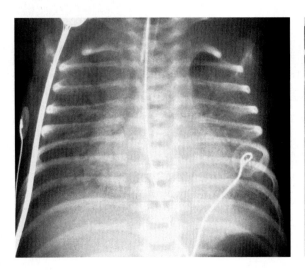

Fig. 7.4. One-week-old infant with typical non-specific changes of diffuse air-space disease from group B streptococcal pneumonia

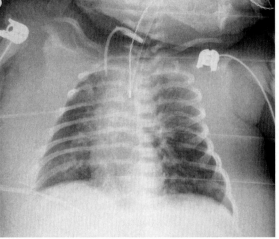

Fig. 7.5. Twelve-day-old infant with severe interstitial pneumonitis and diffuse anasarca from viral sepsis secondary to herpes

CNS malformations. Respiratory infection can be acquired by the infant in the neonatal period from a mother who is actively shedding the virus. In order for the mother to be actively shedding the virus, maternal infection must have occurred within 3 weeks of delivery. The severity of neonatal disease acquired from a prenatally infected mother varies with the time of delivery. Maternal shedding is most active in the first few days of appearance of the rash. At this time, maternal antibody response is still developing, and little significant antibody crosses the placenta. Birth in this time period, therefore, results in a more severely infected neonate, with fatality rates quoted at between 20–40% (ALBRITTON 1998). Administration of varicella-zoster immunoglobulin (VZIG) in this period has been shown to ameliorate the severity of neonatal infection (KEYSERLING 1997). As well, it should be remembered that neonatal infection not uncommonly occurs via nosocomial or familial exposure.

Neonatal varicella pneumonia is a severe complication of disseminated varicella infection and is a major cause of neonatal mortality from this infection. There is, however, a paucity of published reports concerning the radiographic manifestations of neonatal varicella pneumonia. The classically described radiographic manifestation in older individuals is that of a diffuse interstitial reticulonodular pattern (Fig. 7.6), which characteristically appears a little more nodular than reticular (ALBRITTON 1998).

Case reports of neonatal pulmonary infections from adenovirus (ABZUG and LEVIN 1991), RSV (BERKOVICH and TARANKO 1964; KEYSERLING 1997; MEISSNER et al. 1984), parainfluenza (MEISSNER et al. 1984) and enteroviruses (KEYSERLING 1997) have been published which provide only anecdotal descriptions of the radiographic patterns of these viruses in the neonate. Most describe bilateral perihilar "infiltrates" as the predominant radiographic pattern.

Human metapneumovirus has recently been implicated as a relatively common cause of bronchiolitis in infants and children. It appears to be less common than RSV, yet 10% of all cases are in children less than 1 month of age. It appears to clinically act in a fashion similar to other respiratory viruses, in that younger children and those with respiratory co-morbidities are more severely affected. The radiographic findings described are similar to other viral causes of bronchiolitis (FOULONGNE et al. 2006).

7.4.2.3.3
Others

Chlamydia Trachomatis
Chlamydial pneumonia is caused by Chlamydia trachomatis, an obligate intracellular parasite which is a common, sexually transmitted infection. Approximately 4 million new cases of maternal chlamydial

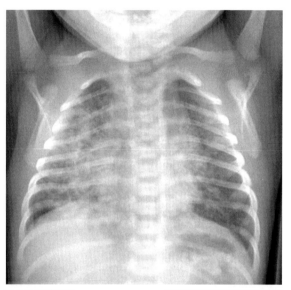

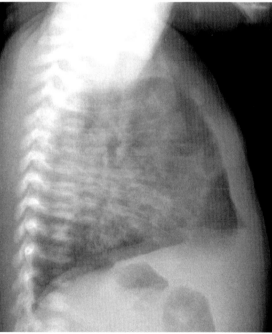

Fig. 7.6. This infant died at 12 days of life after developing disseminated varicella from a mother who manifested active skin lesions 1 week before delivery

infection are reported in the United States annually to the Centers for Disease Control (HAMMERSCHLAG 1994). Approximately 30% of infants born to infected mothers will have positive nasopharyngeal cultures, but only 30% of these will develop pneumonia. Clinically, the infant typically demonstrates an initial conjunctivitis between 5–14 days after birth. This tends to resolve and the pulmonary infection only becomes manifest after 4–12 weeks of age. Clinical manifestations are mild, and fever is characteristically absent (HAMMERSCHLAG 1994). The radiographic manifestations are typically non-specific, but the pattern described is that of hyperinflation with bilateral diffuse reticular perihilar infiltrates (Fig. 7.7) (HAMMERSCHLAG 1994; HARRISON et al 1978; HESS 1993; RADKOWSKI et al. 1981; RETTIG 1988). Interestingly, STAGNO et al. (1981) reviewed a series of infants with pneumonia caused by CMV, chlamydia, ureaplasma and pneumocystis and found the radiographic patterns to be indistinguishable. Chlamydial infection is generally mild and even untreated infants usually improve over 4–8 weeks (RETTIG 1988). There is some evidence, however, that these children demonstrate long-term obstructive changes on pulmonary function tests, with a significantly greater incidence of physician diagnosed asthma in later childhood (WEISS et al. 1986).

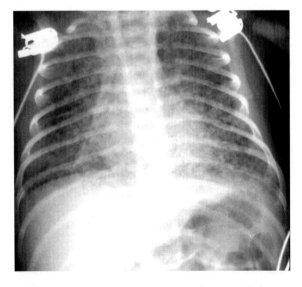

Fig. 7.7. Two-week-old with extensive interstitial and alveolar changes from Chlamydia pneumonia. The young age of this infant is atypical, most cases presenting after 1 month of life

Ureaplasma Urealyticum

Ureaplasma urealyticum is a micro-organism which is similar to the mycoplasma species in that it is a unicellular organism without a cell wall. Asymptomatic colonisation of the maternal genital tract with Ureaplasma urealyticum is common, affecting over half of all pregnant women. It has, however, recently been proposed that it has a pathogenic potential in neonates (DWORSKY and STAGNO 1981; WANG et al. 1997). A significant association and causation has been established between maternal colonisation with U. urealyticum and chorioamnionitis, spontaneous abortion and early neonatal death (DWORSKY and STAGNO 1981; WANG et al. 1997). There is an increasing volume of literature demonstrating an association between neonatal pneumonia and the isolation of this organism from endotracheal aspirates, pleural fluid, lung tissue and/or blood, especially in pre-term infants (PINNA et al. 2006). In addition, the radiographic changes of ureaplasma infection were evaluated in one study (CROUSE et al. 1993), where it was found that abnormalities were diagnosed by an appropriately blinded radiologist twice as frequently in ureaplasma infected babies, than in those who were culture negative. Unfortunately, the radiographic findings, which correlated with tracheal aspirate isolation of ureaplasma, were broad and non-specific. The radiographic findings, which were taken to be indicative of ureaplasma infection, included any radiographic manifestation of bronchopulmonary dysplasia (BPD), as well as a series of non-specific findings of mixed interstitial and air space changes (Fig. 7.8). The study did confirm that radiographic changes do occur in the presence of ureaplasma infection; however, the relative frequency or specificity of the findings were, unfortunately, not addressed. They concluded, however, that radiographic manifestations of typical type III or IV BPD are associated with ureaplasma infection, especially when these changes are seen at a chronological age that is slightly earlier (2 weeks postnatally) than expected from the usual findings of BPD in neonates (CROUSE et al 1993). Interestingly, there is strong evidence which demonstrates a significantly higher incidence of chronic lung disease in infants who previously demonstrated culture-proven Ureaplasma urealyticum pneumonitis (WANG et al 1997; PINNA et al 2006).

The global HIV epidemic warrants comment on the neonatal manifestations of this particular infection. Although there has been a progressive de-

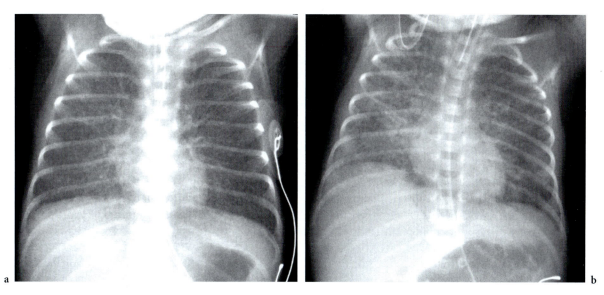

Fig. 7.8. a Baseline state of mild chronic lung disease of 1-month-old premature infant born at 25 weeks of gestational age. **b** Same infant 1 week later, after respiratory deterioration requiring significantly higher ventilatory settings. Cultures of endotracheal tube aspirates were positive for Ureaplasma, and the infant responded well to appropriate antibiotics

cline in incidence of vertically and perinatally acquired infection from HIV in recent years due to a combination of educational programs and routine use of anti-retroviral therapies in developed countries, these interventions have not been as widely available in developing countries. As a result, 90% of worldwide perinatally acquired HIV infection is now seen in Africa alone (GRAHAM 2003). The clinical presentation of HIV infection in the neonatal period is still somewhat uncommon, and most neonates with HIV are relatively asymptomatic for the first few months of life (MARQUIS and BARDEGUEZ 1994). As HIV testing may be inaccurate in the neonatal period, prophylaxis against Pneumocystis jiroveci (previously known as Pneumocystis carinii) is started when HIV-exposed infants are approximately 6 weeks old (KRIST et al 2002). Those few cases that manifest early respiratory symptoms usually do so from infection with an opportunistic organism, most commonly due to P. jiroveci. The described radiographic pattern is that of a fine interstitial diffuse pattern that rapidly progresses to diffuse bilateral air-space disease (MARQUIS and BARDEGUEZ 1994). Early presentation of changes of tuberculous disease or CMV pneumonitis in either the neonatal or infantile period should also raise the suspicion of underlying HIV infection (MARQUIS and BARDEGUEZ 1994; GRAHAM 2003).

7.4.3
Postnatal/Nosocomial Infections

Although the medical care of sick and premature infants has improved to a remarkable extent in recent decades, the problem of nosocomial spread of infection remains a significant cause of morbidity and mortality in neonatal intensive care units. The topic is very broad, encompassing all infections acquired from any source while still in the NICU. This includes fungal complications related to the administration of broad-spectrum antibiotics. As mentioned previously, at least one study has documented an incidence rate of 17% of all low birth weight infants who will acquire at least one nosocomial infection during their stay in the nursery (THOMPSON et al. 1992). HEMMING et al. (1976) reviewed all nosocomially acquired infections in a 3-year period and discovered that 30% of them resulted in pulmonary infection. In that study, the most common pathogens discovered were Staphylococcus aureus (47%) and gram-negative enteric bacilli (45%) (Fig. 7.9). A more recent review (THOMPSON et al. 1992) found Streptococcus epidermidis to be the most common organism responsible for secondary infection in infants with birth weights less than 750 g. Interestingly, aside from low birth weight, the other significant risk factor for acquisition of a nosocomial infection was prolonged ventilation.

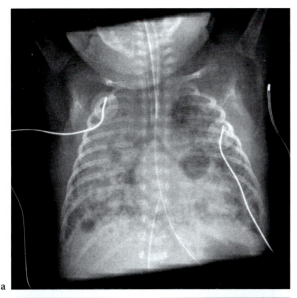

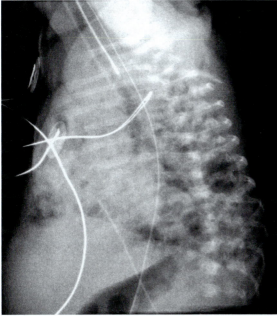

Fig. 7.9a,b. Frontal and lateral chest radiographs of a 3-week-old ventilated premature infant who was born at 25 weeks of gestation demonstrate multifocal areas of airspace consolidation with several air-filled cysts representing developing pneumatoceles. Tracheal aspirates grew Staphylococcus aureus

should instigate an early and aggressive response to diagnosis and treatment of a potential pneumonitis. An aggressive approach is especially needed when some of the potential causes of pneumonia in these infants are fungal in origin. Laboratory identification of fungal organisms is frequently difficult and often delayed. In a review of fungal infections in very low birth weight infants (BALEY et al. 1984), a mean of 33 days was required to diagnose the presence of a fungal infection. Clinically evident respiratory deterioration was present in all ten infants, and eight of these demonstrated worsening pulmonary infiltrates. The chest radiograph, therefore, becomes an integral part of the early clinical investigation of these infants. A systematic review of previous films must be performed to permit recognition of new changes superimposed on the complex chronic abnormalities that are frequently present.

7.5
Conclusion

Neonatal pneumonia remains a significant risk to the health and well being of the newborn, despite contemporary advances in the quality and complexity of medical care. Ironically, the risk of iatrogenic infection is rising with the level of sophistication of neonatal medicine. Both the clinical and radiographic appearances of many of these infections are disappointingly non-specific. The role of the appropriate interpretation of diagnostic images in these children with multi-system disease becomes critical in those cases for which the radiographic pattern is sufficiently specific to be diagnostic. In cases with non-specific radiographic manifestations, the paediatric imager has a critical role, not only in helping to identify a pulmonary site of disease, but also in following the childs' response to therapeutic interventions.

One key to the diagnosis of a nosocomially acquired respiratory tract infection appears to be the presence of deteriorating radiographic changes after an initial period of stability or improvement. The radiographic pattern of deterioration may be non-specific, but the presence of any deterioration

References

Ablow RC, Driscoll SG, Effmann EL et al (1976) A comparison of early-onset group B streptococcal neonatal infection and the respiratory-distress syndrome of the newborn. N Engl J Med 294:65–70

Abzug MJ, Levin MJ (1991) Neonatal adenovirus infection: four patients and review of the literature. Pediatrics 87:890–896

Albritton WL (1998) Varicella pneumonia. In: Chernick V, Boat TF, Kendig EL (eds) Kendig's disorders of the respiratory tract in children. Saunders, Philadelphia, pp 999–1003

Arvin A, Maldonado Y (2001) Other viral infections of the fetus and newborn. In: Remington J, Klein J (eds) Infectious diseases of the fetus and newborn infant, 5th edn. Saunders, Toronto, pp 858–878

0Belady PH, Farkouh LJ, Gibbs RS (1997) Intra-amniotic infection and premature rupture of the membranes. Clin Perinatol 24:43–57

Berkovich S, Taranko L (1964) Acute respiratory illness in the premature nursery associated with respiratory syncytial virus infections. Pediatrics 34:753–760

Bohin S, Field DJ (1994) The epidemiology of neonatal respiratory disease. Early Hum Dev 37:73–90

Bortolussi R, Schlech W (2001) Listeriosis. In: Remington J, Klein K (eds) Infectious diseases of the fetus and newborn infant. Saunders, Toronto, pp 1157–1177

Burko H (1962) Considerations in the roentgen diagnosis of pneumonia in children. AJR Am J Roentgenol [Radium Ther Nucl Med] 88:555–565

Cheeseman SH, Hirsch MS, Keller EW et al (1977) Fatal neonatal pneumonia caused by echovirus type 9. Am J Dis Child 131:1169

Crouse DT, Odrezin GT, Cutter GR et al (1993) Radiographic changes associated with tracheal isolation of ureaplasma urealyticum from neonates. Clin Infect Dis 17 [Suppl 1]: S122–S130

Currarino G, Silverman FN (1957) Roentgen diagnosis of pulmonary disease of the newborn infant. Pediatr Clin North Am 1957:27–52

Dennehy PH (1987) Respiratory infections in the newborn. Clin Perinatol 14:667–682

Document #LFWK 73 (2003)

Dominguez R, Rivero H, Gaisie G et al (1984) Neonatal herpes simplex pneumonia: radiographic findings. Radiology 153:395–399

Duke T (2005) Neonatal pneumonia in developing countries. Arch Dis Child Fetal Neonatal Ed:90:F211–F219

Dworsky ME, Stagno S (1982) Newer agents causing pneumonitis in early infancy. Pediatr Infect Dis 1:188–195

Foulongne V, Guyon G, Rodière M, Segondy M (2006) Human metapumovirus infection in young children hospitalized with respiratory tract disease. Pediatr Defect Dis 25:354–359

Graham SM (2003) HIV and respiratory infection in children. Curr Opin Pulm Med 9:215–220

Hammerschlag MR (1994) Chlamydia trachomatis in children. Pediatr Ann 23:349–353

Haney PJ, Bohlman M, Chen-Chih JS (1984) Radiographic findings in neonatal pneumonia. AJR Am J Roentgenol 143:23–26

Harris GBC (1963) The newborn with respiratory distress: some roentgenographic features. Radiol Clin North Am 1:497–518

Harrison HR, English MG, Lee CK et al (1978) Chlamydia trachomatis infant pneumonitis: comparison with matched controls and other infant pneumonitis. N Engl J Med 298:702–708

Hemming VG, Overall JC Jr, Britt MR et al (1976) Nosocomial infections in a newborn intensive-care unit. Results of forty-one months of surveillance. N Engl J Med 294:1310–1316

Hess DL (1993) Chlamydia in the neonate. Neonatal Netw 12:9–12

Hubbell C, Dominguez R, Kohl S (1988) Neonatal herpes simplex pneumonitis. Rev Infect Dis 10:431–438

Keyserling HL (1997) Other viral agents of perinatal importance: varicella, parvovirus, respiratory syncytial virus, and enterovirus. Clin Perinatol 24:193–211

Kirkpatrick B, Mueller DG (1998) Respiratory disorders in the newborn. In: Chernick V, Boat TF, Kendig EL (eds) Disorders of the respiratory tract in children. Saunders, Philadelphia, pp 338–340

Kohl S (1997) Neonatal herpes simplex virus infection. Clin Perinatol 24:129–150

Krist AH, Crawford-Faucher A (2002) Mangement of Newborns exposed to maternal HIV infection. American Family Physicians 65:2049–2056

Leonidas JC, Hall RT, Beatty EC et al (1977) Radiographic findings in early onset neonatal group B streptococcal septicemia. Pediatrics 59 [Suppl]:1006–1011

Lilien LD, Harris VJ, Pildes RS (1977) Significance of radiographic findings in early-onset group B streptococcal infection. Pediatrics 60:360–363

Marquis JR, Bardeguez AD (1994) Imaging of HIV infection in the prenatal and postnatal period. Clinics in Perinatology 21:125–142

Meissner HC, Murray SA, Kiernan MA et al (1984) A simultaneous outbreak of respiratory syncytial virus and parainfluenza virus type 3 in a newborn nursery. Pediatrics 104:680–684

Papageorgiou A, Bauer CR, Fletcher BD et al (1973) Klebsiella pneumonia with pneumatocele formation in a newborn infant. Can Med Assoc J 109:1217–1219

Payne NR, Burke BA, Day DL et al (1988) Correlation of clinical and pathologic findings in early onset neonatal group B streptococcal infection with disease severity and prediction of outcome. Pediatr Infect Dis J 7:836–847

Potter B, Philipps AF, Bierny JP et al (1995) Neonatal radiology. Acquired diaphragmatic hernia with group B streptococcal pneumonia. J Perinatol 15:160–162

Pinna GS, Skevaki CL, Kafetzis DA. Current Opinion infectious Diseases 2006, 19:283–289

Radkowski MA, Kranzler JK, Beem MO et al (1981) Chlamydia pneumonia in infants: radiology in 125 cases. AJR Am J Roentgenol 137:703–706

Rettig PJ (1988) Perinatal infections with Chlamydia trachomatis. Clin Perinatol 15:321–350

Roberton NRC (1996) Pneumonia. In: Milner AD, Richerton NR (eds) Neonatal respiratory disorders. Oxford University Press, New York, pp 286–312

Sanchez PJ, Wendel GD (1997) Syphilis in pregnancy. Clin Perinatol 24:71–90

Speck WT, Fanaroff AA, Klaus M (1979) Neonatal infections. In: Klaus M, Fanaroff AA (eds) Care of the high risk neonate. Saunders, Philadelphia, pp 267–279

Stagno S, Pifer LL, Hughes WT et al (1980) Pneumocystis carinii pneumonitis in young immunocompetent infants. Pediatrics 66:56–62

Stagno S, Brasfield DM, Brown MB et al (1981) Infant pneumonitis associated with cytomegalovirus, chlamydia, pneumocystis, and ureaplasma: a prospective study. Pediatrics 68:322–329

Starke JR (1997) Tuberculosis: an old disease but a new threat to the mother, fetus, and neonate. Clin Perinatol 24:107–127

Starke JR, Smith M (2001) Tuberculosis. In: Remington J, Klein J (eds) Infectious diseases of the fetus and newborn infant. Saunders, Toronto, pp 1179–1193

Thompson PJ, Greenough A, Nicolaides KH (1992) Nosocomial bacterial infections in very low birth weight infants. Eur J Pediatr 151:451–454

Wang EEL, Matlow AG, Ohlsson A (1997) Ureaplasma urealyticum infections in the perinatal period. Clin Perinatol 24:91–105

Webber S, Wilkinson AR, Lindsell D et al (1990) Neonatal pneumonia. Arch Dis Child 65:207–211

Weiss SG, Newcomb RW, Beem MO (1986) Pulmonary assessment of children after chlamydial pneumonia of infancy. J Pediatr 108:659–664

Whitsett JA, Pryhuber GS, Rice WR (1999) Acute respiratory disorders. In: Avery BB, Fletcher MA, MacDonald MG (eds) Neonatology – pathophysiology and management of the newborn. Williams and Wilkins, Philadelphia, pp 485–508

Wiesenberg RI (1973) Neonatal pneumonia and pulmonary hemorrhage. In: Wiesenberg RI (eds) The newborn chest. Harper and Row, New York, pp 71–83

Willich E (1967) The roentgenological appearance of pulmonary listeriosis. Prog Pediatr Radiol 1:160–176

Antenatal Imaging of Chest Malformations

8

Laurent Garel

CONTENTS

L. Garel MD
Clinical Professor of Radiology, University of Montreal, Hopital Sainte-Justine, 3175 Cote Sainte-Catherine, Montreal, Quebec H3T1C5, Canada

Primum non nocere. (Attributed to Hippocrates or Galen)
Education: The path from cocky ignorance to miserable uncertainty.
Mark Twain

8.1 Introduction

Congenital chest anomalies were considered rare lesions prior to the era of fetal imaging (Cloutier 1993). Routine obstetrical sonograms have contributed to a sharp increase in the number of diagnosed cases in the last decades (Tables 8.1, 8.2). The antenatal recognition of congenital lung malformations and anomalies has consequently raised the controversial issue of their management in asymptomatic newborns (Pilling 1998; Aziz 2004; Davenport 2004)

8.2 General Concepts

8.2.1 Basics of Lung Embryology, Fetal Lung Development and Pathology

The anatomical concept underlying the standardization of terminology of all lung malformations takes into account the normal lung as being composed of several tubes (the bronchopulmonary airway, the arterial supply, the venous drainage, the lymphatic system), with the establishment of communications among the blood vessels, the alveoli and the bronchi (Clements and Warner 1987, Langston 2003, Newman 2006).

The abnormal connection of the tubular components of the lung forms the basis of all congenital malformations. Congenital lung anomalies would then result from an insult to the developing lung bud, the major determining factor of the lesion being the timing and severity of the insult rather than its nature. Accordingly the wheel theory of Clements and Warner displays the end results of this initial insult (Fig. 8.1).

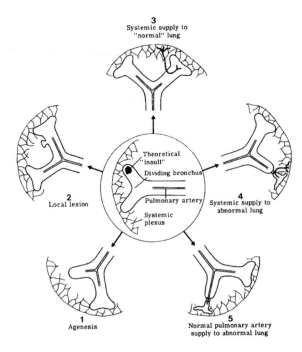

Fig. 8.1. The wheel theory (reprint from Clements and Warner 1987)

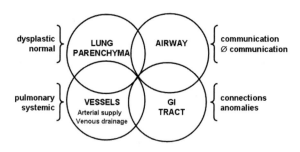

Fig. 8.2. Venn diagram displaying the various components of congenital lung lesions

Congenital lung lesions (CLL) represent a continuum of interrelated abnormalities that can present in isolation or in association. A Venn diagram (Fig. 8.2) outlines the various features of CLL and the possible association among these components. For example, an extra-lobar pulmonary sequestration (ELPS) is made of normal lung parenchyma, without normal communication to the tracheobronchial tree, with a systemic blood supply and a complete covering of visceral pleura. Congenital pulmonary airway malformations (CPAM) are described as hamartous tissue, with communication to the airway, normal arterial supply and venous drainage. CPAM features coexist (CONRAN and STOCKER 1999) in 40 to 50% of cases of ELPS at pathology and are then called hybrid lesions (CASS 1997).

If we switch from a Venn diagram to a longitudinal axis, we can place along the way the classics from congenital lobar overinflation to pulmonary arteriovenous malformations (Fig. 8.3). In addition to the embryologic sequential steps of bronchi formation, alveoli development and vascular connections, several factors are needed for a normal fetal lung development: (1) an adequate amount of amniotic fluid, (2) an adequate thoracic space, (3) the presence of fluid within the lungs and (4) fetal breathing movements.

Pulmonary hypoplasia can therefore result from the various causes of oligohydramnios, from the presence of an intrathoracic mass compressing the lungs, from skeletal dysplasias, from neuromuscular or chromosomal disorders.

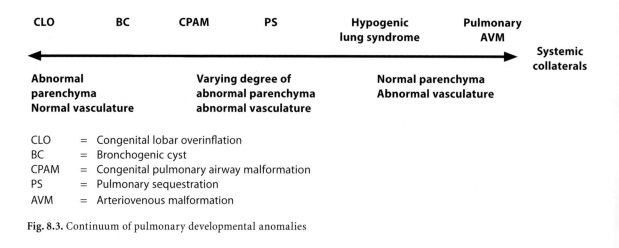

Fig. 8.3. Continuum of pulmonary developmental anomalies

8.2.2
Pathogenesis, Nosology and Classification

According to recent pathological reports of CLL (LANGSTON 2003; RIEDLINGER 2006), the initial insult to the lung bud is an airway obstruction. Such a common pathogenesis, in addition to the better recognition of hybrid lesions, has resulted in an evolving terminology and classification of congenital pulmonary anomalies. CPAM has replaced CCAM (STOCKER 2002); from the three initial histological subtypes (STOCKER 1977), the classification expanded to five types indicating lesions located on progressively distal airways (STOCKER 2002).

1) Involvement of all lobes – incompatible with life;
2) Large cyst(s) (>2 cm) –
   pseudostratified columnar epithelium;
3) Medium size cyst(s) –
   cuboidal or columnar epithelium;
4) Small cyst(s) (<0.5 cm) – cuboidal epithelium;
5) Large air-filled cysts, lined by flattered epithelial cells.

Such a classification can only apply to pathology (resected specimens) and is not appropriate for use in fetal lung lesion imaging. Conversely, sonographic characterization into macrocystic and microcystic subtypes of CPAM has proved practical and useful (ADZIK 1985).

CLL are nowadays classified as follows:
1) Bronchopulmonary malformations
   (CPAM, PS, BC, bronchial atresia (BA));
2) Pulmonary hyperplasia and related conditions
   (CHAOS, polyalveolar lobe);
3) Congenital lobar overinflation and related conditions
   (Congenital lobar emphysema (CLE), bronchial obstruction/compression);
4) Systemic arterial connections to normal lung;
5) Other cystic lesions.

Airway obstruction is considered the common pathogenesis of BP malformations, pulmonary hyperplasia and congenital hyperinflation (LANGSTON 2006). The previous concepts result in defining ground rules for the radiologists regarding CLL (BUSH 2002):
1. Histological features may overlap
   (e.g., hybrid lesions).
2. Nomenclature is evolving (CPAM/CCAM).
3. Natural history is sometimes more complicated than once thought.
4. Describe what is actually seen. Keep clinical description and pathological diagnoses separate.
5. Use a systematic approach (parenchyma/airway/arterial supply/venous drainage/GI connection).

8.3
Prenatal Imaging

8.3.1
Sonography of the Fetal Chest

Routine fetal imaging has resulted in a spectacular increase in the number of diagnosed cases. Over the last 14 years, 900 cases of CLL have been reported in the literature (Tables 8.1, 8.2). In our institution, we see approximately ten cases per year. The four-chamber view of the fetal thorax (Fig. 8.4) is routinely obtained in all obstetrical sonograms. Normally the heart occupies 25 to 30% of the volume of the fetal thorax. In regard to the midline, the axis of the heart is approximately 45°, and most of the right ventricle, the left atrium and the left ventricle are located into the left chest.

Table 8.1. Some series of prenatally diagnosed CCAM/CPAM

Ref/year	Author	Cases
1992	Budorick et al.	14
1993	Revillon et al.	32
1994	McCullagh et al.	13
1994	Thorpe-Beeston et al.	58
1995	Bromley et al.	25
1996	Miller et al.	17
1997	Cacciari et al.	16
1997	Sapin et al.	18
1998	Adzick et al.	134
1999	Waszak et al.	21
1999	van Leeuwen et al.	14
2000	Roggin et al.	12
2000	De Santis et al.	17
2000	Bunduki et al.	18
2001	Laberge et al.	48
2003	Sauvat et al.	29
2003	Pumberger et al.	35
2004	Davenport et al.	67
2004	Khosa et al.	30
2004	Usui et al.	28
2005	Shanmugam et al.	13
2005	Ierullo et al.	34
2005	Illanes et al.	43
2005	Kim et al.	8
2006	Calvert et al.	28
Total:		**772**

Table 8.2. Some series of prenatally diagnosed pulmonary sequestration

Ref/year	Author	Cases
1995	King et al.	5
1998	Becmeur et al.	10
1998	Adzick et al.	41
1999	Lopoo et al.	16
2001	Bratu et al.	13
2003	Dhingsa et al.	9
2005	Illanes et al.	5 (pictorial essay)
2005	Shanmugam et al.	6
2005	Ruano et al.	8
Total:		**113**

CLL will present early in pregnancy (mid-2nd trimester) as an area of abnormal echogenicity exerting a mass effect on adjacent structures. The induced cardiac shift (position and/or axis of the heart) is best recognized on the transverse four-chamber view (Fig. 8.5). The mass is hyperechoic either homogeneously (Fig. 8.5a) or with coexisting cysts of various size (Fig. 8.5b). The mass effect due to the malformation can also take place on the adjacent lung that can be considered falsely as being part of the lesion because of its compression-induced hyperechogenicity.

A great deal of information regarding the natural history of fetal CLL has been gathered thanks to the widespread use of routine mid-2nd trimester ultrasound and follow-up sonograms. Such knowledge has significantly shaded the various prognostic

The lungs appear homogeneous and symmetrical in appearance throughout gestation with a medium-level echogenicity slightly greater in the 3rd trimester than in the 2nd trimester. The fetal diaphragm is seen on longitudinal or oblique scans as a hypoechoic band, concave inferiorly, interposed between the lungs and the liver or spleen. The abdominal position of the liver and stomach is indeed assessed routinely. The thymus is sometimes displayed, anterior to the heart and great vessels root and slightly less echoic than the lung. Fetal

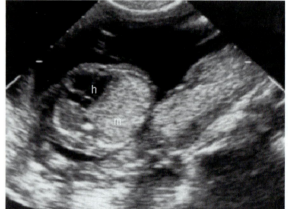

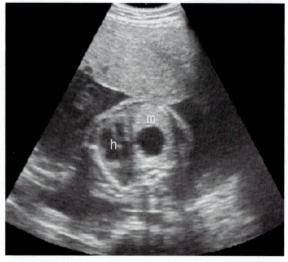

Fig. 8.5a,b. Transverse scans of fetal lung malformation (four-chamber view). The heart is displaced to the right by a left pulmonary mass effect (*h* heart, *m* mass) (**a**) that appears homogeneously hyperechoic in a case of pulmonary sequestration (**b**) with coexisting cysts in a case of CCAM

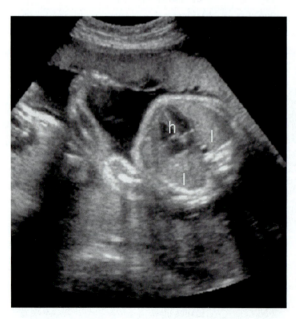

Fig. 8.4. Transverse scan of the normal thorax of an 18-week-old fetus (four-chamber view). The cardiac apex is heading toward the left with a 45-degree axis. Both lungs display uniform echogenicity (*h* heart, *l* lung)

predictors at presentation that were reported in the literature, such as early gestational age at diagnosis, large size of the lesion, importance of the mediastinal shift, polyhydramnios, subtypes of lesions, associated anomalies and hydrops fetalis. Among these historical predictors at presentation, only the presence of hydrops fetalis remains as indicator of a dismal prognosis (ADZICK 1998, 2003) (Fig. 8.6).

8.3.2
Bronchopulmonary Malformations

Because CLLs encompass a spectrum of anomalies with associated pathological features, it seems more appropriate to describe the various imaging patterns rather than insisting on distinct, clear-cut specific entities (BARNES 2003).

The pattern recognition is usually simple, although, at times, not straightforward. Because CPAM are the most frequent CLL and because macrocystic CPAM represent at least 90% of cases, a practical diagnostic rule is that an early-in-pregnancy fetal pulmonary lesion with macrocysts is a CPAM (Fig. 8.7). In large fetal series, CPAMs account for 76 to 85% of all detected fetal lung masses. In over 95% of cases, CPAM involves only a lobe or part of a lobe. Bilateral lesions are rare (1 to 2%).

Without visible macrocysts, the pattern recognition is less reliable; the hyperechoic lung can then be due to several underlying entities (PS, CPAM type III, CLE, bronchial compression or obstruction).

Exlobar PS is very likely when the lesion is posterobasal in location (especially on the left side), triangular in shape and supplied by an arterial feeder (Fig. 8.8). However, the arterial feeder is not always demonstrated prenatally (Fig. 8.9). In Lopoo's series of 14 cases (LOPOO 1999), the systemic arterial feeder was demonstrated by CDU in all cases, whereas in

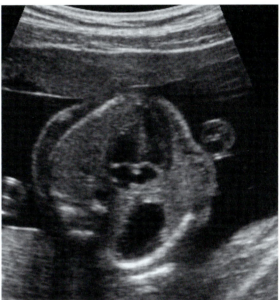

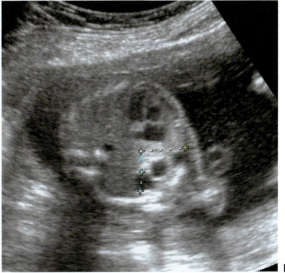

Fig. 8.7a,b. CPAM as displayed on a four-chamber view of the fetal thorax. **a** Right monocystic CPAM in a 20-week-old fetus. **b** Right pleuricystic CPAM in a 19-week-old fetus

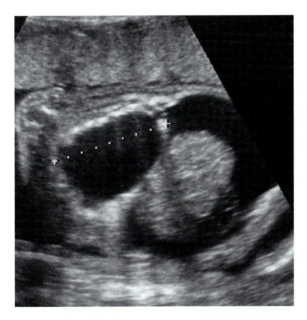

Fig. 8.6. Hydrops fetalis in a case of right lung CPAM in a 22-week-old fetus. The large macrocystic lesion (in between calipers) impaired the venous return with massive ascites surrounding the liver

Becmeur's material only four out of ten cases were displayed prenatally (BECMEUR 1998). Ipsilateral effusion is occasionally seen in PS (6 to 10% of cases) (Fig. 8.10).

CPAM type III presents also as a hyperechoic lung lesion in utero (Fig. 8.11). Hyperechoic fetal lung due to bronchial compression or obstruction is better recognized nowadays and cases of pulmonary sling (SEMPLE 2003), CLE (OLUTOYE 2000), tracheal bronchus, bronchial plug and others, as well as extrinsic bronchial compression (Fig. 8.12) fit into the CLO framework.

As already mentioned, fetal CLLs encompass a spectrum of anomalies with associated pathological features; hybrid lesions are made of coexisting ELPS and CPAM type II (Fig. 8.13). These hybrid lesions can also be located below the diaphragm, usually above the left kidney (Fig. 8.14). In the AFIP material, 50% of ELPS were associated with coexisting CPAM type II (CONRAN-STOCKER 1999). Thirty percent of hybrid lesions in the latter series were beneath the diaphragm.

The various series of antenatally recognized CPAM and PS (Tables 8.1, 8.2) have outlined very different figures in terms of natural history, complications and outcome. These differences are most likely related to the type of practice of the reporting institutions; fetal therapy centers obviously deal with the most severe referred cases, hence the high percentage of fetal hydrops, prenatal intervention and lethality in the corresponding series. Hydrops fetalis superimposed on CLL ranges from 7 to 16% in the literature; hydrops fetalis is rare (2%) in our own material of a low-risk, general population (Fig. 8.6). Interestingly, most survivors are asymptomatic at birth (60 to 90 % of cases), and that is especially the case when the lesions decreased in size in utero (50 to 75% of reported cases). Sonographic monitoring is of utmost importance, because the regression of the mass will often be documented during the 3rd trimester (Fig. 8.15). This regression in utero is partial or complete, absolute (i.e., decrease in lesion volume) or relative (i.e., growth of the chest exceeding growth of the mass) and is demonstrated by the improvement and resolution of cardiac shift on follow-up sonograms. Such reduction of the cardiac shift throughout pregnancy was almost invariably displayed in our material in the absence of hydrops fetal. (Fig. 8.16)

Bronchogenic cysts (BC) are exceptionally detected in utero either as a unicameral or a multilocular cystic mass in the lung (MAYDEN 1984) or the mediastinum (YOUNG 1989). Fetal bronchial compression can also be induced by a hilar BC (Fig. 8.12).

8.3.3
Pulmonary Hyperplasia (CHAOS)

Extremely rare lesions, laryngeal and tracheal obstructions (atresia, cyst and web) are very characteristic on fetal sonogram. Both lungs appear markedly symmetrically enlarged and diffusely echogenic (Fig. 8.17). The diaphragms are flattened. The fluid-filled main bronchi and trachea can be demonstrated (CHOONG 1992). Fetal ascites and polyhydramnios are sometimes present. Anomalies associated with laryngeal atresia are frequent and can be part of Fraser syndrome (tracheal atresia-renal agenesis polysyndactyly).

8.3.4
Congenital Lobar Overinflation

CLE is rarely recognized in utero (OLUTOYE 2000). Sonographically, CLE appears as a diffusely echogenic mass, initially large, without aberrant systemic arterial supply at CDU. Upper lobe (especially left) or right middle lobe involvement can be an additional diagnostic hint. Like most CLL, serial sonograms monitor the gradual involution of fetal CLE in the 3rd trimester. Respiratory distress at birth due to air trapping makes neonatal lobectomy necessary. The differential diagnosis of CLE in utero includes microcystic CPAM (Fig. 8.11) and bronchial obstruction/compression (Fig. 8.12).

Indeed bronchial obstruction also appears antenatally as an echogenic pulmonary mass (Fig. 8.18), most often in the LUL, sometimes in the RUL or RML. In some cases, complete resolution of the echogenic lesion is documented during gestation, suggesting the relief of a relative, transient bronchial obstruction (ACHIRON 1995; MEIZINER 1995).

8.3.5
Pleural Effusion

Pleural effusion in a fetus is always abnormal. Fetal hydrothorax is either primary or a sign of hydrops fetalis. The anechoic effusion is easily detected sonographically (Fig. 8.19). Fetal primary pleural effusion is often of chylous origin, without a precise underlying cause in most instances.

We have already mentioned the occurrence of ipsilateral effusion in 6 to 10% of the cases of ELP (Fig. 8.10). As a general rule, pleural effusions in hydrops fetalis are bilateral and symmetric (Fig. 8.20).

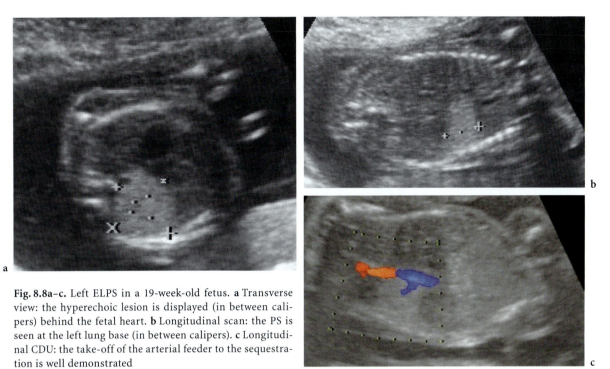

Fig. 8.8a–c. Left ELPS in a 19-week-old fetus. **a** Transverse view: the hyperechoic lesion is displayed (in between calipers) behind the fetal heart. **b** Longitudinal scan: the PS is seen at the left lung base (in between calipers). **c** Longitudinal CDU: the take-off of the arterial feeder to the sequestration is well demonstrated

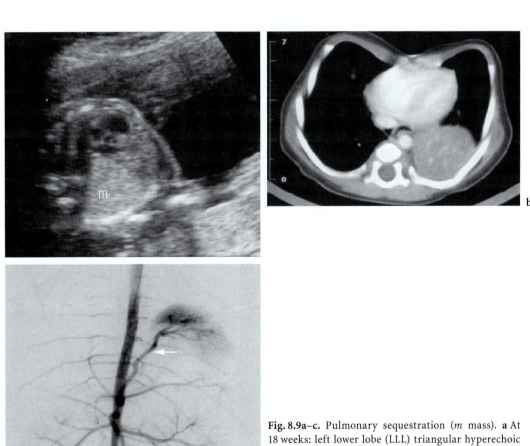

Fig. 8.9a–c. Pulmonary sequestration (*m* mass). **a** At 18 weeks: left lower lobe (LLL) triangular hyperechoic anomaly. **b** CT at birth, showing the sequestration. **c** Pre-embolization angiogram at 5 months of age, outlining the systemic arterial supply (*arrow*)

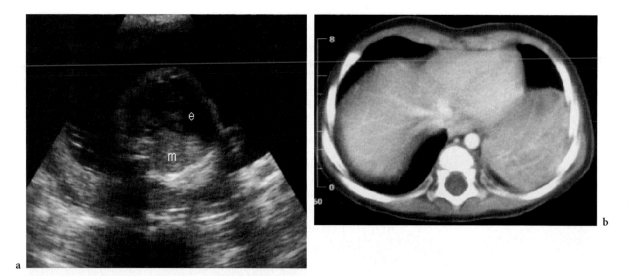

Fig. 8.10a,b. Left pulmonary sequestration associated with antenatal ipsilateral hydrothorax (*e* effusion, *m* mass). **a** In utero at 20 weeks (transverse scan). **b** Post-natal CT at 8 months of age, showing the sequestration

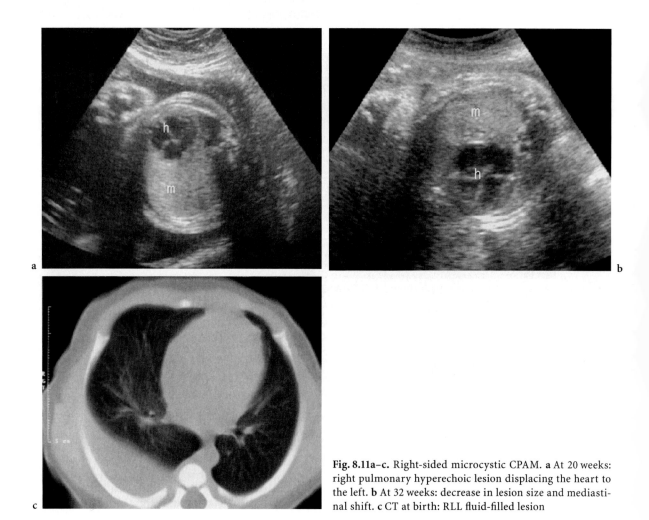

Fig. 8.11a–c. Right-sided microcystic CPAM. **a** At 20 weeks: right pulmonary hyperechoic lesion displacing the heart to the left. **b** At 32 weeks: decrease in lesion size and mediastinal shift. **c** CT at birth: RLL fluid-filled lesion

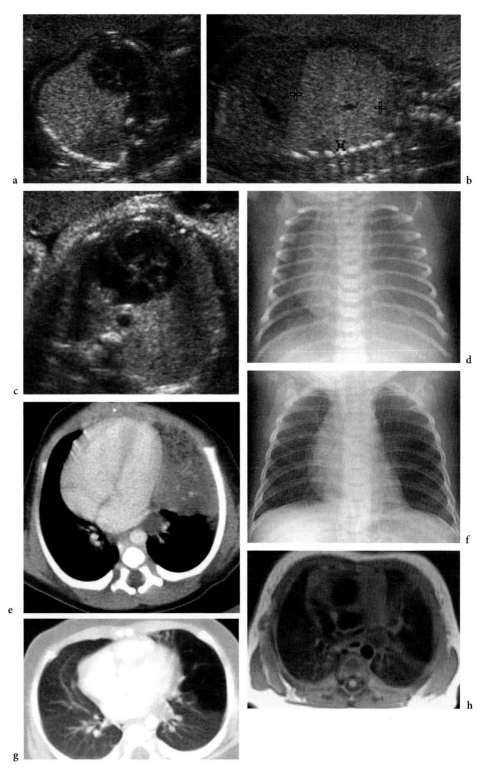

Fig. 8.12a–h. Hyperechoic lung due to bronchial compression (left hilar BC). **a** Transverse scan at 19 weeks: the hyperechoic left lung shifts the fetal heart to the right. **b** Longitudinal scan at 19 weeks: the hyperechoic left lung (in between calipers) is shown above the fetal stomach. **c** Transverse scan at 32 weeks: there has been a marked decrease in the heart shift. **d** Chest X-ray at birth: evidence of alveolar fluid retention is shown in the left lung. **e** CT scan on day 2: the alveolar fluid within the left lung is seen along with the small left hilar mass. **f** Chest X-ray at 6 months: air trapping in the left lung is obvious. **g** Chest CT and **h** MRI at 6 months: same findings of left air trapping and left hilar mass. The left hilar BC was easily removed surgically at 6 months

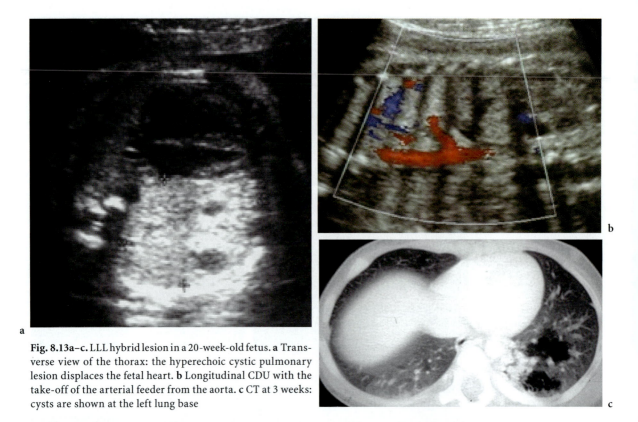

Fig. 8.13a–c. LLL hybrid lesion in a 20-week-old fetus. **a** Transverse view of the thorax: the hyperechoic cystic pulmonary lesion displaces the fetal heart. **b** Longitudinal CDU with the take-off of the arterial feeder from the aorta. **c** CT at 3 weeks: cysts are shown at the left lung base

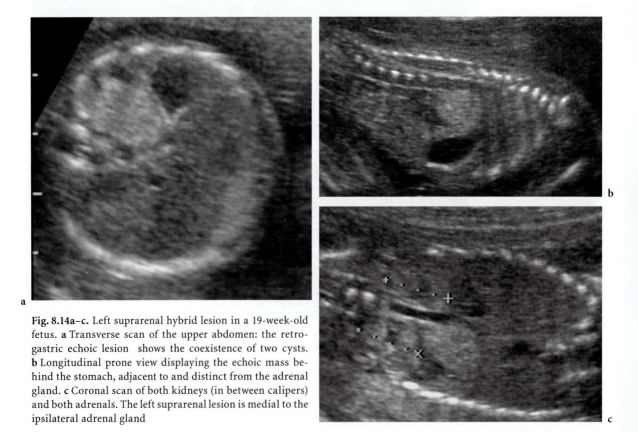

Fig. 8.14a–c. Left suprarenal hybrid lesion in a 19-week-old fetus. **a** Transverse scan of the upper abdomen: the retrogastric echoic lesion shows the coexistence of two cysts. **b** Longitudinal prone view displaying the echoic mass behind the stomach, adjacent to and distinct from the adrenal gland. **c** Coronal scan of both kidneys (in between calipers) and both adrenals. The left suprarenal lesion is medial to the ipsilateral adrenal gland

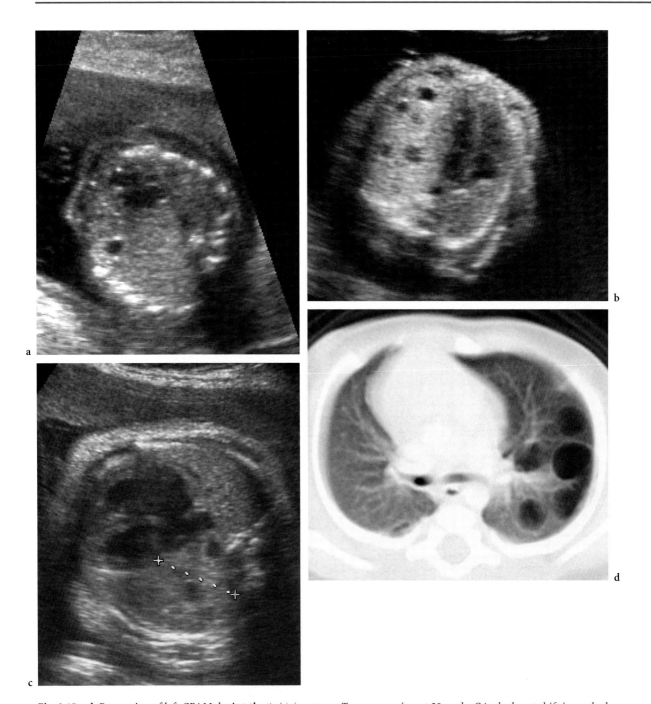

Fig. 8.15a–d. Regression of left CPAM during the 3rd trimester. **a** Transverse view at 20 weeks GA: the heart shift is marked due to an echoic left lung with a visible cyst. **b** Transverse four-chamber view at 30 weeks GA: the heart shift is still visible, in relation to the multicystic CPAM. **c** Transverse four-chamber view at 33 weeks GA: the heart is already back to is normal position, the remaining CPAM (*in between calipers*) smaller in volume. **d** Chest CT at 3 months: the patient was asymptomatic at birth and subsequently

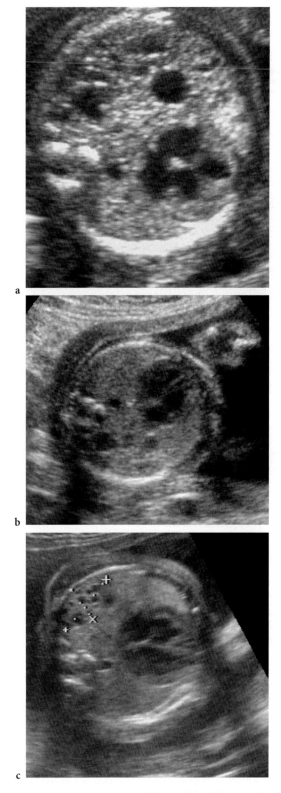

The prognostic predictors of fetal hydrothorax are mainly related to laterality (unilateral vs. bilateral effusion), the presence or absence of associated anomalies, a coexisting hydrops and the evolution. The natural history of primary fetal pleural effusion is variable; spontaneous resolution is seen in 10 to 20% of cases (WEBER and PHILIPSON 1992; AUBARD 1998) and implies a favorable outcome. Fetal karyotyping is recommended by some authors (ACHIRON 1995) who outline a risk of aneuploidy of approximately 5%.

Fetal intervention (thoracocentesis and/or thoracoamniotic shunt) is indicated in large or increasing effusions and in cases of hydrops (NICOLAIDES and AZAR 1990; MUSSAT 1995). In all series, hydrops remains the single most important predictor of a poor outcome (LONGAKER 1989; AUBARD 1998).

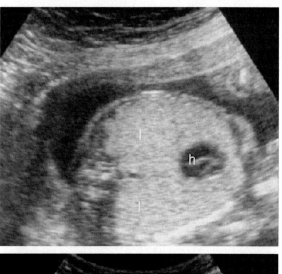

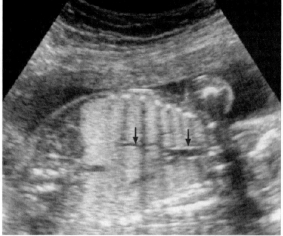

Fig. 8.16a–c. Regression of the cardiac shift throughout pregnancy in a case of right CPAM as shown by sequential transverse scans. **a** At 21-weeks GA. **b** At 25-weeks GA. **c** At 30-weeks GA

Fig. 8.17a,b. Laryngeal atresia in a 20-week fetus (*h* heart, l lung). **a** Transverse scan: the lungs are massively enlarged and are compressing the heart on the midline. **b** Longitudinal scan: fluid is seen within the trachea and bronchi (*arrows*)

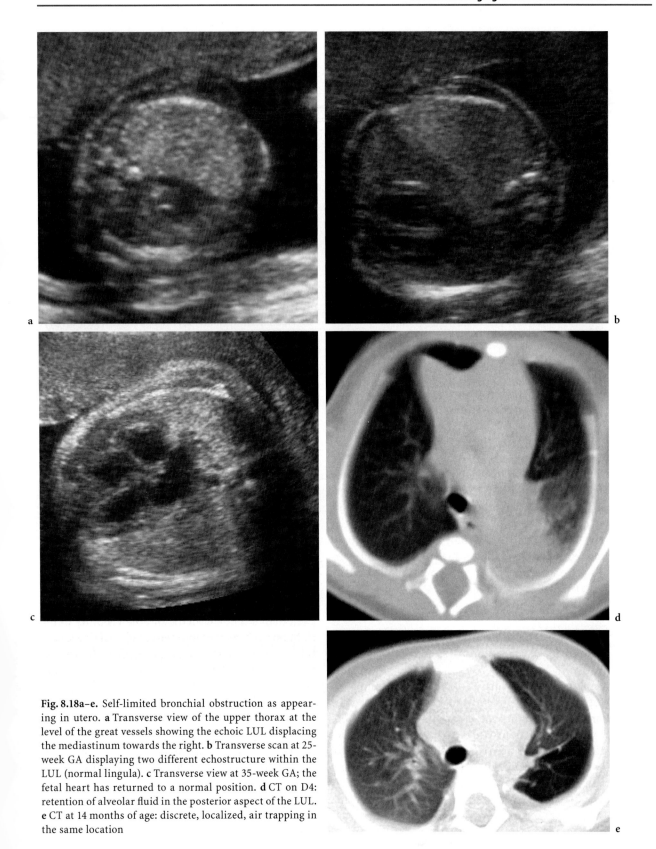

Fig. 8.18a–e. Self-limited bronchial obstruction as appearing in utero. **a** Transverse view of the upper thorax at the level of the great vessels showing the echoic LUL displacing the mediastinum towards the right. **b** Transverse scan at 25-week GA displaying two different echostructure within the LUL (normal lingula). **c** Transverse view at 35-week GA; the fetal heart has returned to a normal position. **d** CT on D4: retention of alveolar fluid in the posterior aspect of the LUL. **e** CT at 14 months of age: discrete, localized, air trapping in the same location

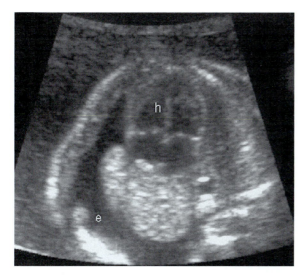

Fig. 8.19. Right pleural effusion in a 19-week fetus without cardiac shift (transverse scan). The effusion subsides spontaneously on follow-up sonograms (*e* effusion, *h* heart)

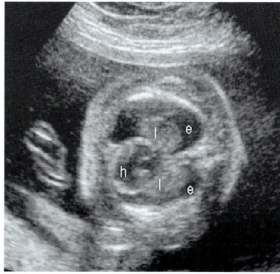

Fig. 8.20. Bilateral pleural effusions associated with hydrops in a 21-week fetus (transverse scan) (*e* effusion, *h* heart, *l* lung)

8.3.6
Mediastinal Abnormalities

Various mediastinal lesions such as pericardial teratomas (TODROS 1991), thymic cyst (DE MIGUEL CAMPOS 1997), bronchogenic cyst (Young 1989) or neurenteric cyst (MACAULAY 1997) have been occasionally reported in utero. Lymphangioma can also be demonstrated prenatally in the mediastinum (Fig. 8.21). Cardiac rhabdomyomas are seen more frequently in the fetus, especially in cases of tuberous sclerosis where the masses are multiple (GREEN 1991; GUSHIKEN 1999).

8.3.7
Congenital Diaphragmatic Hernia (CDH)

Diaphragmatic herniation is observed in approximately 1/5,000 live births and results from the abnormal partitioning of the celomic cavity. The more common herniation is through a postero-lateral defect (Bochdalek's hernia), left-sided in 80 to 85% of cases, right-sided in 10 to 15% and bilateral in less than 5%. Anterior parasternal hernia (Morgagni's hernia), septum transversum defect, hiatal hernia and diaphragmatic eventration are more exceptionally seen in the fetus.

The sonographic hallmark of CDH is the mediastinal shift, opposite to the intrathoracic location of abdominal viscera (KASALES 1998) (Fig. 8.22). In left-sided CDH, the heart is displaced toward the right by the fluid-filled stomach (Fig. 8.23a). The common herniation of the spleen appears less echoic than a CPAM or a PS. The herniated bowel (Fig. 8.22) can sometimes demonstrate evidence of peristalsis. The thoracic herniation of the left lobe of the liver is indicated by the posterior displacement of the stomach (Fig. 8.23b) and the demonstration of the left portal vein on CDU. The diagnosis of right-sided CDH is more difficult because the stomach is usually in an abdominal location and the herniated liver can be confused with a lung abnormality. The high position of the gallbladder (Fig. 8.24), the absence of the right diaphragm landmark and the visibility of the right portal branches into the chest at CDU are useful diagnostic hints. The cardiac shift is often markedly apparent. Bilateral CDH can be overlooked because there is no mediantinal shift.

Once identified, fetal CDH must be evaluated in terms of prognosis. Overall the antenatally diagnosed CDHs have a worse prognosis than the ones recognized after birth (hidden mortality concept) (BERESFORD and SHAW 2000). The prognostic predictors of CDH are the following: associated anomalies, bilaterality, lung hypoplasia, intrathoracic herniation of the liver, size of the hernia and early diagnosis. Chromosomal anomalies, seen in 5 to 15% of CDH, make karyotyping mandatory. Associated anomalies are found in 20 to 45% of cases and

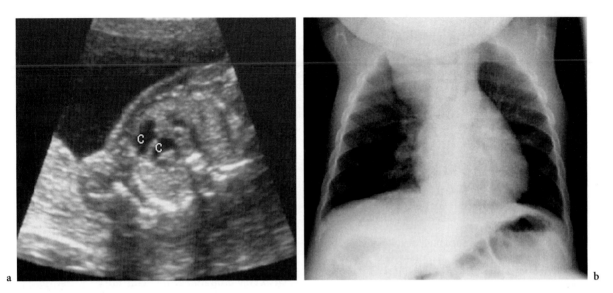

Fig. 8.21a,b. Mediastinal lymphangioma (*c* cyst). **a** In utero (19 weeks): traverse scan of the upper thorax, showing two cysts immediately lateral to the SVC. **b** Chest X-ray at 7 months: the obvious mediastinal lesion is displacing the trachea to the left. The parents were reluctant to allow surgery until the patient became symptomatic

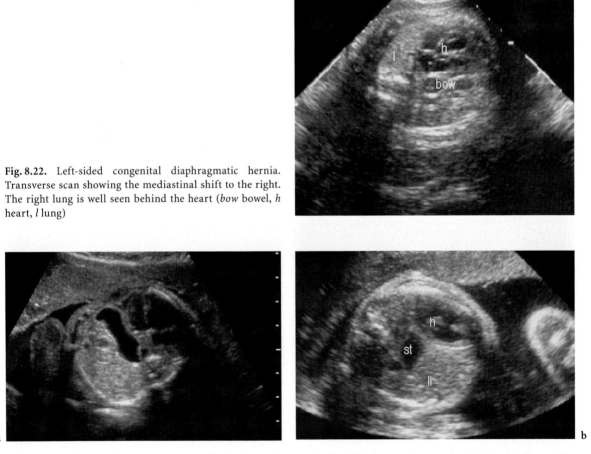

Fig. 8.22. Left-sided congenital diaphragmatic hernia. Transverse scan showing the mediastinal shift to the right. The right lung is well seen behind the heart (*bow* bowel, *h* heart, *l* lung)

Fig. 8.23. a Left side CDH transverse four-chamber view showing the fluid filled stomach at the level of the fetal heart that is displaced towards the right. **b** Left-sided congenital diaphragmatic hernia. Transverse sonogram displaying the cardiac shift, the posterior stomach, and the more anterior left lobe of the liver (*h* heart, *li* liver, *st* stomach)

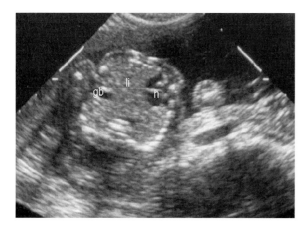

Fig. 8.24. Right-sided congenital diaphragmatic hernia (transverse scan). The heart is displaced to the left. The herniated liver is identified with the uplifted gallbladder (*h* heart, *gb* gallbladder, *li* liver)

are mainly cardiac, cerebral and renal. At times, the associated anomalies are part of a syndrome (e.g., Fryn's syndrome). The evaluation of the size of the controlateral lung is of paramount importance (Fig. 8.25). The lung area is assessed on a transverse four-chamber view and expressed as a ratio: initially, the lung area was compared to the area of the hemithorax (survival rate of 86% when the ratio lung/hemithorax is equal or superior to 50%) (GUIBAUD 1996). Most centers nowadays have adopted the lung/head ratio (LIPSHUTZ 1997): the survival rate is 100% if the lung/head ratio is superior to 1.4. The prognosis of left CDH is worse when the liver is herniated in the thorax (survival rate: 43% vs. 93% when the liver remains within the abdomen) (ALBANESE 1998). The selection of poor prognosis cases (Fig. 8.26) is crucial when contemplating fetal surgery (fetoscopic

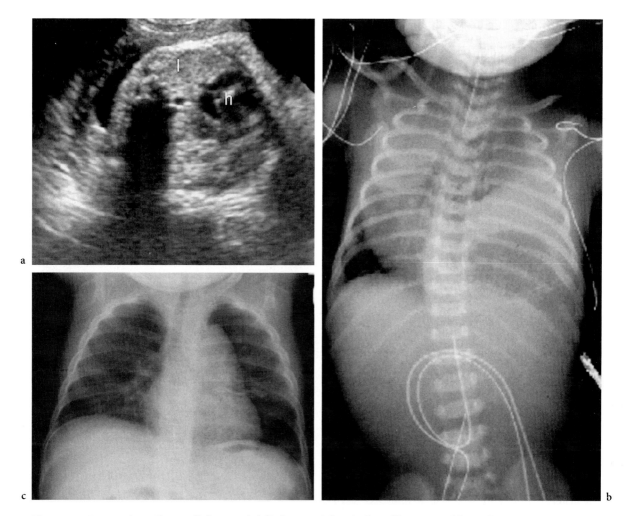

Fig. 8.25a–c. Prognostic predictors of left congenital diaphragmatic hernia: favorable outcome (*h* heart, *l* lung). **a** A 22-week transverse sonogram, showing a well-preserved right lung behind the heart. **b** Post-natal chest X-ray, showing the herniated stomach with the nasogastric tube and the remaining right lung. **c** Chest X-ray at 10 months of age, showing the development of both lungs

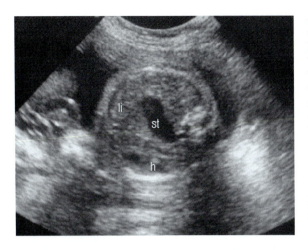

Fig. 8.26. Prognostic predictors of congenital diaphragmatic hernia: poor prognosis case. Transverse sonogram in a 20-week-old fetus: the mediastinal shift is severe, almost without visible lung on the right, and the liver is herniated, anterior to the stomach. The baby died at birth (*h* heart, *li* liver, *st* stomach)

tempory tracheal occlusion) (Harrison 1998), especially in the light of recent technical improvements (Deprest 2006).

MRI proved useful in providing reliable information about associated anomalies, intrathoracic liver herniation (Hubbard 1997) and lung volumetry (Paek 2001; Ward 2006; Cannie 2006). Similarly, volumetric ultrasound shows promising results (Gerards 2006; Peralta 2006).

8.3.8
Pulmonary Hypoplasia

Unilateral lung agenesis has been detected in utero (Bromley and Benacerraf 1997) (Fig. 8.27). Bilateral pulmonary hypoplasia is usually secondary to a persistent oligohydramnios, an intrathoracic mass or a small thorax. Normograms are available for fetal thoracic circumference measurements from 16 to 40 weeks of pregnancy, or for ratios of thoracic circumference to various fetal growth parameters (e.g., thoracic circumference/abdomen circumference). Interestingly, the latter ratio (TC/AC) is fairly stable normally throughout pregnancy (Chitkara 1987; Vintzileos 1989; D'Alton 1992). The sonographic evaluation of the lung area has also proved to be clinically useful (Yoshimura 1996). MRI shows interesting potential in assessing fetal lung volume (Coakley 2000; Rypens 2001). Similarly, volumetric

ultrasound shows promising results (Gerards 2006; Peralta 2006). The most common causes of oligohydramnios are preterm premature rupture of the amniotic membranes, renal abnormalities (agenesis, dysplasia, obstruction and polycystic disease) and intrauterine growth restriction. As a general rule, pulmonary hypoplasia is worse in early prolonged and severe oligohydramnios (Fig. 8.28).

8.4
Post-Natal Issues

Fetal imaging has provided crucial insights regarding the natural history of CLL. CLLs are visible early in pregnancy (routine mid-2nd trimester), they decrease in size in utero (Figs. 8.11, 8.15, 8.16), and most newborns with CLL are asymptomatic (50 to 85%).

8.4.1
Post-Natal Investigations

Post-natal investigations are thus based upon prenatal findings in the majority of cases. The spontaneous resolution of CLL has been addressed unequivocally in the literature for subdiaphragmatic suprarenal hybrid lesions (Daneman 1997; Chowdhury 2004) (Fig. 8.29). It has been well demonstrated also that CT is far superior to chest X-ray in showing residual lesions in asymptomatic newborns with CLL (Fig. 8.30), and subsequently (Winters 1997; Blau 2002). CT should not be performed too early because of the prolonged retention of alveolar fluid within CLL at birth. Post-natal management is dictated by clinical status at birth. In symptomatic newborns with CLL (15% of cases in our material), immediate surgery is indicated; a simple preoperative chest X-ray with a NG tube in place is then sufficient to differentiate a CPAM from a CDH (Fig. 8.31).

8.4.2
Management of Asymptomatic Patients with Prenatally Recognized CLL

Most authors in the surgical literature still recommend the systematic early removal of CLL (Adzick 1998, 2003; Laberge 2001, 2005; Waszak 1999;

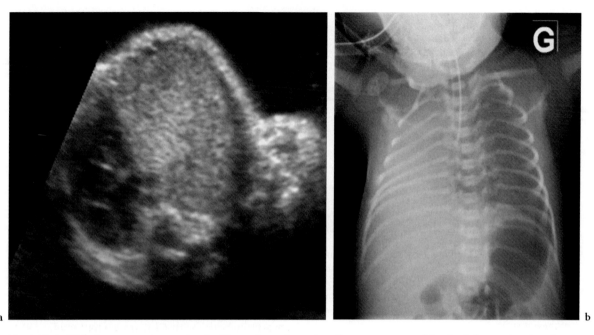

Fig. 8.27a,b. Right lung agenesis associated with esophageal atresia. **a** Transverse scan of the fetal thorax showing the extreme shift of the heart by the left lung. **b** Chest X-ray at birth

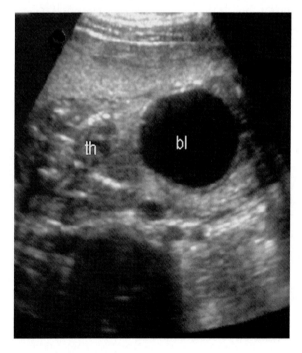

Fig. 8.28. Pulmonary hypoplasia and oligoamnios in a case of urethral atresia in an 18-week-old fetus. The bladder is markedly enlarged, and the thorax very small. There is no amniotic fluid around the fetus (*bl* bladder, *th* thorax)

DUNCOMBE 2002; DAVENPORT 2004; STANTON and DAVENPORT 2006). Their recommendations for surgery are based upon the following rationale:
1) Pulmonary compensatory growth is optimal when surgery is early;
2) Post-natal hazards (infection, malignancy) are ineluctable and severe and should, accordingly, be prevented.

In our experience of antenatally recognized CLL, pulmonary compensatory growth does not only follow the rule of age at surgery (Fig. 8.32). Adequate vascularization is also needed to allow alveoli multiplication and growth. Accordingly, lung hypoplasia following surgery for CLL can be equally encountered in patients operated upon prior to or after 2 years of age.

Infection of CLL does occur (Fig. 8.33), but not as often as some report (Fig. 8.34). The only available prospective study of prenatally diagnosed asymptomatic CPAM (AZIZ 2004) reports an incidence of infection of 10%. The same authors emphasize also that there was no increase in the postoperative complication rate if surgery was delayed until onset of infectious symptoms.

Regarding malignant degeneration of CPAM, some previously reported assumptions [rhabdomyosarcoma or blastoma coexisting with or arising from

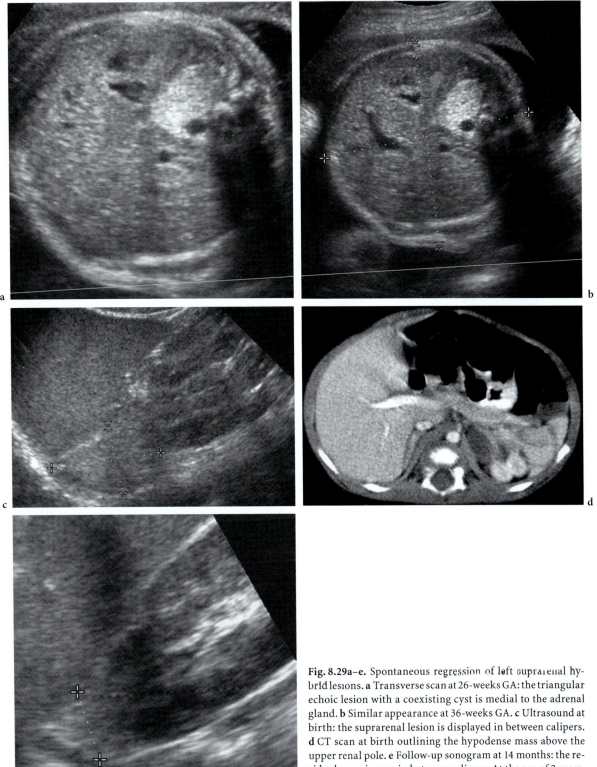

Fig. 8.29a–e. Spontaneous regression of left suprarenal hybrid lesions. **a** Transverse scan at 26-weeks GA: the triangular echoic lesion with a coexisting cyst is medial to the adrenal gland. **b** Similar appearance at 36-weeks GA. **c** Ultrasound at birth: the suprarenal lesion is displayed in between calipers. **d** CT scan at birth outlining the hypodense mass above the upper renal pole. **e** Follow-up sonogram at 14 months: the residual mass is seen in between calipers. At the age of 2 years, the lesion had completely regressed

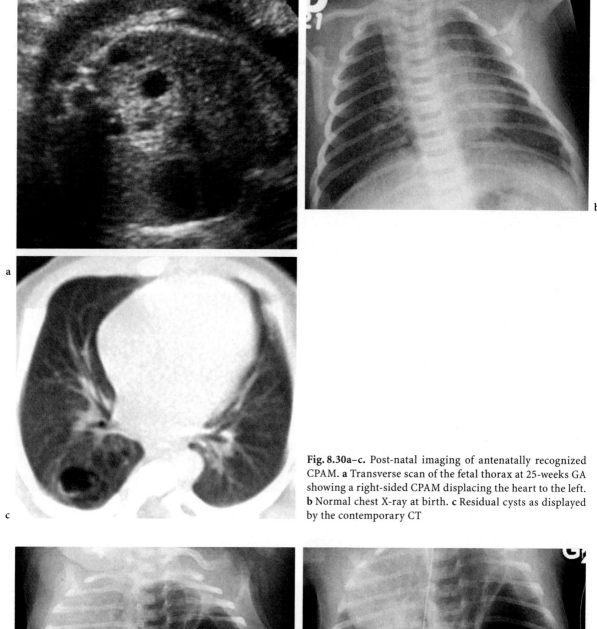

Fig. 8.30a–c. Post-natal imaging of antenatally recognized CPAM. **a** Transverse scan of the fetal thorax at 25-weeks GA showing a right-sided CPAM displacing the heart to the left. **b** Normal chest X-ray at birth. **c** Residual cysts as displayed by the contemporary CT

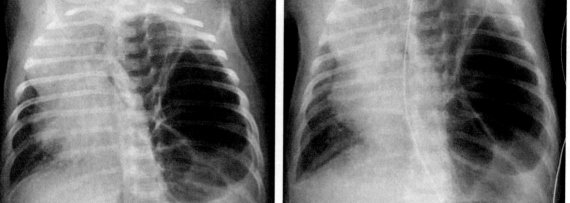

Fig. 8.31a,b. Symptomatic newborn with prenatally recognized left CLL. **a** Chest X-ray: left chest lucencies shifting the heart to the right. **b** Same patient after placement of a NG tube; the normal position of the stomach makes the diagnosis of CPAM very likely. Surgery was immediately performed via a left thoracotomy

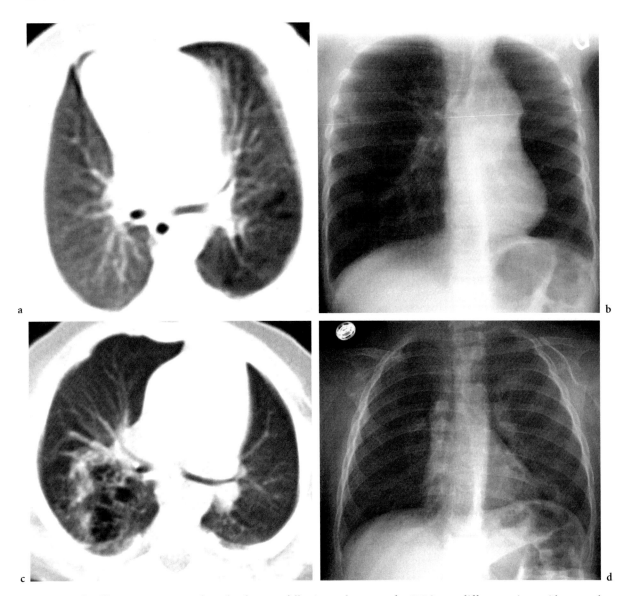

Fig. 8.32a–d. Different compensatory lung development following early surgery for CLL in two different patients with prenatal diagnosis. **a** CT at birth in patient 1 with left cystic lung lesion. Surgery took place at 3 months. **b** Chest X-ray at 5 years of age in the same patient showing a small hypovascular left lung. **c** CT at 3 weeks in patient 2 with a right-sided CPAM. Surgery was performed at 5 months of age. **d** Chest X-ray in the same patient at 3 years; the operated lung has almost a normal volume

CPAM (Murphy 1992; D'Agostino 1997; Granata 1998)] are not valid anymore; congenital lung cysts do not degenerate to become pleuropulmonary blastomas (PPB), and cystic PPBs are blastomas at presentation (Dehner 2005; Langston 2003, 2006). Post-natally, there is no distinguishable imaging feature between macrocystic CPAMs and cystic PPBs. However, besides their relative frequency (CPAMs are common, and cystic PPBs rare), the prenatal timing is a key differential feature. CPAMs occur early in pregnancy and are always demonstrated on the routine 18–20-week GA sonogram. On the other hand, cystic PPBs are exceedingly rare occurrences in utero (Miniati 2006) in the 3rd trimester. Most cystic PPBs (Fig. 8.35) are recognized post-natally (mean age at presentation: 10 months). A similar prenatal timing is also helpful in differentiating the subdiaphragmatic suprarenal hybrid lesions (2nd trimester) and the congenital neuroblastomas (3rd trimester) (Rubinstein 1995).

It is fair to acknowledge that, at the present time, the long-term malignant potential of non-operated CPAM is impossible to quantify. Some case reports

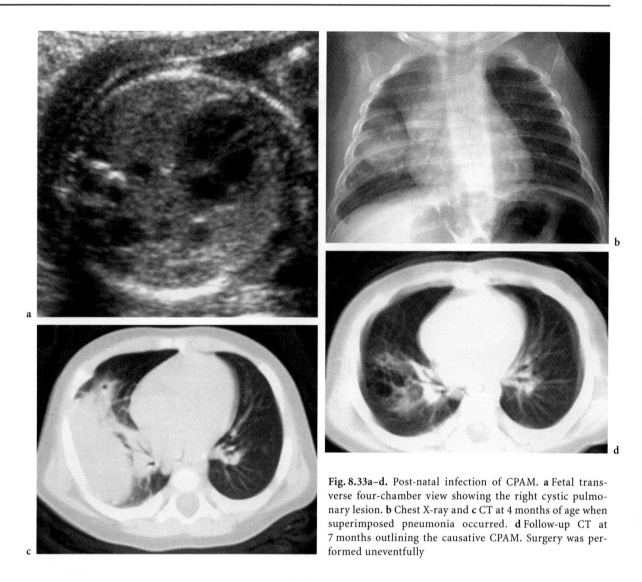

Fig. 8.33a–d. Post-natal infection of CPAM. **a** Fetal transverse four-chamber view showing the right cystic pulmonary lesion. **b** Chest X-ray and **c** CT at 4 months of age when superimposed pneumonia occurred. **d** Follow-up CT at 7 months outlining the causative CPAM. Surgery was performed uneventfully

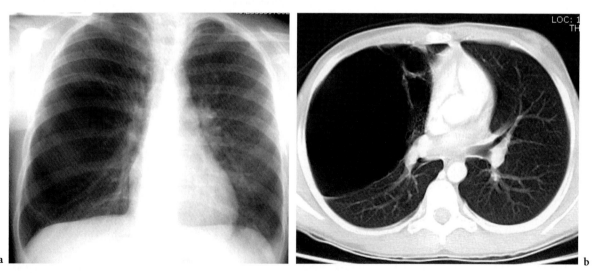

Fig. 8.34a,b. Late-discovery right CPAM in an asymptomatic 11-year-old female without past medical history. **a** Chest X-ray. **b** CT

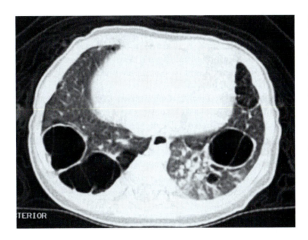

Fig. 8.35. Bilateral cystic PPBs in a 6-month-old infant. Mid-second trimester fetal ultrasound was normal

of carcinomas occurring with CCAM have been described in the adult literature (Benjamin and Cahill 1991; Ribet 1995). However, the link between oncogenesis and teratogenesis is not restricted to the lungs. Similarly, renal cell carcinomas also have been reported in regressed multicystic dysplastic kidneys without leading to routine nephrectomy in asymptomatic newborns with prenatally diagnosed renal dysplasia. Apart from the controversy regarding the post-natal management of asymptomatic patients with antenatally recognized CPAM, there is a trend toward the conservative management of small and/or regressing bronchopulmonary malformations (Sauvat 2003; Chowdhury 2004; Stanton and Davenport 2006) (Fig. 8.29).

8.5
Conclusion

1) Fetal cystic lung anomalies without hydrops fetalis have a good outcome in most instances, and this should be addressed when providing parental counseling.
2) In asymptomatic patients, post-natal imaging consists of chest X-ray and CT within 4 weeks after birth even in the cases with prenatal regression/resolution of lesions.
3) At the present time, most authors still advise elective resection (lobectomy or segmentectomy) of all prenatally recognized CPAM.

References

Achiron R, Weissman A, Lipitz S, Maschiach S, Goldman B. Fetal pleural effusion: the risk of fetal trisomy. Gynecol Obstet Invest 1995;39(3):153–156

Achiron R, Staruss S, Seidman DS, Lipitz S, Mashiach S, Goldman B. Fetal lung hyperechogenicity: prenatal ultrasonographic diagnosis, natural history and neonatal outcome. Ultrasound Obstet Gynecol 1995;6:40–42

Adzick NS, Harrison MR, Glick PL, Golbus MS, Anderson RL, Mahony BS, Callen PW, Hirsch JH, Luthy DA, Filly RA et al. Fetal cystic adenomatoid malformation: prenatal diagnosis and natural history. J Pediatr Surg 1985;20(5):483–488

Adzick NS, Harrison MR, Crombleholme TM, Flake AW, Howell LJ. Fetal lung lesions: Management and outcome. Am J Obstet Gynecol 1998;179:884–889

Adzick NS, Flake AW, Crombleholme TM. Management of congenital lung lesions. Semin Ped Surg 2003;12(1):10–16

Albanese CT, Lopoo J, Goldstein RB, Filly RA, Feldstein VA, Calen PW, Jennings RW, Fattell JA, Harrison MR. Fetal liver position and perinatal outcome for congenital diaphragmatic hernia. Prenat Diagn 1998;18:1138–1142

Aubard Y, Derouineau I, Aubard V, Chalifour V, Preux PM. Primary fetal hydrothorax: a litterature review and proposed antenatal clinical strategy. Fetal Diagn Ther 1998;13:325–333

Aziz D, Langer JC, Tuuha SE, Ryan G, Ein SH, Kim PCW. Perinatally diagnosed asymptomatic congenital cystic adenomatoid malformation: To resect or not? J Pediatr Surg 2004;39(3):329–334

Barnes NA, Pilling DW. Bronchopulmonary foregut malformations: embryology, radiology and quandary. Eur Radiol 2003;13(12):2659–2673

Becmeur F, Horta-Geraud P, Donato L, Sauvage P. Pulmonary sequestrations: prenatal ultrasound diagnosis, treatment, and outcome. J Pediatr Surg 1998;33:492–496

Benjamin DR, Cahill JL. Bronchiolalveolar carcinoma of the lung and congenital cystic adenomatoid malformation. Am J Clin Pathol 1991;95:889–892

Beresford MW, Shaw NJ. Outcome of congenital diaphragmatic hernia. Pediatr Pulmonol 2000;30:249–256

Blau H, Barak A, Karmazyn B, Mussaffi H, Ben Ari J, Schoenfeld T, Aviram M, Vinograd Y, Lotem Y, Meizner I. Postnatal management of resolving fetal lung lesions. Pediatrics 2002;109(1):105–108

Bratu I, Flageole H Chen MF, Di Lorenzo M, Yazbeck S, Laberge JM. The multiple facets of pulmonary sequestration. J Pediatr Surg 2001;36(5):784–790

Bromley B, Benacerraf BR. Unilateral lung hypoplasia: report of three cases. J Ultrasound Med 1997;16:599–601

Bromley B, Parad R, Estroff JA, Benacerraf BR. Fetal lung masses: prenatal course and outcome. J Ultrasound Med 1995;14(12):927–936

Budorick NE, Pretorius DH, Leopold GR, Stamm ER. Spontaneous improvement of intrathoracic masses diagnosed in utero. J Ultrasound Med 1992;11(12):653–662

Bunduki V, Ruano R, Da Silva MM, Miguelez J, Miyadahira S, Maksoud JG, Zugaib M. Prognostic factors associated with congenital cystic adenomatoid malformation of the lung. Prenat Diagn 2000;20(6):459–464

Bush A. Malformations. In: Gibson J et al (ed) Respiratory medicine (3rd edn). Saunders 2002, p 2192

Cacciari A, Ceccarelli PL, Pilu GL, Bianchini MA, Mordenti M, Gabrielli S, Milano V, Zanetti G, Pigna A, Gentili A. A series of 17 cases of congenital cystic adenomatoid malformation of the lung: management and outcome. Eur J Pediatr Surg 1997;7(2):84–89

Calvert JK, Boyd PA, Chamberlain PC, Syed S, Lakhoo K. Outcome of antenatally suspected congenital cystic adenomatoid malformation of the lung: 10 years' experience 1991–2001. Arch Dis Child Fetal Neonatal Ed 2006;91(1): F26–28

Cannie M, Jani JC, De Keyzer F, Devlieger R, Van Schoubroeck D, Witters I, Marchal G, Dymarkowski S, Deprest JA. Fetal body volume: use at MR imaging to quantify relative lung volume in fetuses suspected of having pulmonary hypoplasia. Radiology 2006;241(3):847–853

Cass DL, Crombleholme TM, Howell LJ, Stafford PW, Ruchelli ED, Adzick NS. Cystic lung lesions with systemic arterial blood supply: a hybrid of congenital cystic adenomatoid malformation and bronchopulmonary sequestration. J Pediatr Surg 1997;32(7):986–990

Chitkara U, Rosenberg J, Chervenak FA, Berkowitz GS, Levine R, Fagerstrom RM, Walker B, Berkowitz RL. Prenatal sonographic assessment of the fetal thorax: normal values. Am J Obstet Gynecol 1987;156(5):1069–1074

Choong KK, Trudinger B, Chow C, Osborn RA. Fetal laryngeal obstruction: sonographic detection. Ultrasound Obstet Gynecol 1992;2(5):357–359

Chowdury M, Samuel M, Ramsay A, Constantinou J, Mchugh K, Pierro A. Spontaneous postnatal involution of intraabdominal pulmonary sequestration. J Ped Surg 2004;39(8):1273–1275

Clements BS, Warner JO. Pulmonary sequestration and related congenital bronchopulmonary-vascular malformations: nomenclature and classification based on anatomical and embryological considerations. Thorax 1987;42:401–408

Cloutier MM, Schaeffer DA, Hight D. Congenital cystic adenomatoid malformation. Chest 1993; 103(3):761–764

Coakley FV, Lopoo JB, Lu Y, Hricak H, Albanese CT, Harrison MR, Filly RA. Normal and hypoplastic fetal lungs: volumetric assessment with prenatal single-shot rapid acquisition with relaxation enhancement MR imaging. Radiology 2000;216:107–111

Conran RM, Stocker JT. Extralobar sequestration with frequently associated congenital cystic adenomatoid malformation, type 2: Report of 50 Cases. Pediatr Develop Pathol 1999;2:454–463

D'Agostino S, Bonoldi E, Dante S, Meli S, Cappellari F, Musi L. Embryonal rhabdomyosarcoma of the lung arising in cystic adenomatoid malformation: case report and review of the literature. J Pediatr Surg 1997;32:1381–1383

D'Alton M, Mercer B, Riddick E, Dudley D. Serial thoracic versus abdominal circumference ratios for the prediction of pulmonary hypoplasia in premature rupture of the membranes remote from term. Am J Obstet Gynecol 1992;166:658–663

Daneman A, Baunin C, Lobo E, Pracros JP, Avni F, Toi A, Metreweli C, Ho SS, Moore L. Disappearing suprarenal masses in fetuses and infants. Pediatr Radiol 1997;27:675–681

Davenport M, Warne SA, Cacciaguerra S, Patel S, Greenough A, Nicolaides K. Current outcome of antenally diagnosed cystic lung disease. J Pediatr Surg 2004;39(4):549–556

Dehner LP. Beware of "degenerating" congenital pulmonary cysts. Pediatr Surg Int 2005;21(2):123–124

De Miguel Campos E, Casanova A, Urbano J, Delgado-Carrasco J. Congenital thymic cyst: prenatal sonographic and postnatal magnetic resonance findings. J Ultrasound Med 1997;16:365–367

Deprest J, Jani J, Lewi L, Ochsenbein-Kolble N, Cannie M, Done E, Roubliova X, Van Mieghem T, Debeer A, Debuck F, Sbragia L, Toelen J, Devlieger R, Lewi P, Van de Velde M. Fetoscopic surgery: encouraged by clinical experience and boosted by instrument innovation. Semin Fetal Neonatal Med 2006;11(6):398–412

De Santis M, Masini L, Noia G, Cavaliere AF, Oliva N, Caruso A. Congenital cystic adenomatoid malformation of the lung: antenatal ultrasound findings and fetal-neonatal outcome. Fifteen years of experience. Fetal Diagn Ther 2000;15(4):246–250

Dhingsa R, Coakley FV, Albanese CT, Filly RA, Goldstein R. Prenatal sonography and MR imaging of pulmonary sequestration. AJR 2003;180(2):433–437

Duncombe GJ, Dickinson JE, Kikiros CS. Prenatal diagnosis and management of congenital cystic adenomatoid malformation of the lung. Am J Obstet Gynecol 2002;187(4):950–954

Gerards FA, Engels MA, Twisk JW, van Vugt JM. Normal fetal lung volume measured with three-dimensional ultrasound. Ultrasound Obstet Gynecol 2006;27(2):134–144

Granata C, Gambini C, Balducci T, Toma P, Michelazzi A, Conte M, Jasonni V. Bronchioloalveolar carcinoma arising in congenital cystic adenomatoid nancies originating in congenital cystic adenomatoid malformation. Pediatr Pulmonol 1998;25:62–66

Green KW, Bors-Koefoed R, Pollack P, Weinbaum PJ. Antepartum diagnosis and management of multiple fetal cardiac tumors. J Ultrasound Med 1991;10:697–699

Guibaud L, Filiatrault D, Garel L, Grignon A, Dubois J, Miron MC, Dallaire L. Fetal congenital diaphragmatic hernia accuracy of sonography in the diagnosis and prediction of the outcome after birth. AJR Am J Roentgenol 1996;166:1195–1202

Gushiken BJ, Callen PW, Silberman NH. Prenatal diagnosis of tuberous sclerosis in monozygotic twins with cardiac masses. J Ultrasound Med 1999;18:165–168

Harrison MR, Mychaliska GB, Albanese CT, Jennings RW, Farrell JA, Hawgood S, Sandberg P, Levine AH, Lobo E, Filly RA. Correction of congenital diaphragmatic hernia in utero IX: fetuses with poor prognosis (liver herniation and low lung-to-head ratio) can be saved by fetoscopic temporary tracheal occlusion. J Pediatr Surg 1998;33:1017–1022

Hubbard AM, Adzick NS, Crombleholme TM, Haselgrove JC. Left-sided congenital diaphragmatic hernia: value of prenatal MR imaging in preparation for fetal surgery. Radiology 1997;203:636–640

Ierullo AM, Ganapathy R, Crowley S, Craxford L, Bhide A, Thilaganathan B. Neonatal outcome of antenatally diagnosed congenital cystic adenomatoid malformations. Ultrasound Obstet Gyncecol 2005;26:150–153

Illanes S, Hunter A, Evans M, Cusick E, Soothill P. Prenatal diagnosis of echogenic lung: evolution and outcome. Ultrasound Obstet Gynecol 2005;26:145–149

Kasales CJ, Coulson CC, Meilstrup JW, Ambrose A, Botti JJ, Holley GP. Diagnosis and differentiation of congenital diaphragmatic hernia from other noncardiac thoracic fetal masses. Am J Perinatol 1998;15:623–628

Khosa JK, Leong SL, Borzi PA. Congenital cystic adenomatoid malformation of the lung: indications and timing of surgery. Pediatr Surg Int 2004;20(7):505–508

Kim YT, Kim JS, Park JD, Kang CH, Sung SW, Kim JH. Treatment of congenital cystic adenomatoid malformation-does resection in the early postnatal period increase surgical risk? Eur J Cardiothorac Surg 2005;27(4):658–661

King SJ, Pilling DW, Walkinshaw S. Fetal echogenic lung lesions: prenatal ultrasound diagnosis and outcome. Pediatr Radiol 1995;25(3):208–210

Laberge JM, Flageole H, Pugash D, Khalife S, Blair G, Filiatrault D, Russo P, Lees G, Wilson RD. Outcome of the prenatally diagnosed congenital cystic adenomatoid lung malformation: a Canadian experience. Fetal Diagn Ther 2001;16:178–186

Laberge JM, Pulingandla P, Flageole H. Asymptomatic congenital lung malformations. Semin Pediatr Surg 2005;14(1):16–33

Langston C. New concepts in the pathology of congenital lung malformations. Semin Pediatr Surg 2003;12(1):17–37

Langston C. Current concepts in the pathology of congenital lung malformations. Scientific Symposium (Congenital cystic lung lesions: from embryology to pathology), American Thoracic Society May 23, 2006

Lipshutz GS, Albanese CT, Feldstein VA, Jennings RW, Housley HT, Beech R, Farrell JA, Harrison MR. Prospective analysis of lung-to head ratio predicts survival for patients with prenatally diagnosed congenital diaphragmatic hernia. J Pediatr Surg 1997;32:1634–1636

Longaker MT, Laberge JM, Dansereau J, Langer JC, Crombleholme TM, Callen PW, Golbus MS, Harrison MR. Primary fetal hydrothorax: natural history and management. J Pediatr Surg 1989;24:573–576

Lopoo JB, Goldstein RB, Lipshutz GS, Goldberg JD, Harrison MR, Alabanese CT. Fetal pulmonary sequestration: a favourable congenital lung lesion. Obstet Gynecol 1999;94(4):567–571

Macaulay KE, Winters TC III, Shields LE. Neurenteric cyst shown by prenatal sonography. AJR Am J Roentgenol 1997;169:563–565

Mayden KL, Tortora M, Chervenak FA, Hobbins JC. The antenatal sonographic detection of lung masses. Am J Obstet Gynecol 1984;148:349–351

McCullagh M, MacConnachie I, Garvie D, Dykes E. Accuracy of prenatal diagnosis of congenital cystic adenomatoid malformation. Arch Dis Child 1994;71(2):F111–113

Meizner I, Rosenak D. The vanishing fetal intrathoracic mass: consider an obstructing mucous plug. Ultrasound Obstet Gynecol 1995;5(4):275–277

Miller JA, Corteville JE, Langer JC. Congenital cystic adenomatoid malformation in the fetus: natural history and predictors of outcome. J Pediatr Surg 1996;31(6):805–808

Miniati DN, Chintagumpala M, Langston C, Dishop MK, Olutoye OO, Nuchtern JG, Cass DL. Prenatal presentation and outcome of children with pleuropulmonary blastoma. J Pediatr Surg 2006;41(1):66–71

Murphy JJ, Blair GK, Fraser GC, Ashmore PG, LeBlanc JG, Sett SS, Rogers P, Magee JF, Taylor GP, Dimmick J. Rhabdomyosarcoma arising within congenital pulmonary cysts: report of three cases. J Pediatr Surg 1992;27:1364–1367

Mussat P, Dommergues M, Parat S, Mandelbrot L, De Gamarra E, Dumez Y, Moriette G. Congenital chylothorax with hydrops: postnatal care and outcome following antenatal diagnosis. Acta Paediatr 1995;84:749–755

Newman B. Congenital bronchopulmonary foregut malformations: concepts and controversies. Pediatr Radiol 2006;36(8):773–791

Nicolaides KH, Azar GB. Thoraco-amniotic shunting. Fetal Diagn Ther 1990;5:153–164

Olutoye OO, Coleman BG, Hubbard AM, Adzick NS. Prenatal diagnosis and management of congenital lobar emphysema. J Pediatr Surg 2000;35(5):792–795

Paek BW, Coakley FV, Lu Y, Filly RA, Lopoo JB, Qayyum A, Harrison MR, Albanese CT. Congenital diaphragmatic hernia: prenatal evaluation with MR lung volumetry–preliminary experience. Radiology 2001;220:63–67

Peralta CF, Cavoretto P, Csapo B, Falcon O, Nicolaides KH. Lung and heart volumes by three-dimensional ultrasound in normal fetuses at 12–32 weeks' gestation. Ultrasound Obstet Gynecol 2006;27(2):128–133

Pilling D. Fetal lung abnormalities–what do they mean? Clin Radiol 1998;53:789–795

Pumberger W, Hormann M, Deutinger J, Bernaschek G, Bistricky E, Horcher E. Longitudinal observation of antenatally detected congenital lung malformations (CLM): natural history, clinical outcome and long-term follow-up. Eur J Cardiothorac Surg 2003;24(5):703–711

Revillon Y, Jan D, Plattner V, Sonigo P, Dommergues M, Mandelbrot L, Dumez Y, Nihoul-Fekete C. Congenital cystic adenomatoid malformation of the lung: prenatal management and prognosis. J Pediatr Surg 1993;28(8):1009–1011

Ribet ME, Copin MC, Soots JG, Gosselin BH. Bronchioloalveolar carcinoma and congenital cystic adenomatoid malformation. Ann Thorac Surg 1995;60:1126–1128

Riedlinger WF, Vargas SO, Jennings RW, Estroff JA, Barnewolt CE, Lillehei CW, Wilson JM, Colin AA, Reid LM, Kozakewich HP. Bronchial atresia is common to extralobar sequestration, intralobar sequestration, congenital cystic adenomatoid malformation, and lobar emphysema. Pediatr Dev Pathol 2006;9(5):361–373

Roggin KK, Breuer CK, Carr SR, Hansen K, Kurkchubasche AG, Wesselhoeft CW Jr, Tracy TF Jr, Luks FI. The unpredictable character of congenital cystic lung lesions. J Pediatr Surg 2000;35(5):801–805

Ruano R, Benachi A, Aubry MC, Revillon Y, Emond S, Dumez Y, Dommergues M. Prenatal diagnosis of pulmonary sequestration using three-dimensional power Doppler ultrasound. Ultrasound Obstet Gynecol 2005;25(2):128–133

Rubenstein SC, Benacerraf BR, Retik AB, Mandell J. Fetal suprarenal masses: sonographic appearance and differential diagnosis. Ultrasound Obstet Gynecol 1995;5(3):164–167

Rypens F, Metens T, Rocourt N, Sonigo P, Brunelle F, Quere MP, Guibaud L, Maugey-Laulom B, Durand C, Avni FE, Eurin D. Fetal lung volume: estimation at MR imaging-initial results. Radiology 2001;219:236–241

Sapin E, Lejeune V, Barbet JP, Carricaburu E, Lewin F, Baron JM, Barbotin-Larrieu F, Helardot PG. Congenital adenomatoid disease of the lung: prenatal diagnosis and perinatal management. Pediatr Surg Int 1997;12(2–3):126–129

Sauvat F, Michel JL, Benachi A, Emond S, Revillon Y. Management of asymptomatic neonatal cystic adenomatoid malformations. J Pediatr Surg 2003;38(4):548–552

Semple MG, Bricker L, Shaw BN, Pilling DW. Left pulmonary artery sling presenting as unilateral echogenic lung on 20-week detailed antenatal ultrasound examination. Pediatr Radiol 2003;33(8):567–569

Shanmugam G, MacArthur K, Pollock JC. Congenital lung malformations–antenatal and postnatal evaluation and management. Eur J Cardiothorac Surg 2005;27:45–52

Stanton M, Davenport M. Management of congenital lung lesions. Early Human Development 2006;82(5):289–295

Stocker JT, Madewell JE, Drake RM. Congenital cystic adenomatoid malfromation of the lung. Classification and morphologic spectrum. Hum Pathol 1977;8:155–171

Stocker JT. Congenital pulmonary airway malformation (CPAM): a new name and an added classification of CCAM of lung. Histopathology 2002;41:424–431

Thorpe-Beeston JG, Nicolaides KH. Cystic adenomatoid malformation of the lung: prenatal diagnosis and outcome. Prenat Diagn 1994;14(8):677–688

Todros T, Gaglioti P, Presbitero P. Management of a fetus with intrapericardial teratoma diagnosed in utero. J Ultrasound Med 1991;10:287–290

Usui N, Kamata S, Sawai T, Kamiyama M, Okuyama H, Kubota A, Okada A. Outcome predictors for infants with cystic lung disease. J Ped Surg 2004;39(4):603–606

van Leeuwen K, Teitelbaum DH, Hirschl RB, Austin E, Adelman SH, Polley TZ, Marshall KW, Coran AG, Nugent C. Prenatal diagnosis of congenital cystic adenomatoid malformation and ist postnatal presentation, surgical indications, and natural history. J Pediatr Surg 1999;34(5):794–798

Vintzileos AM, Campbell WA, Rodis JF, Nochimson DJ, Pinette MG, Petrikovsky BM. Comparison of six different ultrasonographic methods for predicting lethal fetal pulmonary hypoplasia. Am J Obstet Gynecol 1989;161(3):606–612

Ward VL, Nishino M, Hatabu H, Estroff JA, Barnewolt CE, Feldman HA, Levine D. Fetal lung volume measurements. determination with MR imaging-effect of various factors. Radiology 2006;240(1):187–193

Waszak P, Claris O, Lapillonne A, Picaud JC, Basson E, Chappuis JP, Salle BL. Cystic adenomatoid malformation of the lung: neonatal management of 21 cases. Pediatr Surg Int 1999;15:326–331

Weber AM, Philipson EH. Fetal pleural effusion: a review and meta-analysis for prognostic indicators. Obstet Gynecol 1992;79:281–286

Winters WD, Effmann EL. Congenital masses of the lung: prenatal and postnatal imaging evaluation. J Thorac Imaging 2001;16(4):196–206

Yoshimura S, Masuzaki H, Gotoh H, Fukuda H, Ishimaru T. Ultrasonographic prediction of lethal pulmonary hypoplasia: comparison of eight different ultrasonographic parameters. Am J Obstet Gynecol 1996;175:477–483

Young G, L'Heureux PR, Krueckeberg ST, Swanson DA. Mediastinal bronchogenic cyst: prenatal sonographic diagnosis. AJR Am J Roentgenol 1989;152:125–127

Postnatal Imaging of Chest Malformations

STEPHANIE RYAN

CONTENTS

S. RYAN, FFR, RCSI
Radiology Department, Children's University Hospital,
Temple St., Dublin 1, Ireland and The Rotunda Hospital,
Parnell Square, Dublin 1, Ireland

9.1
Abnormalities of Oesophageal Development

9.1.1
Oesophageal Atresia and Tracheo-Oesophageal Fistula

Oesophageal atresia, with or without tracheoesophageal fistula, is the most common congenital malformation of the oesophagus. Oesophageal atresia and tracheoesophageal fistula represent a complex of congenital anomalies characterised by a failure of formation of the tubular oesophagus and/or an abnormal communication between the oesophagus and trachea. The precise cause is unknown, but it is thought to be due to a developmental disorder in formation and separation of the primitive foregut into trachea and oesophagus. Oesophageal atresia may be suspected if a nasogastric tube cannot be passed in a newborn infant with excessive oral secretions.

The chest radiograph may show the air-filled distended proximal oesophageal pouch or the feeding tube coiled in this pouch. Gas in the abdomen on the abdominal radiograph in such a baby indicates the presence of a tracheo-oesophageal fistula. A gasless abdomen is found in pure oesophageal atresia (Figs. 9.1 and 9.2). No further imaging is needed for diagnosis in these cases.

In pure oesophageal atresia prognosis depends on the distance between the oesophageal segments with short gaps with a distance of two vertebral bodies or shorter being associated with a good outcome. Bridging an oesophageal gap longer than three or more vertebral bodies is very difficult. Measuring the gap requires opacification of the proximal segment by contrast or tube and of the distal segment either by refluxed stomach contrast placed via gastrostomy or by passage of a radio-opaque bougie through the gastrostomy (Fig. 9.3). Serial measurements of this

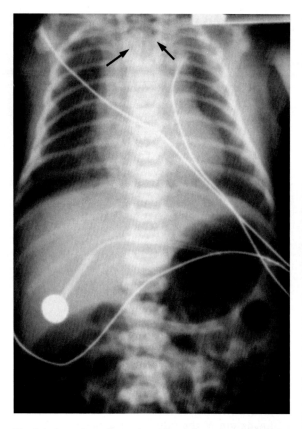

Fig. 9.1. Oesophageal atresia with tracheo-oesophageal fistula. Gas can be seen in the distended proximal oesophageal pouch (*arrows*). Gas in the stomach and intestines indicates the presence of a tracheo-oesophageal fistula

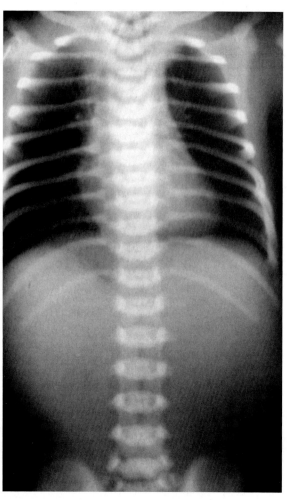

Fig. 9.2. Oesophageal atresia. A coiled feeding tube can be seen in the distended proximal oesophageal pouch. The gasless abdomen indicates the absence of a tracheo-oesophageal fistula

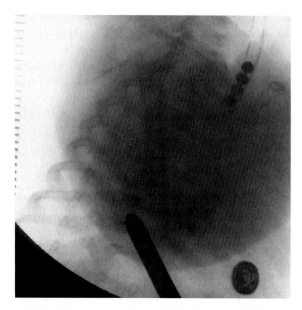

Fig. 9.3. Oesophageal atresia. Measuring the gap between the oesophageal segments. A feeding tube marks the proximal segment and a bougie passed through the gastrostomy marks the distal segment

gap over several weeks by some authors have demonstrated progressive narrowing of the gap. Such oesophageal growth may allow delayed oesophageal anastomosis in some babies in whom the gap at birth had been too long for primary anastomosis (Puri 1992).

Much less commonly, babies with oesophageal atresia have a fistula from both the proximal and distal oesophageal segments or from the proximal segment only (Fig. 9.4). A more important condition is the presence of a tracheo-oesophageal fistula with an intact oesophagus, occurring in 5% of tracheo-esophageal fistulae. This so-called H-type fistula is in fact N-shaped, passing from the oesophagus up to the trachea above the level of the carina, usually between C7 and T2 vertebral levels (Fig. 9.5a). Very

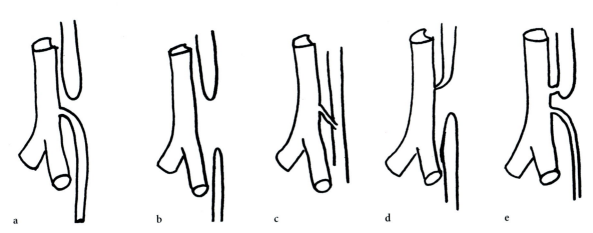

Fig. 9.4a–e. Diagram of oesophageal atresia (OA) and tracheo-oesophageal fistula (TOF) combinations. **a** OA and distal TOF, commonest combination. **b** OA without fistula. **c** TOF without atresia, so-called "H type" fistula, may present after several days or weeks. **d** OA with proximal TOF. **e** OA with proximal and distal TOFs

rarely this fistula may pass in a downward direction from the oesophagus to the trachea (Fig. 9.5b). Babies with this fistula usually become symptomatic in the neonatal period, though not the immediate newborn period. They present with coughing and respiratory distress during feeding.

Radiological demonstration of an H-type fistula can be very difficult. A contrast study should be done in the true lateral position with attention to the first swallows to exclude aspiration of contrast through the larynx. If the fistula cannot be shown on swallowing, a feeding tube should be passed and contrast injected during withdrawal through the oesophagus, especially at the expected site of the fistula above the carina (Fig. 9.5). Injecting in the prone position with lateral fluoroscopy is possible by placing the baby prone on the step of an upright fluoroscopy table (Fig. 9.6).

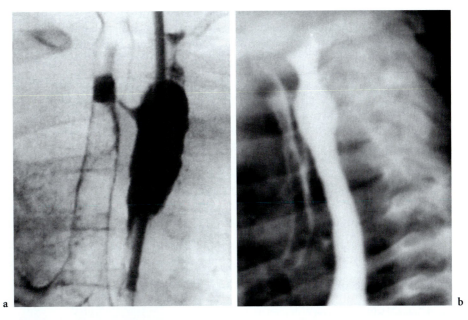

Fig. 9.5a,b. H-type tracheo-oesophageal fistula. **a** A 3-week-old baby with respiratory distress during feeding. Barium from the oesophagus can be seen passing up to the trachea through a fine fistula. **b** Another neonate with feeding difficulties. In this baby the fistula passes inferiorly from the oesophagus to the trachea – an unusual direction

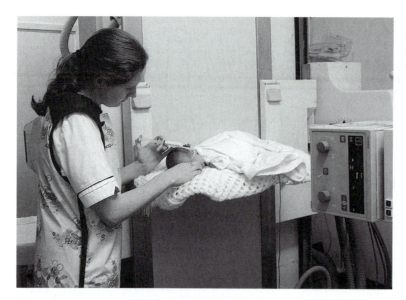

Fig. 9.6. To identify an H-type tracheo-oesophageal fistula – positioning baby on step of upright fluoroscopy table to allow lateral fluoroscopy while baby is prone

Laffan et al. have suggested that tube oesopha-gograms may not be necessary if no contrast passes into the trachea during swallowing (LAFFAN et al. 2006). They reported the detection of the fistula by contrast oesophagram alone in 80% of babies. Contrast was seen passing to the trachea in all of the remainder. Tube oesophagogram was used in only these 20%. Many authors have proposed the use of CT including 3D CT for the detection of fistulae (TAM 1987; ISLAM 2004). More recently, STURLA et al. have modified the CT technique by air distension of the oesophagus and with multiplanar and virtual endoscopic reconstructions (Fig. 9.7) (STURLA 2006). These techniques are not in widespread use however.

Oesophageal atresia and tracheo-oesophageal fistula may be part of the VACTER association. This describes an association of vertebral, anorectal, cardiac, tracheo-oesophageal, renal and radial ray limb abnormalities. These may be diagnosed by appropriate radiological investigations (BARNES 1987). OA and TOF may also be associated with other gastrointestinal atresias. An increased incidence of right-sided aortic arch with TOF is surgically important since such babies would have left rather than right thoracotomy for repair of the oesophagus.

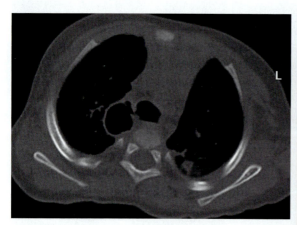

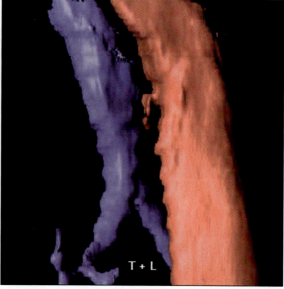

Fig. 9.7a,b. CT with distension of oesophagus with air allows visualisation of air filled tracheoooesopgageal fistula. **a** axial image. **b** 3D reconstruction, trachea blue. oesophagus and fistula pink (images courtesy Dr. M. Sturla, Buenos Aires, Argentina.)

9.1.2
Postoperative Imaging after Repair of Tracheo-Oesophageal Fistula

Imaging after repair of tracheo-oesophageal fistula is aimed at detection of complications such as anastomotic leak, anastomotic stricture and recurrent fistula. Before the baby is given any fluids orally, a contrast oesophagogram using water-soluble contrast should be done. This is usually about 10 days after surgery. The baby is placed in a true lateral position and given the contrast to drink from a bottle and teat. This allows assessment of sucking and swallowing function and possible aspiration as well as assessment of the anastomosis. If no stricture or leak is seen the findings can be confirmed by using barium. Recurrent fistula or the rare missed proximal fistula may be seen on this study or may present later.

There have been several case reports of a communicating bronchopulmonary foregut malformation (see Sect. 9.2.8) associated with type-three oesophageal atresia and tracheo-oesophageal fistula. Such a communication with the distal oesophagus can only be diagnosed on the postoperative imaging when the oesophagus is in continuity (JAMIESON and FISHER 1993).

9.2
Abnormalities of Lung Bud and Vascular Development

9.2.1
Agenesis and Aplasia of the Lung

Complete failure of development of one lung, usually the right lung, is a very uncommon abnormality. It has a high incidence of association with other congenital anomalies, especially congenital heart disease and the VATER association. Pulmonary aplasia is similar except that a blind ending rudimentary bronchus is present.

The radiograph shows a single lung displacing the heart and mediastinum towards the side of the absent lung. The hemi-thorax on the agenetic side is smaller. Confirmation of absence of one lung is not usually necessary, but could be done by CT with assessment of the pulmonary vessels by CT angiography.

9.2.2
Pulmonary Hypoplasia

Pulmonary hypoplasia results in a decrease in volume of one lung or part of one lung, usually the right lung (Fig. 9.8), associated with a small or absent pulmonary artery and a shift of the mediastinum to the affected side (see Fig. 9.7). This may be an incidental finding and does not usually present in the neonatal period (SWISHCHUK 1979; CURRARINO 1985; PORTER 1999).

The radiograph shows that the affected lung is smaller with a smaller hilum and that the other lung is expanded. On the lateral radiograph a band of density anteriorly is thought to be due to extrapleural areolar connective tissue on the hypoplastic side. This may however be no more than the displaced mediastinum anterior to the hypoplastic lung. Fluoroscopy on inspiration and expiration excludes air trapping by showing no paradoxical movement of the diaphragm or mediastinum. Expiratory CT may show patchy air trapping in the bigger lung. CT angiography will identify those babies with absent pulmonary artery, but is not always necessary. Pulmonary hypoplasia may be associated with an accessory diaphragm (see Sect. 9.3.4).

Secondary pulmonary hypoplasia is an important feature of congenital diaphragmatic hernia (see Sect. 9.3) and of oligohydramnios, such as in the Potter sequence. Bilateral pulmonary hypoplasia may also be secondary to chest wall abnormality such as skeletal dysplasias with short ribs (see Chap. 18) or to neuromuscular disorders that result in reduced respiratory motion. Lung size as seen on antenatal ultrasound and on postnatal chest radiographs is used as an indicator of prognosis in these conditions. Persistent pulmonary hypertension may occur secondary to primary or secondary pulmonary hypoplasia. The prognosis is poorer when this is a feature.

In pulmonary hypoplasia a reduction in the number, size and branching of the pulmonary arteries and veins compared to normal may be appreciated on CT (CURRARINO 1985). In some babies, however, the pulmonary hypoplasia is secondary to an abnormality of the pulmonary vessels rather than vice versa. Pulmonary hypoplasia may therefore be a feature of

- Alveolar capillary dysplasia
- Absent pulmonary artery
- Absent pulmonary vein
- Pulmonary artery sling
- Scimitar or venolobar syndrome

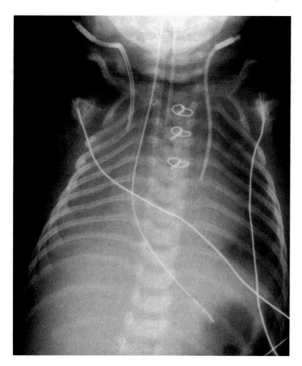

Fig. 9.8. Hypoplasia of right lung. Note the sternotomy due to related congenital heart disease. Note also the position of the left jugular venous line which indicates the presence of a left-sided superior vena cava

9.2.2.1
Alveolar Capillary Dysplasia

This is a congenital abnormality of the terminal airspaces and the pulmonary capillary formation. The chest radiographs show bilateral pulmonary hypoplasia. Clinically there is persistent pulmonary hypertension with a curiously variable period of hours, days or even weeks after birth before symptoms begin (NEWMAN 1990). There is no treatment for this condition and the prognosis is very poor.

9.2.2.2
Absent Pulmonary Artery

When one pulmonary artery is absent this is usually the right, in which case the main pulmonary artery continues directly into the left hilum supplying only one lung. On the chest radiograph the affected lung is small with a small hilum. There may be rib notching visible because of collateral systemic supply to the affected lung. CT or MRI will demonstrate the abnormality of the main pulmonary arteries and usually also shows a small hilar pulmonary artery

on the affected side (usually the right) which has been reconstituted by collaterals. This finding is very important since it raises the surgical possibility of graft insertion between the main pulmonary artery and this hilar vessel to improve blood flow to the affected lung (ELLIS 1991).

9.2.2.3
Absent Pulmonary Vein

Pulmonary vein atresia is usually unilateral or affects the upper or lower pulmonary vein on one side. Chest radiograph shows a small lung with a small hilum. There may be a unilateral reticular pattern in the affected lung. The cause of this is unknown, but it may represent dilated lymphatics in the lung with the compromised venous return. The absence of the vein or a small vein may be detectable by CT. There is no treatment for this condition. Because of this and because of the high incidence of associated congenital heart disease (50%), the prognosis is poor (SWISCHUK 1980).

9.2.2.4
Pulmonary Artery Sling

The left pulmonary artery may arise from the posterior aspect of the right pulmonary artery and reach the left hilum by passing between the trachea and oesophagus. The aberrant vessel may compress the distal or the right main bronchus. Compression of the right main bronchus may result in right lung hypoplasia or in right lung hyperaeration which are detectable on radiographs. The abberant left pulmonary artery may be visible on lateral chest radiograph or more likely on an oesophagogram between the trachea and the oesophagus, with or without compression of these. CT or MR may be used to show the aberrant left pulmonary artery directly (Fig. 9.9).

9.2.2.5
Pulmonary Venolobar Syndrome
(Scimitar Syndrome)

Pulmonary hypoplasia associated with anomalous pulmonary venous return of all or part of the right lung is called pulmonary venolobar syndrome. The anomalous pulmonary vein may drain to the right atrium, the coronary sinus, the inferior vena cava, the hepatic or portal veins. The anomalous vein as it passes inferiorly may be visible on the radiograph as a crescent-shaped density, the wider part inferiorly, parallel to the right heart border (Fig. 9.10). The appearance of this vein has been likened to a Turkish sword, a scimitar, giving the condition the name scimitar syndrome (FOLGER 1976). The small right lung may be bilobar with a left lung type bronchial branching pattern. This may present in the neonatal period especially if associated with congenital heart disease such as Fallot's tertralogy or truncus arteriosus. There is an associated atrial septal defect in 25% of these babies and there is also an increased incidence of vertebral and rib abnormalities. There may be an associated absence of the right pulmonary artery, systemic arterial supply of the right lung, with or without sequestration, absence of IVC or accessory hemidiaphragm (CURRARINO 1985; KONEN 2003). Systemic arterial supply of the affected lung causes a left to right shunt which may worsen the clinical picture. Conventional angiography and more recently magnetic resonance angiography will demonstrate the anomalous vein and its drainage (KIVELITZ 1999).

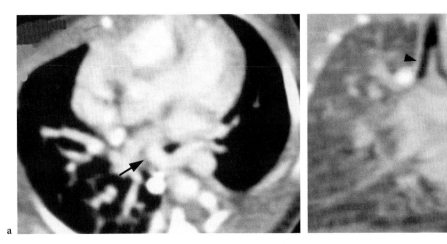

Fig. 9.9a,b. Pulmonary sling. A 10-day-old baby with respiratory distress. **a** Axial CT with contrast shows left pulmonary artery (*arrow*) arising from the posterior aspect of the right pulmonary artery and reaching the left hilum by passing posterior to the trachea which is narrowed. **b** Cor CT reconstruction shows a relatively large bronchus to the right upper lobe arising from the trachea (*arrowhead*). The remainder of the trachea (*arrow*) and the right and left main bronchi are very narrow

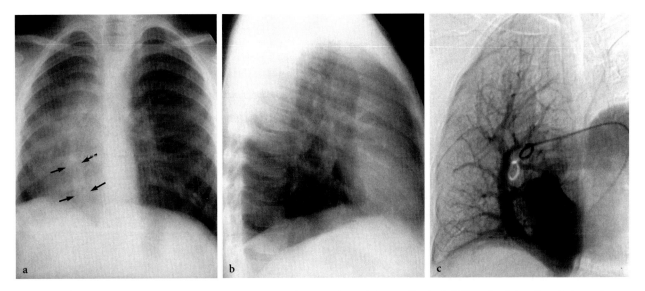

Fig. 9.10a–c. Venolobar syndrome. **a** The right lung is hypoplastic with resulting mediastinal shift to the right. The scimitar vein can be seen passing inferiorly (*arrows*). **b** Lateral view shows density anteriorly (see text). **c** Angiogram (venous phase of a pulmonary angiogram) in another patient shows the scimitar vein draining the right lung to the inferior vena cava

9.2.3
Horseshoe Lung

This is usually associated with hypoplasia and anomalous venous return of the right lung and is probably a variant of the venolobar syndrome. An isthmus of the right lung inferiorly passes between the oesophagus and the heart and abuts or is fused to the lower left lung. Lung tissue behind the heart may be visible on the lateral radiograph (FRANK 1986). CT to demonstrate continuity of the pulmonary parenchyma and vasculature behind the heart is diagnostic.

9.2.4
Congenital Lobar Emphysema (CLE)

Air-filled distension of one lobe of the lung, congenital lobar emphysema, may cause respiratory distress in the neonatal period. This is three times commoner in boys than girls. Congenital lobar emphysema most commonly affects the left upper lobe (50%). The next commonest sites are the right middle (30%) and right upper lobes (20%) in that order. Lower lobe involvement is rare (<1%). There is an associated ventricular septal defect or patent ductus arteriosus in 15% of patients. The aetiology of this condition is unclear, but it probably results from an abnormality of the lobar bronchus which may have an obstructive cartilage abnormality. Since the alveoli are overdistended but the alveolar walls are preserved, this condition might be more correctly referred to as congenital lobar hyperinflation rather than emphysema. Lobar emphysema may also be caused by compression of the left upper lobe bronchus by a persistent patent ductus arteriosus, by an aberrant left pulmonary artery or by hugely dilated pulmonary arteries such as in tetralogy of Fallot with absent pulmonary valves. This secondary lobar emphysema typically is less severe and with less compression of the lower lobe than in idiopathic congenital lobar emphysema.

Since the air gets into the affected lobes by diffusion more slowly than air fills the remainder of the lungs, the radiograph immediately after birth may show opacification of the affected lobe and also often the adjacent compressed but otherwise normal lobes (Table 9.1). Once air filled, the affected lobe is seen to be hyperexpanded. The most typical appearance is of an expanded, hyperlucent left upper lobe with a compressed, dense left lower lobe and the mediastinum displaced to the right (Fig. 9.11). CT may be useful to determine which lobe is involved (Fig. 9.12). Treatment involves resection of the affected lobe in all symptomatic cases (KARNAK 1999).

Table 9.1. Opaque hemithorax with mediastinal shift in a newborn: differential diagnosis

Congenital diaphragmatic hernia
Congenital lobar emphysema
Cystic adenomatoid malformation
Pleural fluid, usually chylothorax

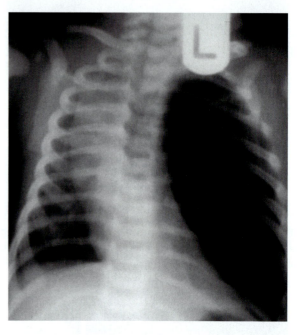

Fig. 9.11. Congenital lobar emphysema expanding the left upper lobe and compressing the left lower lobe

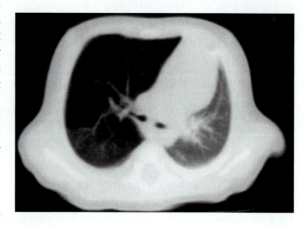

Fig. 9.12. CT showing congenital lobar emphysema of right middle lobe

9.2.5
Bronchial Atresia

Bronchial atresia may be considered a variant of lobar emphysema. Though congenital, this condition seldom presents in the neonatal period (Schuster 1987). Congenital focal obliteration of a proximal segmental or subsegmental bronchus is associated with normal development of the distal structures of the lung. One bronchus is affected, typically in the apical posterior segment of the left upper lobe. The lung distal to the atresia is hyperinflated by collateral air drift. The bronchus distal to the atresia is filled with mucous or debris and is visible on a chest radiograph as an oval density surrounded by hyperlucent lung. These features can be seen on the radiograph, but are more clearly seen on CT (Ward 1999; Winters 2001).

9.2.6
Congenital Cystic Adenomatoid Malformation (CCAM)

Hamartomatous development of the terminal respiratory structures may result in a multicystic mass, a congenital cystic adenomatoid malformation. The cysts may communicate with each other, but seldom with the airway. Seventy percent present as a symptomatic mass with respiratory distress in the neonatal period. Increasingly these are being diagnosed antenatally resulting in an increasing proportion of smaller asymptomatic masses being diagnosed shortly after birth (Marshall 2000).

The commonest form, type I CCAM, has multiple air-filled cysts more than 2 cm in diameter. In the less common type II, the cysts are smaller and there may be solid components. A completely solid form, type III, is rare. Types II and III carry a poorer prognosis because of increased incidence of associated severe congenital abnormalities including bilateral renal agenesis. The use of the term congenital pulmonary airway malformation (CPAM) has been proposed as preferable to CCAM since not all are cystic and only type III is adenomatoid (Newman 2006). This term has not yet achieved widespread use however. Types II and III have pathological lung findings similar to those of other cases of in utero airway obstruction. This supports the hypothesis of a common pathological mechanism of airway obstruction during development in this and other congenital lung abnormalities (Langston 2003).

The radiograph after birth usually shows a dense mass which, if large and extending to the diaphragm, may be difficult to distinguish from a congenital diaphragmatic hernia, a lobar emphysema or a pleural effusion (Table 9.1). A radiograph a few hours later usually shows air-filled cysts (Fig. 9.13). Differentiation from a hernia is easy if there is normal lung between the CCAM and the diaphragm. If not, including the abdomen in the film may help by showing the presence or absence of a normal amount of bowel loops in the abdomen. CT has a role in defining the extent of the lesion and which lobes are involved (Fig. 9.14).

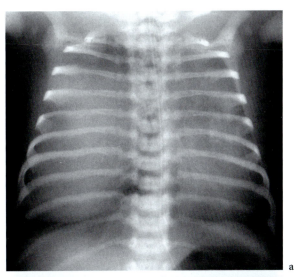

a

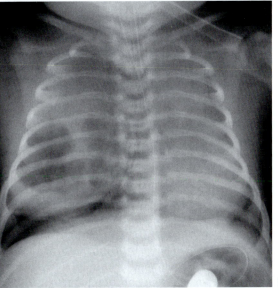

b

Fig. 9.13a,b. Cystic adenomatoid malformation. **a** Chest radiograph immediately after birth shows fluid-filled mass in the right lung. **b** Two hours later air has filled some of the cysts within the mass

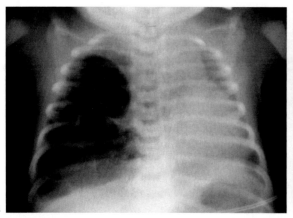
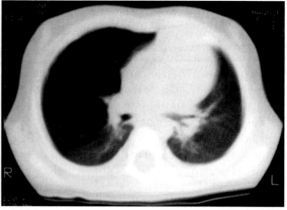

Fig. 9.14a,b. Cystic adenomatoid malformation. **a** Multiple cysts expand part of the right middle lobe. **b** CT same baby shows mass with multiple air-filled cysts

Pulmonary sequestrations (see Sect. 9.2.7) may be associated with areas of cystic adenomatoid malformation and both conditions are probably in a spectrum of related lung abnormalities (Cass 1997; Samuel 1999) (Figs. 9.15, 9.16 and Sect. 9.2.11 Hybrid lesions). CT with CT angiography is recommended therefore in the evaluation of CCAM because of the possibility of systemic arterial supply which is very important information to the surgeon if resection is planned.

There are several reports of foetal cystic lung masses resolving spontaneously or reducing in size on antenatal scanning. Winter et al. (1999) report seven such babies who had a normal or near normal radiograph after birth. CT scan showed an abnormality however in each case. All were CCAM with features of intralobar sequestration in four of these. Van Leeuwan and co-workers reported 8 of 14 CCAMS had normal CXR (Van Leeuwan 1999). It is therefore important to do a CT scan shortly after birth in all babies in whom an antenatal diagnosis of lung mass was made even if this appeared to resolve on serial antenatal scans or if the postnatal chest radiograph appears normal.

Management of symptomatic CCAM is surgical excision. The decision and timing of an excision in an asymptomatic patient remains controversial (Van Leeuwan 1999). The risk of infection, malignant transformation, pneumothorax and haemorrhage has been reported as justification for removal of all lesions including small asymptomatic involuting lesions (Fig. 9.16) (Aziz 2004). Aziz reported 10% incidence of infection in 35 asymptomatic CCAMs on conservative management.

The premalignant potential of CCAMs is not clearly known. There have been several reports of malignancy coexisting with CCAM or bronchial cysts (Cohen 1991; Murphy 1992; D'Agostino 1997; Granata 1998). In a review of pathological findings in 28 CCAMS, Mac Sweeney et al. found five with foci of bronshioloalveolar carcinoma while another with focal stromal hypercellularity went on to develop pleuropulmonary blastoma (Mac Sweeney et al. 2003). Several studies report successful conservative management of CCAM without malignancy, but none of these are randomised, prospective, big enough or have adequate follow-up to completely eliminate the concept of malignant transformation of these lesions (Van Leeuwan 1999; Roggin 2000; Aziz 2004). Two reports of three children describe the development of pleuropulmonary blastoma within an area of lung where there had been previous resection of cystic lung abnormality suggesting that even surgical excision does not protect from malignant transformation (Papagiannopoulos 2001; Hasiotou 2004).

Some cases previously described as malignant transformation of CCAM may have been cystic pleuropulmonary blastoma (PPB) which can be indistinguishable from CCAM radiologically. This is a dysontogenetic neoplasm that may be pulmonary or pleural based (Priest 1997). Many previously described mesenchymal scarcomas or rhabdomyosarcomas are probably forms of PPB. Pneumothorax at presentation is commoner in PPB than in CCAM. The difficulty differentiating PPB from CCAM may of itself however be a case for resection of congenital cystic lung masses.

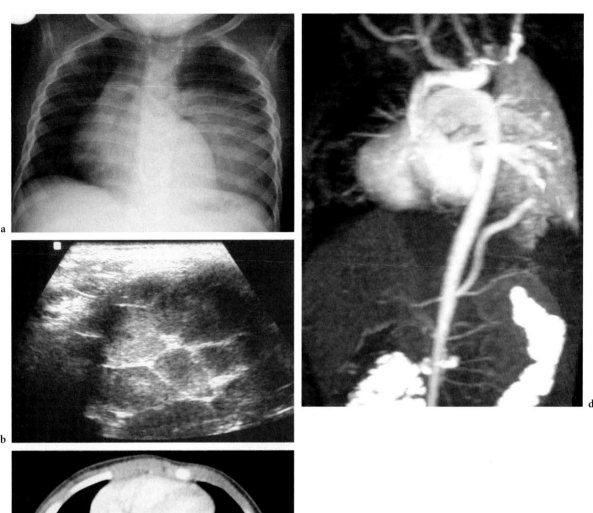

Fig. 9.15a–d. Cystic adenomatoid malformation with sequestration. **a** Chest radiograph shows large lung mass that persisted despite 8 days of antibiotic treatment. **b** Ultrasound of the lesion shows that it is a multilocular cystic mass. **c** CT with contrast confirms multilocular cystic mass. Large vessel anterior to mass here (*arrow*) and on lower cuts was seen to pass through mass and towards abdominal aorta. **d** MR angiogram confirms large vessel arising from the abdominal aorta supplying the mass. Pathological examination of the excised specimen confirmed intralobar sequestration with features of cystic adenomatoid malformation

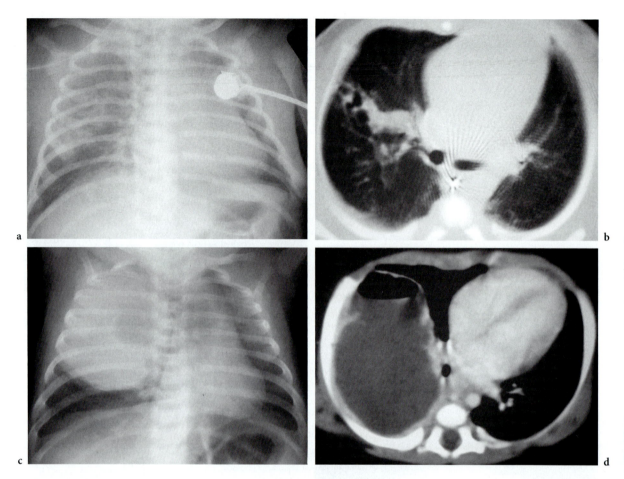

Fig. 9.16a–d. Cystic adenomatoid malformation complicated by infection. Antenatal diagnosis of lung abnormality. **a** Chest radiograph shows poorly defined right lung mass. **b** CT day 2 shows cystic adenomatoid malformation. **c** At 6 weeks of age she represented with sepsis. Chest radiograph shows large right lung mass with single air bubble. **d** CT with contrast shows a large fluid-filled cyst right lung with air fluid level. This was drained and found to be pus

9.2.7
Sequestration

Pulmonary sequestration is a mass of pulmonary tissue that is supplied by systemic arteries rather than pulmonary arteries. The systemic arterial supply is usually from the thoracic aorta, often by a large vessel. Supply may be from the abdominal aorta and pass through the diaphragm. Awareness of this vessel is of value prior to thoracotomy since extreme care must be taken to control such a vessel lest it retract bleeding into the abdomen, out of the operative field. Sequestrations may also receive their blood supply from other systemic arteries including the intercostal, subclavian or coronary arteries or from the coeliac or splenic arteries (ITO 2003; SILVERMAN 1994; GRIGORYANTS 2000; CURROS 2000). There may even be dual sup-

ply – a feature very important to the surgeon for resection or to the interventional radiologist for embolisation.

Venous drainage may be to the pulmonary or systemic veins or there may be drainage to both systems. Most sequestrations are not connected to the bronchial tree, but sources differ as to whether sequestrated lung can ever be connected to the bronchial system.

Extralobar sequestrations drain primarily to the systemic veins such as the azygous system and have a separate pleural covering. Though less common than the intralobar form, extralobar sequestration is more likely to present in the neonatal period. Ninety percent are found in the left lower lobe adjacent to the diaphragm. There is 50% incidence of associated congenital abnormalities, especially diaphragmatic hernias.

Intralobar sequestrations usually (95%) drain to the pulmonary veins and do not have a separate pleural covering. These are commoner than extralobar sequestrations by three to one, but more than 50% remain asymptomatic throughout childhood. They may present later in childhood with a history of recurrent respiratory tract infections. They have a lower incidence of associated congenital abnormalities, about 6%. Some authors believe that all intralobar sequestrations are acquired and result from obstruction of bronchi by infection or other causes leading to reduction in pulmonary blood flow and parasitisation of bronchial systemic arteries (STOCKER 1986; GEBAUER and MASON 1959) or, more likely, of normally occurring branches of the thoracic aorta that supply the oesophagus and pass through the pulmonary ligament to the visceral pleura of the lower lobes (STOCKER 1984). Chronic inflammatory change, abscess and multicystic change can be seen in resected sequestrations and are felt by some to be primary rather than secondary findings (FRAZIER 1997). However several reports of antenatal ultrasound diagnosis and of neonatal diagnosis of intralobar sequestrations confirm that many of these are in fact congenital (LAURIN 1999). Some suggest that the location and type of sequestration reflect the timing of outpouching of an accessory lung bud. If this outpouching develops early it will be closer to the normal lung bud and be intralobar. A later outpouching will result in an extralobar sequestration. Others suggest that sequestration is a form of bronchial atresia. An atretic or obstructed bronchus may be identifiable pathologically (see Fig. 9.15) and the pathological appearances of the lung in a sequestration are similar to those of the lung distal to an atresia (LANGSTON 2003). Reports of intralobar sequestration secondary to carcinoid tumour or foreign body obstructing a bronchus would support the latter theory (EUSTACE 1996; SCULLY 1983). I have seen a baby with an in utero diagnosis of a lung abnormality who had an intralobar sequestration that appears to be secondary to an in utero pulmonary artery thrombosis (personal communication). These findings support the theory of a common origin of sequestration and other bronchopulmonary foregut malformation as parts of an obstructive malformation complex (NEWMAN 2006) (see Sect. 9.2.10 Hybrid lesions).

Sequestrations are visible on radiographs as masses, usually dense, in the lower lobes, especially the medial basal segment of the left lower lobe. Two thirds are on the left side. One-third occur on the right side. If they present with clinical respiratory infection, the density persists after the infection

resolves. Identification of the diagnostic systemic arterial supply may be by ultrasound, CT angiography, MR angiography or conventional angiography (Figs. 9.16–9.18) (KOUCHI 2000). Many are picked up during evaluation of congenital heart disease. Fifteen percent of extralobar sequestrations are intrabdominal, usually above the left kidney. Sequestrations in the neck, mediastinum and pericardium have been described (NEWMAN 2006).

Up to 50% of sequestrations may be associated with areas of cystic adenomatoid malformation and both conditions are probably in a spectrum of related lung abnormalities (CASS 1997; SAMUEL 1999). In a review of 39 patients with pulmonary sequestration, BRATU et al. (2001) found 17 were atypical or associated with other pulmonary lesions such as cystic adenomatoid malformation, bronchogenic cysts, bronchopulmonary foregut malformation or scimitar syndrome (see Sect. 9.2.10 Hybrid lesions).

Management of the symptomatic baby with sequestration is by resection. Successful management of pulmonary sequestration in babies by endovascular embolisation has been described (CURROS 2000).

As with cystic adenomatoid malformation, an increasing number of pulmonary sequestrations are being diagnosed antenatally leading to a diagnosis of this condition in asymptomatic neonates. The optimal management of the asymptomatic sequestration is not known. Serial antenatal and postnatal imaging may show gradual shrinkage of these lesions and support non-surgical management (GARCIA-PENA 1998). Some promote resection or embolisation in the asymptomatic baby to prevent possible complications including the risk of infection and the rare but documented risk of cardiac failure secondary to a left to right shunt. Lobar emphysema, haemoptysis, pleural effusion and haemothorax have been also described as complications of sequestration. Coexistence of sequestration and CCAM has been reported to be unlikely to involute and to be an indication for surgical resection (SAMUEL 1999). Successful management of pulmonary sequestration in babies with endovascular embolisation has been described (CURROS 2000).

An area of normal lung may have a systemic blood supply. This rare condition is probably in the spectrum of sequestration. This may present as an incidental finding on a radiograph or as a left to right shunt. The affected area of lung has an increased amount of blood supply, but is otherwise normal on CXR or CT.

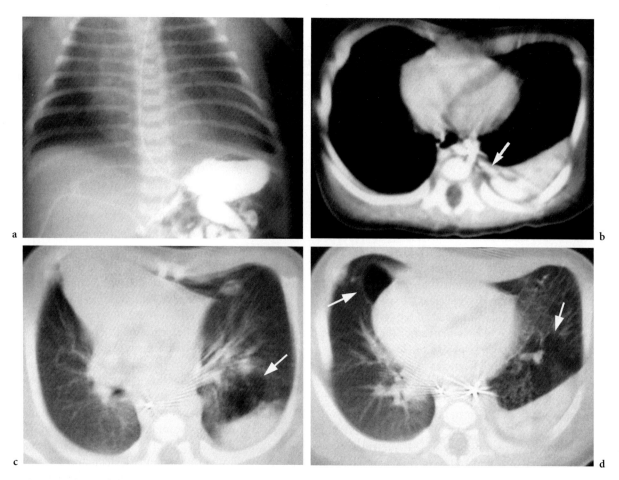

Fig. 9.17a–d. Extralobar sequestration. **a** Chest radiograph 2 h after birth shows a very poorly defined density in the left lower lobe. This was not visible on an earlier less rotated view. **b** CT scan with contrast shows the sequestration and its aortic arterial supply (*arrow*). The contrast was injected through an umbilical arterial line with its tip in the thoracic aorta. This line causes some streak artefact. **c,d** Lung windows reveal areas of air-filled cysts (*arrows*) consistent with cystic adenomatoid malformation anterior to sequestration and in right middle lobe. Both were confirmed at surgery

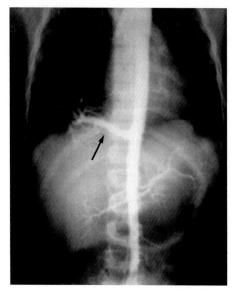

Fig. 9.18. Pulmonary sequestration. An aortic angiogram demonstrates a large vessel feeding a sequestration in the right lower lobe. A large dense mass was visible here on chest radiograph. (Images courtesy of Godfrey Gaisie MD, Children's Hospital, Akron, OH)

9.2.9
Oesophageal Bronchi

A segment of lung may be connected to the oe-sophagus or the fundus of the stomach. Such lung usually has a systemic blood supply and represents a form of sequestration (LEITHISER 1986). Rarely a lobe or an entire lung, usually the right lung, which is otherwise anatomically normal, is sup-plied by an oesophageal bronchus. This usually presents in the neonatal period with a relatively dense lung. The radiograph shows a density in the lungs, usually in the left lower lobe which may have tubular or cyst-like lucencies within it. Air-filled bronchi within the density as seen on CT should alert one to do a contrast oesophagogram to demonstrate the oesophageal or stomach com-munication (Fig. 9.19).

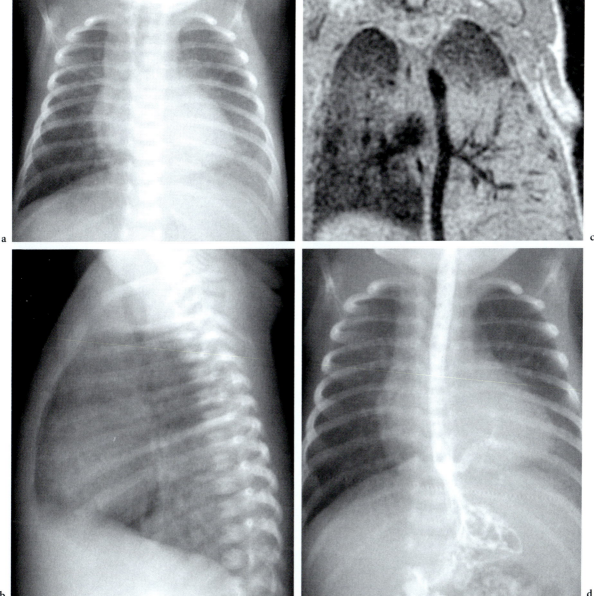

Fig. 9.19a–d. Oesophageal bronchus to a pulmonary sequestration. Newborn with an antenatal diagnosis of lung abnormal-ity. **a** AP and (**b**) lateral chest radiographs show density in left posterior basal aspect of the left lung. **c** MRI shows supply to the segment by a large branch of the thoracic aorta. **d** Contrast oesophagogram shows an oesophageal bronchus within the lesion. (Images courtesy of Godfrey Gaisie MD, Children's Hospital, Akron, OH)

9.2.10
Bronchogenic Cysts

These cysts are thought to be due to abnormal bronchial budding during lung development. If they occur early in lung development, the cyst will be mediastinal, often carinal, and those that occur later in development will be intraparenchymal.

The cysts are round or oval, lined by bronchial mucosa with or without cartilage in their walls. Many are incidental findings and are not commonly detected in the neonatal period. Table 9.2 lists the differential diagnosis of cystic mediastinal masses.

Chest radiographs show a dense round mass, either subcarinal, elsewhere in the mediastinum or in the pulmonary parenchyma. CT or MRI shows the characteristic fluid centre (McAdams 2000). Mediastinal lesions may also be shown to be cystic by oesophageal or conventional echocardiography (Fig. 9.20). Bronchogenic cysts are sometimes associated with sequestration, lobar emphysema or bronchial atresia (see Sect. 9.2.10 Hybrid lesions)

Table 9.2. Mediastinal cysts

Bronchogenic cyst
Neuroenteric cyst
Oesophageal duplication cyst

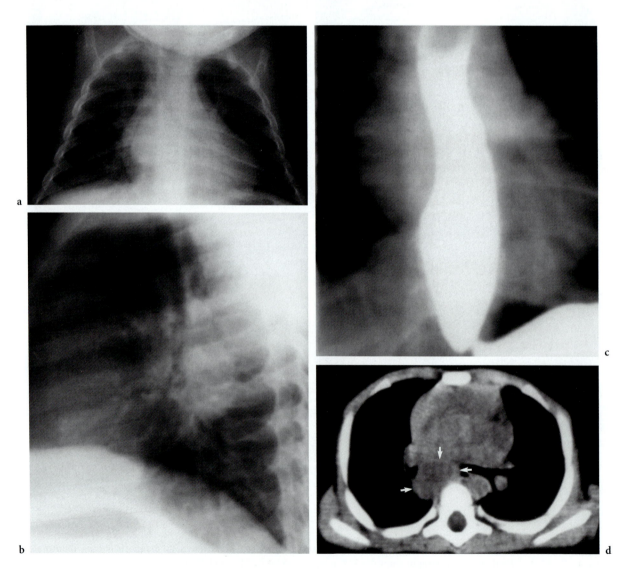

Fig. 9.20a–d. Bronchogenic cyst. **a** AP and (**b**) lateral chest radiograph shows subcarinal mass. **c** Oesophagogram shows extrinsic mass deviating mid oesophagus. **d** CT confirms that the mass (*arrows*) is cystic

9.2.11
Hybrid lesions–Bronchopulmonary Foregut Malformation

The term bronchopulmonary foregut malformation used to have a narrow definition of a lung abnormality associated with an oesophageal bronchus. Now the term is used to include a variety of lung abnormalities that may occur singly, or in any combination in any given patient, including CCAM, sequestration, bronchogenic cyst, bronchial atresia and congenital lobar emphysema (Figs. 9.15, 9.16 and 9.18). The conditions of tracheal atresia, pulmonary agenesis, scimitar syndrome, oesophageal cysts, neuroenteric cysts and even oesophageal atresia and tracheo-oesphageal fistula are probably also related conditions that should be included within this umbrella group. Langston and Newman and others have suggested that many, if not all of these conditions have a common aetiology of bronchial obstruction leading to secondary pulmonary dysplasia (Langston 2003; Newman 2006).

Some of the conditions with small lungs or lung segments may have a vascular aetiology (see Sect. 9.2.2). These conditions, especially extralobar sequestration, have a strong association with congenital heart disease. The conditions, especially oesophageal atresia and tracheo-oesophaeal atresia, have an association with renal, anorectal, rib, radial ray limb abnormalities and vertebral abnormalities in the VACTERL association.

9.2.12
Neuroenteric Cysts

Neuroenteric cysts result from failure of separation of the lung bud from the notochord. A posterior mediastinal cystic lesion associated with vertebral abnormalities strongly suggests this diagnosis (Fig. 9.21). This cyst may communicate with the oesophagus or spinal canal.

9.2.13
Pulmonary Vascular Malformation

Pulmonary arteriovenous malformations may be single or multiple, but are unusual in the neonatal period. Most patients (60%) with pulmonary arteriovenous malformations have Osler Weber Rendu syndrome. Children may present with cyanosis, dyspnoea, clubbing, haemoptysis or be asymptomatic. CXR shows single or multiple round pulmonary densities. Large feeding vessels or draining veins may be visible on CXR. CT and CT angiography or MR angiography confirms the vascular nature of the lesions which may be amenable to embolisation.

9.2.14
Chylothorax

Congenital pleural effusions other than those associated with cardiac disease or hydrops are most likely to be due to chylothorax. Aspirated fluid will have a high lymphocyte count, but will not have a milky appearance until after the baby has had a feed containing fat. The cause of the chylothorax is unknown. Birth trauma to the thoracic duct is unlikely since the effusion may be seen antenatally by ultrasound. Late maturation of the thoracic duct has been proposed and may explain the resolution of the effusion after several aspirations and recurrences.

The initial radiograph will show the effusion (Fig. 9.22). If large enough to opacify the hemithorax the radiographic appearance may be indistinguishable from large diaphragmatic hernia, cystic adenomatoid malformation or congenital lobar emphysema (Table 9.1). Once aspirated the effusion may recur, but typically resolves after a few aspirations.

9.2.15
Abnormalities in Situs

Abnormalities of visceral and atrial situs are associated with abnormalities of the branching pattern of the bronchi. In asplenia syndrome the lungs are bilaterally trilobed and both have eparterial bronchi (i.e., the bronchi are above the pulmonary arteries at the hilum). In polysplenia, the lungs are bilaterally bilobed with bilateral hyparterial bronchi (i.e., the bronchi are below the pulmonary arteries at the hilum).

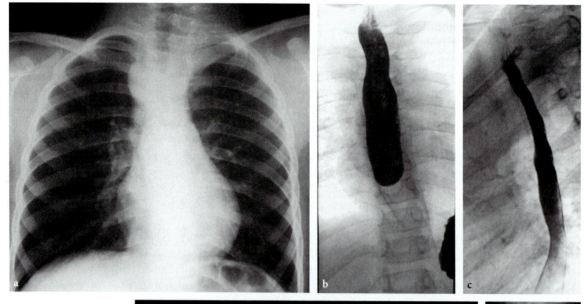

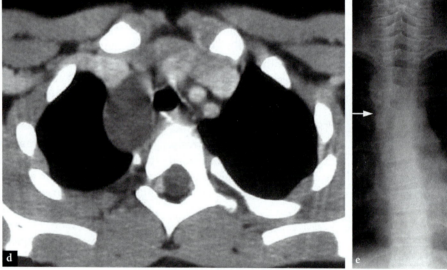

Fig. 9.21a–e. Neuroenteric cyst. **a** Chest radiograph shows a right upper mediastinal mass originally thought to be a right-sided aortic arch. **b** AP oesophagogram shows right indentation of oesophagus but (**c**) lateral shows no evidence of abnormal vessel. **d** CT shows that the mass is cystic. **e** Thoracic spine radiograph shows associated right hemibutterfly vertebra (*arrow*) at level below cyst

9.3
Abnormalities of the Diaphragm

9.3.1
Congenital Diaphragmatic Hernia: Bochdalek Type

A defect in the diaphragm in the fetus called the pleuroperitoneal canal allows abdominal contents including bowel into the thorax. The closure of the pleuroperitoneal canal of the foetus occurs close to the time of return of the bowel into the abdomen. If closure is delayed or if the bowel returns before closure is complete a defect will result. The presence of bowel loops in the thorax causes hypoplasia of the ipsilateral lung. The prognosis for the baby depends on the degree of hypoplasia of one or both lungs, which in turn depends on the volume of abdominal contents in the thorax and for how long it has been there. The diagnosis may be made antenatally and the baby usually presents with early and severe respiratory distress. The hernia is on the left side in 90% of cases.

The radiograph initially shows an opaque mass on the left side. There is little or no aeration of the ipsilateral lung. The mediastinum is displaced to the contralateral side (Fig. 9.23). The initial radiograph may thus be similar to that of a baby with a large cystic adenomatoid malformation, a congenital lobar emphysema or a large amount of pleural fluid (see Table 9.1). Over the following hours, air passes into the gastrointestinal tract giving the characteristic appearance of air-filled bowel loops in the thorax. It is helpful to include the abdomen on this second radiograph because absence of bowel gas in the abdomen helps to distinguish a congenital diaphragmatic hernia from a large cystic adenomatoid malformation (Fig. 9.23b). A nasogastric tube passing into the thorax also confirms the diagnosis. The use of barium to confirm that gastrointestinal contents are in the thorax is seldom necessary.

Prognosis depends on the degree of hypoplasia of the lungs. This in turn depends principally, but not solely on the size of the herniated contents (Fig. 9.24). Donnelly et al. (1999) addressed the value of the initial radiograph in predicting survival in babies with congenital diaphragmatic hernia. When the radiograph was scored for factors including the percentage of aerated ipsilateral and contralateral lung,

mediastinal shift and hernia contents, poor prognosis was related to a higher score. A worse prognosis has also been related to the presence of the stomach in the thorax since this indicates that the diaphragmatic defect is big.

Right-sided diaphragmatic hernias tend to present later, often beyond the neonatal period. These may contain part of liver or kidney in addition to bowel (Fig. 9.25).

After repair of a Bochdalek hernia the radiograph shows the volume of the underlying lung. This may expand immediately to completely fill the hemithorax. A very hypoplastic lung however is unable to fill the thorax. The radiograph may show a large air-filled pleural space with small lungs and residual mediastinal shift mimicking a tension pneumothorax (Fig. 9.23c). It is important to recognise that the problem is the volume of the lungs since attempts to suction the "tension pneumothorax" could result is severe mediastinal shift, kinking of the inferior vena cava and dangerous obstruction to venous return.

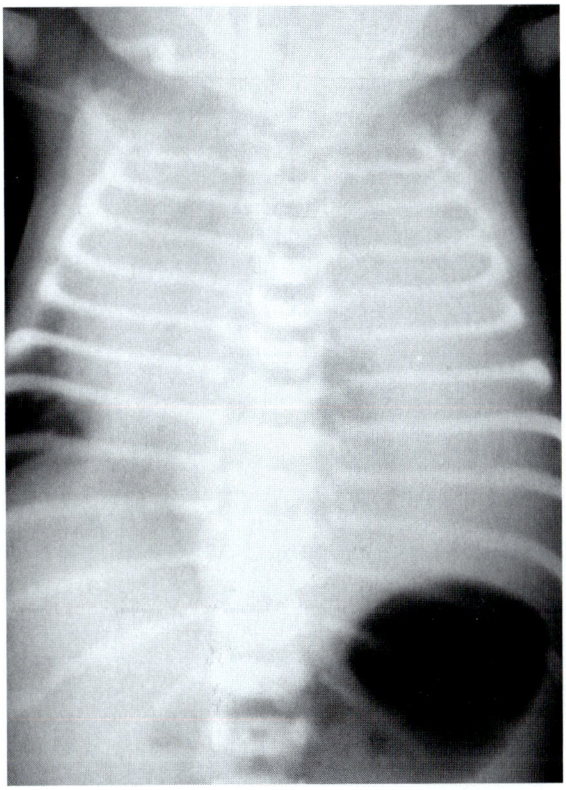

Fig. 9.22. Chylothorax. Radiograph immediately after birth shows opacification of the entire left hemithorax with mediastinal shift to the right side and downward displacement of the stomach. This recurred twice after aspiration and then resolved after the third aspiration

9.3.2
Congenital Diaphragmatic Hernia: Morgagni Type

Herniation of abdominal contents through an anterior defect in the diaphragm is less common and much less likely to present in the neonatal period. This type of diaphragmatic hernia, known as Morgagni hernia, may be multiple, right and left of the midline and usually contains colon.

The radiograph shows a midline cyst-like lucency projected over the heart. A lateral radiograph shows that this lies anterior to the heart. A barium study shows the involved bowel (Fig. 9.26).

9.3.3
Eventration of the Diaphragm

A localised bulge of part of one hemidiaphragm may occasionally cause or exacerbate neonatal respiratory distress because of a combination of ineffective diaphragmatic function and the mass effect of the upwardly displaced diaphragm and the structures beneath it. Surgical repair of the eventration may be necessary (Fig. 9.27). More commonly the eventration is an asymptomatic finding on a neonatal radiograph that may need to be distinguished from a right lower lobe pulmonary mass or atelectasis.

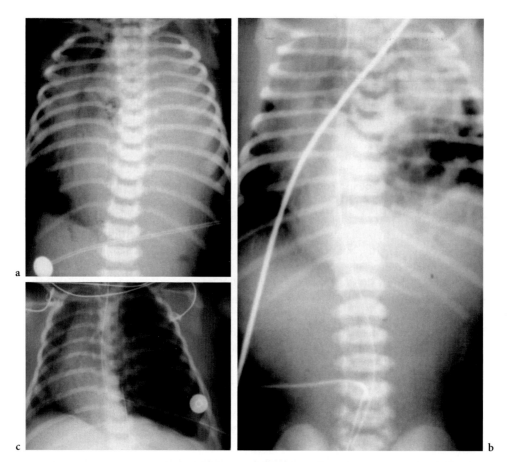

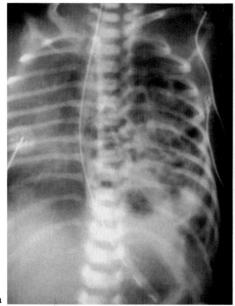

Fig. 9.23a–c. Congenital diaphragmatic hernia. **a** Initial newborn radiograph shows dense left hemi-thorax with mediastinal shift. **b** Two hours later air-filled bowel loops can be seen in the left thorax while there are none in the abdomen. **c** Postoperative radiograph shows very hypoplastic lung and a large pneumothorax

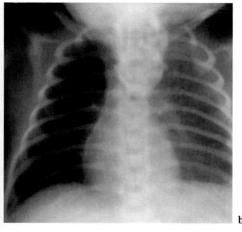

Fig. 9.24a,b. Another baby with congenital dia-phragmatic hernia. **a** Diaphragmatic hernia is as big as in baby of Figure 9.19. **b** Postoperative radio-graph 2 days after surgery shows near normal volume of both lungs

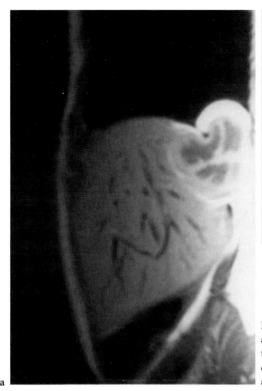

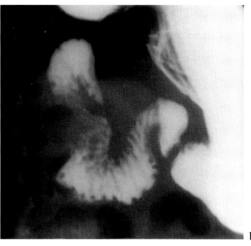

Fig. 9.25a,b. Small right-sided diaphragmatic hernia. **a** Sagittal MRI shows herniation of the upper part of the right kidney through the small defect in the right diaphragm. **b** Barium study shows that the hernia also contains duodenum

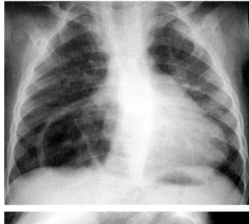

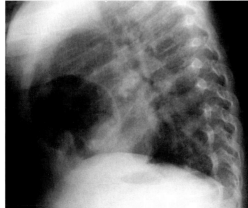

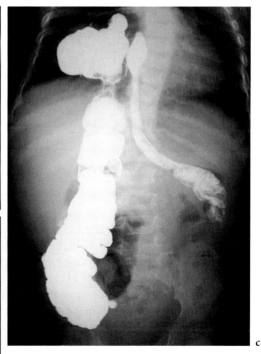

Fig. 9.26a–c. Morgagni hernia. **a** CXR shows air-filled cyst-like structures to right of heart. **b** The lateral view showed that the abnormality is anterior to the heart. **c** Barium studies showed that this is due to herniation of colon through an anterior diaphragmatic defect

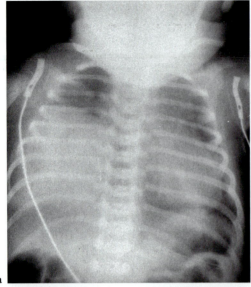

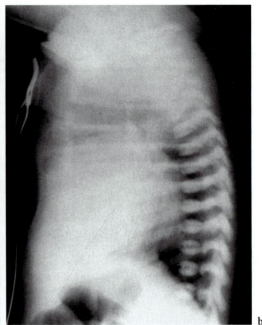

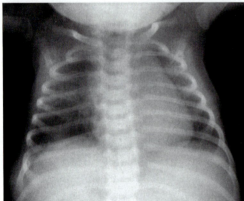

Fig. 9.27a–c. Eventration of the right hemidiaphragm. **a** AP chest radiograph shows opacification of more than half of the left hemithorax. **b** The lateral view shows that this is due to a diaphragmatic defect or eventration. Surgery performed in the neonatal period because of respiratory distress showed a thin but intact diaphragm eventrating into the right hemithorax. **c** Postoperative chest radiograph shows normal right lung volume

9.3.4
Accessory Diaphragm

An accessory diaphragm usually occurs on the right side. It lies above the right hemidiaphragm, separating part of the right lower lobe from the remainder of the right lung. It is usually fused anteriorly with the diaphragm and passes postero-superiorly to the posterior chest wall above the level of the remainder of the diaphragm. A defect medially allows bronchovascular structures from the hilum to pass inferior to the accessory diaphragm. Depending on the size of the defect the lung below the accessory hemidiaphragm may be hyperinflated, collapsed and solid or normal. The right lung is usually hypoplastic. The accessory diaphragm may be visible as a linear or broad density on the chest radiograph, but radiographic findings are more usually those of the pulmonary hypoplasia.

References

Aziz D, Langer JC, Tuuha SE et al (2004) Perinatally diagnosed asymptomatic congenital cystic adenomatoid malformation: to resect or not? J Pediatr Surg 39:329–334

Barnes JC, Smith WL (1987) The VATER association. Radiology 126:445–449

Bratu I, Flageole H, Chen M et al (2001) The multiple facets of pulmonary sequestration. J Pediatr Surg 36(5):784–790

Cass DL, Crombleholme T, Howell LJ et al (1997) Cystic lung lesions with systemic arterial supply: A hybrid of congenital cystic adenomatoid malformation and bronchopulmonary sequestration. J Pediatr Surgery 32 (7):986–990

Cohen M, Emms M, K, Kaschula RO (1991) Childhood pulmonary blastoma: a pleuropulmonary variant of the adult-type pulmonary blastoma. Pediatr Pathol 11(5):737–49

Currarino G (1985) Causes of unilateral pulmonary hypoplasia: a study of 33 cases. Pediatr Radiol 15:15–24

Curros F, Chigot V, Emond S et al (2000) Role of embolisation in the treatment of bronchopulmonary sequestration. Pediatr Radiol 30:769–773

d'Agostino S, Bonoldi E,Dante S et al (1991) Embryonal rhabdomyosarcoma of the lung arising in cystic adenomatoid malformation: case report and review of the literature. J Pediatr Surg 32(9):1381–1383

Donnelly LF, Sakurai M, Klosterman LA et al (1999) Correlation between findings on chest radiography and survival in neonates with congenital diaphragmatic hernia. AJR 173:1589–1593

Ellis K (1991) Developmental abnormalities in the systemic blood supply to the lungs. AJR 156:669–679

Eustace S, Valentine S, Murray J (1996) Acquired intralobar bronchopulmonary sequestration secondary to occluding endobronchial carcinoid tumor. Clin Imaging 20(3):178–80

Folger GM (1976) The scimitar syndrome. Angiology 27:373–407

Frank JL, Poole CA, Rosas G (1986) Horseshoe lung: Clinical, pathological and radiological features and a new plain film finding. AJR 143:217–226

Frazier AA, Rosado de Christenson ML, Stocker JT, Templeton PA (1997) **Intralobar sequestration: radiologic-pathologic correlation**. Radiographics 17:725–745

Garcia-Pena P, Lucaya J, Hendry GMA, McAndrew PT, Duran C (1998) Spontaneous involution of pulmonary sequestration in children: report of two cases and review of the literature. Pediatr Radiol 28:266–270

Gebauer PW, Mason CB (1959) Intralobar pulmonary sequestration associated with anomalous pulmonary vessels: A non-entity. Dis Chest 35:282–288

Grigoryants V, Sargent S, Shorter N (2000) Extralobar pulmonary sequestration receiving its arterial blood supply from the innominate artery. Pediatr Radiol 30:696–698

Granata C, Gambini C, Balducci T et al (1998) Bronchioloalveolar carcinoma arising in congenital cystic adenomatoid malformation in a child: a case report and review on malignancies originating in congenital cystic adenomatoid malformation. Pediatr Pulmonol 25(1):62–66

Hasiotou M, Polyviou P, Strantzia CM et al (2004) Pleuropulmonary blastoma in the area of a previously diagnosed congenital lung cyst: report of two cases. Acta Radiol 45:289–292

Islam S, Cavanaugh E, Honeke R et al (2004) Diagnosis of a proximal tracheoesophageal fistula usin 3-D CT scan: a case report. J Pediatr Surg 39:100–102

Ito F, Asaoka M, Nagai N et al (2003) Upper thoracic extralobar pulmonary sequestration with anomalous blood supply from the subclavian artery. J Pediatr Surg 38:626–628

Jamieson DH, Fisher RM (1993) Communicating bronchopulmonary foregut malformation associated with oesophageal atresia and tracheo-oesophageal fistula. Pediatr Radiol 23:557–558

Konen E, Raviv-Zilka L, Cohen A et al (2003) Congenital pulmonary venolobar syndrome: spectrum of helical CT findings with emphasis on computerized reformatting. Radiographics 23:1175–1184

Karnak I, Senocak ME, Ciftci AO et al (1999) Congenital lobar emphysema: diagnostic and therapeutic considerations. J Pediatr Surg 34(9):1347–1351

Kivelitz DE, Scheer I, Taupitz M (1999) Scimitar syndrome: diagnosis with MR angiography. AJR Am J Roentgenol 172(6):1700

Kouchi K, Yoshida H, Ohtsuka Y et al (2000) Intralobar bronchopulmonary sequestration evaluated by contrast enhanced three-dimensional MR angiography. Pediatr Radiol 30:774–5

Laffan EE, Daneman A, Ein SH et al (2006) Tracheoesophageal fistula without esophageal atresia: are pull-back tube esophagograms needed for diagnosis? Pediatr Radiol 36:1141–1147

Langston C (2003) New concepts in the pathology of congenital lung malformations. Semin Pediatr Surg 12:17–37

Laurin S, Hagerstrand I (1999) Intralobar bronchopulmonary sequestration in the newborn–a congenital malformation. Pediatr Radiol. 29(3):174–178

Leithiser RE, Capitanio MA, MacPherson RI, Wood BP (1986) Communicating bronchopulmonary foregut malformations. AJR 146:227–231

MacSweeney F, Papagiannopoulos K, Goldstraw P et al (2003) An assessment of the expanded classification of congenital cystic adenomatoid malformations and their relationship to malignant transformation. Am J Surg Pathol 27:1139–1146

Marshall KW, Blaine CE, Teitelbaum DH et al (2000) Congenital cystic adenomatoid malformation: Impact of prenatal diagnosis and changing strategies in the treatment of the asymptomatic patient. AJR 175:1551–1554

McAdams HP, Kiejczyk WM, Rasado-de-Christenson ML et al (2000) Bronchogenic cyst: Imaging features with clinical and histopathological correlation. Radiology 217:441–446

Murphy JJ, Blair GK, Fraser GC et al (1992) Rhabdomyosarcoma arising within congenital pulmonary cysts: report of three cases. J Pediatr Surg. 27(10):1364–1367

Newman B, Yunis E (1990) Primary alveolar capillary dysplasia. Pediatr Radiol 21:20–22

Newman B (2006) Congenital bronchopulmonary foregut malformations: concepts and controversies. Pediatr Radiol 36:773–791

Papagiannopoulos KA, Sheppard M, Bush AP et al (2001) Pleuropulmonary blastoma: is prophylactic resection of congenital lung cysts effective? Ann Thorac Surg 72:604–605

Roggin KK, Breuer CK, Carr SR et al (2000) The unpredictable character of congenital cystic lung lesions. J Pediatr Surg. 35(5):801–805

Puri P, Ninan GK, Blake NS, Fitzgerald RJ, Guiney EJ, O'Donnell B (1992) Delayed primary anastomosis for esophageal atresia: 18 months' to 11 years' follow-up. J Pediatr Surg 27(8):1127–1130

Poerter HJ (1999) Pulmonary hypoplasia. Arch Dis Child Fetal Neonatal 81(2):F81–83

Priest JR, Mc Dermott MB, Watterson J et al (1997) Pleuropulmonary blastoma. Cancer 80:147–160

Samuel M, Burge DM (1999) Management of antenatally diagnosed pulmonary sequestration associated with congenital cystic adenomatoid malformation. Thorax 54:701–706

Schuster SR, Harris GBC, Williams A et al (1978) Bronchial atresia: A recognisable entity in the pediatric age group. J Pediatr Surg 13: 682–689

Scully RE, Mark EJ, McNeely BU (1983) Case records of the Massachusetts General Hospital. A 14-year-old boy with recurrent hemoptysis. N Engl J Med 309:1374–1381

Silverman ME, White CS, Ziskind AA (1994) Pulmonary sequestration receiving arterial supply from the left circumflex coronary artery. Chest 106:948–949

Stocker JT, Malczak HT (1984) A study of pulmonary ligament arteries. Relationship to intralobar pulmonary sequestration. Chest 86(4):611–615

Stocker JT (1986) Sequestrations of the lung. Semin Diagn Pathol. 3(2):106–121

Sturla M, Picco G, San Roman JL, Inon AE, Garcia-Monaco R (2006) Spiral CT with Air Distension of the Esophagus Helps the Detection of Tracheoesophageal Fistula in Pediatric Patients. Abstract VP11–14 2006 Pediatric Radiology Series: Chest Radiology II. RSNA annual meeting program

Swischuk LE, Richardson CJ, Nichols NM et al (1979) Bilateral pulm hypoplasia in the neonate (a classification). AJR 233:1057–1063

Swischuk LE, Heureux PL (1980) Unilateral pulmonary vein atresia. AJR 135:667–672

Tam PKH, Chan FL, Saing H (1987) Diagnosis and evaluation of esophageal atresia by direct sagittal CT. Pediatr Radiol 17(1):68–70

Van Leeuwen K, Teielbaum DH, Hirschl RB et al (1999) Prenatal diagnosis of congenital cystic adenomatoid malformation and its postnatal presentation, surgical indications and natural history. J Pediatr Surg 34(5):794–799

Ward S, Morcos SK (1999) Congenital bronchial atresia–presentation of three cases and a pictorial review. Clin Radiol 54:144–148

Winters WD, Effman EL, Nghiem HV, Nyberg DA (1997) Disappearing fetal lung masses: importance of postnatal imaging studies. Pediatr Radiol 27:535–539

Winters WD, Effman EL (2001) Congenital masses of the lung: prenatal and post natal imaging evaluation. J Thorac Imaging 16:196–206

Congenital Anomalies of the Neonatal Upper Airway

David Manson

10.1
Introduction

Anomalies of the upper airway constitute a relatively uncommon cause of neonatal respiratory distress. Unfortunately, the clinical presentations of some of these malformations are nonspecific, yet potentially life threatening. As well, many of these anomalies require advanced airway management skills in order to secure a functional and patent airway. Early radiological recognition of the type of malformation can direct subsequent investigation and airway management into an effective and efficient course. This chapter reviews the imaging manifestations of some of the more common or classic malformations, in conjunction with the usual clinical presentations with which each is associated.

D. Manson, MD, FRCP
Department of Diagnostic Imaging, The Hospital for Sick Children, 555 University Avenue, Toronto, Canada
Assistant Professor and Division Head, Paediatric Radiology, Department of Medical Imaging, University of Toronto, Toronto, Ontario, M5G IX8, Canada

10.2
Nasal Anomalies

Choanal atresia was first identified as a cause of neonatal respiratory distress in the late eighteenth century, with the first repair described in 1851 (Keller and Kacker 2000). The incidence of this disorder ranges from 1:5,000 to 1:10,000 live births, with a male:female ratio of 1:2 (Keller and Kacker 2000; Kirkpatrick and Mueller 1998). Unilateral atresia may present with mild respiratory distress or inability to pass a nasogastric tube. More commonly, however, symptoms of unilateral atresia will not be present until later in life, frequently manifesting as a chronic nasal discharge. The disorder is bilateral in approximately one-third of cases, resulting in clinical symptoms of significant respiratory distress in the neonatal period. The anatomic positioning of the neonatal tongue with respect to the posterior pharynx results in the neonate being an obligate nose breather. Any cause of nasal obstruction will, therefore, produce significant symptoms in the neonatal period (Keller and Kacker 2000). The resultant respiratory distress is frequently accompanied by cyclical cyanosis, which is relieved by crying. Feeding difficulties are common, since the nipple will occlude the oral airway while the atresia occludes the nasal airway. The theory of embryogenesis of this disorder is still a topic of debate, but failure of resorption of the fetal nasobuccal membrane in the posterior portion of the primary palate is a commonly accepted mechanism (Keller and Kacker 2000; Jones et al. 1998). A more global disorder of mesenchymal migration has also been proposed, which would explain the ancillary findings in the CHARGE (coloboma, heart disease, choanal atresia, growth and/or mental retardation, and ear malformations) association, which is seen in approximately 50% of cases (Keller and Kacker 2000; Jones et al. 1998).

The diagnosis is made clinically by the inability to pass a soft, small (6 F) catheter through the nares into the hypopharynx (KELLER and KACKER 2000). Radiographically, computed tomography (CT) has replaced the previously described method of contrast injection under fluoroscopic guidance. CT has become the modality of choice (KELLER and KACKER 2000; JONES et al. 1998; KIRKPATRICK and MUELLER 1998) for noninvasive demonstration of the bony and/or membranous bridge across the posterior nasopharynx (Fig. 10.1). CT can also demonstrate nasal aperture stenosis and bony nasal cavity stenosis (JONES et al. 1998), similar deformities which may lie in the spectrum of this disorder. Surgical repair, frequently followed by a period of nasal stenting, is the only definitive therapy (KELLER and KACKER 2000).

A variety of congenital abnormalities of the midface can result in the formation of solid tissue masses or cystic malformations, which may cause a varying degree of nasal obstruction in the neonatal period. These are, fortunately, rare, and include nasal meningo-encephaloceles, dermoids, mucoceles, and/or hemangiomas. While these may be appreciated at prenatal sonography, their imaging characteristics are best visualised by "three-dimensional" imaging modalities such as helical CT with 3D reconstruction or magnetic resonance imaging (MRI), due to the complexity of the normal craniofacial anatomy and potential involvement of central nervous system (CNS) structures. Surgical planning for some of these lesions may well require both modalities (DINWIDDIE 2004).

10.3
Oral Airway Anomalies

The anatomy of the neonatal pharyngeal tissues is unique in that the combination of a relatively small oral airway, large tongue, and superiorly positioned larynx predisposes the infant to oral airway obstruction. When micrognathia and/or macroglossia are found in conjunction with these normal anatomic factors, oral airway obstruction becomes a significant clinical problem. There are over 50 described syndromes which manifest either macroglossia or micrognathia, and which can result in respiratory compromise in the neonatal period (KIRKPATRICK and MUELLER 1998). Many of the micrognathia syndromes have been grouped into the "Pierre Robin sequence" of disorders; however, others include Goldenhar syndrome, mandibulofacial dysostosis, and some trisomies. Approximately 60% will have an associated "U"-shaped cleft palate, as well as mandibular hypoplasia and glossoptosis. This combination of anatomic abnormalities results in blockage of the oral airway, which is most pronounced in the supine position and/or with feeds. It is thought that the disorder originates from arrest in normal mandibular development somewhere between 7 and 11 weeks of gestational age, causing the tongue to sit abnormally high in the developing oropharynx. This prevents the normal midline fusion at 11 weeks of age of the two palatal shelves, resulting in the frequently associated cleft palate.

Approximately 80% of infants with the Pierre–Robin sequence will manifest some degree of symptomatic airway obstruction (TOMASKI et al. 1995). While conservative therapy involves frequent use of prone positioning and special feeding nipples, approximately 30% will require some form of artificial airway (TOMASKI et al. 1995). The problem can improve with age as the oral airway and mandible grow, and the larynx assumes a more adult, inferiorly located, anatomic configuration. However, some infants will require tracheostomy or definitive surgical correction (LERNER and PEREZ FONTAN 1998; KIRKPATRICK and MUELLER 1998; TOMASKI et al. 1995).

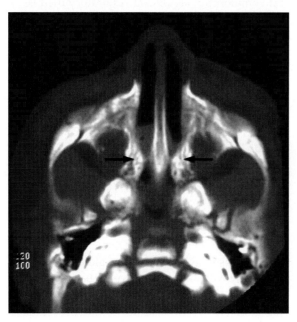

Fig. 10.1. Choanal atresia. CT scan of the head in a 2-week-old with recurrent cyanotic spells reveals bilateral membrano-osseous choanal atresia (*arrows*) with a visible fluid level in the right nasopharynx

The initial radiographic investigation is the lateral view of the facial bones, which can readily demonstrate the generalized underdevelopment of the mandible compared with the maxilla (Fig. 10.2). However, CT is the investigation of choice in surgical planning for more definitive repair. Distraction osteotomy of the mandible has recently been described for use in the early neonatal period in severe cases (KATZEN et al. 2001). In these cases, volumetrically acquired craniofacial CT imaging with subsequent 3D reconstruction has been shown to be useful in the preoperative planning for the mandibular corrective surgery.

10.4
Laryngomalacia

Laryngomalacia, also known in the literature as "congenital laryngeal stridor," is a relatively common cause of neonatal stridor. It is generally mild and clinically insignificant, yet in up to 10% of cases it can be severe enough to produce significant respiratory compromise (THURMOND and COTE 1996).

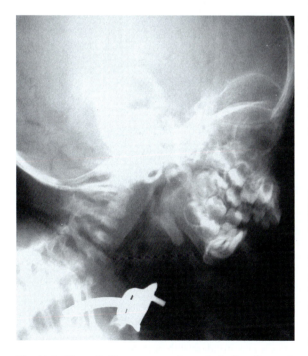

Fig. 10.2. Pierre-Robin sequence. Lateral skull radiograph of a 1-year-old who required tracheostomy in the neonatal period for airway obstruction secondary to micrognathia

There are many proposed causes of this problem, such that it appears that the true cause is probably multifactorial. The most commonly proposed mechanism is derived from what is observed at laryngoscopy. In most of these children, the aryepiglottic folds are noted to prolapse into the laryngeal airway during inspiration. It has, therefore, been proposed that the neonate may have more compliant soft tissues, more immature and pliable arytenoid cartilages, and shorter aryepiglottic folds (THURMOND and COTE 1996; CHUNG et al. 2000). These factors may predispose the aryepiglottic folds to prolapse more easily when the intra-laryngeal pressure is more negative than that in the surrounding tissues, as occurs in normal inspiration. However, immature neuromuscular factors have also been implicated, possibly due to the frequent association of laryngomalacia and gastro-oesophageal reflux (LANDAU 1999). As well, laryngomalacia has a higher incidence in some chromosomal anomalies, most notably the "cri-du-chat" of the 5p- chromosome deletion syndrome.

The diagnosis of laryngomalacia is frequently made laryngoscopically. Radiologically, excessive motion of the aryepiglottic folds at fluoroscopy has been described (STRIFE 1988; KIRKPATRICK and MUELLER 1998). When this becomes significant, relative obstruction of the laryngeal airway causes nonspecific distension of the hypopharyngeal airway on the standard, lateral soft-tissue neck examination. The initial treatment is a relatively conservative approach of infant positioning. When the problem persists, nasal continuous positive airway pressure (CPAP) has been beneficial, and definitive surgery or laser therapy is reserved for only the most severe cases (LANDAU 1999).

10.5
Laryngeal Malformations

Primary congenital laryngeal malformations are rare causes of neonatal respiratory compromise. There is a spectrum of these disorders, ranging from the most severe form, laryngeal atresia, to the more variable forms of posterior laryngeal cleft and laryngo-oesophageal cleft. Laryngeal atresia is, in itself, incompatible with life unless an immediate tracheostomy is performed in the delivery room. As this diagnosis can now be made with careful prenatal sonographic examination, sporadic case reports of immediate postnatal management and tracheostomy are being reported (BUI et al. 2000; DECOU et al. 1998). Laryngeal clefts, however, are relatively well described in the literature. These anomalies occur when a variable segment of the normal posterior tracheo-oesophageal septum fails to fuse, resulting in a persistent posterior defect in the larynx (MOUNGTHONG and HOLINGER 1997). In its mildest form, there may be a small, barely symptomatic residual posterior cleft in the larynx, which may not clinically present until adulthood with persistent hoarseness (MOUNGTHONG and HOLINGER 1997). However, more severe forms may present in the neonatal period with cyanosis associated with feedings, and severe and/or recurrent episodes of aspiration, which may require endotracheal intubation (ROTH et al. 1983; MOUNGTHONG and HOLINGER 1997). Polyhydramnios is seen in approximately one-third of cases, and 20% will have other congenital anomalies (CHUNG et al. 2000; MANCUSO 1996). As well, 20% of cases will have an associated tracheo-oesophageal fistula in its usual intra-thoracic location (MANCUSO 1996).

Documentation of the persistent cleft can be extremely difficult. The most definitive evaluation is through a laryngoscopic examination, yet the cleft may be small and easily overlooked, even at direct visualization. The radiographic evaluation must also be meticulous, and will depend on the presence of a tracheo-oesophageal communication. The fluoroscopic findings during contrast oesophagography include a decrease in the usual soft-tissue distance between the larynx and the upper oesophagus, and the documentation of spill of contrast into the trachea at the level of the larynx and/or upper cervical trachea (MOUNGTHONG and HOLINGER 1997; MANCUSO 1996) (Fig. 10.3). Unfortunately, this spill of contrast is easily misinterpreted as aspiration from above due to poor pharyngeal coordination. As well, differentiation of a "high" tracheo-oesophageal fistula from a true laryngo-oesophageal cleft can be difficult, yet crucial to surgical planning. The above-noted association of laryngo-oesophageal cleft with a second, more typically located tracheo-oesophageal fistula mandates that the examination includes an evaluation of the whole length of the tracheo-oesophageal relationship.

Despite early detection and definitive laryngeal reconstruction, mortality from a laryngo-oesopha-

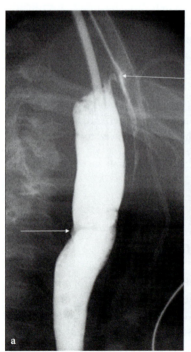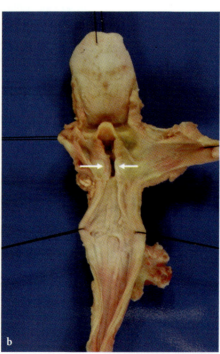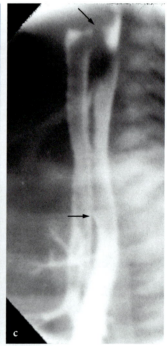

Fig. 10.3a–c. Posterior laryngeal defect. Water-soluble oesophagogram on an infant with persistent feeding difficulties. **a** There is spill of contrast from the upper oesophagus into the upper trachea at a level just below the larynx. **b** At autopsy, a small defect in the posterior wall of the larynx was seen. **c** An "H"-type tracheo-oesophageal fistula is also noted more inferiorly (*arrow*) in a second child with a small laryngeal cleft

geal cleft is as high as 50%, which is probably related to difficulties in diagnosis as well as surgical repair (ROTH et al. 1983). Even after definitive surgical correction, most children will have persistent swallowing dysfunction.

10.6
Upper Airway Cysts/Masses

Upper airway obstruction in the neonatal period is not necessarily caused by intrinsic abnormalities in the airway itself. Many neonates have significant respiratory compromise due to large, extrinsic masses or malformations, which may produce symptoms by an extrinsic mass effect causing airway compression. These include laryngeal cysts, subglottic haemangiomas, cervical teratomas and cervical vascular/lymphatic malformations. These may be initially appreciated in the fetal life through the development of polyhydramnios from interference with fetal swallowing. At birth, these can predispose to an increased risk of tracheomalacia and neonatal asphyxia from initial airway management difficulties.

Laryngeal cysts in the paediatric population are frequently congenital in origin, with up to 60% presenting within the first 2 weeks of life (MITCHELL et al. 1987). Their pathogenesis is unclear, although either obstruction of the collecting ducts (MITCHELL et al. 1987), or isolation of laryngeal embryonic cells from the larynx (WEBER et al. 1993) seem to be the most plausible explanations. When large enough, they produce symptoms by obstructing the airway, resulting in inspiratory stridor in 90% of cases. Up to 50% will have associated feeding difficulties (MITCHELL et al. 1987). They may occur in a wide variety of locations within the larynx, demonstrating no particular site preference. Radiographic manifestations include the presence of a soft-tissue, laryngeal mass, best seen when using a high-kVp, filtered, frontal airway view (JOSEPH et al. 1976; MITCHELL et al. 1987) or during contrast oesophagogram. CT, MRI and even sonographic examinations (WEBER et al. 1993) have been sporadically used to demonstrate the cystic nature of these laryngeal masses.

Subglottic haemangioma is a well-described cause of neonatal respiratory compromise, constituting approximately 1.5% of all congenital laryngeal anomalies and carrying a female:male ratio of approximately 2:1 (PHIPPS et al. 1997; SHIKHANI et al. 1986). The characteristic appearance is of an eccentrically located mass in the subglottic region, usually resulting in airway compromise. These children demonstrate an associated cutaneous haemangioma in approximately 50% of cases (CHUNG et al. 2000). As with all neonatal haemangiomas, they may grow and become more manifest over the first few months of life, only to regress spontaneously over the first few years. Approximately 80%–90% will present before 6 months of age, with the mean age at presentation being approximately 3.6 months (SHIKHANI et al. 1986). Most present with stridor and cough, which can proceed to overt cyanosis if there is significant obstruction. Swallowing is characteristically normal (SHIKHANI et al. 1986).

At high-kVp, filtered, frontal radiographic examination, an eccentrically located soft-tissue mass is typically seen (JOSEPH et al. 1976; CHUNG et al. 2000). At CT, the lesion is characteristically a polypoid, enhancing, eccentrically located subglottic mass, with variable involvement of the regional soft tissues (Fig. 10.4). The presence of phleboliths can be extremely useful in establishing a diagnosis. At MRI examination, a similarly enhancing, eccentric subglottic mass may be seen in association with tortuous signal voids representing the increased vascularity sometimes seen with these malformations (FAERBER and SWARTZ 1991).

Treatment includes exogenous administration of systemic steroids, which can accelerate the involution of the mass. Alpha interferon has been used in refractory cases (PHIPPS et al. 1997). Laser therapy can be used, although increased incidences of subsequent subglottic stenosis have been described with laser therapy (PHIPPS et al. 1997).

Large cystic lymphangiomas and cervical teratomas occur in the late fetal and neonatal period, which can result in significant respiratory compromise. As with other cervical masses, they may result in fetal polyhydramnios and may complicate fetal extraction at delivery, especially if not detected at prenatal sonographic examination.

Lymphatic malformations are relatively common vascular malformations, and approximately 80% of these will occur in the head and neck region. Only a small minority, however, are massive enough to result in significant airway compromise in the neonatal period. As such, they are usually appreciated at prenatal sonographic examination as a multicystic mass with thin septations (KOELLER et al. 1999).

The vast majority of congenital cervical teratomas are histologically benign, with a malignancy rate of only approximately 10% (ELMASALME et al. 2000). Most cases do not, therefore, produce an increase in serum alpha fetoprotein. Conventional radiographs may demonstrate internal calcification in large teratomas in up to 16% of cases (JORDAN and GAUDERER 1988). CT, however, demonstrates internal calcification to a much better extent, and should be used for definitive investigation and staging due to the small malignant potential (JORDAN and GAUDERER 1988).

Ultrasound and CT usually demonstrate multiple thin-walled, water density, cystic spaces in both teratomas and lymphangiomas (Fig. 10.5), but the presence of calcification or fat in a teratoma is more easily appreciated at CT (FAERBER and SWARTZ 1991) (Fig. 10.6). Limited case reports of the use of MRI

in the evaluation of these cervical masses have been published to date, primarily emphasizing the role that multiplanar imaging can play in evaluating the anatomic extent of these lesions in an area of such anatomic complexity (GREEN et al. 1998). Prenatal MRI has most recently been used for prenatal evaluation, as well as for planning perinatal management, in cases of large cervical teratomas and lymphangiomas (KATHARY et al. 2001, TEKSAM et al. 2005, SICHEL et al. 2002). This modality can demonstrate the extent of the mass as it relates to regional anatomy, and the extent of airway compromise that can be expected at birth. Current use of EXIT (ex utero intrapartum) therapy, where the fetal head and neck are delivered and the airway is secured before severing the placental circulation, requires extensive prenatal planning and coordination.

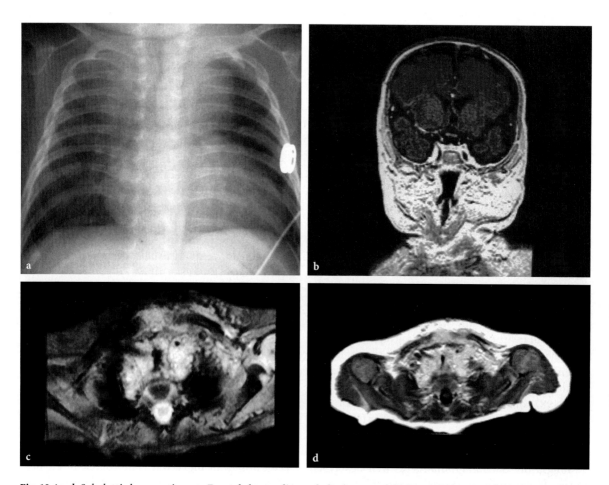

Fig. 10.4a–d. Subglottic haemangioma. **a** Frontal chest radiograph; **b–d** post-gadolinium MRI images of a 1-month-old after a respiratory arrest, demonstrating a large cervico-thoracic enhancing haemangioma that is causing diffuse tracheal lumen compromise

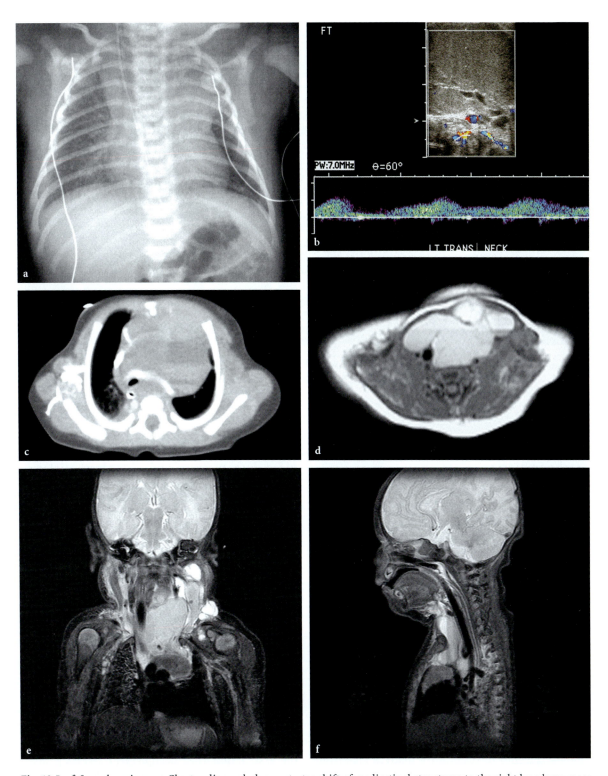

Fig. 10.5a–f. Lymphangioma. **a** Chest radiograph demonstrates shift of mediastinal structures to the right by a large mass compromising the airway. **b** Doppler ultrasound demonstrates an avascular, cystic and septated mass containing fine internal echoes, suggesting internal haemorrhage. **c** Axial enhanced CT demonstrates the cystic mass with internal fluid – fluid levels compromising the airway. **d–f** T2-weighted MRI demonstrate a multiplanar display of the extent of this lymphangioma and its relative effects on the regional anatomy

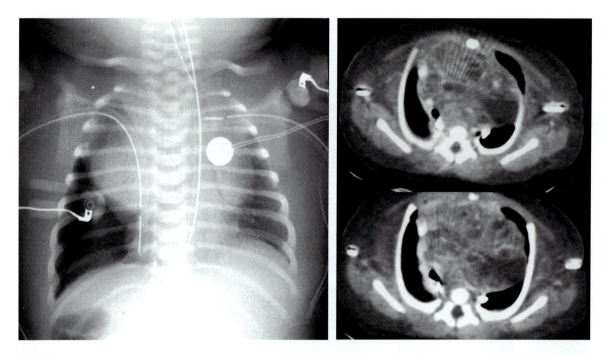

Fig. 10.6. Teratoma. Frontal chest radiograph and enhanced CT examination in the neonatal period on an infant with a large mediastinal mass, pulmonary hypoplasia, and fetal hydrops. Biopsy revealed the mediastinal mass to be an immature teratoma

10.7
Tracheomalacia

Tracheomalacia is characterized by abnormal compliance of the tracheal wall. This creates the potential for the tracheal air column to collapse when intrathoracic pressures exceed intratracheal pressures. The tracheal air column is normally supported by a network of tissues that include "U"-shaped, organized, fibrocartilaginous rings and fibromuscular supportive soft tissues. Any disturbance in the in-utero formation of these structures can result in increased tracheal wall compliance. Clinically, this increased compliance can result in varying degrees of luminal compromise, resulting in respiratory distress. The symptoms are classically exacerbated when the pressure outside the trachea exceeds intratracheal pressures. This occurs during forced expiration, agitation, crying or feeding, which precipitate episodes of respiratory distress classically characterized by expiratory stridor or even wheezing. The majority of cases are mild and improve with growth. However, tracheomalacia can uncommonly present with severe respiratory distress in the neonatal period (CHEN and HOLINGER 1994; BAXTER and DUNBAR 1963).

The causes of tracheomalacia are usually divided into primary and secondary etiologies. Primary tracheomalacia is less common, usually resulting from an isolated malformation of the tracheal cartilage rings or hypotonia of the myoelastic elements (CHEN and HOLINGER 1994; BAXTER and DUNBAR 1963). Secondary tracheomalacia is much more common, usually related to the associated presence of oesophageal atresia. WAILOO and EMERY (1979) demonstrated that approximately 75% of neonates with oesophageal atresia demonstrate some deficiency in their tracheal cartilage rings, many of which also have abnormal formation of the septum that separates the trachea from the oesophagus. The combination of increased tracheal compliance, dilatation of the proximal oesophageal pouch and the frequently associated gastro-oesophageal reflux can result in significant airway compromise related to feedings. Although the association with oesophageal atresia is common, tracheomalacia can be seen when any entity interferes with normal in utero tracheal growth. Other causes, therefore, include vascular rings, anomalous great vessel formation, and adjacent masses or congenital malformations (MANCUSO 1996).

The diagnosis of tracheomalacia can be made at fluoroscopy or during a carefully performed bronchoscopic examination. Holinger's group (CHEN and HOLINGER 1994) demonstrated that the infant's trachea may normally collapse during forced expiration to 25%–50% of its original antero-posterior diameter. It is, therefore, suggested that collapse of 75% or greater may be considered significant when there is associated respiratory distress (WITTENBORG et al. 1967). This observation can be made easily and safely from a fluoroscopic examination in the awake and, preferably, agitated child who is examined in the lateral decubitus position (Fig. 10.7). Alternatively, the bronchoscopic examination should be performed by a team of physicians with experience in paediatric bronchoscopy. During the bronchoscopic examination, the child must be observed during spontaneous respiration in order to ensure that the tracheal calibre is observed during spontaneous expiration when there is positive intrathoracic pressure relative to intratracheal pressure. A paralysed infant will be ventilated with positive pressure breathing, which does not permit the infant to generate positive extratracheal pressures in expiration. The trachea, therefore, may appear erroneously normal if the bronchoscopic examination is performed improperly. Ultrafast, or electron-beam computerized tomography is optimally designed for rapid sequence imaging of the trachea in a truly physiologic fashion. Subsecond imaging times permit examinations in both inspiration and expiration, and accurate tracheal dimensions can be calculated while the mediastinum is imaged for potential underlying causes (BRASCH et al. 1987). Unfortunately, this highly specialized type of CT equipment is not widely available. As conventional CT equipment is providing progressively faster scan times, it is hoped that this type of dynamic and physiologic scanning will soon be more widely available.

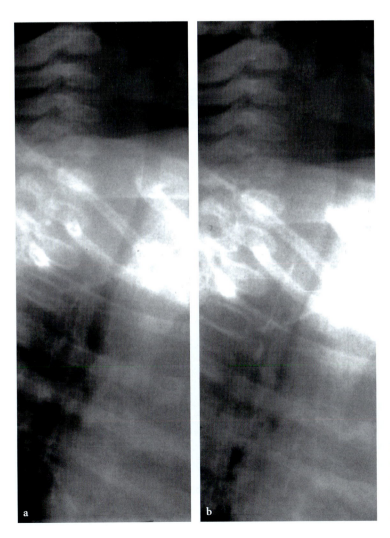

Fig. 10.7a,b. Tracheomalacia. a Inspiratory and b expiratory images at fluoroscopic examination reveal significant collapse in tracheal calibre during expiration from tracheomalacia secondary to oesophageal atresia

10.8
Congenital Tracheal Stenosis

Congenital tracheal stenosis is a rare disorder that demonstrates variable clinical presentation. It is characterized by the presence of a segment of fixed tracheal luminal narrowing of variable length and severity. The narrowing is produced by abnormal tracheal cartilaginous rings, most commonly in the form of complete cartilaginous rings, where the normal posterior fibromembranous wall of the trachea has been replaced by cartilage (CANTRELL and GUILD 1964). Less commonly, the cartilage rings are disorganized and misshapen (GRILLO 1996). In the mid 1960s, CANTRELL and GUILD (1964) produced a hallmark paper on this disorder, describing the three most common patterns seen: a long intrathoracic segment of tracheal narrowing, a short segment of "funnel"-shaped narrowing with the narrowest portion at the inferior aspect of the funnel, and a segmental, distal tracheal narrowing that

is accompanied by an aberrant origin of the right main stem bronchus directly from the distal trachea (the so-called bridging bronchus malformation).

Tracheal stenosis may be seen as an isolated finding, but may also be present in association with a variety of other disorders. In a fairly large review of cases of aberrant origin of the left pulmonary artery creating a "pulmonary sling", DOHLEMANN et al. (1995) found that just over 75% of children with a pulmonary sling will have associated complete ring, tracheal stenosis, the so-called ring–sling complex (BERDON et al. 1984) (Fig. 10.8). Alternatively, in a large review of cases of congenital tracheal stenosis by BENJAMIN et al. (1981), only approximately 5% of children had an associated pulmonary sling, yet approximately 90% of children with congenital tracheal stenosis had some other congenital anomaly. Other associations include oesophageal atresia with fistula, pulmonary hypoplasia, truncus arteriosus, atrial and ventricular septal defect (ASD and VSD, respectively).

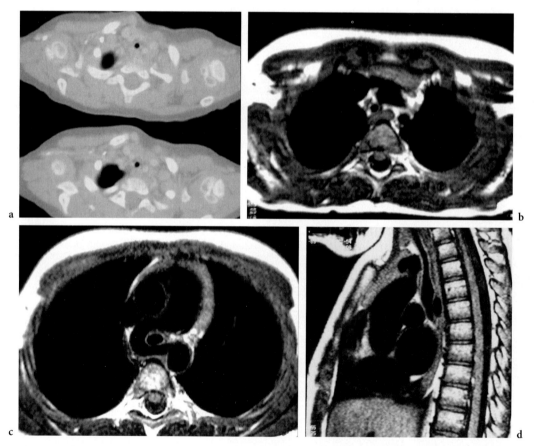

Fig. 10.8a–d. Congenital tracheal stenosis and pulmonary "sling". **a** Axial CT and **b,c** axial and **d** sagittal T1-weighted MRI examination of a long-segment, complete cartilage ring tracheal stenosis in association with a pulmonary sling, completing the "ring-sling" complex

The clinical presentation of this disorder is quite variable. BENJAMIN et al. (1981) described a population in whom 52% presented before 2 months of age. Infants with this disorder characteristically present with biphasic stridor, frequently worse on expiration, depending upon the location of the stenosis and its severity (MANCUSO 1996). The symptoms frequently increase with time. The cause for this worsening is unclear. It was initially thought that the tracheal cartilage did not grow, resulting in the respiratory needs of the infant "outgrowing" the capability of the trachea to transmit sufficient air (MURPHY et al. 1990; CANTRELL and GUILD 1964). Recent studies have shown the capability of tracheal cartilage to grow, allowing some children to undergo a relatively uneventful childhood (BENJAMIN et al. 1981; MANSON et al. 1994, 1996). The rate of growth, however, is still unknown. It is well accepted that the newborn period and first year of life are particularly critical, as respiratory infections in this period tend to cause acute respiratory deterioration (CHIU and KIM 2006).

The diagnosis of congenital tracheal stenosis may be difficult and potentially dangerous. Persistent narrowing of the trachea may be the first sign on conventional chest radiographs performed for respiratory stridor. A particularly helpful examination is the high-kVp, coned frontal view of the trachea with added filtration and/or magnification (JOSEPH et al. 1976). Some children are discovered to have tracheal narrowing during a barium swallow performed in the initial investigation for a potential pulmonary sling. Many of these children then undergo bronchoscopic and bronchographic examination to confirm the presence of complete cartilage rings. Unfortunately, the stenosis is, at times, sufficiently narrow to block the passage of the bronchoscope through the length of the stenosis. This is a critical finding to establish surgical correctability, since potential involvement of the main stem bronchi is associated with a poor prognosis. CT (MANSON et al. 1994, 1996), especially helical CT (TOKI et al. 1997) using computerized reformatting and reconstruction, can be performed without potentially dangerous airway manipulation. This examination can establish the length of stenosis, degree of narrowing, involvement of main stem bronchi, and associated anomalies noninvasively (Fig. 10.9).

Critical congenital stenosis producing significant respiratory compromise probably requires surgical correction. Short segment stenosis (involving ≤5 tracheal rings) can be corrected with a simple seg-

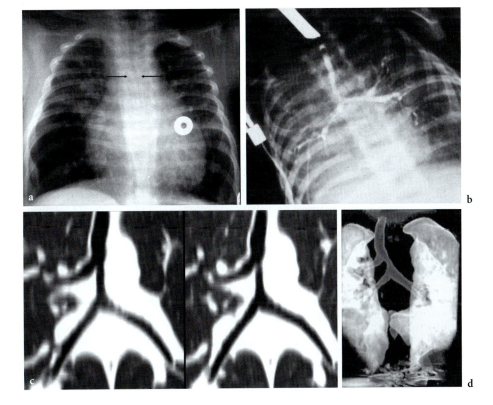

Fig. 10.9a–d. Isolated tracheal stenosis. **a** Frontal chest radiograph of a 1-month-old with respiratory distress demonstrates diffuse intrathoracic tracheal narrowing (*arrows*). **b** Subsequent bronchogram shows involvement of the main stem bronchi. **c, d** Reconstructed CT images of two separate cases of tracheal stenosis with a "bridging bronchus" deformity, demonstrating the noninvasive capability of this modality to image the complete length of the trachea for surgical planning without airway manipulation

mental resection and a primary end-to-end anastomosis (JOHNSON 1991). Longer stenoses require
more extensive surgical repair. Various procedures
have been described, including pericardial or cartilage grafts and the recently described "slide" tracheoplasty (CUNNINGHAM et al. 1998), each with
variable success. As well, recently described postoperative use of intratracheal stents (FILLER et al.
1998; SHIN et al. 2006; VALERIE et al. 2005; Airway
Reconstruction Team 2005) has demonstrated better postoperative outcomes.

10.9
Conclusion

The early radiologic recognition of airway malformations causing airway compromise is the challenging and critical role the paediatric radiologist must
play in the initial evaluation and subsequent imaging management of these children. The knowledge
of the common imaging manifestations of these
disorders and the appropriate subsequent course of
investigation becomes an integral part of the successful management of these children.

References

Airway Reconstruction Team (2005) Recent challenges in the
    management of congenital tracheal stenosis: an individu-
    alised approach. J Pediatr Surg 40:774–780
Baxter JD, Dunbar JS (1963) Tracheomalacia. Ann Otol Rhi-
    nol Laryngol 72:1013–1023
Benjamin B, Pitkin J, Cohen D (1981) Congenital tracheal
    stenosis. Ann Otol Rhinol Laryngol 90:364–371
Berdon WE, Baker DH, Wung JT et al (1984) Complete car-
    tilage-ring tracheal stenosis associated with anomalous
    left pulmonary artery: the ring-sling complex. Radiology
    152:57–64
Brasch RC, Gould RG, Gooding CA et al (1987) Upper air-
    way obstruction in infants and children: evaluation with
    ultrafast CT. Radiology 165:459–466
Bui TH, Grunewald C, Frenckner B et al (2000) Successful
    EXIT (ex utero intrapartum treatment) procedure in a
    fetus diagnosed prenatally with congenital high-airway
    obstruction syndrome due to laryngeal atresia. Eur J Pe-
    diatr 10:328–333
Cantrell JR, Guild HG (1964) Congenital stenosis of the tra-
    chea. Am J Surg 108:297–705
Chen J-C, Holinger LD (1994) Congenital tracheal anoma-
    lies. Pediatr Pathol 14:513–537

Chiu PP, Kim P (2006) Prgnostic factors in the surgical treat-
    ment of congenital tracheal stenosis: a multicenter analy-
    sis of the literature. J Pediatr Surg 41:221–225
Chung CJ, Fordham LA, Mukherji SK (2000) The paediatric
    airway: a review of differential diagnosis by anatomy and
    pathology. Neuroimaging Clin N Am 10:161–180
Cunningham MJ, Eavey RD, Vlahakes GJ et al (1998) Slide
    tracheoplasty for long-segment tracheal stenosis. Arch
    Otolaryngol Head Neck Surg 124:98–103
DeCou JM, Jones DC, Jacobs HD et al (1998) Successful ex
    utero intrapartum treatment (EXIT) procedure for con-
    genital high airway obstruction syndrome (CHAOS) ow-
    ing to laryngeal atresia. J Pediatr Surg 33:1563–1565
Dinwiddie R (2004) Congenital upper airway obstruction.
    Pediatr Respir Rev 5:17–24
Dohlemann C, Mantel K, Vogl TJ et al (1995) Pulmonary
    sling: morphological findings. Pre- and postoperative
    course. Eur J Pediatr 154:2–14
Elmasalme F, Giacomantonio M, Clarke KD et al (2000) Con-
    genital cervical teratoma in neonates. Case report and re-
    view. Eur J Pediatr Surg 10:252–257
Faerber EN, Swartz JD (1991) Imaging of neck masses in infants
    and children. CRC Crit Rev Diagn Imaging 31:283–314
Filler RM, Forte V, Chait P (1998) Tracheobronchial stenting
    for the treatment of airway obstruction. J Pediatr Surg
    33:304–311
Green J, Dickinson FL, Rickett A et al (1998) MRI in the as-
    sessment of a newborn with cervical teratoma. Pediatr
    Radiol 28:709–710
Grillo HC (1996) Pediatric tracheal problems. Chest Surg
    Clin N Am 6:693–700
Hislop A, Reid L (1970) New pathological findings in emphy-
    sema of childhood. 1. Polyalveolar lobe with emphysema.
    Thorax 25:682–690
Johnson DG (1991) Tracheal stenosis. In: Fallis JC, Filler
    RM, Lemoine G (eds) Pediatric thoracic surgery. [Cur-
    rent topics in general thoracic surgery.] Elsevier Science,
    New York, pp 151–160
Jones JE, Young E, Heier L (1998) Congenital bony nasal cav-
    ity deformities. Am J Rhinol 12:81–86
Jordan RB, Gauderer MW (1988) Cervical teratomas: an
    analysis. Literature review and proposed classification.
    J Pediatr Surg 23:583–591
Joseph PM, Berdon WE, Baker DH et al (1976) Upper airway
    obstruction in infants and small children. Improved ra-
    diographic diagnosis by combining filtration, high kilo-
    voltage, and magnification. Radiology 121:143–148
Kathary N, Bulas DI, Newman KD, Schonberg RL (2001) MR
    imaging of fetal neck masses with airway compromise:
    utility in delivery planning. Pediatr Radiol 31:727–731
Katzen JT, Holliday RA, McCarthy JG (2001) Imaging the
    neonatal mandible for accurate distraction osteogenesis.
    J Craniofac Surg 12:26–30
Keller JL, Kacker A (2000) Choanal atresia, CHARGE asso-
    ciation, and congenital nasal stenosis. Otolaryngol Clin
    North Am 33:1343–1351
Kirkpatrick BV, Mueller DG (1998) Respiratory disorders of
    the newborn. In: Churnick V, Boat TF, Kendig EL (eds)
    Kendig's disorders of the respiratory tract in children,
    6th edn. Saunders, Toronto, pp 328–363
Koeller KK, Alamo L, Adair CF, Smirniotopoulas JG (1999)
    Congenital cystic masses of the neck: radiologic-patho-
    logic correlation. Radiographics 19:121–146

Landau LI (1999) Investigation and treatment of chronic stridor in infancy. Monaldi Arch Chest Dis 54:18–21

Lerner DL, Perez Fontan JJ (1998) Prevention and treatment of upper airway obstruction in infants and children. Curr Opin Pediatr 10:265–270

Mancuso RF (1996) Stridor in neonates. Pediatr Clin North Am 43:1339–1356

Manson D, Babyn P, Filler R et al (1994) Three-dimensional imaging of the pediatric trachea in congenital tracheal stenosis. Pediatr Radiol 24:175–179

Manson D, Filler R, Gordon R (1996) Tracheal growth in congenital tracheal stenosis. Pediatr Radiol 26:427–430

Mitchell DB, Irwin BC, Bailey CM et al (1987) Cysts of the infant larynx. J Laryngol Otol 101:833–837

Moungthong G, Holinger LD (1997) Laryngotracheoesophageal clefts. Ann Otol Rhinol Laryngol 106:1002–1011

Murphy P, Lloyd-Thomas A, Elliott M (1990) Management of congenital tracheal stenosis in infants. Br J Hosp Med 44:266–270

Phipps CD, Gibson WS, Wood WE (1997) Infantile subglottic hemangioma: a review and presentation of two cases of surgical excision. Int J Pediatr Otorhinolaryngol 18/41:71–79

Roth B, Rose KG, Benz-Bohm G et al (1983) Laryngo-tracheo-oesophageal cleft. Clinical features, diagnosis and therapy. Eur J Pediatr 140:41–46

Shikhani AH, Jones MM, Marsh BR et al (1986) Infantile subglottic hemangiomas. An update. Ann Otol Rhinol Laryngol 95:336–347

Shin JH, Hong SJ, Song HY, Park SJ, Ko GY, Lee SY, Kim HB Jang JY (2006) Placement of covered retrievable expandable metallic stents for pediatric tracheobronchial obstruction. J Vasc Interv Radiol 17:309–317

Sichel JY, Gomori JM, Ezra Y, Eliashav R (2002) Prenatal magnetic resonance imaging of a cervical cystic lymphangioma for assessment of the upper airway. Ann Otol Rhinol Laryngol 111:464–465

Strife JL (1988) Upper airway and tracheal obstruction in infants and children. Radiol Clin North Am 26:309–322

Teksam M, Ozyer U, McKinney A, Kirbos I (2005) MR imaging and ultrasound of fetal cervical cystic lymphangioma:utility in antepartum treatment planning. Diagn Interv Radiol 11:87–89

Thurmond M, Cote DN (1996) Stridor in the neonate: laryngomalacia. J La State Med Soc 148:375–378

Toki A, Todani T, Watanabe Y et al (1997) Spiral computed tomography with 3-dimensional reconstruction for the diagnosis of tracheobronchial stenosis. Pediatr Surg Int 12:334–336

Tomaski SM, Zalzal GH, Saal HM (1995) Airway obstruction in the Pierre Robin sequence. Laryngoscope 105:111–114

Valerie EP, Durrant AC, Forte V, Chait P, Kim PC (2005) A decade of using tracheal/bronchial stents in the management of tracheomalacia and/or bronchomalacia: is it better than aortopexy? J Pediatr Surg 40:904–907

Wailoo MP, Emery JL (1979) The trachea in children with tracheo-oesophageal fistula. Histopathology 3:329–338

Weber PC, Kenna MA, Casselbrant ML (1993) Laryngeal cysts: a cause of neonatal airway obstruction. Otolaryngol Head Neck Surg 109:129–134

Wittenborg WH, Gyepes MT, Crocker D (1967) Tracheal dynamics in infants with respiratory distress, stridor and collapsing trachea. Radiology 88:653–662

Computed Tomography of the Central and Peripheral Airways

Alistair D. Calder and Catherine M. Owens

A. D. Calder, FRCR; C. M. Owens, FRCR
Department of Radiology, Great Ormond Street, Hospital for
Sick Children, NHS Trust, London, WC1N 3JH, UK

11.1
Introduction

Abnormalities of the airways in neonates may be congenital or acquired, and include both intrinsic airway disorders and disorders of extrinsic tracheo-bronchial compression. Disorders of the larger airways are frequently related to compression by anomalous vessels, and thus imaging techniques producing excellent vascular detail are usually required. Whilst both magnetic resonance imaging (MRI) and multi-detector computed tomography (CT) offer high-quality vascular imaging, CT is often preferred in this setting. This primarily reflects the rapid image acquisition possible with CT; thus fewer patients require sedation, which is frequently hazardous in small children with airway disorders. CT also provides excellent imaging of the lung parenchyma: it is thus able to depict effects of airway lesions on the lung parenchyma, such as overinflation, atelectasis, consolidation and mucus plugging.

In this chapter we review the CT techniques and findings in neonates and infants with abnormalities of the central and peripheral pulmonary airways.

11.2
Central Airways

Central airway disorders (here defined as disorders of the trachea and left and right main bronchi) in the neonate are conveniently divided into extrinsic compression and intrinsic airway disorders. Vascular anomalies producing complete and incomplete vascular rings, or otherwise compressing airways, account for the majority of extrinsic compressive lesions: these are the conditions for which CT is most frequently required and are the main focus of this chapter. Intrinsic airway disorders include tracheobronchomalacia and tracheal stenosis: these are fairly frequent accompaniments to prematurity, particularly following prolonged mechanical ventilation.

Congenital abnormalities affecting the central airways are all rare. Vascular rings comprise approximately 1% of congenital cardiac anomalies (Hernanz-Schulman 2005). Incidences for primary intrinsic airway abnormalities are not known: the incidence of primary tracheomalacia is, however, estimated at approximately 1:1500 live births (Callahan 1998). Acquired tracheal stenosis and tracheomalacia are also rare with a similar overall frequency, but are relatively common in the neonate requiring prolonged intubation.

11.2.1
Indications and Clinical Presentations

Central airway narrowing in neonates typically presents with inspiratory or biphasic (i.e. both inspiratory and expiratory) stridor. Other presentations include a characteristic cough (described as similar to a seal's bark) and recurrent respiratory infection (Turner et al. 2005). Although the oesophagus is frequently also involved in disorders narrowing the trachea, feeding difficulty is a rare presenting feature in the neonate and before the introduction of solid food. Many of these disorders are associated with other anomalies and these will be detailed below. Antenatal diagnosis of vascular tracheobronchial compression syndromes has been described, but is the exception rather than the rule (Patel et al. 2006).

11.2.2
Purposes of Imaging

In neonates with suspected large airways disease, imaging should be focused on identifying the cause of the disorder, and delineating the anatomical relationships of the airways to the major vessels. This is particularly important in vascular compression syndromes requiring surgery, where imaging directs the surgical approach to be utilized (Walters 2005). As an example, a double aortic arch may be approached by either a left-sided or a right-sided thoracotomy depending on which arch is dominant.

11.2.2.1
Non-CT Imaging Techniques

11.2.2.1.1
Chest Radiography

Chest radiography remains an important initial investigation in the child with a suspected airway anomaly. The presence of a right-sided arch in an infant with stridor is certainly suggestive of the presence of a vascular ring, as this is present in the majority of cases. The airway itself may be directly visualized on the chest film. Lung collapse or consolidation relating to the airway problem may also be efficiently demonstrated. Although an entirely normal radiograph makes a vascular ring unlikely (Hernanz-Schulman 2005), it is probably not sensitive enough to exclude the diagnosis.

11.2.2.1.2
Contrast Oesophagography

Contrast oesophagography has long been a useful tool in the investigation of vascular tracheobronchial compression syndromes, on the basis that any vascular anomaly causing tracheal compression will also cause oesophageal compression. Indeed it is believed that a normal contrast oesophagram excludes the presence of a vascular ring. However, the widespread availability of multidetector CT (MDCT) has led to a reduction in use of oesophagography, although some authors still advocate a role as a screening tool, particularly when clinical suspicion for a vascular ring is low (Hernanz-Schulman 2005; Turner et al. 2005).

11.2.2.1.3
Bronchoscopy

Bronchoscopy allows direct visualization of the central airways, and is particularly useful in the identification of intrinsic airway anomalies. Pulsatility of the airway at the level of narrowing suggests vascular compression.

11.2.2.1.4
Contrast Bronchography

Contrast bronchography is still widely practised in the neonatal setting, and is particularly useful in the evaluation of tracheobronchomalacia. The technique can give useful dynamic information such as airway opening pressures, which may be used to guide management.

11.2.2.1.5
Magnetic Resonance Imaging

As discussed earlier, MRI may also be used to evaluate vascular tracheobronchial compression syndromes, but suffers the key disadvantage of prolonged imaging times and the frequent need for sedation or general anaesthesia. It does however avoid the use of ionizing radiation, and may be the technique of choice in the more stable patient (ODDONE et al. 2005). A full discussion of MRI techniques is beyond the scope of this chapter.

11.2.2.2
CT Techniques

Multidetector CT (MDCT) techniques have revolutionized the imaging of vascular tracheobronchial compression syndromes and other airway disorders, and are now the most widely performed advanced imaging techniques in this setting.

Acutely unwell neonates with airway disorders may be intubated and ventilated at the time of examination, and this allows controlled breath-holding for the duration of the acquisition. In order to avoid artefactual "stenting" of a tracheal stenosis by the endotracheal tube, the tip of the tube should be positioned in the most proximal position that is safe, as guided by the attending anaesthetist. This can be confirmed on the scout view. For non-intubated patients, the scan can be acquired during quiet spontaneous respiration. Sedation is generally used sparingly and with caution in patients with airway problems.

To produce exquisite vascular detail requires a large volume of data with thin beam collimation. For a 16-slice scanner, in our institution we use a beam collimation of 0.75 mm with a feed per rotation of 8–12 mm (equates to a pitch of 0.75-1) and a rotation time of 0.5 s. We use a tube voltage of 100 kVp. Diagnostic-quality studies can be obtained using low tube currents to minimize dose (PACHARN et al. 2002): for neonates we use a tube current typically of 15–20 mAs. The effective dose with these parameters for a CT of the entire thorax is of the order of 0.7–0.9 mSv.

We administer intravenous contrast via a large peripheral vein where possible, using at least a 22-g cannula. We use a dose of 2 ml/kg of iodinated contrast material at 300 mmol iodine/l. Contrast administration is timed using a reference scan at the level of the main pulmonary artery following the contrast bolus, triggering the helical acquisition when the bolus reaches the main pulmonary artery. In our experience automated bolus tracking is problematic in neonates, as drawing a region of interest correctly is difficult in these very small patients.

We reconstruct images with two kernels, a soft-tissue algorithm (B30f) and a high spatial frequency algorithm for lungs (B60f). We send 3-mm reconstructions at both kernels to the Picture Archiving and Communication System (PACS). We also reconstruct thin section data at 1 mm thickness with the B30f kernel, which we send to a 3D workstation (Loenardo, Siemens, Erlangen) for post processing.

Post processing is essential to fully clarify the relationship of vascular structures to airways. Multiplanar reformats in axial, coronal and sagittal (and oblique/angled planes as necessary) are an important first step (Fig. 11.1a). Maximal intensity projections (MIPS) in thin and thick sections can help to accentuate vascular structures, but may obscure the airways (Fig. 11.1b). Volume rendered tomogram (VRT) images may be very useful to demonstrate overall arch anatomy (Fig. 11.1c). The airways can also be reconstructed with volume rendering to produce a "virtual bronchogram", which elegantly demonstrates the overall appearance of the main airways (Fig. 11.1d). Finally, a "fly-through" virtual bronchoscopy can help demonstrate abnormalities in a way that is familiar to clinicians (Fig. 11.1e) (HONNEF et al. 2006). MDCT techniques are summarized in Figure 11.2.

11.3
Extrinsic Airway Compression: Vascular Rings

11.3.1
Anatomical and Embryological Considerations

Understanding vascular tracheobronchial compression syndromes is facilitated by an appreciation of the embryological development of the major vessels. This is largely based on the theoretical studies of EDWARDS (1948a, 1948b). The major vessels develop from six primitive aortic arches, of which

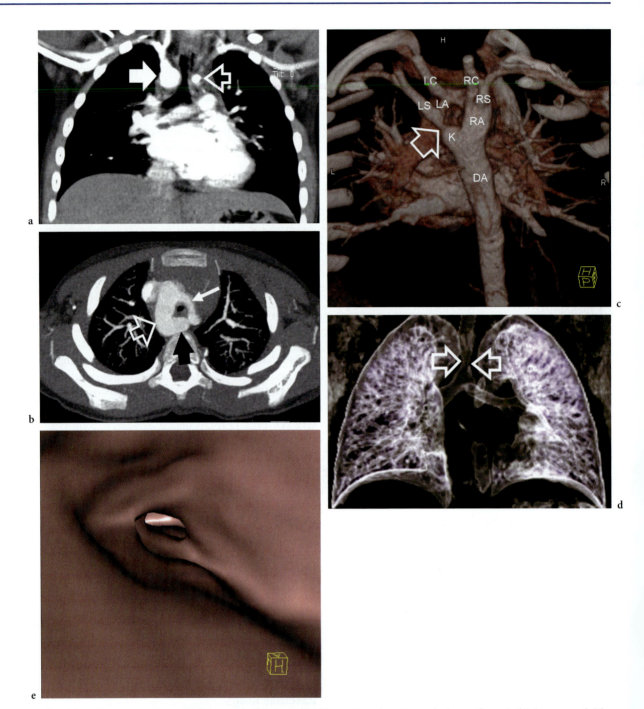

Fig. 11.1a–e. Post processing techniques: right dominant double aortic arch. **a** Coronal-plane reformat: this is very useful for demonstrating tracheal narrowing due to a double arch, in this case a right dominant double arch (*white arrow right arch*, *open arrow left arch*). **b** Axial 10-mm maximal intensity projection: MIPS are useful for accentuating vascular structures. **c** Volume rendered tomogram, posterior cut-away view: this view gives a clear overview of the arch anatomy (*DA* dorsal aorta, *LA* left arch, *RA* right arch, *RC/LC* right/left common carotid, *RS/LS* right/left subclavian artery): the *arrow* indicates a stenosis between the distal left arch, which forms a Kommerell diverticulum (K), and the proximal left arch. **d** Virtual bronchogram view, which gives an overview of bronchial anatomy: there is a narrowing at the level of the double arch. **e** Virtual bronchoscopy: although not particularly useful to the radiologist, this gives the clinician a familiar view of the tracheal anatomy: there is predominantly antero-posterior narrowing at the level of the double arch

no more than four are present at any one time: these connect dorsal and ventral aortas. From this can be derived a hypothetical composite comprising a double aortic arch, the two arches uniting to form the dorsal aorta, with each arch giving off a ductus to the ipsilateral pulmonary artery (Fig. 11.3). Each arch also gives rise to the ipsilateral subclavian and carotid artery. Normal development requires regression of the right arch proximal to the level of the right subclavian, with resorption of the right-sided ductus. Malformations and anatomical variations result from persistence of these normally regressing structures, and/or regression at other sites; for example, the commonest anatomical variant of the aortic arch, the left arch with aberrant right subclavian, arises when the segment of the right arch between the right subclavian and right carotid regresses, with the more proximal right arch persisting as the origin of the aberrant subclavian. When only the proximal aspect of the second arch regresses, the patent remnant can often be distinguished as a posterior aortic diverticulum, also known as a Kommerell diverticulum. This is a frequent finding in vascular rings. A Kommerell diverticulum is frequently the origin of an aberrant subclavian artery (e.g. Fig. 11.7b), but may also be blind ending. A ductus or ligamentum arteriosus may also arise from the diverticulum (e.g. Fig. 11.6). If this is contralateral to the side of the aortic arch, a complete ring will ensue.

11.3.2
Classification and Terminology

The term vascular ring refers to an encirclement of the trachea and oesophagus by an abnormal combination of derivatives of the aortic arch system. The nomenclature of these disorders is somewhat confusing: the current classification system employed by The Society of Thoracic Surgeons divides vascular rings into complete rings, consisting primarily of the double aortic arch and right aortic arch with left ligamentum arteriosus, and incomplete rings, principally the pulmonary artery sling and innominate artery compression syndrome, Fig. 11.4 (BACKER and MAVROUDIS 2000). It might be argued that an incomplete ring is not a ring at all, and some authors prefer "vascular tracheo-bronchial compression syndrome" as an umbrella term, reserving vascular ring to describe complete encirclements only (WALTERS 2005).

CT parameters for 16 slice MDCT	
Beam collimation	0.75mm
Feed per rotation	8-12mm
Rotation time	0.5s
Tube voltage	100kVp
Tube current	15-20mAs
Patient dose	0.7mSv (male)
	0.9mSv (female)

Image reconstruction	
PACS	3mm axial soft tissue (B30f)
	3mm axial lung (B60f)
Workstation	1mm axial soft tissue (B30f)

Post processing	
Technique	Purpose
Multiplanar reformats	To demonstrate anatomical relationships
Maximal intensity projections	To accentuate vascular structures
Virtual rendering tomography	Overview of vascular anatomy
Virtual bronchogram	Overview of tracheo-bronchial anatomy
Virtual bronchoscopy	At clinician request

Fig. 11.2. Summary of MDCT imaging parameters for imaging central airway abnormalities in neonates

11.3.3
Complete Vascular Rings

The original description of a complete vascular ring was made in 1945 by Gross, who was the first to identify and treat a double aortic arch. It is important to note that a vascular ring is not necessarily completed by patent vascular structures: complete vascular rings also occur when a right-sided aortic arch is associated with a left ligamentum arteriosum (i.e. a ligamentous remnant of the ductus arteriosus), often in association with a Kommerell diverticulum. Non-patent vascular structures such as a ligamentum or atretic arch segment are not usually directly visualized with imaging: their presence is inferred from the finding of an appropriate arrangement of the major vessels with a narrowed airway at the level of the ring.

11.3.3.1
Double Aortic Arch

A double arch is the most common type of symptomatic aortic ring: it is characterized by two aortic arches arising from the ascending aorta which unite behind the oesophagus, thus encircling both trachea and oesophagus. Typically, each carotid and subclavian artery has its own independent origin from the two arches.

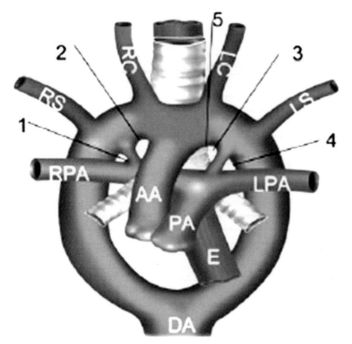

Fig. 11.3. The hypothetical double arch of Edwards. (*AA* Ascending aorta, *DA* dorsal aorta, *E* oesophagus, *PA* pulmonary artery, *R/LPA* right/left pulmonary artery, *R/LC* right/left carotid, *R/LS* right/left subclavian.) A ductus connects each arch to the ipsilateral pulmonary artery. Normal development requires regression of the right arch between dorsal aorta and right subclavian to *point 1*, and regression of the right-sided ductus. The right subclavian and carotid join to become the innominate artery. If regression occurs at *point 2*, a left arch with aberrant right subclavian results. Regression at *point 3* results in right arch with aberrant left subclavian, frequently with a persisting left-sided ductus/ductal ligament. Regression at *point 4* results in right arch with mirror image branching: the left arch may persist as a Kommerell diverticulum with a left-sided duct or ligament completing the vascular ring. Figure from Hernanz-Schulman M. Vascular rings: a practical approach to imaging diagnosis. Pediatr Radiol 2005 Oct;35(10):961–979. Epub 2005 Jul 29. Review. PMID: 16052335

Vascular rings	Complete Rings	Double arch	Balanced double arch
			Right dominant double arch
			Left dominant double arch
		Right arch, left ligamentum	Retro-oesophageal left subclavian artery
			Mirror-image branching
			Circumflex aorta
	Rare rings		Left arch, circumflex aorta
			Others
	Incomplete rings	Innominate artery compression	
		Pulmonary artery sling	

Fig. 11.4. Simplified classification of vascular rings, after the Congenital Heart Surgery Nomenclature and Database Project

In approximately 75% of double arches, the right arch is said to be dominant, being larger and usually slightly higher in position than the left (Fig. 11.1). Most of the remainder are said to be "balanced" with equal sizes of the two arches (Fig. 11.5) (Hernanz-Schulman 2005). Both balanced and right dominant arches are treated through a left-sided thoracotomy. In a minority, the left arch is dominant: it is critical, wherever possible, to identify this minority of patients, as they will require a right-sided thoracotomy to ligate the non-dominant arch. Further variations of double arch occur when one of the arches, almost invariably the left arch, is non-patent and atretic: the left arch persists as a ligamentous remnant. The atretic segment lies between either the left subclavian and descending aorta, or between left carotid and left subclavian,

the patent remnant in this case forming a Kommerell diverticulum. The imaging appearances in these cases are usually indistinguishable from a right arch with mirror image branching and right arch with retro-oesophageal left subclavian, respectively (Hernanz-Schulman 2005; Schlesinger et al. 2005).

11.3.3.2
Right Aortic Arch with Left-Sided Ligamentum

In this, the other main group of complete vascular rings, a right-sided aortic arch is associated with a left-sided ligamentum arteriosus (ductal ligament) connecting the main pulmonary artery to the descending aorta. This primarily occurs in one of two patterns: in approximately two-thirds of cases,

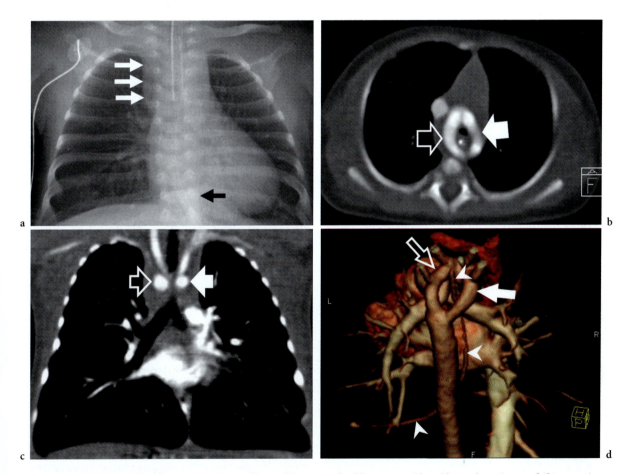

Fig. 11.5a–d. Balanced double aortic. **a** Chest radiograph in a 6-week-old neonate with stridor and respiratory failure requiring intubation. There is abnormal right paratracheal soft tissue (*white arrows*). The descending aorta is left sided (*black arrow*). **b** Axial, and **c** coronal CT reconstructions demonstrating a double aortic arch (*open arrow right arch, white arrow left arch*) of approximately equal size, encircling the narrowed trachea and oesophagus (a nasogastric tube is in situ). **d** Volume rendered 3D reconstruction: view from right postero-superior position: the nasogastric tube (*arrowheads*) runs between the right (*white arrow*) and left (*open arrow*) aortic arches

the left subclavian artery is the final branch of the aortic arch, and follows a retro-oesophageal course. This is analogous to the common variant of aberrant right subclavian with left arch; however, with a right arch, the aberrant subclavian is frequently associated with a left-sided ductus and thus a complete ring. The aberrant subclavian artery frequently arises from a Kommerell diverticulum, from which the ductus or ligamentum arteriosus also usually arises (Fig. 11.6). In most remaining cases, there is "mirror-image" branching, with a left-sided innominate artery arising as the first branch. In general, a right arch with mirror-image branching, although strongly associated with congenital heart disease, is only infrequently associated with a vascular ring. When a ring is present, this is usually due to a left-sided ductal ligament either in association with a left-sided descending aorta (a "circumflex" aorta) or with a blind-ending Kommerell diverticulum (Fig. 11.7c) (HERNANZ-SCHULMAN 2005; ODDONE et al. 2005; TURNER et al. 2005).

11.3.3.3
Other Complete Rings

Rarely, a complete ring is associated with a left-sided aortic arch. In order to produce a complete ring in this setting, a right-sided ductal ligament needs to be present: this most commonly occurs in the presence of a circumflex aorta, i.e. a left arch with a right-sided descending aorta. Typically, the right-sided ductal ligament connects the right pulmonary artery and the descending aorta. This is occasionally associated with an aberrant right subclavian artery arising as the last branch of the aorta from a Kommerell diverticulum (Fig. 11.7d). It should be noted that an aberrant right subclavian artery as the only arch abnormality is almost never associated with a vascular ring, as the ductus is almost invariably left sided in this case (HERNANZ-SCHULMAN 2005; ODDONE et al. 2005; TURNER et al. 2005).

Four examples of arch arrangements associated with complete rings are given in Figure 11.7.

11.3.4
Incomplete Vascular Rings

Incomplete vascular rings consist predominantly of pulmonary artery sling and innominate artery compression syndrome.

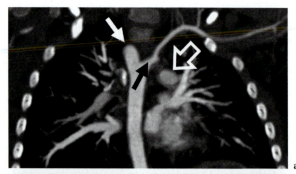

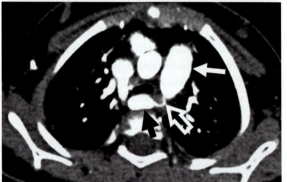

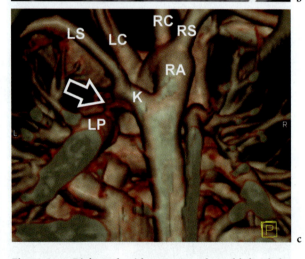

Fig. 11.6a–c. Right arch with retro-oesophageal left subclavian artery, and patent left ductus arteriosus. **a** Coronal MPR image in 18-month-old child with dysphagia following a ventricular septal defect (VSD) repair: there is a right aortic arch (*white arrow*), with a left subclavian artery arising aberrantly off a Kommerell diverticulum (*black arrow*). The left pulmonary artery is in close proximity to this (*open arrow*). **b** Axial thin section demonstrates patent ductus arteriosus (*open arrow*) running between the Kommerell diverticulum (*black arrow*) and the left pulmonary artery (*white arrow*), completing the ring. **c** VRT image. Posterior cut-away view demonstrates overview of arch anatomy. (*K* Kommerell diverticulum, *LP* left pulmonary artery, *LS/LC* left subclavian/common carotid, *RA* right aortic arch, *RS/RC* right subclavian/common carotid.) The left-sided ductus is visible as a thin structure between the Kommerell diverticulum and the left pulmonary artery

11.3.4.1
Pulmonary Sling

A pulmonary artery sling, sometimes known as a retrotracheal left pulmonary artery, is characterized by the left pulmonary artery arising from the right pulmonary artery or distal pulmonary trunk, rather than the main pulmonary trunk as is normal. The left pulmonary artery arches around the trachea, above the right main bronchus, and runs in between trachea and oesophagus. The artery may compress the right main bronchus, the right and posterior walls of the trachea and the anterior wall of the oesophagus. This extrinsic compression is frequently exacerbated by intrinsic tracheobronchial abnormalities: complete cartilaginous rings are particularly common (Fig. 11.8). Other associations include frequent cardiac anomalies and occasionally a tracheal right upper lobe bronchus (BERDON 2000; ODDONE et al. 2005).

11.3.4.2
Innominate Artery Compression

This somewhat controversial entity is the combination of the clinical features of upper airway obstruction with tracheal narrowing related to the position of the innominate artery. Controversy arises as tracheal narrowing at this site may be found in asymptomatic children, and the degree of tracheal narrowing relates poorly to the level of symptoms. Furthermore, it is not clear if the primary abnormality is the extrinsic compression or intrinsic tracheomalacia. Imaging typically demonstrates an abnormally distal origin, or occasionally a dilated or aneurysmal root of the innominate artery and tracheal narrowing of at least 50% of the normal lumen (Fig. 11.9). Treatment is by aortopexy or occasionally reimplantation of the innominate artery (BERDON 2000; FAUST et al. 2002; ODDONE et al. 2005; SHELL et al. 2001).

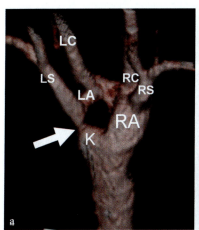 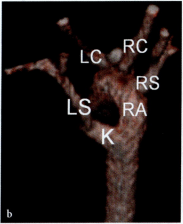 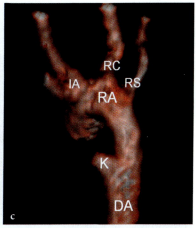

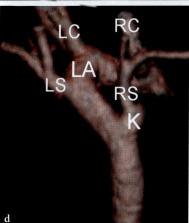

Fig. 11.7a–d. Arch arrangements associated with complete vascular rings: volume rendered posterior views. (*DA* Dorsal aorta, *IA* innominate artery, K Kommerell diverticulum, *RA/LA* right/left aortic arch, *RC/LC* right/left common carotid, *RS/LS* right/left subclavian artery.) **a** Double arch with right arch dominance (3-year-old male): there is narrowing of the left arch between proximal and distal portions (*arrow*) with the distal portion showing dilatation (a Kommerell diverticulum). Carotid and subclavian branches arise from each ipsilateral arch. **b** Right arch with retro-oesophageal left subclavian artery (4-year-old male): the aberrant subclavian arises from a Kommerell diverticulum. This arrangement resembles a double arch with atresia of the left proximal arch segment. The vascular ring is completed by a ligamentous remnant of a left-sided ductus arteriosus between the Kommerell diverticulum and left pulmonary artery. **c** Right arch with mirror-image branching and Kommerell diverticulum (2-month-old female). Again a ligament from the Kommerell diverticulum to the left pulmonary artery completes the ring. **d** Left arch with circumflex aorta (right-sided dorsal aorta) and aberrant right subclavian artery (4-month-old female). This is almost a mirror image of case **b**: unlike most cases of left arch with aberrant subclavian, the ductus arteriosus is right sided, and thus forms a complete ring

11.3.4.3
Other

There are a number of other congenital great arch anomalies associated with airway compromise all of which are rare. The most notable of these is a cervical aortic arch, where the top of the arch crosses the sternum: this typically presents as a pulsatile mass in the suprasternal notch, but occasionally presents with tracheo-oesophageal compression.

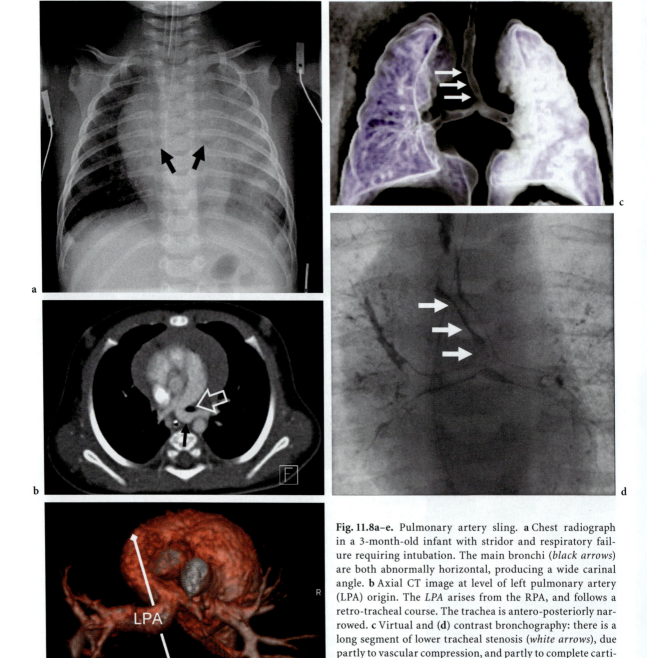

Fig. 11.8a–e. Pulmonary artery sling. **a** Chest radiograph in a 3-month-old infant with stridor and respiratory failure requiring intubation. The main bronchi (*black arrows*) are both abnormally horizontal, producing a wide carinal angle. **b** Axial CT image at level of left pulmonary artery (LPA) origin. The *LPA* arises from the RPA, and follows a retro-tracheal course. The trachea is antero-posteriorly narrowed. **c** Virtual and (**d**) contrast bronchography: there is a long segment of lower tracheal stenosis (*white arrows*), due partly to vascular compression, and partly to complete cartilaginous rings. **e** Volume rendered 3D reformat, postero-superior view of the heart and pulmonary arteries. The course of the trachea is indicated by the *arrow*

11.4
Extrinsic Airway Compression: Other Vascular Anomalies

The preceding disorders all feature anatomically anomalous vessels as a primary abnormality. In some circumstances, hypertrophy and dilatation of normally originating vascular structures result in tracheobronchial compression.

11.4.1
Absent Pulmonary Valve Syndrome

This is a disorder characterized by massive pulmonary arterial dilatation secondary to profound pulmonary valve insufficiency. It is almost always associated with other cardiac anomalies, usually tetralogy of Fallot. Chromosome 22.q11 deletion and

DiGeorge syndrome are other occasional accompaniments. Airway obstruction is an early and dominant feature: the dilated arteries may narrow the trachea or either main bronchus (Fig. 11.10). Surgical treatment typically consists of a homograft valve conduit and reduction arterioplasty of the dilated vessels. Tracheobronchial stenting is also occasionally employed (Norgaard et al. 2006; Taragin et al. 2006).

11.4.2
Major Aortico-Pulmonary Collateral Artery (MAPCA)

Major aorto-pulmonary collateral arteries (MAPCA) are a frequent finding in cyanotic congenital heart disease associated with pulmonary valve atresia. Extrinsic bronchial compression by MAPCA is not infrequent in these patients, and may contribute to poor cardiorespiratory function (Fig. 11.11) (Yamagishi et al. 2002).

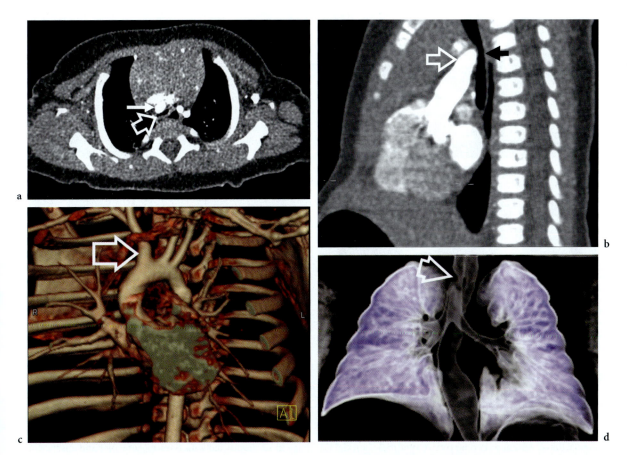

Fig. 11.9a–d. Innominate artery compression in a 2-month-old infant with stridor. **a** Axial CT demonstrates eccentric tracheal narrowing at the level of the innominate artery origin. **b** Sagittal reformat demonstrates narrowing of >50% of upper tracheal diameter. **c** The aortic arch anatomy is normal. **d** Virtual bronchogram demonstrates eccentric narrowing of the right side of the trachea

11.5
Extrinsic Airway Compression: Non-Vascular

Non-vascular causes account for a minority of extrinsic airway compression in neonates and infants, but encompass a range of congenital and neoplastic entities. Commoner causes include bronchogenic cyst (Fig. 11.12), mediastinal teratoma (Fig. 11.13) and congenital neuroblastoma.

11.6
Intrinsic Airway Abnormalities

Intrinsic abnormality of the central airways as a solitary finding accounts for a minority of neonatal airway abnormalities, but frequently occurs in association with extrinsic compression. Airway abnormalities can be conveniently divided into dynamic airway narrowing, or tracheobronchomalacia, and fixed tracheobronchial stenoses.

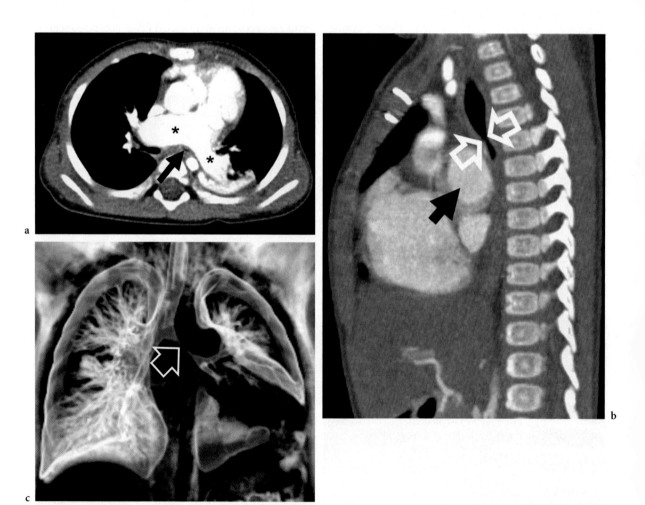

Fig. 11.10a–c. Absent pulmonary valve syndrome. **a** Axial CT image in 10-month-old with tetralogy of Fallot and absence of the pulmonary valve. The main pulmonary arteries (*asterisks*) are massively dilated, producing marked narrowing of the left main bronchus (*arrow*) as it passes between them. **b** Sagittal reformat demonstrates massive main pulmonary artery dilatation (*black arrow*) with marked antero-posterior narrowing of the left main bronchus (*between open arrows*). **c** Virtual bronchogram demonstrates almost complete occlusion of the left main bronchus (*open arrow*)

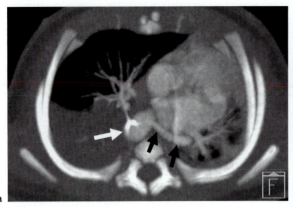
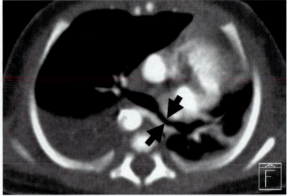

Fig. 11.11a–c. Major aortico-pulmonary collateral artery. **a** Axial 10-mm maximal intensity projection image from CT study in 2-day-old neonate with complex congenital heart disease including hypoplastic right ventricle, pulmonary atresia and tricuspid stenosis. The lungs are predominantly supplied by aorto-pulmonary collateral arteries. This image demonstrates a large collateral (*black arrows*) arising from the descending aorta (*white arrow*). **b** Axial CT image demonstrates the close relationship of the collateral artery to the left main bronchus, which is narrowed at this level (*between arrows*). **c** Virtual bronchogram demonstrates narrowing of left main bronchus (*white arrow*)

11.6.1
Tracheobronchomalacia

Tracheobronchomalacia (TBM) refers to a weakness of the central airway walls resulting from deficient elastic or cartilaginous components. This results in softer airways that are more compliant, and which undergo exaggerated changes in luminal diameter during inspiration and expiration. The pathological consequence is expiratory airway collapse. In its primary form, TBM represents the commonest intrinsic tracheal abnormality. Whilst occasionally seen in term infants, TBM most typically occurs in the premature neonate. Primary TBM also occurs in congenital cartilage disorders such as chondro-malacia, chondrodysplasia and polychondritis, and a range of other genetic conditions including the mucopolysaccharidoses and various chromosomal anomalies. The acquired or secondary form occurs in three principal settings: in association with tracheo-oesophageal fistula (many consider this primary), following prolonged intubation and in association with any of the causes of extrinsic compression already described (CARDEN et al. 2005).

The essence of TBM is its dynamic nature, and this renders imaging evaluation challenging in the neonate. The most widely practised imaging technique is conventional bronchography: contrast is injected via an endotracheal tube at various airway pressures, allowing definition of opening pressures for the airways. This allows optimal management. Whilst in principal, CT can also demonstrate airway opening at different pressures (Fig. 11.14), this is not currently a widely used strategy in neonates and infants (MOK et al. 2001). CT in these children maintains a role, however, in identifying extrinsic causes of TBM.

11.6.2
Tracheal Stenosis

11.6.2.1
Congenital Tracheal Stenosis

Congenital tracheal stenosis describes a spectrum of disorders characterized by fixed narrowing of the trachea. These narrowings may involve a

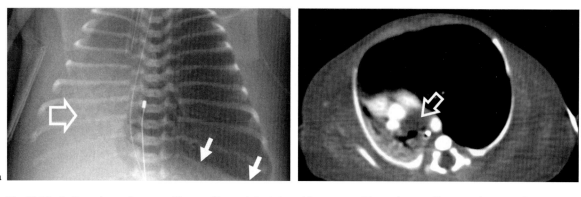

Fig. 11.12a, b. Bronchogenic cyst. **a** Chest radiograph in 1-day-old neonate with respiratory distress. There is collapse of the right lung (*open arrow*) and overinflation of the left lung with flattening of the diaphragm (*white arrows*). **b** Axial CT in same patient just below level of the carina. There is a water density structure anterior to the carina: this is causing obstructive atelectasis of the right lung and overinflation of the left lung. Histological examination confirmed a bronchogenic cyst

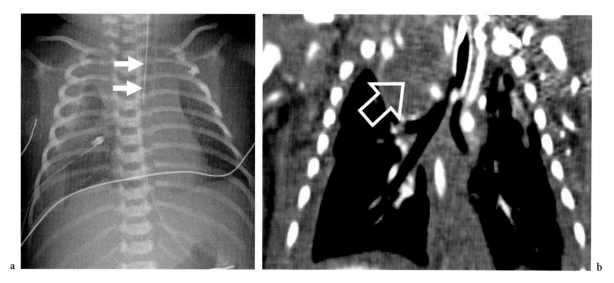

Fig. 11.13a,b. Teratoma. **a** Chest radiograph in 7-day-old neonate requiring emergency intubation. There is a moderate right pleural effusion. There is pronounced displacement of the trachea to the left (*white arrows*). **b** Coronal CT reformat demonstrating right superior mediastinal soft-tissue mass displacing trachea (*open arrow*). Histological evaluation demonstrated intra-thyroidal immature teratoma

short segment or extend over the entire length of the trachea and involve one or both main bronchi. They are typically characterized by the presence of a complete tracheal cartilaginous ring or rings. Congenital stenoses are frequently associated with other anomalies, the commonest being tracheal bronchus, pulmonary artery sling and agenetic lung. Tracheomalacia often co-exists. As with tracheomalacia, contrast bronchography and bronchoscopy are the principle investigations in identifying and characterizing these disorders. The main role of CT again is to identify associated anomalies, particularly vascular anomalies such as pulmonary artery sling. The presence of a complete cartilaginous ring typically produces a very rounded appearance to the airway on axial section at the level of narrowing, as opposed to the normal ovoid appearance (Fig. 11.15). Short stenoses may be managed by simple resection and end-to-end anastomosis, although balloon dilatation combined with laser therapy, and stenting have also been used. Longer stenoses are typically treated by slide tracheoplasty (ANTON-PACHECO et al. 2006; ELLIOTT et al. 2003).

11.6.2.2
Acquired Tracheal Stenosis

Tracheal stenosis also occurs as a complication of prolonged endotracheal intubation, particularly in the setting of prematurity and tracheal infection. Presentation may be delayed beyond infancy. Imaging strategies and management are similar to those for congenital stenoses.

11.7
Peripheral Airway

11.7.1
Congenital Bronchial Anomalies

11.7.1.1
Anatomical Variants

Anatomical variants and anomalies of tracheobronchial division are common, being identified in as many as 12% of diagnostic studies, but are frequently asymptomatic. The most commonly encountered are the tracheal bronchus and the accessory cardiac bronchus.

11.7.1.1.1
Tracheal Bronchus

The term tracheal bronchus is used to encompass a range of conditions whereby a bronchial structure arises anomalously from the trachea, carina or proximal main bronchi and is directed towards the upper lobes. These occur much more commonly on the right. The bronchus may replace the normal upper lobe bronchus, in which case it is called a replaced tracheal bronchus, or pig bronchus (Fig. 11.16). Alternatively, the tracheal bronchus may be present in addition to a normal upper lobe bronchial supply, termed an accessory tracheal bronchus: this may be blind ending. A tracheal bronchus is frequently an isolated and incidental finding; however, it may occasionally be symptomatic if drainage is impaired, usually manifesting as recurrent respiratory infection. A tracheal bronchus is also found with increased frequency in association with other anomalies, including partial anomalous pulmonary venous drainage, and pulmonary artery sling (GHAYE et al. 2001).

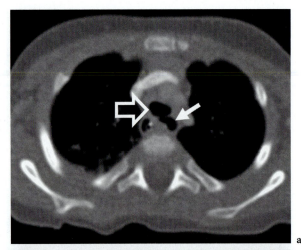

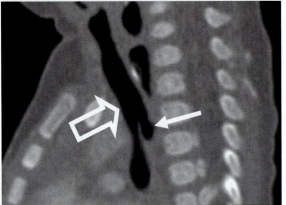

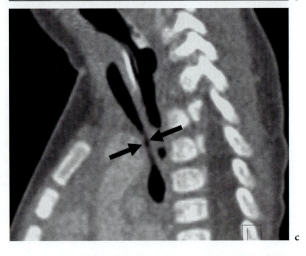

Fig. 11.14a–c. Tracheomalacia. Axial (**a**) and sagittal planar reformatted (**b**) CT in inspiration at the level of the upper trachea in 6-month-old infant with stridor following repair of oesophageal atresia and tracheo-oeophageal fistula. The trachea has an irregular contour (*open arrow*), with a large tracheal diverticulum at the site of repair (*white arrow*). **c** Sagittal plane reformat in expiration demonstrates almost complete collapse of the trachea

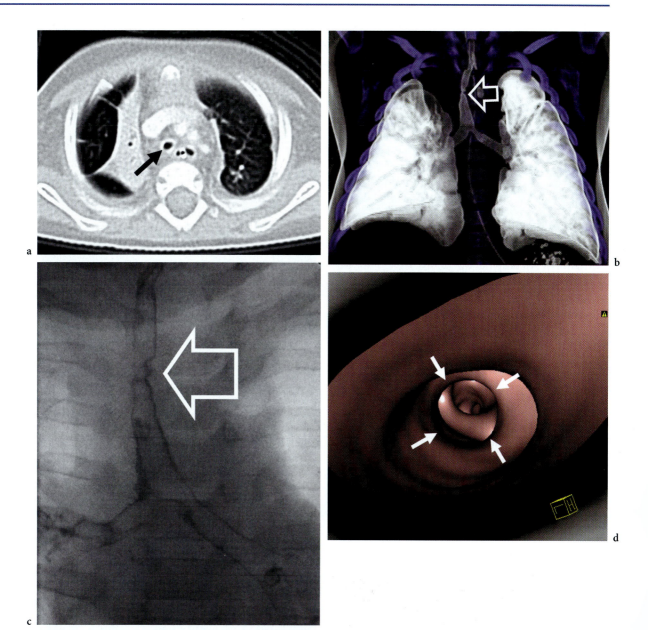

Fig. 11.15a–d. Congenital tracheal stenosis. **a** Axial CT image in 6-month-old infant with stridor, and complete tracheal rings on bronchoscopy. The trachea adopts a very rounded morphology at the level of a stenosis (*black arrow*). **b** Virtual and **c** contrast bronchography demonstrate area of stenosis (*open arrows*). **d** Virtual bronchoscopy shows the rounded morphology of the tracheal lumen at the level of tracheal stenosis (*arrows*) suggestive of a complete ring

11.7.1.1.2
Accessory Cardiac Bronchus

An accessory cardiac bronchus is a supernumerary bronchus arising from the medial wall of the right main bronchus or bronchus intermedius, opposite the origin of the right upper lobe bronchus. It is usually blind ending. Again this anomaly is typically asymptomatic but may act as a focus for recurrent infection.

11.7.1.2
Bronchial Atresia

This condition, which typically presents beyond the neonatal period, results from abnormal development of a segmental bronchus. This results in accumulation of mucoid secretions in the bronchus distal to the obstruction, and obstructive overinfla-

tion of the lung parenchyma supplied by that bronchus, as a result of collateral air drift. The typical imaging appearance is of an overinflated lung segment or lobe, with a tubular or nodular mass, sometimes containing an air-fluid level, at the apex of the overinflated lung (Fig. 11.17). The condition is also known as a congenital bronchocoele. Although often asymptomatic, there is a pathological and radiological overlap with the more frequently symptomatic conditions of congenital lobar emphysema and congenital cystic adenomatoid malformations (MORIKAWA et al. 2005).

11.7.2
Lung Malformations

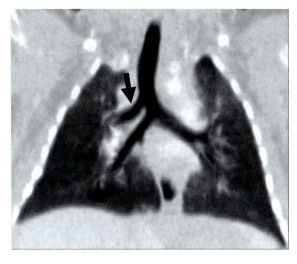

Fig. 11.16. Tracheal bronchus. Minimal intensity projection image in the coronal plane in a 3-month-old infant with congenital spinal anomalies. The right upper lobe bronchus arises from the trachea: this exclusively supplies the whole right upper lobe, a true "pig bronchus"

Many of the disorders, which are conventionally defined as pulmonary parenchymal malformations, also involve the peripheral airway; whilst these are considered in detail elsewhere (see Chaps. 8 and 9), we will review two of these conditions here.

11.7.2.1
Congenital Lobar Overinflation

Congenital lobar overinflation (CLO, or congenital lobar emphysema: the former term is preferred as there is no destruction of alveolar walls in this condition) is not traditionally considered a neonatal airway anomaly, and is considered in detail in Chapter 9. However, there is considerable evidence that the primary abnormality in most cases of CLO is an abnormality of the lobar bronchus: this may be focal bronchomalacia, bronchial atresia or a web, or extrinsic compression. Indeed, many of the conditions causing extrinsic airway compression that we

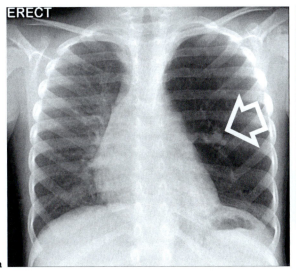

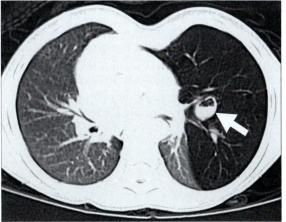

Fig. 11.17a,b. Bronchial atresia. **a** Chest radiograph in 5-year-old child with recurrent respiratory infections. The left upper lobe is overinflated and hypertransradiant. A tubular structure is projected adjacent to the left hilum. **b** Axial CT in the same patient: the left upper lobe is overinflated and there is a dilated segment of the left upper lobe bronchus containing a fluid level – a congenital bronchocoele

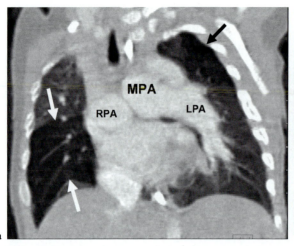 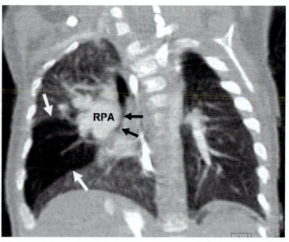

Fig. 11.18a,b. Lobar overinflation in extrinsic bronchial compression. **a** Coronal MPR in 4-month-old child with absent pulmonary valve syndrome: the main pulmonary artery (*MPA*) and left and right pulmonary arteries (*LPA/RPA*) are massively dilated. The right middle lobe is hypertransradiant and overinflated due to air trapping (*white arrows*). There is segmental overinflation within the left upper lobe (*black arrow*). **b** More posterior coronal MPR shows narrowing of the right middle lobe bronchus by the dilated *RPA* (*black arrows*) and overinflation of the right middle lobe Legends

have already considered may result in air-trapping and overinflation, which, for all intents and purposes, is a form of congenital lobar overinflation (Fig. 11.18).

11.7.2.2
Congenital Cystic Adenomatoid Malformation

Similarly, congenital cystic adenomatoid malformation (CCAM) is typically considered a lung malformation rather than an airway abnormality (see Chap. 9). There is, again, evidence that CCAM also results from a bronchial abnormality: bronchial atresia was identified in 69% of resected specimens of CCAM in a recent study (KUNISAKI et al. 2006). It is hypothesized that the insult to lung development occurs at an earlier stage in CCAM than in CLO or bronchial atresia.

11.8
Conclusions

Multidetector CT plays a central role in the modern evaluation of the neonate or infant with suspected airway abnormalities. It is particularly useful in assessing vascular tracheobronchial compression syndromes, allowing simultaneous detailed vascular imaging along with imaging of the airways and pulmonary parenchyma, with short imaging times.

References

Anton-Pacheco JL, Cano I, Comas J, Galletti L, Polo L, Garcia A, Lopez M, Cabezali D (2006) Management of congenital tracheal stenosis in infancy. Eur J Cardiothorac Surg 29(6):991–996

Backer CL, Mavroudis C (2000) Congenital heart surgery nomenclature and database project: vascular rings, tracheal stenosis, pectus excavatum. Ann Thorac Surg 69 [4 Suppl]:S308–S318

Berdon WE (2000) Rings, slings, and other things: vascular compression of the infant trachea updated from the midcentury to the millennium – the legacy of Robert E. Gross, MD, and Edward B. D. Neuhauser, MD. Radiology 216(3):624–632

Callahan CW (1998) Primary tracheomalacia and gastroesophageal reflux in infants with cough. Clin Pediatr (Phila) 37(12):725–731

Carden KA, Boiselle PM, Waltz DA, Ernst A (2005) Tracheomalacia and tracheobronchomalacia in children and adults: an in-depth review. Chest 127(3):984–1005

Edwards J (1948a) Vascular rings related to anomalies of aortic arch system. Mod Concepts Cardiovasc Dis 17:19–20

Edwards J (1948b) Anomalies of the derivatives of the aortic arch system. Med Clin North Am 32:925–949

Elliott M, Roebuck D, Noctor C, McLaren C, Hartley B, Mok Q, Dunne C, Pigott N, Patel C, Patel A, Wallis C (2003) The management of congenital tracheal stenosis. Int J Pediatr Otorhinolaryngol 67 [Suppl 1]:S183–192

Faust RA, Rimell FL, Remley KB (2002) Cine magnetic resonance imaging for evaluation of focal tracheomalacia: innominate artery compression syndrome. Int J Pediatr Otorhinolaryngol 65(1):27–33

Ghaye B, Szapiro D, Fanchamps JM, Dondelinger RF (2001) Congenital bronchial abnormalities revisited. Radiographics 21(1):105–119

Gross RE (1945) Surgical relief for tracheal obstruction from a vascular ring. N Engl J Med 233:586–590

Hernanz-Schulman M (2005) Vascular rings: a practical approach to imaging diagnosis. Pediatr Radiol 35(10):961–979

Honnef D, Wildberger JE, Das M, Hohl C, Mahnken AH, Barker M, Gunther RW, Staatz G (2006) Value of virtual tracheobronchoscopy and bronchography from 16-slice multidetector-row spiral computed tomography for assessment of suspected tracheobronchial stenosis in children. Eur Radiol 16(8):1684–1691

Kunisaki SM, Fauza DO, Nemes LP, Barnewolt CE, Estroff JA, Kozakewich HP, Jennings RW (2006) Bronchial atresia: the hidden pathology within a spectrum of prenatally diagnosed lung masses. J Pediatr Surg 41(1):61–65

Mok Q, Negus S, McLaren CA, Rajka T, Elliott MJ, Roebuck DJ, McHugh K (2005) Computed tomography versus bronchography in the diagnosis and management of tracheobronchomalacia in ventilator dependent infants. Arch Dis Child Fetal Neonatal Ed 90(4):F290–F293

Morikawa N, Kuroda T, Honna T, Kitano Y, Fuchimoto Y, Terawaki K, Kawasaki K, Koinuma G, Matsuoka K, Saeki M (2005) Congenital bronchial atresia in infants and children. J Pediatr Surg 40(12):1822–1826

Norgaard MA, Alphonso N, Newcomb AE, Brizard CP, Cochrane AD (2006) Absent pulmonary valve syndrome. Surgical and clinical outcome with long-term follow-up. Eur J Cardiothorac Surg 29(5):682–687

Oddone M, Granata C, Vercellino N, Bava E, Toma P (2005) Multi-modality evaluation of the abnormalities of the aortic arches in children: techniques and imaging spectrum with emphasis on MRI. Pediatr Radiol 35(10):947–960

Pacharn P, Poe SA, Donnelly LF (2002) Low-tube-current multidetector CT for children with suspected extrinsic airway compression. AJR Am J Roentgenol 179(6):1523–1527

Patel CR, Lane JR, Spector ML, Smith PC (2006) Fetal echocardiographic diagnosis of vascular rings. J Ultrasound Med 25(2):251–257

Schlesinger AE, Krishnamurthy R, Sena LM, Guillerman RP, Chung T, DiBardino DJ, Fraser CD Jr. (2005) Incomplete double aortic arch with atresia of the distal left arch: distinctive imaging appearance. AJR Am J Roentgenol 184(5):1634–1639

Shell R, Allen E, Mutabagani K, Long F, Davis JT, McCoy K, Castile R (2001) Compression of the trachea by the innominate artery in a 2-month-old child. Pediatr Pulmonol 31(1):80–85

Taragin BH, Berdon WE, Printz B (2006) MRI assessment of bronchial compression in absent pulmonary valve syndrome and review of the syndrome. Pediatr Radiol 36(1):71–75

Turner A, Gavel G, Coutts J (2005) Vascular rings – presentation, investigation and outcome. Eur J Pediatr 164(5):266–270

Walters HL (2005) Vascular tracheoesophageal compressive syndromes: a surgeon's view. Pediatr Radiol 35(10):945–946

Yamagishi H, Maeda J, Higuchi M, Katada Y, Yamagishi C, Matsuo N, Kojima Y (2002) Bronchomalacia associated with pulmonary atresia, ventricular septal defect and major aortopulmonary collateral arteries, and chromosome 22q11.2 deletion. Clin Genet 62(3):214–219

Ultrasound of the Neonatal Thorax

12

Ingmar Gassner and Theresa E. Geley

12.1 Introduction

As reflected by the other issues in this volume diseases of the newborn chest are commonly evaluated by means of the three dominant imaging modalities: conventional chest radiographs, computed tomography (CT) and magnetic resonance (MR).

Thorax ultrasound is not often performed mainly because bone and air are traditionally considered natural barriers for the ultrasound beam. However, the unique thoracic anatomy of the neonate as well as certain pathologic conditions provides many acoustic windows into the chest. Little effort is needed to evaluate and diagnose a wide range of clinical problems in the thorax without the radiation exposure from frequent chest radiographs and CT, or the need for sedation sometimes required for CT and MR imaging. In particular, ultrasound is quickly implemented in the remote intensive care situation where patients can be examined in any given position and location minimizing the need to move or transfer patients who are on life support devices.

Ultrasound is particularly useful in differentiating pulmonary from pleural lesions, in visualizing diseased parenchyma hidden by a pleural effusion on chest radiographs, and in detecting and characterizing pleural fluid collections. It can also delineate anomalies of mediastinum and great vessels and, last but not least, assess malposition and complications of central vein catheters.

12.2 Technique

To correlate findings it is always helpful to review the patient's most recent chest radiograph prior to ultra-

I. GASSNER, MD; T. E. GELEY, MD
Department of Pediatrics, University Hospital Innsbruck, Anichstrasse 35, 6020 Innsbruck, Austria

sound examination. In general transducers are selected according to the size of the patient and position of the lesion being evaluated. Small infants and neonates are easily examined with high-frequency linear or sector transducers. Small transducers are valuable to insonate from the supraclavicular or suprasternal notch. Manoeuvring the patient into different positions will delineate the position dependency of a lesion and can help to move intestinal air out of sight. It may be helpful for the abdominal approach to feed the pa-

tient prior to or during examination, since a fluid-filled stomach provides an excellent acoustic window.

12.2.1
Imaging Approach to the Mediastinum

To analyse mediastinal structures a supraclavicular, suprasternal, transsternal, parasternal, subcostal and subxiphoidal approach is used (Fig. 12.1).

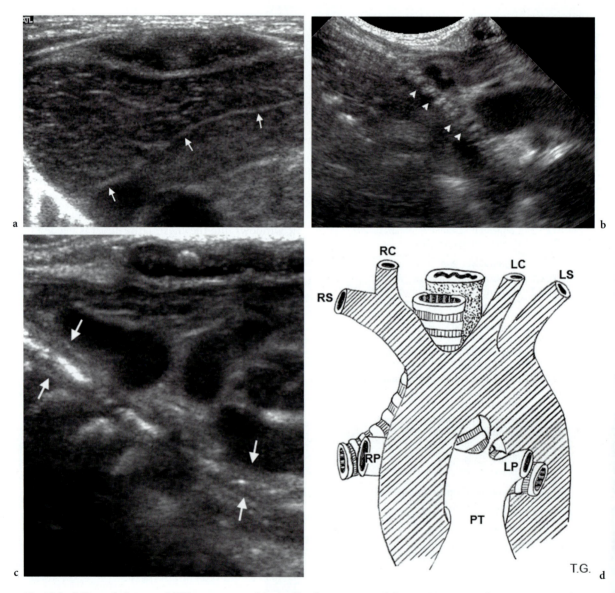

Fig. 12.1a–i. Normal ultrasound (US) appearance of the mediastinum. **a** Normal thymus. Transsternal transverse scan shows the normal echo pattern with multiple linear echogenic lines and foci. *Arrows* Border of the two thymic lobes. **b** Suprasternal longitudinal scan shows the trachea with the echo-poor cartilages (*arrowheads*). **c** Transsternal longitudinal scan demonstrates the oesophagus (*arrows*) with echogenic mucosa and submucosa, sonolucent muscle and intraluminal air. **d** Normal left aortic arch. Schematic diagram.

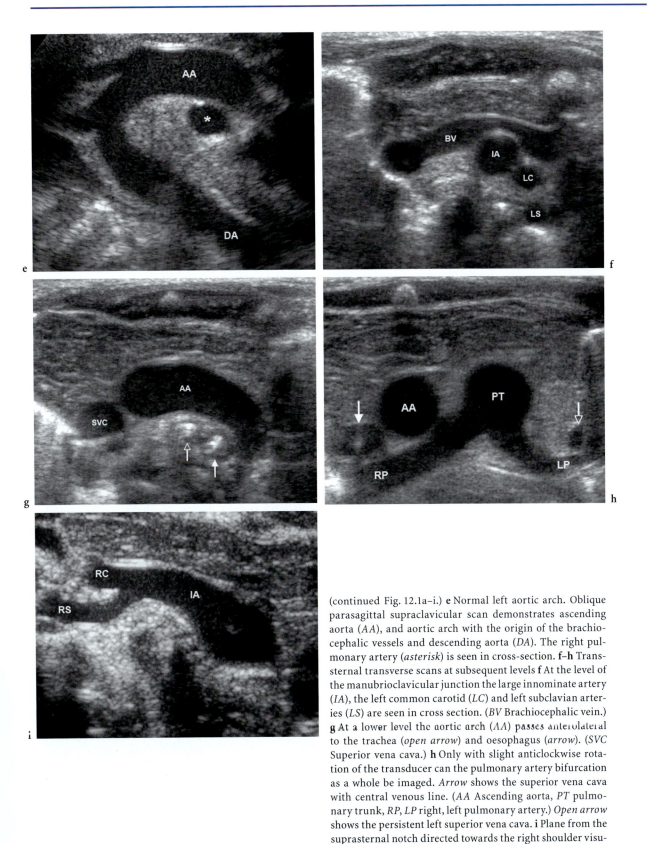

(continued Fig. 12.1a–i.) **e** Normal left aortic arch. Oblique parasagittal supraclavicular scan demonstrates ascending aorta (*AA*), and aortic arch with the origin of the brachiocephalic vessels and descending aorta (*DA*). The right pulmonary artery (*asterisk*) is seen in cross-section. **f–h** Transsternal transverse scans at subsequent levels **f** At the level of the manubrioclavicular junction the large innominate artery (*IA*), the left common carotid (*LC*) and left subclavian arteries (*LS*) are seen in cross section. (*BV* Brachiocephalic vein.) **g** At a lower level the aortic arch (*AA*) passes anterolateral to the trachea (*open arrow*) and oesophagus (*arrow*). (*SVC* Superior vena cava.) **h** Only with slight anticlockwise rotation of the transducer can the pulmonary artery bifurcation as a whole be imaged. *Arrow* shows the superior vena cava with central venous line. (*AA* Ascending aorta, *PT* pulmonary trunk, *RP*, *LP* right, left pulmonary artery.) *Open arrow* shows the persistent left superior vena cava. **i** Plane from the suprasternal notch directed towards the right shoulder visualizes the innominate artery (*IA*) and its bifurcation into the right subclavian (*RS*) and right carotid (*RC*) artery

Transsternal views are obtained with the transducer placed directly over the sternum. In neonates and small infants sternum as well as ribs are predominantly cartilaginous and, therefore, allow ultrasound transmission.

A supraclavicular or suprasternal approach is best performed with a helping hand lifting the patient's shoulders to extend the neck naturally. If no helper is available, the patient's head is turned to the contralateral side to free access to the region. The transducer is placed above the sternum or clavicle and tilted posteriorly. This position offers high flexibility for documenting mediastinal structures in different planes.

Axial and sagittal parasternal views are acquired with the transducer positioned next to the sternum as the patient lies in the supine position.

Subcostal or subxiphoidal ultrasound access is a transducer position immediately below the xiphoid process and along the lower border of the thoracic cage. Transverse, coronal and sagittal scans image intrathoracic pathology, the spine, inferior vena cava and the aorta, and determine the situs.

12.2.2
Imaging Approach to Pleura, Diaphragm and Lung

Most of the pleura is superficial and readily examined by subcostal, intercostal or subxiphoidal scans. Liver and spleen provide good through transmission and are used as acoustic windows. The air-filled lung covered by visceral pleura blocks sound penetration deeper into the chest and produces a bright, linear interface that moves with respiration ("gliding sign") (TARGHETTA et al. 1992).

Horizontal artefacts are often seen when studying the pleura. They are caused by reflection of the sound waves at the pleura–lung interface surface and are seen as a series of echogenic parallel lines equidistant from one another below the pleural line. In addition, vertically oriented "comet tail" artefacts can be seen created by the fluid-rich subpleural interlobular septae, which are surrounded by air (LICHTENSTEIN et al. 1997, 1999). When the lung above the diaphragm is air filled the curved surface of the diaphragm-lung interface acts as a mirror-like reflector. Longitudinal subcostal images through the liver therefore show an artefactual mirror-image reflection of the liver or spleen above the diaphragm. Changing the transducer position will de-

lineate the artefact. Retrohepatic hyperechogenicity in newborns that does not change with transducer position, however, is a pathognomic sign of hyaline membrane disease (AVNI et al. 1990).

The diaphragm is imaged by intercostal, subcostal, or subxiphoidal approaches that use liver, spleen and fluid-filled stomach as acoustic windows. The examination is performed with the child in quiet respiration. For comparison of movements in cases of diaphragmatic paralysis, a subxiphoidal approach with the transducer tilted cephalad will document both diaphragms within the same scan (Fig. 12.2).

12.3
Mediastinum

12.3.1
Thymus, Trachea, Oesophagus

12.3.1.1
Thymus

The thymus is the most dominant noncardiac structure in the infant chest (Fig. 12.1a). Although changes in size, configuration and position occur with patient age, recognition of the thymus on ultrasound is easy due to its characteristic appear-

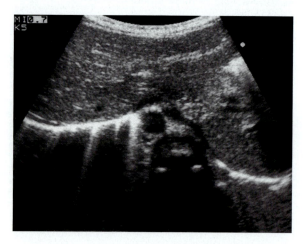

Fig. 12.2. Paralysis of the left hemidiaphragm in a 1-day-old boy with brachial plexus injury (Erb's palsy) at birth (breech delivery). Transverse scan with the transducer angled cephalad allows comparison of the movement of both hemidiaphragms. During inspiration the left hemidiaphragm moves cranially (paradoxical motion)

ance (FRANCO et al. 2005). It is bilobulated, with homogenous echogenicity slightly less than that of the thyroid gland and isoechoic to the liver, with some regular linear and punctate echogenicities most likely representing connective tissue (HAN et al. 2001). It is hypovascular on Doppler imaging and has a well-defined margin. Even when large, the thymus does not compress or displace neighbouring vascular structures. One important characteristic of the thymus is that the gland responds to acute physiologic stress with rapid and severe involution (BENDON and COVENTRY 2004). It regenerates weeks to months after the cessation of the stress and may then be enlarged due to "rebound growth".

Thymic aplasia or hypoplasia is found with 22q11.2 deletion syndrome, a disorder caused by the deletion of a small piece of chromosome 22. The syndrome is characterized by cardiac defects, abnormal facial features, thymic hypoplasia, cleft palate, and hypocalcemia. It is not a simple disease and the features of the syndrome vary widely. Because of this symptom variety, different groupings of features were once described as separate conditions. Authors refer to these as the CATCH 22 syndrome and include anomalies such as velo-cardio-facial syndrome, DiGeorge syndrome, hearing loss with craniofacial syndromes and conotruncal anomaly face syndrome (YONEHARA et al. 2002). Mediastinal ultrasound will document agenesis or hypoplasia of the thymus and associated cardiac and aortic arch anomalies.

In hypocalcemic newborns the thymus may be small from perinatal stress alone. The lack of associated malformations in these cases speaks against CATCH 22 syndrome as a differential diagnosis (BEN-AMI et al. 1993).

Congenital position anomalies of the thymus are classified as aberrant or ectopic. The normal pathway of the thymic descent is from the angle of the mandible to the superior mediastinum. Rarely the thymus fails to descend or descends incompletely. In this case, entire or partial thymus remains in the cervical region (BEN-AMI et al. 1993; TOVI and MARES 1978). Remnants of thymic tissue can be found in any location along the normal pathway of descent (aberrant thymus) or in any other location (ectopic thymus), i.e. posterior neck or mediastinum, pharynx, larynx, trachea, or oesophagus, occasionally causing compression or displacement of adjacent mediastinal structures (BAYSAL et al. 1999). Aberrant thymus predominantly presents as a bulging cervical or suprasternal mass. Ultrasound documents similar echogenicity and often shows continuity to the normally positioned thymus (SPIGLAND et al. 1990).

Thymic haemorrhage causes sudden widening of the mediastinal shadow on chest radiographs and is associated with haemorrhagic disease of the newborn or complicating cardiac surgery. Ultrasound features closely resemble those of haemorrhage in liver or spleen (LEMAITRE et al. 1989).

12.3.1.2
Trachea

On a longitudinal scan the wall of the trachea has the appearance of a necklace due to the echopoor cartilages and is, therefore, easily identified (Fig. 12.1b). The trachea and the oesophagus run together in the midline and both can be used to determine the midline of the mediastinum. A significant shift of the trachea to one side of the chest may be a due to hypoplasia or agenesis of the lung as well as atelectasis of lung parenchyma on the ipsilateral side of the shift or a mass on the contralateral side.

Of clinical relevance in the neonatal period is congenital short or long segment tracheal stenosis, a rare disorder characterized by the presence of focal or diffuse complete tracheal cartilage rings (BERROCAL et al. 2004). Neonates with congenital tracheal stenosis present with respiratory distress and either cannot be intubated or cannot be weaned off a ventilator. Ultrasound may reveal complete cartilage rings on axial scans. Long segment tracheal stenosis may be associated with pulmonary artery sling and ultrasound can delineate this association as described below (Fig. 12.3).

Haemangioma, a congenital anomalous proliferation of blood vessels, can occur in isolation or in groups anywhere in the body, most frequently in the skin and subcutaneous tissue. A localization within the epithelial and subepithelial lining of the trachea is rare but may result in tracheal stenosis (Fig. 12.4) (RAHBAR et al. 2004). When large, the haemangioma infiltrates the soft tissue around the trachea or the thyroid gland. Ultrasound documents the characteristic features of haemangioma with rather homogenous ultrasonographic echogenicity with varying numbers of hypoechoic sinusoids. Draining and feeding vessels may be identified. Blood flow, documented with colour flow Doppler, varies between exuberant and barely detectable.

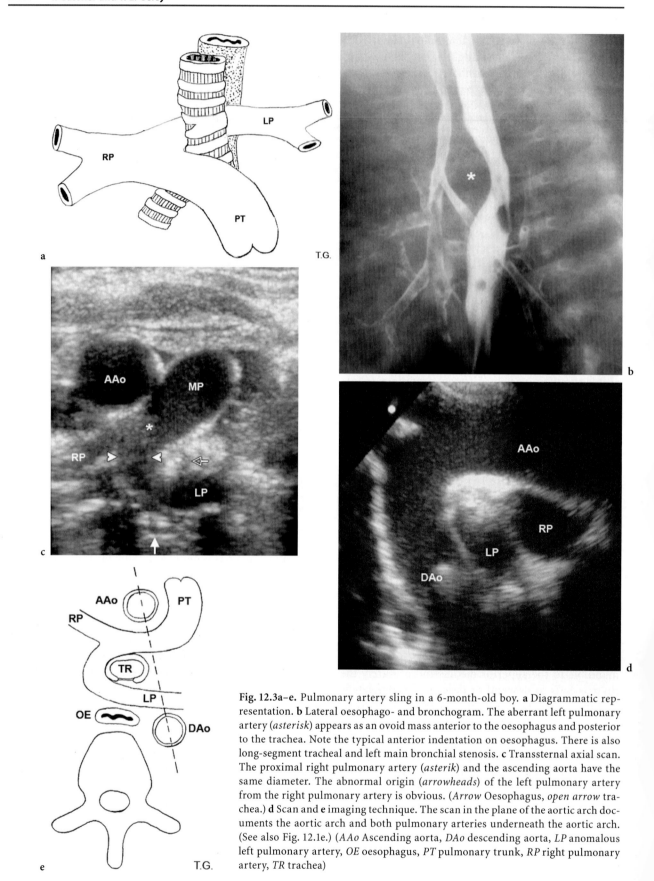

Fig. 12.3a–e. Pulmonary artery sling in a 6-month-old boy. **a** Diagrammatic representation. **b** Lateral oesophago- and bronchogram. The aberrant left pulmonary artery (*asterisk*) appears as an ovoid mass anterior to the oesophagus and posterior to the trachea. Note the typical anterior indentation on oesophagus. There is also long-segment tracheal and left main bronchial stenosis. **c** Transsternal axial scan. The proximal right pulmonary artery (*asterik*) and the ascending aorta have the same diameter. The abnormal origin (*arrowheads*) of the left pulmonary artery from the right pulmonary artery is obvious. (*Arrow* Oesophagus, *open arrow* trachea.) **d** Scan and **e** imaging technique. The scan in the plane of the aortic arch documents the aortic arch and both pulmonary arteries underneath the aortic arch. (See also Fig. 12.1e.) (*AAo* Ascending aorta, *DAo* descending aorta, *LP* anomalous left pulmonary artery, *OE* oesophagus, *PT* pulmonary trunk, *RP* right pulmonary artery, *TR* trachea)

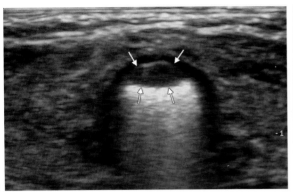

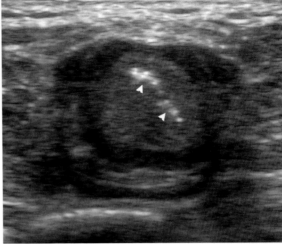

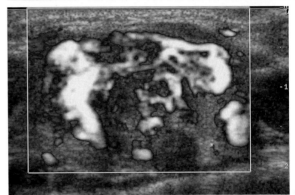

Fig. 12.4a–c. Subglottic hemangioma in a 2-month-old girl with stridor. **a** Subglottic transverse scan at the age of 2 months reveals narrowing of the tracheal lumen by a polypoid anterior intratracheal mass (*arrows*). Tracheostomy was performed. **b** Six months later, the size of the haemangioma has dramatically increased and it compresses the tracheal lumen to a small gap (*arrowheads*). **c** Colour Doppler shows the high vascularity and the involvement of the adjacent soft tissues (i.e. thyroid)

12.3.1.3
Oesophagus

The oesophagus is a muscular tube with echogenic mucosa and submucosa and sonolucent muscle (Fig. 12.1c). It usually contains a mixture of liquid and air whose movement can be visualized by ultrasound imaging. Visualization of the oesophagus can be enhanced when the patient swallows fluid. Retrograde flow of fluid and air bubbles, seen as echogenic reflections, into the oesophageal lumen demonstrates gastro-oesophageal reflux. Oesophageal anomalies of clinical relevance during the neonatal period are oesophageal atresia and tracheo-oesophgeal fistula and oesophageal duplication.

Oesophageal atresia and tracheo-oesophageal fistula (TEF) are the most common congenital malformations of the oesophagus (Figs. 12.5, 12.6) (McCook and Felman 1978). Associated anomalies such as right aortic arch, congenital heart disease, gastrointestinal anomalies and the VA(C)TER(L) complex (vertebral defects, anal atresia, TEF, radial aplasia, renal dysplasia and cardiac and limb anomalies) are frequent and significantly influence prognosis. Isolated TEF are less frequent and present later than those with atresia. Antenatal ultrasound diagnosis of oesophageal atresia is possible in one-third of patients. All others may have a tracheo-oesophageal communication that is large enough to allow passage of amniotic fluid resulting in normal gastric fluid and absent polyhydramnios (Stringer et al. 1995). In the majority of patients the atresia is between the proximal and middle third of the oesophagus in association with a distal fistula.

Ultrasound allows documentation of the length, configuration and wall condition of the blind upper pouch. Instillation of a small amount of fluid may be used to distend the pouch. The same feature of moving air bubbles during fluoroscopy ("atomiser" sign) (Deffrenne et al. 1970) may be documented with ultrasound, reflected in tiny hyperechoic spots that move in the soft tissue between the trachea and the oesophagus or ascend within the oesophagus. In addition, ultrasound may delineate features of the fistula's wall (Gassner and Geley 2005).

Oesophageal duplication is caused by abnormal embryological development in which islands of cells are sequestered from the primitive foregut (Fig. 12.7). Most often duplications are spherical cysts and symptoms in the newborn and infant are due to pressure on the adjacent lung or oesophagus leading to respiratory difficulties or dysphagia and vomiting (Eichmann et al. 2001; Sodhi et al. 2005). Association of oesophageal duplication cysts with pulmonary cystic malformations, oesophageal atresia and vertebral defects have been described (Narasimharao and Mitra 1987; Snyder et al. 1996). Ultrasound demonstrates a fluid-filled cystic structure and continuity of the muscularis propria of the oesophagus with the muscle layer of the cyst wall (Bhutani et al. 1996).

Differentiation between oesophageal duplication cysts and neuroenteric cysts may at times be difficult. Neuroenteric cysts, however, are frequently associated with anomalies of the vertebral column and the spinal canal and its contents. Therefore, we strongly recommend sonography of the spinal cord.

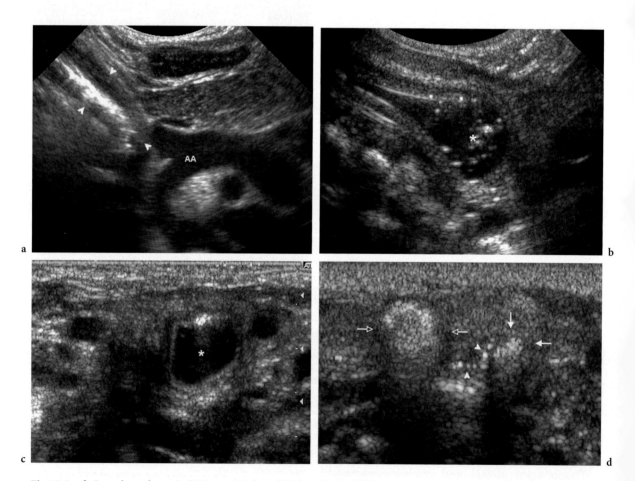

Fig. 12.5a–d. Oesophageal atresia (*OA*). **a–c** A 1-day-old boy with type III b OA: **a** Suprasternal longitudinal scan shows the nondistended proximal pouch (*arrowheads*) ending at the level of the aortic arch (*AA*). After filling with saline solution **a** the suprasternal longitudinal scan and the **c** transverse scan clearly demonstrate the distended oesophageal pouch (*asterisk*). **d** A 1-day-old girl with type III OA with two proximal and no distal tracheo-oesophageal fistulae (*TEF*). Suprasternal transverse scan shows moving air bubbles (*arrowheads*) between the trachea (*open arrows*) and oesophagus (*arrows*) indicating a proximal TEF (see also Fig. 12.6b)

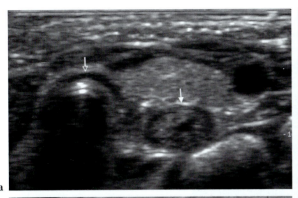

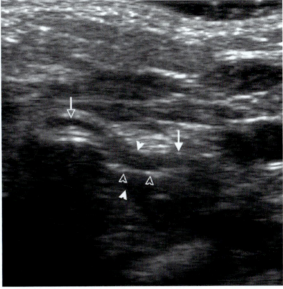

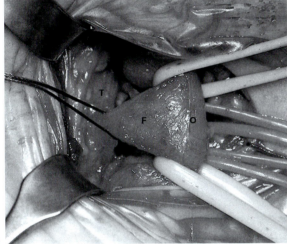

Fig. 12.6a–c. H-type tracheo-oesophageal fistula (*TEF*) in a 3-week-old girl. **a** Suprasternal transverse scan. The trachea (*open arrow*) and proximal oesophagus (*arrow*) lie side by side. **b** Suprasternal transverse scan. Moving air bubbles (*open arrowheads*) between the trachea (*open arrow*) and oesophagus (*arrow*) indicate a tracheo-oesophageal fistula. The wall of the fistula is also clearly visible (*arrowheads*). **c** Photograph taken at time of surgery shows the fistula (*F*), oesophagus (*O*), and trachea (*T*) (by courtesy of Dr. Murat Sanal, Innsbruck)

12.3.2
Heart and Great Vessels

12.3.2.1
Imaging Approach

The cardiovascular structures in the middle mediastinum can be well assessed with the suprasternal, supraclavicular, transsternal, parasternal, subcostal, and subxiphoidal approaches (Fig. 12.1).

Ultrasound assessment of cardiovascular structures identifies on a high transverse scan the aortic arch branches in cross-section: the large innominate artery, and two smaller vessels, the left common carotid and left subclavian artery (Fig. 12.1f). Directly anterior runs the left brachiocephalic vein. At a lower level the left-sided aortic arch passes from right to left, anterolateral to trachea and oesophagus (Fig. 12.1g). A transverse scan just below visualizes simultaneously the right superior vena cava, ascending aorta, main pulmonary artery and right pulmonary artery. Because the left pulmonary artery runs more cephalad than the right, the pulmonary artery

bifurcation as a whole can only be imaged by slight anticlockwise rotation of the transducer (Fig. 12.1h). On a coronal scan from the suprasternal fossa the aortic arch is cut in cross-section. Above it is the left innominate vein that joins the superior vena cava. The right pulmonary artery runs beneath the aortic arch and behind the superior vena cava. Oblique sagittal images demonstrate the ascending aorta, aortic arch with commonly three brachiocephalic branches and proximal descending aorta on a single image (Fig. 12.1e). The right pulmonary artery runs below the arch and is seen in cross-section. A midline marker such as the trachea or the oesophagus must be identified to determine the side of the aortic arch (Fig. 12.1b,c). In cases of oesophageal atresia the proximal oesophageal pouch is unreliable for determining the midline, and the trachea must be used instead. The side of the aortic arch may also be determined by visualization of a right or left innominate artery. A plane that is directed towards the right shoulder from the suprasternal notch will visualize the innominate artery and its bifurcation into the right subclavian and carotid artery (Fig. 12.1i).

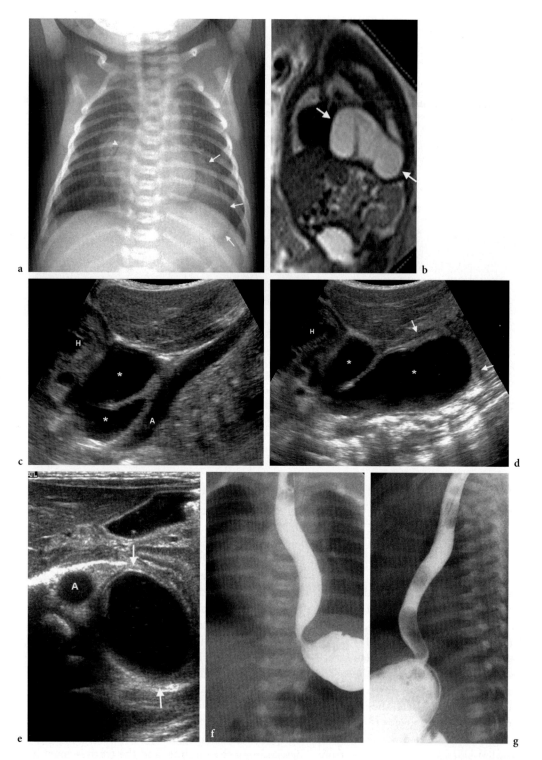

Fig. 12.7a–g. Oesophageal duplication cyst in a 1-day-old boy detected in utero. **a** Chest radiograph reveals a large retrocardial soft tissue mass (*arrow*) compressing the right bronchus (*arrowhead*). **b** Sagittal T$_2$-weighted magnetic resonance image at 33 weeks shows a large retrocardial cyst (*arrows*). **c,d** Sagittal scans and **e** axial scan through liver show a large bilobed cyst (*asterisks*) posterior to the heart (*H*) and in front of the aorta (*A*) which markedly depresses the left hemidiaphragm (*arrows*). **e** The cyst has a well-defined hypoechoic muscular and echogenic mucosal layer and contains multiple echoes (which is seen in duplication cysts). There was no abnormality of the spine and spinal cord. **f** Frontal and **g** lateral oesophagram. The oesophagus is deviated to the left and ventrally by the cyst. There is no communication between the cyst and the gastrointestinal tract

A right innominate artery implies a left aortic arch and vice versa. With an anomalous right subclavian artery only the right carotid branch is seen.

In the sagittal right parasternal scan the ascending aorta, superior vena cava and azygos vein entering the posterior aspect of the superior vena cava are visualized.

Subcostal transverse and sagittal scans image the spine, inferior vena cava and the entire thoracic aorta. In addition, azygos continuation of the inferior vena cava can be diagnosed.

When studying patients with vascular anomalies it is of great importance to delineate deviations from the norm. Only three ultrasound scans are needed to reliably document normal anatomy. The first scan has to document the aortic arch to be left-sided, i.e. left to trachea and oesophagus and gives rise to three main vessels. This feature excludes a right aortic arch and a double aortic arch. The second scan has to show a normal pulmonary artery bifurcation and thus excludes a pulmonary artery sling and anomalies of the proximal pulmonary arteries. The third scan finally delineates either normal branching of the right innominate artery or three main vessels leaving the aortic arch with the first being the largest and thus excludes an aberrant subclavian artery. Patient presenting with clinical signs of stridor, however, should always undergo additional barium swallow fluoroscopy if there are any doubts about the present vascular anatomy. MR imaging and/or CT should be only used to further delineate an existing anomaly.

12.3.2.2
Congenital Vascular Anomalies

Congenital vascular anomalies such as right aortic arch with aberrant left subclavian artery, double aortic arch, aberrant left pulmonary artery and anomalous pulmonary venous return including scimitar syndrome are known to have a great impact on related extra cardiac systems (BERROCAL et al. 2004). Not only cardiologists but also the paediatric radiologists are, therefore, compelled to acquire profound knowledge about normal as well as aberrant vascular anatomy of the mediastinum.

Because this section is focused on ultrasound we ask the kind reader to refer to other articles in this volume for a more detailed insight into the subject.

In right aortic arch with aberrant left subclavian artery, a right aortic arch is present together with a right descending aorta (Fig. 12.8), in contrast to the commonly asymptomatic left aortic arch with aberrant right subclavian artery (Fig. 12.9). The aberrant left subclavian artery originates from a Kommerell diverticulum, an enlargement of the take off of the subclavian artery (MOES and FREEDOM 1993). The ductus arteriosus is commonly on the left side and extends from this diverticulum to the left pulmonary artery leading to a vascular ring that may cause tracheo-oesophageal compression in cases where the ductus or ligamentum arteriosum is tight (BERDON 2000). The trachea is displaced to the left. Ultrasound evaluation reveals a right aortic arch and a left carotid artery as a solitary vessel. The presence of an aberrant left subclavian artery is then suspected and demonstrated on a slightly oblique transverse scan. The retro-oesophageal Kommerell diverticulum can be confirmed by delineating the oesophagus.

A double aortic arch shows two arches with the right arch usually being a little larger and slightly higher than the left (Fig. 12.10). The upper descending aorta may be right- or left-sided. Suprasternal sagittal scans demonstrate both arches and their common carotid and subclavian arteries. A clue to diagnosis is that each arch gives rise to only two main vessels. One will notice that the carotid and subclavian arteries are symmetrically arranged on a high transverse scan. With slight clockwise rotation of the transducer the left arch is imaged on the left side of the oesophagus. Rotation of the transducer in the other direction will reveal the right arch on the right side of the oesophagus. Both arches are displayed in cross-section in a suprasternal coronal plane. The complete vascular ring may be shown on a transsternal axial scan.

In anomalous left pulmonary artery also known as pulmonary artery sling, the left pulmonary artery arises from the posterior aspect of the right pulmonary artery and courses behind the trachea and in front of the oesophagus to reach the left lung (Fig. 12.3). Pulmonary artery sling may either be found in association with a basically normal trachea and a normal bronchial branch pattern (Type I) or, more often, with an anomalous tracheal and bronchial structure as well as an anomalous bronchial branching pattern (Type II). In these cases a bridging bronchus that supplies the middle and lower lobes of the right lung arises from the left main bronchus (BERDON 2000; WELLS et al. 1988, 1990). In Type II, chest radiographs show the increased bronchial angle of the bridging bronchus leading to the "inverted T" bronchial pattern of the abnormal low-lying pseudocarina. Both types present clinical signs of airway obstruction which are caused by simple extrinsic compression in Type I, and abnormal tracheal (complete cartilage rings) and bronchial cartilages in Type II. Ultrasound evaluation in the plane of the aortic arch shows both right and aberrant left pulmonary artery in cross-section beneath the aortic arch. In this scan the slightly larger right pulmonary artery is found ventral to the smaller left pulmonary artery. In the axial transsternal scan an abnormal bifurcation of the main pulmonary artery is found. The origin of the left pulmonary artery from the right is found directly or slightly to the left behind the ascending aorta.

In total anomalous pulmonary venous return the pulmonary veins form a single vessel due to abnormal development of the common pulmonary vein (Figs. 12.11, 12.12). The pulmonary veins unite posterior to the heart to join the right-sided circulation (Harris and Valmorida 1997). According to the drainage four types of lesions are described: Type I (supracardiac connection), the common pulmonary vein joins the persistent left superior vena cava on the left or the azygos vein on the right; Type II (cardiac connection), the common pulmonary vein drains into the right atrium; Type III (infracardiac connection), the common pulmonary vein inserts into a systemic abdominal vein, most frequently into the portal vein; and Type IV, a mixture of the first three types. Type I and Type III have characteristic radiological features that guide the paediatric radiologist through subsequent ultrasound analyses. In Type I the line up of venous connections (common vein, persistent left superior vena cava, innominate vein, superior vena cava) forms an inverted U-shaped vessel that can be demonstrated on ultrasound, as can the unusual enlargement of the azygos vein seen with Type I anomaly draining into the azygos vein (Fig. 12.11). Type III is frequently associated with life-threatening clinical symptoms related to interstitial pulmonary oedema caused by pulmonary venous obstruction. Abdominal ultrasound will demonstrate the large infra-diaphragmatic connection of the common pulmonary vein into the portal venous system (Fig. 12.12). When pulmonary oedema is present on a neonatal chest radiograph we, therefore, strongly recommend performing an abdominal ultrasound to rule out Type III anomaly.

12.3.2.3
Cardiac Tumours

Cardiac tumours in neonates are extremely rare. The most common cardiac tumour of this age group is rhabdomyoma (Fig. 12.13). Cardiac rhabdomyomas often present in patients with tuberous sclerosis and have been shown to undergo spontaneous regression (Wang et al. 2003; Wu et al. 2002). Their clinical manifestations vary widely from asymptomatic presentations to life-threatening cardiac events. Ultrasound shows multiple echogenic tumour masses of varying size within the myocardium.

12.4
Diaphragm

Characteristically, the diaphragm appears as a relatively smooth, slightly moving echogenic linear structure on both longitudinal and transverse scans. A sagittal scan will show the crural parts as relatively prominent, band-like structures in front of the spine. When documented on an axial scan their hypoechoic feature must not be mistaken for abdominal lymph nodes. In the presence of pleural effusion the muscular component of the diaphragm is clearly seen as a hypoechoic band-like structure, a feature that is normally obscured by the high echogenicity of the aerated lung (Fig. 12.14b).

12.4.1
Diaphragmatic Hernias

Congenital diaphragmatic hernias result from abnormal partitioning of the coelomic cavity and are usually isolated and sporadic (Figs. 12.15, 12.16). It may also be associated with chromosomal anomalies or be part of a polymalformation syndrome (Manni et al. 1994). The most common herniation, known as Bochdalek's hernia, is through a posterolateral defect on the left (80%–85%) side of the diaphragm. Bilateral (less than 5%) or right-sided (10%–15%) defects are less common.

Major complications associated with Bochdalek's hernia are pulmonary hypoplasia and persistent foetal circulation (Fig. 12.15). Left-sided defects may contain the left lobe of the liver, the spleen, the stomach, the large or small bowel, or the kidney. In right-sided defects the large right lobe of the liver and occasionally other abdominal viscera are found, and the stomach is usually in an abdominal location. Ultrasound demonstrates a mediastinal shift to the contralateral side, the relative size of the lung, the presence of pleural fluid collection, and the abdominal contents such as

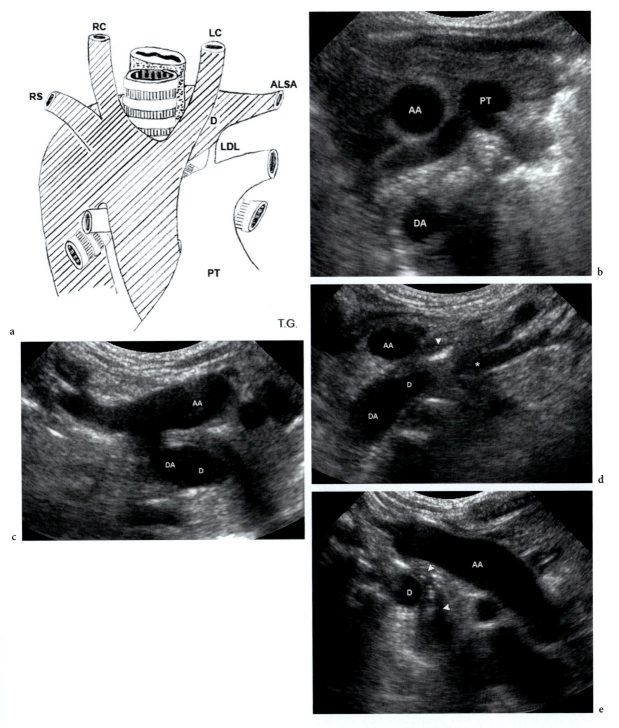

Fig. 12.8a–e. Right aortic arch with aberrant left subclavian artery (*ALSA*) in a 5-day-old girl. **a** Diagrammatic representation. **b** Transsternal axial scans at the level of the pulmonary artery and transsternal axial scans at the level of the aortic arch show a right aortic arch and right descending aorta (*DA*) and the large Kommerell diverticulum (*D*). **d** A slightly oblique transsternal section demonstrates the ALSA (*asterisk*) arising from the diverticulum (*D*) and passing behind the trachea (*arrowhead*) and oesophagus. **e** Suprasternal parasagittal scan shows the diverticulum (*D*) in cross-section with posterior indentation of the oesophagus (*arrowheads*). (*AA* Ascending aorta, *LC*, *RC* left, right common carotid artery, *RS* right subclavian artery, *PT* pulmonary trunk, *LDL* left ductus ligament)

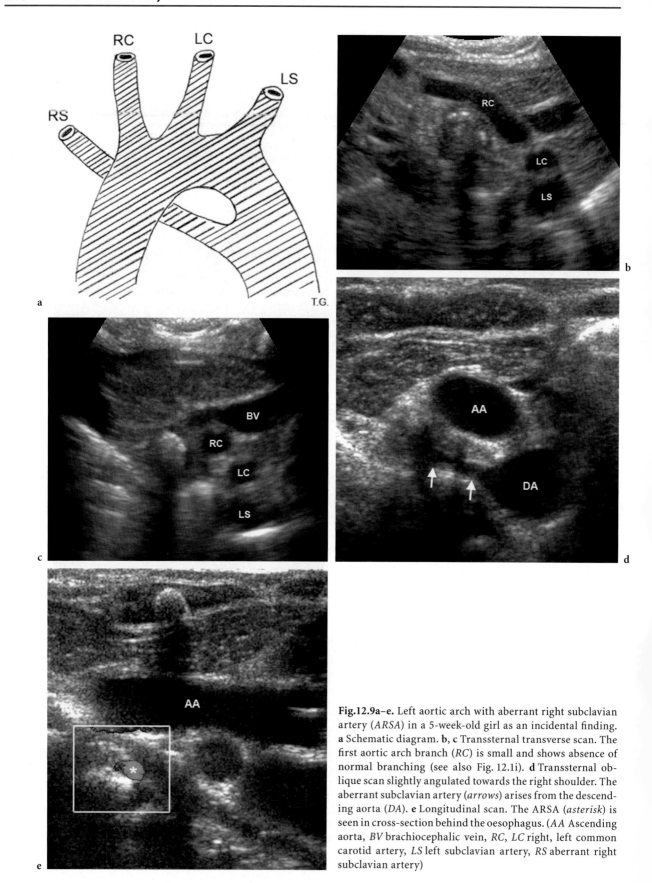

Fig.12.9a–e. Left aortic arch with aberrant right subclavian artery (*ARSA*) in a 5-week-old girl as an incidental finding. **a** Schematic diagram. **b, c** Transsternal transverse scan. The first aortic arch branch (*RC*) is small and shows absence of normal branching (see also Fig. 12.1i). **d** Transsternal oblique scan slightly angulated towards the right shoulder. The aberrant subclavian artery (*arrows*) arises from the descending aorta (*DA*). **e** Longitudinal scan. The ARSA (*asterisk*) is seen in cross-section behind the oesophagus. (*AA* Ascending aorta, *BV* brachiocephalic vein, *RC*, *LC* right, left common carotid artery, *LS* left subclavian artery, *RS* aberrant right subclavian artery)

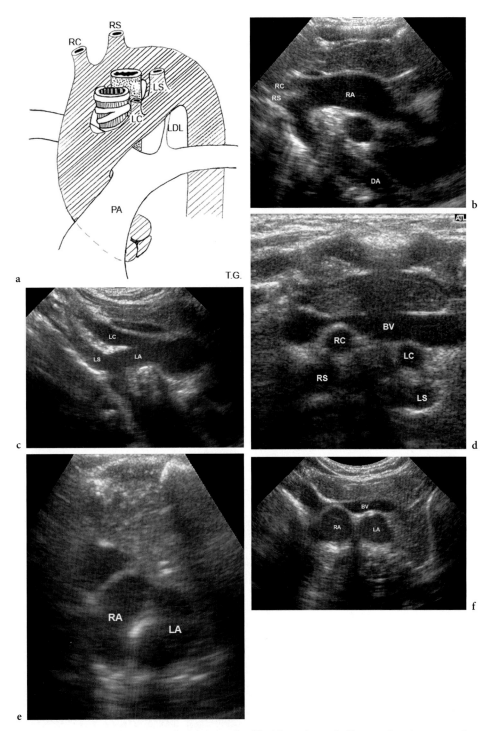

Fig. 12.10a–f. Double aortic arch in a 6-month-old-girl. **a** Schematic diagram. **b, c** Suprasternal right and left parasagittal scans demonstrate the right (**b**) and left (**c**) aortic arches and their common carotid and subclavian arteries. The aorta descends on the right side. (*DA* Descending aorta.) **d** Transsternal axial scan. The right and left common carotid and subclavian arteries are symmetrically arranged! **e** Transsternal axial scan. The complete vascular ring is shown at once surrounding the severely narrowed trachea and oesophagus. **f** Suprasternal coronal plane. Both arches are displayed in cross section. (*BV* Brachiocephalic vein, *LDL* left ductus ligament, *PA* pulmonary artery, *RA, LA* right, left aortic arch, *RC, LC* right, left common carotid artery, *RS, LS* right, left subclavian artery,)

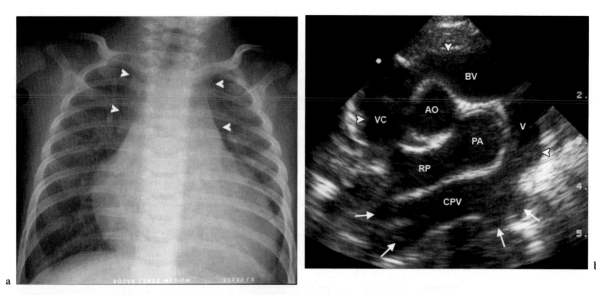

Fig. 12.11a,b. Total anomalous pulmonary venous connection to the left innominate vein via the vertical vein in a 3-month-old boy. **a** Frontal view demonstrates marked right atrial and right ventricular dilatation and increased pulmonary blood flow. The "snowman" configuration (*arrowheads*) is barely visible. **b** Suprasternal coronal view. All of the pulmonary veins (*arrows*) drain into the common pulmonary vein (*CPV*). The vertical vein (*V*) enters a dilated left brachiocephalic vein (*BV*), which in turn joins the right-sided superior vena cava (*VC*). These connections form an inverted U-shaped vessel (*arrowheads*). Within the encircling venous structures, the aortic arch (*Ao*) and main pulmonary artery (*PA*) are seen in cross-section. (*RP* Right pulmonary artery)

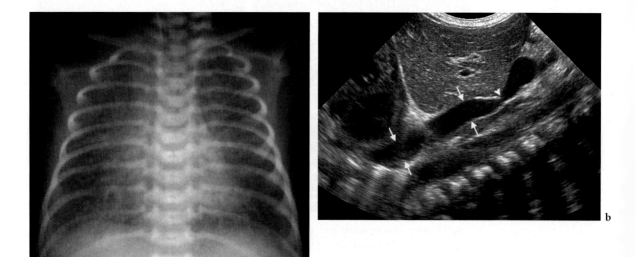

Fig. 12.12a, b. Total anomalous pulmonary venous return below the diaphragm in a girl 4 h after birth. **a** AP chest radiograph. Small cardiac size. Both lung fields show diffuse reticular vascularity characteristic of passive vascular engorgement. Haziness results from associated pulmonary interstitial oedema. Note the fluid in the minor fissure. **b** Longitudinal scan shows the large common pulmonary vein (*arrows*) with intrinsic stenosis (*arrowhead*) crossing the diaphragm and draining into the portal vein

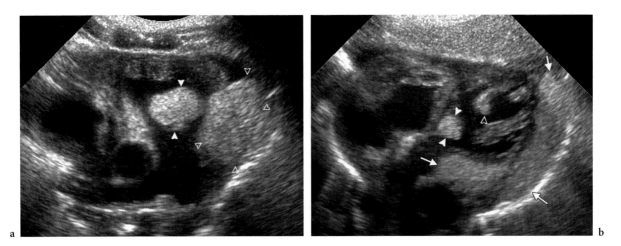

Fig. 12.13a, b. Multiple intracardiac rhabdomyomas in a 1-day-old boy with tuberous sclerosis. **a** High parasternal axial scan shows highly echogenic rhabdomyomas in (*arrowheads*) and adjacent to (*open arrowheads*) the right ventricular outflow tract. **b** Subxiphoidal scan: a large rhabdomyoma surrounds the left ventricular wall from the base of the heart to the apex (*arrows*). Smaller rhabdomyomas in the left ventricular outflow tract (*arrowheads*) and in the papillary muscle (*open arrowhead*)

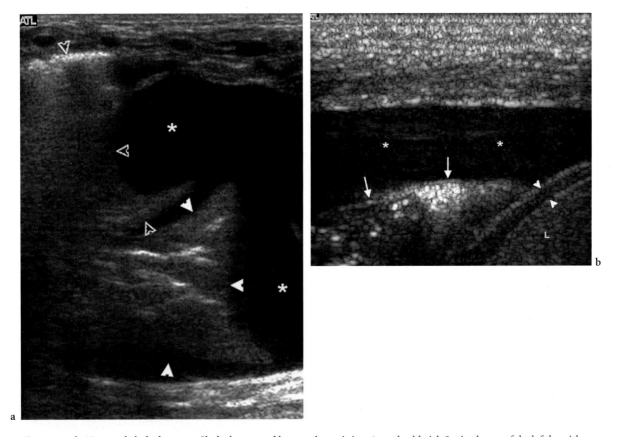

Fig. 12.14a, b. Neonatal chylothorax. **a** Chylothorax and lung atelectasis in a 4-week-old girl. Sagittal scan of the left hemithorax shows large pleural effusion (*asterisks*). The lower lobe (*arrowheads*) is compressed with internal branching bright echogenicities representing air bronchograms. The upper lobe (*open arrowheads*) is only partially atelectatic. **b** Chylothorax in a 2-week-old boy. Coronal scan of the right hemithorax shows the fairly echo-poor chylous content within the pleural space (*stars*). Note the effusion acts as an acoustic window and allows clear delineation of the muscular part of the diaphragm (*arrowheads*). (*Arrows* Lung, *L* liver)

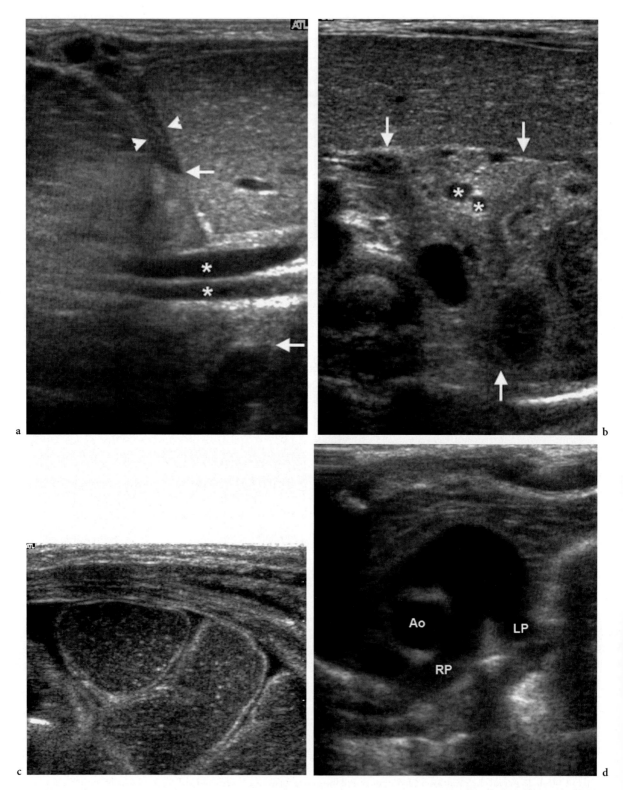

Fig. 12.15a–d. Congenital diaphragmatic hernia (Bochdalek's hernia) in a 1-day-old girl. **a** Longitudinal sonograms of the upper left abdomen and **b** transverse sonograms of the upper left abdomen show the diaphragmatic defect (*arrows*) and the anterior remnant of the diaphragm (*arrowheads*). The mesenteric artery and vein (*asterisks*) course cranially into the chest. **c** Low transverse sonogram and **d** high transverse sonograms of the chest demonstrate fluid-filled bowel loops and a small amount of free fluid. There is a well-developed left pulmonary artery (*LP*). (*Ao* Aorta, *RP* right pulmonary artery)

liver or bowel within the thoracic cavity (CAMPBELL and LILLY 1982; KASALES et al. 1998; YOKOYAMA et al. 1984). The echogenicity varies according to content and intestinal aeration. The airless lung and the liver have fairly similar features on ultrasound. The typical vascular anatomy helps to differentiate between them. Doppler ultrasound may be used to document vascular anatomy of the airless lung and delineates the mesenteric vessels coursing cephalad into the thoracic cavity. In cases where there is doubt that the ultrasound findings of abdominal content within the thoracic cavity are caused by agenesis of the lung with subsequent eventration, documentation of the ipsilateral pulmonary artery confirms the presence of a diaphragmatic hernia (Fig. 12.17). The muscular components of the anterior diaphragmatic remnants may be documented as hypoechoic bands.

Anterior parasternal herniation (Morgagni's hernia) is found with failure of fusion of the costal and xiphoid fibrotendinous components of the diaphragm, which results in herniation of abdominal content through the hiatus for the internal mammary artery (Fig. 12.16) (SARIHAN et al. 1996). Morgagni's hernias are commonly right-sided because the left-sided defects are covered by the heart and pericardium. Morgagni's hernia usually contains omentum, transverse colon and liver and is frequently associated with malformations of the heart. Except for a central diaphragmatic defect sonographic findings are similar to Bochdalek's hernia.

12.4.2
Diaphragmatic Eventration

Eventration is the result of congenital weakness or thinness of the diaphragmatic muscle. The defect can be focal or complete and is more often right-sided than left-sided. Sonographic findings are a thinned but intact diaphragm that bulges cephalad and is adjacent to the liver or spleen. In cases of a rather thinned diaphragm sonographic findings alone may not be able to distinguish between eventration and diaphragmatic hernia (Fig. 12.16) (MERTEN et al. 1982; YANG 2003).

12.4.3
Diaphragmatic Palsy

Diaphragmatic palsy or dysfunction is a failure of normal diaphragmatic motion related to complete or incomplete injury at various levels such as the respi-ratory centre, the upper or lower motor nerve or to the diaphragm itself (Fig. 12.2). In neonates injury of the phrenic nerve is commonly secondary to obstetric trauma, occurs after thoracic or abdominal surgery or follows insertion of an internal jugular venous catheter. For ultrasound evaluation of diaphragmatic palsy B-mode and sometimes time-motion-mode (TM-mode) ultrasound is used. B-mode ultrasound shows para-doxical motion of the paralysed hemidiaphragm and decreased motion of the affected hemidiaphragm in diaphragmatic dysfunction. Determining the wrong direction of motion is at times difficult in the latter. Due to the small size of the neonate both hemidia-phragms can be documented on the same transverse scan using the subxiphoidal approach with the trans-ducer tilted cephalad. This scan can be used to assess whether diaphragmatic movements are synchronized and equal in dimension. TM-mode may be used to visualize and record diaphragmatic motion as a func-tion of time (EPELMAN et al. 2005; URVOAS et al. 1994). One has to bear in mind, however, that the patient needs to be disconnected from an assisting ventilator for a short time to achieve reliable results.

12.5
Lung and Pleura

12.5.1
Congenital Lung Disease

The lung is composed of the bronchopulmonary air-way, the arterial supply, the venous drainage, and the lymphatic system. The establishment of proper com-munication between all four systems is essential in the development of the normal lung parenchyma. An insult to the developing lung results in congenital anomalies. The timing and severity of the insult rather than the nature of the insult itself is the major determining fac-tor and leads to a continuum of malformations between congenital cystic adenomatoid malformation (CCAM), pulmonary sequestration (PS), congenital lobar emphy-sema (CLE), bronchogenic cysts and bronchial atresia, which may even coexist (PANICEK et al. 1987).

12.5.1.1
Congenital Cystic Adenomatoid Malformation

CCAM is the most common lung malformation characterized by abnormal growth of the terminal

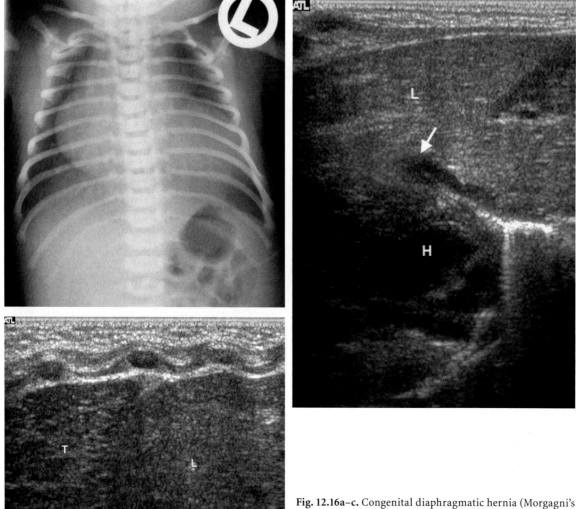

a

b

c

Fig. 12.16a–c. Congenital diaphragmatic hernia (Morgagni's hernia) in a 1-day-old-girl. **a** Frontal chest film shows a large well-defined mass in the left chest with displacement of the heart to the right. **b, c** Longitudinal scans demonstrate herniation of the liver (*L*) through an anterior diaphragmatic defect into the chest. The liver is lying partially anterior to the heart (*H*) and is in contact with the thymus (*T*). *Arrow* shows the edge of the diaphragm. Differentiation between hernia and eventration is not possible with certainty

bronchioles without alveolar differentiation. There is communication between the individual cysts within the CCAM and also with the bronchial tree. Three types of CCAM are classified according to the size of cystic components (PATERSON 2005). Type I has cysts larger than 2 cm in size, and Type II and III contain progressively smaller cystic components. CCAM is increasingly being diagnosed on antenatal ultrasound examinations where it is seen as an echogenic mass of variable size that may or may not contain cysts. The sonographic classification of CCAM follows the his-

tological typing and describes a macrocystic CCAM (Type I and II) and a microcystic CCAM, with the latter accounting for only 10% of cases. In the first hours of life cysts are filled with retained fetal lung fluid reflected in the sonographic feature of a complex mass containing fluid-filled cysts. This tends to clear over the first few days of life. Acoustic shadowing is found when the cysts contain air. Colour flow Doppler shows a relatively avascular structure. Differential diagnostic considerations have to include congenital diaphragmatic hernia and all above-mentioned

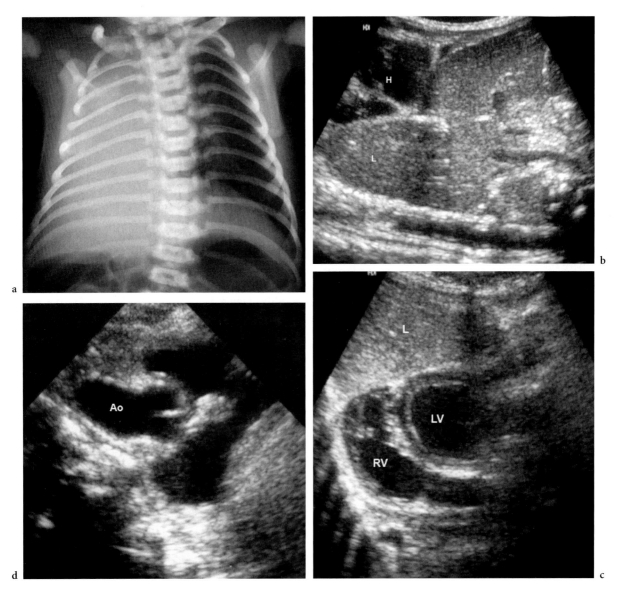

Fig. 12.17a–d. Right lung aplasia in a 3-day-old boy. **a** AP chest radiograph shows opaque right hemithorax with marked mediastinal shift to the right and levoscoliosis. **b** Longitudinal scan. The liver (*L*) bulges superiorly into the right hemithorax. (*H* Heart.) **c** Transverse cranially angulated scan. The heart is completely displaced into the right hemithorax. (*L* Liver, *LV* left ventricle, *RV* right ventricle.) **d** Right parasternal longitudinal scan. There is no right pulmonary artery visible behind the ascending aorta (*Ao*) (see also Fig. 12.1e)

members of the malformation continuum (BRATU et al. 2001; NEWMAN 2006).

12.5.1.2
Congenital Lobar Emphysema

Congenital lobar emphysema (CLE), also called congenital lobar overinflation, is a condition characterized by hyperinflation of a lobe without destruction of alveolar septa (BERROCAL et al. 2004). Although CLE has specific imaging characteristics in neonates it is not a specific disease. Several intrinsic and extrinsic pathologic causes are described in detail in other chapters of this issue. CLE either shows a normal number of hyperinflated alveoli or an increased number of normally inflated alveoli (polyalveolar lobe). Immediately after birth fetal lung fluid may be trapped in the affected lobe producing an opaque hemithorax on chest radiography and a homogenous, hypoechoic lobe with enhanced sound transmission on ultrasound.

12.5.1.3
Bronchogenic Cyst

Bronchogenic cysts are the commonest intra-thoracic cysts and are thought to arise secondary to abnormal budding of the primitive ventral foregut. Most commonly bronchogenic cysts are incidental findings. Symptoms depend on the location and size of the cysts and may be severe or entirely absent. They are usually located in the mediastinum close to the carina, but may be found in the right paratracheal region, alongside the oesophagus, the hilum of the lung or even within the lung parenchyma (BERROCAL et al. 2004; MAYDEN et al. 1984; YOUNG et al. 1989). Apart from these locations, where the aerated lung blocks sound transmission, ultrasound delineates the cyst as a round or oval mass with sharply marginated smooth walls. The internal appearance varies according to its content. Most cysts are fluid filled and do not connect with the bronchial tree. Predominantly fluid-filled cysts are hypoechoic. A complex pattern with hypoechoic and echoic reverberations suggests a combination of fluid and air. Bronchogenic cysts are differentiated from other foregut malformation cysts by histological evaluation (Fig. 12.7). The appearance of CCAM may be mimicked when the cyst compresses a bronchus and the sound transmission through the adjacent hypoinflated lung is increased.

12.5.1.4
Bronchial Atresia

Bronchial atresia seldom presents in the neonatal period (SCHUSTER et al. 1978). This congenital condition results from failure of a segmental or subsegmental bronchus to develop or maintain its communication with the central airways. Subsequently the bronchus distal to the obstruction becomes dilated and mucus-impacted and the affected lung is overaerated due to collateral air drift. Ultrasound is limited due to this hyperinflation but, after infection has occurred, may demonstrate a consolidated lobe with dilated hypoechoic bronchi filled with moving mucus.

12.5.1.5
Pulmonary Sequestration

Pulmonary sequestration consists of non-functioning lung tissue that does not communicate normally with the tracheobronchial tree and is supplied by an anomalous systemic artery (Fig. 12.18). Most of the masses occur at the lung bases. The two types of pulmonary sequestration described are intralobar sequestration (contained within visceral pleura) and extralobar sequestration (covered by their own pleura) (BERROCAL et al. 2004; ROSADO-DE-CHRISTENSON et al. 1993). The feeding artery usually arises from the descending aorta. The draining vein connects to systemic veins in extralobar sequestration and to pulmonary veins in intralobar sequestration. Overlaps of both types are described. The sonographic appearance of the pulmonary parenchyma depends on the degree of aeration of the sequestered lung. A sequestration that does not communicate with the airway appears as a rather homogeneous echogenic mass containing vessels of various sizes. When the sequestration communicates with the remainder lung, a complex or cystic mass with reverberation artefacts is found usually after being infected. Small fluid-filled bronchi or cystic areas may be noted on occasion. Doppler demonstration of the systemic artery feeding the lesion from the descending aorta is diagnostic. Neuroblastoma, however, may mimic this sonographic finding by encasing a regional vessel, which then appears as a systemic feeding artery. Therefore, one has to further investigate any questionable findings (MANSON and DANEMAN 2001).

12.5.1.6
Scimitar Syndrome

Scimitar syndrome or congenital venolobar syndrome is a form of hypoplasia of the right lung in association with anomalous ipsilateral venous return, commonly into the inferior vena cava (Fig. 12.19) (BERROCAL et al. 2004; HOLT et al. 2004). Other possible terminations are the right atrium, superior vena cava, azygos vein, portal vein, or hepatic vein. Anomalous arterial supply from the abdominal aorta to part or all of the hypoplastic lung, cardio-vascular or ipsilateral diaphragmatic anomalies, pulmonary isomerism resulting in a left bronchial branching pattern, or horseshoe lung may be seen (DIKENSOY et al. 2006). Ultrasound demonstrations of a slender right pulmonary artery, anomalous venous drainage and a feeding artery commonly arising from the abdominal aorta are indicative of the diagnosis. Any patient who presents with an unexplained shift of the mediastinum to the right should carefully be examined for the presence of a scimitar vein.

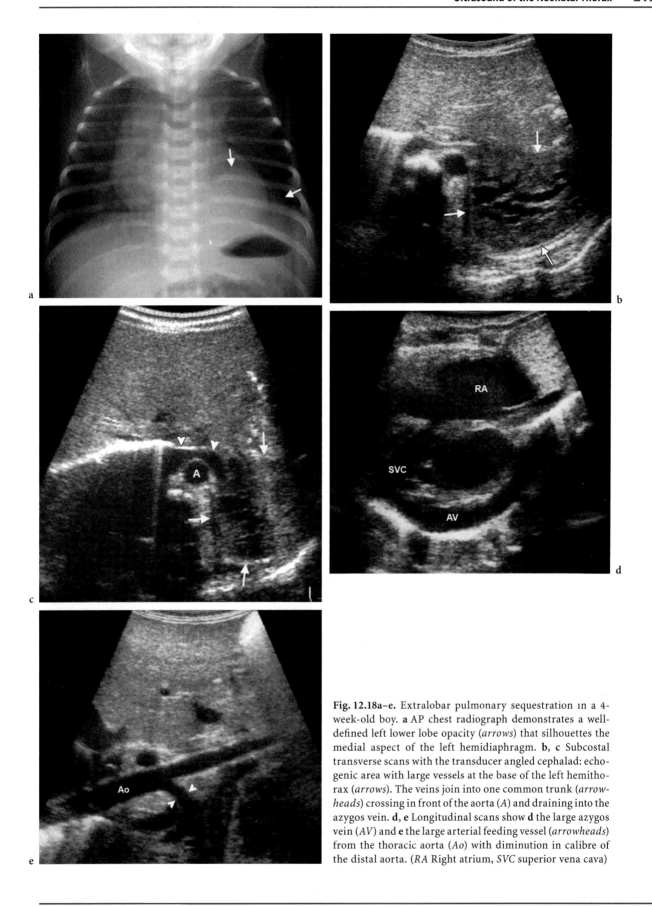

Fig. 12.18a–e. Extralobar pulmonary sequestration in a 4-week-old boy. **a** AP chest radiograph demonstrates a well-defined left lower lobe opacity (*arrows*) that silhouettes the medial aspect of the left hemidiaphragm. **b, c** Subcostal transverse scans with the transducer angled cephalad: echogenic area with large vessels at the base of the left hemithorax (*arrows*). The veins join into one common trunk (*arrowheads*) crossing in front of the aorta (*A*) and draining into the azygos vein. **d, e** Longitudinal scans show **d** the large azygos vein (*AV*) and **e** the large arterial feeding vessel (*arrowheads*) from the thoracic aorta (*Ao*) with diminution in calibre of the distal aorta. (*RA* Right atrium, *SVC* superior vena cava)

12.5.2
Pleura

12.5.2.1
Pleural Fluid

The main role of ultrasound in the study of pleural fluid is to document whether a collection is simple or complicated (Fig. 12.14). An anechoic free-flowing appearance is considered to be simple. An effusion is complicated when features such as echogenic debris, mobile fibrin strands, septations or a honeycomb appearance are present.

The sonographic appearance of pleural fluid can be related to the biochemical division of pleural fluid into exudate or transudate. On sonography both transudate and exudate can be anechoic, but collections presenting features of complicated effusions are always exudates or haemorrhages.

Pleural effusions are rare in the neonate and usually occur as hydrops or congenital chylothorax (Riccabona 2003). Isolated pleural effusion, so-called primary pleural effusion, denotes a pleural effusion without documented aetiology. Chromosomal anomaly such as Down syndrome and Noonan syndrome may be associated. The content of the isolated pleural effusion is mostly chylous. Secondary pleural effusion is associated with several clinical conditions such as cardiac, inflammatory or iatrogenic problems, disorders of connective tissue or fetal hydrops. On ultrasound most neonatal effusions appears as anechoic collections just above the diaphragm and adjacent to it which alter with changes in the patient's position (Rocha et al. 2006).

Useful sonographic signs described in literature are the "displaced crus sign" and the "bare area sign". Interposition of the fluid between the crus and the vertebral column displaces the crus away from the spine ("displaced crus sign"). The posterior aspect of the right lower lobe of the liver is directly attached to the posterior diaphragm without peritoneum. In contrast to pleural fluid, ascites cannot extend behind the liver at the level of the bare area ("bare area sign") (Halvorsen and Thompson 1986).

Due to compression, the underlying lung is usually atelectatic. With atelectasis vessels become crowded together and have a more parallel orientation. Their orderly linear and branching structure, however, is preserved. Abdominal ultrasound should always be performed to reveal associated ascites.

Pneumonia in its early stages often causes a small pleural transudate. If antimicrobial therapy fails the effusion subsequently develops features of complicated pleural fluid collection. Purulent as well as haemorrhagic fluid collection is a rare finding in the neonatal period. Colour flow Doppler signals are seen within the effusion ("fluid colour sign") related to the moveable debris in both entities (Wu et al. 1995).

12.5.2.2
Pneumothorax

When air is introduced into the pleural space a gap is created between the two pleural layers disrupting the normal acoustic interface. On ultrasound the gliding sign can no longer been seen, and the normal reverberation as well as comet tail artefacts are replaced by static posterior acoustic shadowing. The pneumothorax has a defined volume, however, and a point of sudden change to normal pleural features has to be expected, unless the pneumothorax is major leading to a total collapse of the lung. This point of change moves with inspiration and expiration and can be documented with ultrasound. The sonographic sign that documents a sudden change of pattern suggestive of pneumothorax into a pattern of lung gliding and comet tail artefacts during inspiration and a return to pneumothorax pattern on expiration is named "lung point" (Lichtenstein et al. 2000). All above-mentioned features together allow the reliable diagnosis of even a very small pneumothorax and we, therefore, favour ultrasound as the method of choice for examining neonates with questionable pneumothorax in the intensive care setting. One must always be aware, however, that intrapleural air will always be located at the highest level in the thorax.

12.6
Use of Chest Ultrasound in Neonatal Intensive Care

Ultrasound can be used to detect the endotracheal tube position (Hsieh et al. 2004). The non-intubated airway produces a broken linear dense echo whereas the endotracheal tube produces a continuous linear density. The tip of the tube can easily be identified. Optimal tube position is obtained when the tip is 1 cm above the aortic arch.

Sonography is an excellent method for guiding pleural fluid aspiration. It is particularly helpful

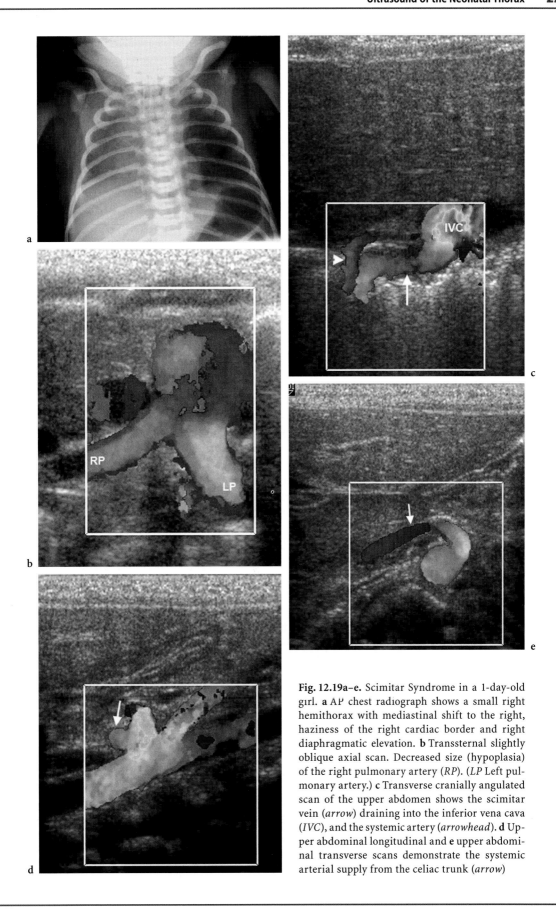

Fig. 12.19a–e. Scimitar Syndrome in a 1-day-old girl. **a** AP chest radiograph shows a small right hemithorax with mediastinal shift to the right, haziness of the right cardiac border and right diaphragmatic elevation. **b** Transsternal slightly oblique axial scan. Decreased size (hypoplasia) of the right pulmonary artery (*RP*). (*LP* Left pulmonary artery.) **c** Transverse cranially angulated scan of the upper abdomen shows the scimitar vein (*arrow*) draining into the inferior vena cava (*IVC*), and the systemic artery (*arrowhead*). **d** Upper abdominal longitudinal and **e** upper abdominal transverse scans demonstrate the systemic arterial supply from the celiac trunk (*arrow*)

in determining whether a fluid collection will respond to drainage (anechoic, without septation) or not. The gliding sign changes into a "curtain sign" in hydropneumothorax, created by movement of an air-fluid level.

The placement of a venous catheter has become an integral component of neonatal intensive care. Peripheral intravenous lines can provide the majority of fluid and nutritional needs. However, neonates, who require higher caloric supplementation, need central venous access achieved by peripherally inserted central venous catheters or standard central venous lines. Insertion of a venous catheter has been associated with both immediate and long-term complications (Fig. 12.20). The immediate complications include catheter malposition, extraluminal placement with infusate extravasation, pneumothorax, and haemothorax usually secondary to the insertion procedure. Late complications are occlusion, thrombosis, sepsis and catheter tip migration. Catheter tip migration may lead to pericardial effusion, cardiac tamponade, or hydrothorax. Various explanations have been given for the leakage of fluid through the vessel or the very thin atrial wall, such as perforation or endothelial damage and the subsequent increase in permeability caused by hyperosmolar parenteral infusate (Hogan 1999; Kidney et al. 1998). Ultrasound may be used to guide insertion through direct visualization and allows documentation of optimal tip placement. Any chest radiograph that reveals an unusual catheter position or a catheter position that is closer to the midline than expected should be further analysed by ultrasound to exclude catheter malposition in the aorta (Sridhar et al. 2005). Furthermore catheter malposition should be suspected if an acute pleural collection is seen on the same side as the catheter. Malfunction of the central line may be due to incorrect catheter position, clot formation around the catheter or thrombosis of the subclavian vein or superior vena cava. Thrombosis of the superior vena cava may lead to lymphatic duct blockage and subsequently chylothorax. Thrombosis of the inferior vena cava may extend into the renal veins, causing symptoms such as haematuria, hypertension or renal failure (Cartwright 2004).

Ultrasound may visualize the location of the catheter tip close to the vessel wall, an echogenic clot around or at the end of the catheter, or an echogenic clot within the vein and the lack of a normal response of the vein to respiratory movements. A fibrin deposit around the catheter is frequently formed, but does not necessarily cause malfunction of the catheter.

Ultrasound evaluation after catheter removal may show the remaining fibrin sheath which may mimic a catheter fragment (Fig. 12.20c) (Konen et al. 2004). Doppler ultrasound can be used to demonstrate the lack of jet flow in an obstructed catheter and the lack of blood flow in an obstructed vessel.

References

Avni EF, Braude P, Pardou A, Matos C (1990) Hyaline membrane disease in the newborn: diagnosis by ultrasound. Pediatr Radiol 20:143–146

Baysal T, Kutlu R, Kutlu O, Yakinci C, Karaman I (1999) Ectopic thymic tissue: a cause of emphysema in infants. Clin Imaging 23:19–21

Ben-Ami TE, O'Donovan JC, Yousefzadeh DK (1993) Sonography of the chest in children. Radiol Clin North Am 31:517–531

Bendon RW, Coventry S (2004) Non-iatrogenic pathology of the preterm infant. Semin Neonatol 9:281–287

Berdon WE (2000) Rings, slings, and other things: vascular compression of the infant trachea updated from the midcentury to the millennium – the legacy of Robert E. Gross, MD, and Edward BD. Neuhauser, MD. Radiology 216:624–632

Berrocal T, Madrid C, Novo S, Gutierrez J, Arjonilla A, Gomez-Leon N (2004) Congenital anomalies of the tracheobronchial tree, lung, and mediastinum: embryology, radiology, and pathology. Radiographics 24:e17

Bhutani MS, Hoffman BJ, Reed C (1996) Endosonographic diagnosis of an esophageal duplication cyst. Endoscopy 28:396–397

Bratu I, Flageole H, Chen MF, Di LM, Yazbeck S, Laberge JM (2001) The multiple facets of pulmonary sequestration. J Pediatr Surg 36:784–790

Campbell DN, Lilly JR (1982) The clinical spectrum of right Bochdalek's hernia. Arch Surg 117:341–344

Cartwright DW (2004) Central venous lines in neonates: a study of 2186 catheters. Arch Dis Child Fetal Neonatal Ed 89:F504–F508

Deffrenne P, Beraud C, Saint D (1970) Isolated tracheoesophageal fistulas. Arch Fr Pediatr 27:657–665

Dikensoy O, Kervancioglu R, Bayram NG, Elbek O, Uyar M, Ekinci E (2006) Horseshoe lung associated with scimitar syndrome and pleural lipoma. J Thorac Imaging 21:73–75

Eichmann D, Engler S, Oldigs HD, Schroeder H, Partsch CJ (2001) Radiological case of the month. Denouement and discussion: congenital esophageal duplication cyst as a rare cause of neonatal progressive stridor. Arch Pediatr Adolesc Med 155:1067–1068

Epelman M, Navarro OM, Daneman A, Miller SF (2005) M-mode sonography of diaphragmatic motion: description of technique and experience in 278 pediatric patients. Pediatr Radiol 35:661–667

Franco A, Mody NS, Meza MP (2005) Imaging evaluation of pediatric mediastinal masses. Radiol Clin North Am 43:325–353

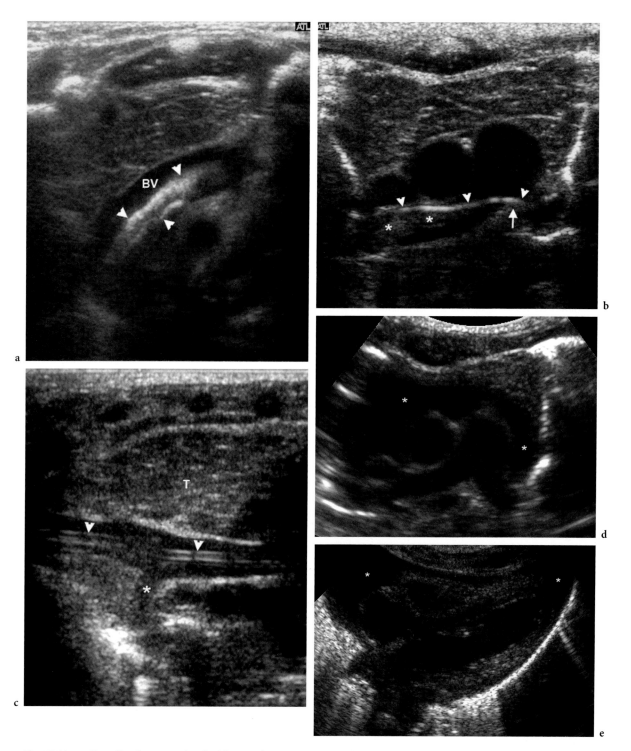

Fig. 12.20a–e. Complications associated with central venous access. **a** Thrombus in the brachiocephalic vein around a central venous catheter in a 5-week-old girl. Transsternal axial scan. (*Arrowheads* Thrombus, *BV* brachiocephalic vein.) **b** Embolization of a broken catheter fragment into the pulmonary artery in a 1-week-old boy. Transsternal axial scan. The fragment (*arrowheads*) with adherent thrombus (*asterisks*) overrides the pulmonary artery bifurcation (*arrow*). **c** The fibrin sheath of a catheter left behind in the superior vena cava after removal of a central venous line in a 10-day-old boy. Right parasternal longitudinal scan: *arrowheads*, fibrin sheath; *asterisk*, azygos vein; *T*, thymus. **d, e** Pericardial effusion related to the catheter tip in the right atrium in a 3-day-old girl. Transsternal high (**d**) and low (**e**) axial scans demonstrate a significant amount of pericardial echo-free fluid (*asterisks*)

Gassner I, Geley TE (2005) Sonographic evaluation of oesophageal atresia and tracheo-oesophageal fistula. Pediatr Radiol 35:159–164

Halvorsen RA Jr., Thompson WM (1986) Ascites or pleural effusion? CT and ultrasound differentiation. CRC Crit Rev Diagn Imaging 26:201–240

Han BK, Suh YL, Yoon HK (2001) Thymic ultrasound. I. Intrathymic anatomy in infants. Pediatr Radiol 31:474–479

Harris MA, Valmorida JN (1997) Neonates with congenital heart disease, Part IV: Total anomalous pulmonary venous return. Neonatal Netw 16:63–66

Hogan MJ (1999) Neonatal vascular catheters and their complications. Radiol Clin North Am 37:1109–1125

Holt PD, Berdon WE, Marans Z, Griffiths S, Hsu D (2004) Scimitar vein draining to the left atrium and a historical review of the scimitar syndrome. Pediatr Radiol 34:409–413

Hsieh KS, Lee CL, Lin CC, Huang TC, Weng KP, Lu WH (2004) Secondary confirmation of endotracheal tube position by ultrasound image. Crit Care Med 32:S374–S377

Kasales CJ, Coulson CC, Meilstrup JW, Ambrose A, Botti JJ, Holley GP (1998) Diagnosis and differentiation of congenital diaphragmatic hernia from other noncardiac thoracic fetal masses. Am J Perinatol 15:623–628

Kidney DD, Nguyen DT, Deutsch LS (1998) Radiologic evaluation and management of malfunctioning long-term central vein catheters. AJR Am J Roentgenol 171:1251–1257

Konen O, Daneman A, Traubici J, Epelman M (2004) Intravascular linear thrombus after catheter removal: sonographic appearance mimicking retained catheter fragment. Pediatr Radiol 34:125–129

Lemaitre L, Leclerc F, Dubos JP, Marconi V, Lemaire D (1989) Thymic hemorrhage: a cause of acute symptomatic mediastinal widening in an infant with late haemorrhagic disease. Sonographic findings. Pediatr Radiol 19:128–129

Lichtenstein D, Meziere G, Biderman P, Gepner A, Barre O (1997) The comet-tail artifact. An ultrasound sign of alveolar-interstitial syndrome. Am J Respir Crit Care Med 156:1640–1646

Lichtenstein D, Meziere G, Biderman P, Gepner A (1999) The comet-tail artifact: an ultrasound sign ruling out pneumothorax. Intensive Care Med 25:383–388

Lichtenstein D, Meziere G, Biderman P, Gepner A (2000) The "lung point": an ultrasound sign specific to pneumothorax. Intensive Care Med 26:1434–1440

Manni M, Heydanus R, Den Hollander NS, Stewart PA, De VC, Wladimiroff JW (1994) Prenatal diagnosis of congenital diaphragmatic hernia: a retrospective analysis of 28 cases. Prenat Diagn 14:187–190

Manson DE, Daneman A (2001) Pitfalls in the sonographic diagnosis of juxtadiaphragmatic pulmonary sequestrations. Pediatr Radiol 31:260–264

Mayden KL, Tortora M, Chervenak FA, Hobbins JC (1984) The antenatal sonographic detection of lung masses. Am J Obstet Gynecol 148:349–351

McCook TA, Felman AH (1978) Esophageal atresia, duodenal atresia, and gastric distension: report of two cases. AJR Am J Roentgenol 131:167–168

Merten DF, Bowie JD, Kirks DR, Grossman H (1982) Anteromedial diaphragmatic defects in infancy: current approaches to diagnostic imaging. Radiology 142(2):361–365

Moes CA, Freedom RM (1993) Rare types of aortic arch anomalies. Pediatr Cardiol 14:93–101

Narasimharao KL, Mitra SK (1987) Esophageal atresia associated with esophageal duplication cyst. J Pediatr Surg 22:984–985

Newman B (2006) Congenital bronchopulmonary foregut malformations: concepts and controversies. Pediatr Radiol 36:773–791

Panicek DM, Heitzman ER, Randall PA, Groskin SA, Chew FS, Lane EJ Jr., Markarian B (1987) The continuum of pulmonary developmental anomalies. Radiographics 7:747–772

Paterson A (2005) Imaging evaluation of congenital lung abnormalities in infants and children. Radiol Clin North Am 43:303–323

Rahbar R, Nicollas R, Roger G, Triglia JM, Garabedian EN, McGill TJ, Healy GB (2004) The biology and management of subglottic hemangioma: past, present, future. Laryngoscope 114:1880–1891

Riccabona M (2003) Thoracic sonography in infancy and childhood. Radiologe 43:1075–1089

Rocha G, Fernandes P, Rocha P, Quintas C, Martins T, Proenca E (2006) Pleural effusions in the neonate. Acta Paediatr 95:791–798

Rosado-De-Christenson ML, Frazier AA, Stocker JT, Templeton PA (1993) From the archives of the AFIP. Extralobar sequestration: radiologic-pathologic correlation. Radiographics 13:425–441

Sarihan H, Imamoglu M, Abes M, Soylu H (1996) Pediatric Morgagni hernia. Report of two cases. J Cardiovasc Surg (Torino) 37:195–197

Schuster SR, Harris GB, Williams A, Kirkpatrick J, Reid L (1978) Bronchial atresia: a recognizable entity in the pediatric age group. J Pediatr Surg 13:682–689

Snyder CL, Bickler SW, Gittes GK, Ramachandran V, Ashcraft KW (1996) Esophageal duplication cyst with esophageal web and tracheoesophageal fistula. J Pediatr Surg 31:968–969

Sodhi KS, Saxena AK, Narasimha Rao KL, Singh M, Suri S (2005) Esophageal duplication cyst: an unusual cause of respiratory distress in infants. Pediatr Emerg Care 21:854–856

Spigland N, Bensoussan AL, Blanchard H, Russo P (1990) Aberrant cervical thymus in children: three case reports and review of the literature. J Pediatr Surg 25:1196–1199

Sridhar S, Thomas N, Kumar ST, Jana AK (2005) Neonatal hydrothorax following migration of a central venous catheter. Indian J Pediatr 72:795–796

Stringer MD, McKenna KM, Goldstein RB, Filly RA, Adzick NS, Harrison MR (1995) Prenatal diagnosis of esophageal atresia. J Pediatr Surg 30:1258–1263

Targhetta R, Bourgeois JM, Chavagneux R, Marty-Double C, Balmes P (1992) Ultrasonographic approach to diagnosing hydropneumothorax. Chest 101:931–934

Tovi F, Mares AJ (1978) The aberrant cervical thymus. Embryology, pathology, and clinical implications. Am J Surg 136:631–637

Urvoas E, Pariente D, Fausser C, Lipsich J, Taleb R, Devictor D (1994) Diaphragmatic paralysis in children: diagnosis by TM-mode ultrasound. Pediatr Radiol 24:564–568

Wang JN, Yao CT, Chen JS, Yang YJ, Tsai YC, Wu JM (2003) Cardiac tumors in infants and children. Acta Paediatr Taiwan 44:215–219

Wells TR, Gwinn JL, Landing BH, Stanley P (1988) Reconsideration of the anatomy of sling left pulmonary artery: the association of one form with bridging bronchus and imperforate anus. Anatomic and diagnostic aspects. J Pediatr Surg 23:892–898

Wells TR, Stanley P, Padua EM, Landing BH, Warburton D (1990) Serial section-reconstruction of anomalous tracheobronchial branching patterns from CT scan images: bridging bronchus associated with sling left pulmonary artery. Pediatr Radiol 20:444–446

Wu RG, Yang PC, Kuo SH, Luh KT (1995) "Fluid color" sign: a useful indicator for discrimination between pleural thickening and pleural effusion. J Ultrasound Med 14:767–769

Wu SS, Collins MH, de Chadarevian JP (2002) Study of the regression process in cardiac rhabdomyomas. Pediatr Dev Pathol 5:29–36

Yang JI (2003) Left diaphragmatic eventration diagnosed as congenital diaphragmatic hernia by prenatal sonography. J Clin Ultrasound 31:214–217

Yokoyama T, Ichikawa T, Hiyama E, Okita M, Miyoshi N (1984) Bochdalek's hernia in the newborn – 6 years' experience. Hiroshima J Med Sci 33:697–702

Yonehara Y, Nakatsuka T, Ichioka S, Sasaki N, Kobayashi T (2002) CATCH 22 syndrome. J Craniofac Surg 13:623–626

Young G, L'Heureux PR, Krueckeberg ST, Swanson DA (1989) Mediastinal bronchogenic cyst: prenatal sonographic diagnosis. AJR Am J Roentgenol 152:125–127

Ultrasound in Congenital Heart Disease

13

COLIN J. MCMAHON and BENJAMIN W. EIDEM

C. J. MCMAHON, FRCPI, FAAP
Department of Paediatric Cardiology, Our Lady's Hospital for
Sick Children, Crumlin, Dublin 12, Ireland
B. W. EIDEM, MD
Department of Paediatric Cardiology, Mayo Clinic, Rochester,
Minnesota, USA

13.1
Introduction

Over the last two to three decades with the advent of two-dimensional echocardiography and colour Doppler, echocardiography has evolved as the primary imaging modality in the evaluation of children with congenital heart disease (SNIDER et al. 1997; ALLEN et al. 2000). Increasingly cardiac catheterization is solely used for interventional purposes and although cardiac magnetic resonance imaging is increasingly utilized, echocardiography remains the primary imaging modality (BOXT 1996). The echocardiogram in children with congenital heart disease is not complete until the segmental anatomy has been fully delineated.

13.2
History of Ultrasound

Pierre and Jacques Curie discovered the piezoelectric effect, namely that mechanical distortion of crystals produces electric potential and conversely that stimulation of crystals results in tissue distortion, 130 years ago. Although early pioneers developed amplitude-mode (A-mode) imaging and brightness-mode (B-mode) imaging, Edler and Hertz of Lund University in Sweden were first credited with the application of ultrasound to cardiac diagnosis in 1953 (GOLDBERG and KIMMELMAN 1988). They developed continuous moving images of the heart in M-mode echocardiograms. Subsequently two-dimensional (2-D) echocardiography allowed the complete evaluation of cardiac anatomy in a segmental logical approach (GEVA 1975).

13.3
Physics of Ultrasound

If one applies an electric current to a piezoelectric crystal this generates ultrasound waves which will travel through tissue at 1540 m per second or through air at 330 m/s. The echocardiographic probe emits rapid frequent pulses of ultrasound and subsequently acts as a receiver of the same emitted pulses. Some of the energy of the pulse will be reflected back to the transmitter depending on the characteristics of the tissue from which it is reflected. The axial resolution along the axis of the ultrasound beam is equivalent to its wavelength and the lateral resolution is the ability to differentiate objects perpendicular to the axis of the beam, equivalent to the beam width.

13.4
Echocardiographic Planes in Congenital Heart Disease

13.4.1
Subcostal Views

The subcostal coronal imaging plane (Figs. 13.1, 13.2) first defines the cardiac situs (SILVERMAN 1983). The heart should occupy the left side of the chest, termed levocardia. In cases where it occupies the right side of the chest with the apex pointing to the right this is dextrocardia. A central location of the cardiac mass within the thorax is termed mesocardia. Visceral situs solitus is defined by the stomach and aorta to the left of the spine and the liver and inferior vena cava (IVC) to the right of the spine. Situs inversus represents the opposite position of these structures. Situs ambiguus, usually in the setting of isomeric hearts, may demonstrate an interrupted IVC with azygous continuation to a persistent left superior vena cava (SVC) (RUSCAZIO et al.

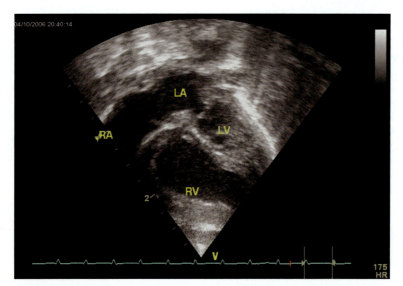

Fig. 13.1. Subcostal coronal view demonstrating hypoplastic left heart syndrome

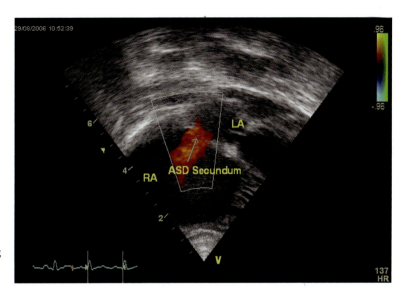

Fig. 13.2. Subcostal coronal view using color flow Doppler demonstrating a secundum atrial septal defect

1998). The sagittal subcostal view demonstrates the SVC and IVC draining to the right atrium and the aorta along its length. Demonstration of normal pulsatility in the descending aorta is an important finding when one is concerned about the possibility of coarctation of the aorta. Further scanning along the subcostal coronal plane from posterior to anterior will demonstrate the atrio-ventricular connections, ventriculoarterial connections and allow evaluation of both the inflow and outflow tracts. The subcostal views are among the most important in defining the cardiac segmental anatomy.

13.4.2
Four-Chamber View

This view (Figs. 13.3, 13.4, 13.5) allows clear delineation of the atria, ventricles, and inflow and outflow tracts. Scanning from posterior to anterior defines the coronary sinus within the right atrium, the mitral and tricuspid valves, the ventricular septum, the left ventricular outflow tract and finally the right ventricular outflow tract. Two-dimensional imaging, colour Doppler imaging and pulse wave (PW) or continuous wave (CW) Doppler interrogation of the tricuspid, mitral, aortic and pulmonary valves is mandatory for complete echocardiographic evaluation. Mitral or tricuspid stenosis may be missed unless Doppler interrogation is performed at the annulus, at the leaflets tips and below the leaflet tips in the atrioventricular valves. Likewise Doppler interrogation across the aortic and pulmonary valves is important to assess the presence of a significant gradient and outflow tract obstruction.

13.4.3
Parasternal Views

For the parasternal long-axis (Figs. 13.6, 13.7) imaging plane, the probe transducer is lined up along the long axis of the heart. Slight movements of the echocardiographic transducer anterior and posterior allow interrogation of several structures in this region. The mitral valve, aortic valve and interventricular septum should be studied first. Tilting the transducer anterior will demonstrate the right ventricular outflow tract. Posterior movement of the transducer allows assessment of the tricuspid valve.

For the parasternal short-axis (Fig. 13.8) imaging plane the transducer is positioned 90° or perpendicular relative to the parasternal long-axis plane. This allows clear assessment of the aortic valve morphology, interventricular septum and right ventricular outflow tract. The atrial septum can also be studied in this plane. Posterior scanning will reveal the interventricular septum down to the apex of the heart. The location and number of mitral valve papillary muscles and the presence of a mitral cleft or regurgitation can be evaluated in this plane. Anterior scanning will reveal the branch pulmonary arteries and the presence of a patent ductus arteriosus (PDA).

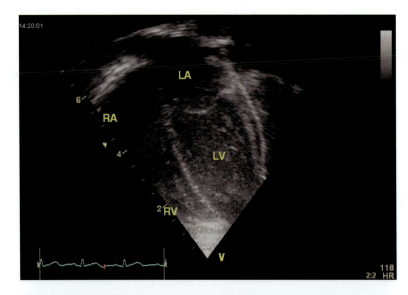

Fig. 13.3. Apical four-chamber view in a normal patient

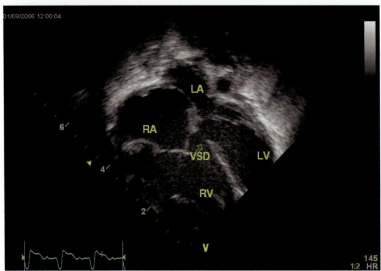

Fig. 13.4. Apical four-chamber view demonstrating an inlet ventricular septal defect

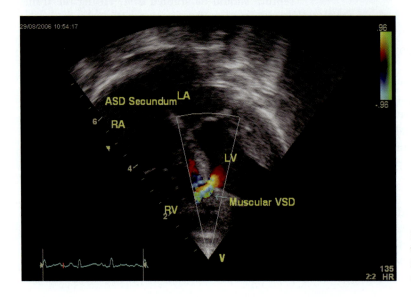

Fig. 13.5. Apical four-chamber view with color flow Doppler demonstrating a mid-muscular ventricular septal defect (*VSD*)

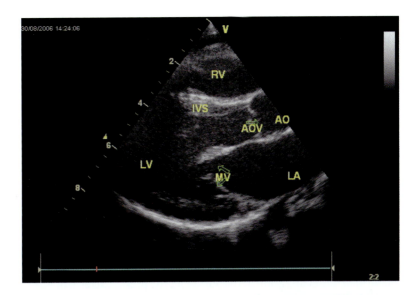

Fig. 13.6. Parasternal long axis view in a normal patient

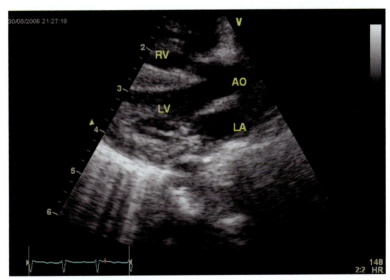

Fig. 13.7. Parasternal long axis view demonstrating moderate malalignment VSD with aortic override in a patient with Tetralogy of Fallot

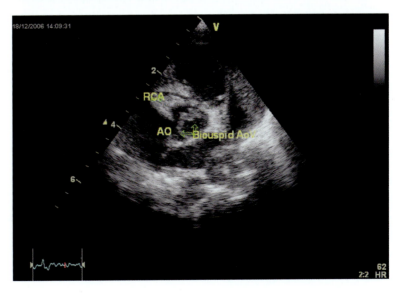

Fig. 13.8. Parasternal short-axis view demonstrating a bicuspid aortic valve

13.4.4
Suprasternal Views

The suprasternal coronal view is a useful view for evaluating aortic arch sidedness. Typically, in the absence of an aberrant left subclavian artery, the first branch arising from the aorta represents the innominate artery, which passes in the opposite direction to that of the arch. The pulmonary veins can be seen to drain to the left atrium in the suprasternal short-axis view also. If all four pulmonary veins are not seen to drain to the left atrium, the course of each one must be investigated.

In the suprasternal sagittal views (Fig. 13.9) the aortic arch is scanned along its length in the so-called candy-cane view. This is a useful scanning plane to define coarctation of the aorta and the presence of a PDA or aorto-pulmonary collaterals.

13.4.5

Right Parasternal Window
(the Fifth Imaging Plane)

This is used with the patient in a right lateral decubitus position and allows estimation of a gradient across the left ventricular outflow tract. This window is also excellent to image the atrial septum, especially in adult patients with poor subcostal windows.

13.5
Segmental Cardiac Anatomy

The performance of an echocardiogram is incomplete until the entire cardiac segmental anatomy has been defined. In order to do so the logical sequential approach outlined above needs to be adhered to rigidly in each patient studied. The following components of segmental anatomy require definition. Thoraco-abdominal situs is solitus, inversus or ambiguus. Cardiac location is levocardia, dextrocardia or mesocardia. Atrial location is solitus, inversus or isomeric (right or left atrial isomerism). The relation of the atria to the ventricles, termed the atrioventricular connection, is either concordant, discordant, atresia of one or other atria, double inlet, straddling or rarely criss-cross. The ventricles are termed D-looped or L-looped. The position of the conus is either subpulmonic, subaortic, bilateral or rarely absent. The relationship of the ventricles to the outlet chambers is concordant, discordant, double outlet or single outlet (ICARDO and SANCHEZ DE VEGA 1991). Finally the great vessel arrangement is solitus, inversus, transposed or side-by-side great vessels. Only when all these details have been clearly defined is the echocardiographic study complete. Persons not trained in cardiology or echocardiography risk missing crucial cardiac details. Incomplete interrogation of the heart in children and particularly sick

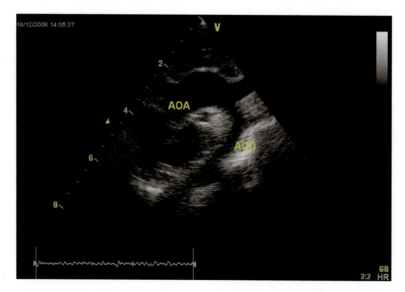

Fig. 13.9. Suprasternal sagittal view demonstrating the normal aortic arch "candy-cane" view

neonates may give rise to poor patient management and potentially morbidity and mortality.

13.5.1
Abdominal Situs – Cardiac Location

Transverse scanning directly inferior to the xiphisternum allows delineation of the stomach, liver and cardiac mass. In abdominal situs solitus the stomach is left-sided, the liver right-sided. In visceral situs inversus the stomach is right-sided and the liver left-sided. Ambiguus visceral situs describes a midline liver and the stomach may be left, right or central in position. Levocardia describes the heart in the left chest; dextrocardia, in the right chest with the apex pointing to the right; and mesocardia describes the heart in the centre of the chest. Dextroversion is a term used for the heart being positioned in the right chest with the apex pointing to the left. Levocardia with visceral situs inversus is associated with a high prevalence of congenital heart disease (90%) while situs inversus totalis with dextrocardia is associated with a much lower incidence of congenital heart disease (10%) (Anjos et al. 1990).

13.5.2
The Cava and the Atria

The IVC when intact nearly always drains to the right atrium; the SVC, however, may drain to either the left or right atrium, or both in cases with persistence of a left SVC. The IVC is interrupted with an absence of the hepatic portion of the IVC in left atrial isomerism. In this instance there is an azygous continuation of the IVC which typically drains to the left SVC.

Identification of the atria may prove a challenge. Specific morphological features however define each atrium. The right atrium is characterized by the eustachian and thebesian embryonic valves, a broad short atrial appendage and the presence of musculi pectinati. The left atrium has a long narrow atrial appendage. However, the atrial appendages may be juxtaposed and appendage identification may not help define the atria in such instances (Bevilacqua et al. 1991). In left atrial isomerism there are two left atria; in right atrial isomerism, two right atria. The atrioventricular valve does not help identify the atrium above it as it remains faithful to the ventricle it

fills rather than the atria it drains. In cases of ventricular inversion this would result in a misinterpretation of the anatomy.

13.5.3
Caval Veins and Right Atrium

The right SVC, innominate vein and when present the left SVC can be imaged in the suprasternal short-axis views. A bridging vein should be looked for in cases with bilateral SVCs. The IVC is best viewed in the subcostal long-axis and coronal views. When the IVC is absent the azygous continuation is best viewed from the transverse abdominal views. The coronary sinus may be seen posteriorly passing through the left atrium and draining into the right atrium.

13.5.4
Atrial Septum

The subcostal sagittal and coronal views provide the best views for examining this structure. The parasternal short-axis view may also provide images of the septum. Multiple views should be used to assess the size and location of atrial septal defects (ASDs). The presence of a superior or inferior sinus venosus defect is best detected from the sagittal subcostal images. Primum ASDs are typically seen in the four-chamber apical view.

13.5.5
Left Atrium and Pulmonary Veins

The pulmonary venous drainage is best viewed from a combination of suprasternal short-axis, apical four-chamber and subcostal views. All four pulmonary veins should be detected to rule out a partial anomalous pulmonary venous drainage. Partial anomalous drainage is common in the setting of a sinus venosus ASD, isomeric hearts and Scimitar syndrome. Total anomalous pulmonary drainage may be supracardiac (most commonly to the innominate vein), cardiac (to the coronary sinus) or infra-cardiac (draining to the inferior vena cava). Defining the pulmonary venous confluence and the drainage pattern of an anomalous connection may require novel views. The left atrium is best identified from the apical four-chamber and the parasternal long-axis views.

13.5.6
Atrioventricular Arrangement

The atrioventricular valve defines the ventricle to which it is attached. The tricuspid valve has three leaflets, is hinged more apical than the mitral valve, and is septophilic, i.e. has septal attachment to the interventricular septum. In contrast the mitral valve has two leaflets and is septophobic, i.e. only has attachments to the left ventricular free wall. The mitral valve is more apical in location. The prominent moderator band also defines the right ventricle.

AV concordance describes when the atrium is attached to the corresponding ventricle, i.e. right atrium attaches to right ventricle and left atrium to left ventricle, and discordance when the atrium attaches to the contralateral ventricle, e.g. left atrium to right ventricle. Double inlet occurs when both AV valves drain into one ventricle, either double inlet left or right ventricle (RICE et al. 1985). Atresia describes an absent AV valve connection, either tricuspid or mitral atresia. A straddling AV valve describes when one AV valve traverses a ventricular septal defect and has attachments into the contralateral ventricle (DANIELSON et al. 1979). Criss-cross AV connection describes when each AV valve drains into the contralateral ventricle, often seen in association with superior-inferior orientation of the ventricles (SOTO et al. 1980).

13.5.7
Ventricular Morphology

The right ventricle has a prominent moderator band, is triangular in shape and has coarse trabeculations. The left ventricle is ovoid in shape with an absence of trabeculations. D-looping of the ventricles describes the rightward anterior relation of the right ventricle, and L-looping describes leftward and anterior right ventricle. The RV has three components: inlet, trabecular and outlet portions.

13.5.8
Ventricular Septum

The interventricular septum consists of the muscular and membranous septum (ANDERSON and FREEDOM 2005). Muscular ventricular septal defects (VSDs) comprise inlet, trabecular and outlet

VSDs. Inlet VSDs typically occur in association with atrioventricular septal defects and often are associated with clefts in the mitral valve. Trabecular VSDs are within the muscular septal wall extending from the membranous to the apical septum. Outlet defects may be sub-aortic, subpulmonary or doubly committed subarterial defects. The membranous portion of the septum is between the tricuspid and aortic valves and is located directly below the aortic valve. This region is clearly seen from the parasternal long-axis view. Delineation of the location, number and size of VSDs is crucial particularly prior to surgical intervention.

13.5.9
Conal Morphology

The segment or space connecting the ventricles to the great arteries is termed the infundibulum or the conus. Several cardiac defects including tetralogy of Fallot and transposition of the great arteries are associated with abnormalities in conal development (ANDERSON et al. 2001). The subpulmonary conus is present in the normal heart and best viewed from the subcostal views. In tetralogy of Fallot there is a narrowing of the conus although debate continues as to whether the conus is lengthened or shortened. In d-transposition of the great arteries there is a subaortic conus. Double outlet right ventricle is characterized by bilateral subarterial coni.

13.5.10
Ventriculo-Arterial Relationship

The aortic annulus is rightward and posterior relative to the pulmonary annulus, termed situs solitus of the great vessels. When the aortic annulus is leftward and posterior to the pulmonary annulus this is situs inversus of the great vessels and occurs in dextrocardia. When the aorta arises from the right ventricle and the pulmonary artery from the left ventricle this is termed ventriculo-arterial discordance as opposed to ventriculo-arterial concordance in the normal heart. When both great vessels arise from the right ventricle, this is termed double-outlet right ventricle (DORV) (HATLE and ANGELSEN 1995). DORV is also associated with fibrous discontinuity between the mitral valve and aorta in normally related great vessels or between the mitral valve and pulmonary artery in DORV with the aorta anterior

and rightward. Transposition of the great arteries may be termed d-transposition when the aorta is anterior and rightward, and l-transposition with the aorta leftward and anterior. The orientation of the great vessels is best appreciated from the parasternal short-axis views.

13.5.11
The Aortic Arch and Coronary Arteries

The aortic arch is best viewed from the suprasternal and subcostal views. The arch sidedness is determined from the side of the trachea over which the aorta passes. In the normal left aortic arch, the innominate artery branches to the right. The suprasternal long- and short-axis views allow delineation of coarctation, PDA and aorto-pulmonary collaterals.

The origins of both left and right coronary arteries are viewed arising from the appropriate coronary sinuses in the parasternal short-axis and the apical four-chamber views.

13.6
Doppler Echocardiography

Christian Johann Doppler first described the fact that the frequency of transmitted sound is altered when the source of sound is moving (SNIDER and RITTER 2000). The Doppler equation describes the relationship between shift in frequency, velocity and direction of blood, angle of intercept of the ultrasound beam and velocity of sound in tissue:

$$f_d = \frac{2fo}{c} V \cos \Phi$$

where fd = observed Doppler velocity shift, fo = the transmitted frequency, c = the velocity of sound in tissue, V = velocity of sound in human tissue (1560 m/s), and Φ = the intercept angle between ultrasound beam and blood flow (HENRY et al. 1980).

There are three types of Doppler flow mapping: pulse Doppler (PW), continuous wave Doppler (CW) and colour Doppler mapping. Pulsed wave Doppler is characterized by a single ultrasound crystal alternately transmitting and receiving the ultrasound signal. A short burst of ultrasound is transmitted to a selected depth called the pulse repetition frequency (PRF). PW Doppler has range resolution but limited maximum frequency shifts that can be unambiguously displayed at a given depth. The maximum detectable frequency is called the Nyquist limit and this is equal to ±PRF/2. In CW Doppler there are two crystals, one which transmits the ultrasound signal and the other receiving the signal. There is no range resolution but its advantage is there are no limits to the velocities that can be mapped. Colour flow mapping is based upon the reflected ultrasound pulses being separated into two parts, the first to form a conventional 2-D echocardiogram and the second composed of reflections from the blood flow. Mean velocity is calculated by autocorrection and then converted into a colour display. Typically 120 time gates are sampled along the scan plane. Accurate determination of Doppler frequency shifts requires multiple successive sampling interrogations. Autocorrelation is a computational technique that allows an estimate of the mean Doppler shift. Flow pixels are assigned a colour based upon direction and velocity of flow: red being towards the transducer and blue away from the transducer. Aliasing may occur at higher Doppler velocities.

13.7
Echocardiographic Tools Available for Analysis of Ventricular Function

Accurate assessment of ventricular function is crucial in children with and without congenital heart disease. There are inherent differences between such echocardiographic assessments in adults and children with acquired or congenital heart disease. Age and body size spectrum in children is considerably larger and this creates inherent difficulties in assessing myocardial function, as changes occur during maturation of the heart (CINTRON et al. 1993). Most children with congenital heart disease and palliative or corrective repair of such lesions (such as patches for VSD) often have ventricles with a nongeometric shape, which makes assessment of right and left ventricular function more difficult. Postoperative residual physiologic abnormalities may complicate the echocardiographic evaluation. Lastly, many children have only one functional ventricle, which hampers serial assessment of myocardial performance.

Although Doppler ultrasound is the mainstay of diagnostic examinations for assessing ventricular function, a preliminary thorough two-dimensional examination with colour Doppler interrogation is essential to assess congenital cardiac anatomy and evaluate postoperative residua. As systolic dysfunction is often preceded by diastolic dysfunction, quantitative assessment of diastolic function may be predictive of eventual systolic dysfunction in these patients.

13.8
Left Ventricular Systolic Dysfunction

Left ventricular dimensions are often abnormal in children with congenital heart disease, and in patients with associated heart failure there is an increase in end-diastolic as well as end-systolic dimensions. It is important to understand the pathophysiology of various lesions in the interpretation of both increased dimensions as well as shortening fraction. For example, a shortening fraction in the normal range in a patient with aortic or mitral regurgitation would be indicative of deteriorating function (as one would expect such a patient to possess a supranormal shortening fraction). The progression of findings in regurgitant lesions prior to heart failure is usually an increase in end-diastolic dimension, followed by an increase in end-systolic dimension, and lastly a decrease in shortening fraction as the heart decompensates and fails.

Left ventricular (LV) systolic dysfunction has long been recognized to be a powerful predictor of the development of cardiac symptoms and poor long-term outcome in adults with heart failure (COHN et al. 1993; ROWLAND and GUTGESELL 1995; CORTI et al. 2001). In children with congenital heart lesions decreased LV systolic function has also been shown to predict poor outcome in many disease states (HAENDCHEN et al. 1983; JINDAL et al. 2000). Echocardiographic measures of LV systolic function include M-mode and two-dimensional examinations for dimension and volume changes as well as Doppler-derived ejection indices (RAINES et al. 1976). Quantitation of blood flow such as cardiac output and stroke volume, however, has generally not been used for assessment of cardiac performance as cardiac output can be preserved until myocardial dysfunction is severe.

The majority of echocardiographic measures of LV systolic function represent ejection phase indices such as shortening fraction, ejection fraction, velocity of circumferential fibre shortening, peak dP/dt, and systolic time intervals that rely upon geometric assumptions inherent in the elliptical shape of the LV. These measurements are significantly influenced by a variety of hemodynamic factors including altered ventricular preload and afterload, heart rate, LV mass and myocardial contractility. Unfavourable loading conditions can therefore mimic depressed contractility and, conversely, contractility can be falsely assessed to be normal in certain situations. The emergence of Doppler-derived measures of ventricular performance has circumvented many of the geometric challenges inherent in the global assessment of ventricular performance, especially in the evaluation of right ventricular (RV) performance as well as quantitative assessment of systolic function in patients with complex ventricular morphologies (JIANG et al. 1994; TEI et al. 1996a; EIDEM et al. 1998; SEBBAG et al. 2001).

13.8.1
Dimension-Derived Indices

One-dimensional wall motion analysis, or M-mode echocardiography, has traditionally been the most common method used to measure the extent of LV shortening fraction. There are limitations with this relatively crude methodology of assessing ventricular function. First, contraction of the left ventricle cannot be assumed to be entirely uniform or symmetrical. In addition, regional differences in wall motion and wall thickening should be taken into account in the interpretation of shortening fraction. Lastly, a flattened interventricular septum (as observed in patients with a right ventricular volume or pressure overload) invalidates such a measurement.

Shortening fraction represents the change in LV short axis diameter (with the cursor between the papillary muscles apical to the mitral valve leaflets):

$$SF(\%) = \frac{[LVEDD - LVESD]}{LVEDD} \times 100$$

where LVEDD represents the LV end-diastolic minor axis dimension and LVESD represents the LV end-systolic minor axis dimension. Normal values for

shortening fraction range between 28% and 44% with variation for age.

Determination of LV ejection fraction is somewhat more tedious than the calculation for LV shortening fraction described above but recent improvements in technology, including automated border detection or acoustic quantification, have simplified this procedure. Two-dimensional echocardiography allows measurement of LV ejection fraction (LVEF) by quantifying changes in ventricular volume during the cardiac cycle. The geometric model most commonly used to measure LV ejection fraction is the modified Simpson's biplane method. By utilizing orthogonal apical four-chamber and two-chamber views of the LV, this geometric model calculates LVEDV and LVESV by summing equal sequential slices of LV area from each of these scan planes (Fig. 13.3). LVEF can then be calculated as:

$$EF(\%) = \frac{[LVEDV - LVESV]}{LVEDV} \times 100$$

Recent studies have validated the ability of 3-D echocardiography to obtain accurate and reproducible estimates of LV and RV volumes and ejection fraction (ISAAZ et al. 1989a). Normal values for LV ejection fraction range between 56% and 78%. Similar to shortening fraction, LV ejection fraction has been shown to be dependent on changes in ventricular loading conditions.

13.8.1.1
Doppler-Derived Indices

Much information can be derived from the aortic velocity curve including peak aortic velocity, acceleration time, ejection time, velocity time integral, peak rate of acceleration, mean acceleration, and the acceleration-to-ejection time ratio. Because these indices are dependent on load conditions, they have the same limitations as shortening and ejection fraction determinations described above.

Non-invasive Doppler measurements of peak aortic velocity and peak aortic acceleration time have been shown to correlate with other measures of LV systolic function. Previous studies have demonstrated that LV ejection force correlated better than peak aortic velocity and peak aortic acceleration time with invasive angiographically derived LV ejection fraction in patients with heart failure (SAHN et al. 1974; STODDARD et al. 1989). Serial changes in peak aortic acceleration time have also shown promise in

demonstrating the extent and rate of recovery of LV systolic function in patients after an acute myocardial infarction and were predictive of the development of congestive heart failure in these patients (GARDIN et al. 1983). In patients with dilated cardiomyopathy, peak aortic Doppler velocity, aortic time velocity integral, and aortic acceleration time have all been shown to be decreased compared to normal controls (HARRISON et al. 1989a). Both aortic time intervals and Doppler peak velocities, however, are impacted by heart rate and loading conditions; studies have documented decreased peak aortic acceleration time and peak aortic velocity with increased heart rate as well as increased afterload (BARGIGGIA et al. 1989; HARRISON et al. 1989b).

Mitral regurgitation (MR) is a common finding in patients with heart failure; if mitral regurgitation is present, the peak and mean rate of change in LV systolic pressure can be derived from the ascending portion of the continuous-wave MR velocity curve signal (BESSEN and GARDIN 1990). Utilizing the simplified Bernoulli equation, two velocity points along the MR Doppler envelope during the isovolumic contraction period are selected from which a corresponding LV pressure change (rate of pressure rise) can be derived. This change in LV pressure can then be divided by the change in time between the two Doppler velocities (1 and 3 m/s) to derive the LV dP/dt [so that LV dP/dt=$(4\times3^2-4\times1^2)$/time in seconds or 32 mmHg/s]. Normal mean dP/dt is >1200 mmHg/s.

While more time consuming to perform, the MR velocity curve and the calculated peak dP/dt correlate accurately with invasive cardiac catheterization measurements (CHEN et al. 1991). To ascertain peak LV dP/dt noninvasively, the MR signal is digitized to obtain the first derivative of the pressure gradient curve (GONZALEZ-VILCHEZ et al. 1999). Similar to other ejection phase indices, LV dP/dt is affected by changes in loading conditions, most notably by increased afterload.

13.8.2
The Stress–Velocity Index

There are considerable limitations to the Doppler-derived ejection indices in estimating myocardial performance. Possible sources of error include equating the anatomical area with area of flow, circular or elliptical cross-section models, temporal constancy of the areas as well as the velocities, and lack of correction for angular deviations (SCHILLER et al. 1989).

The rate of LV fibre shortening (average rate of change of the left ventricular circumference in diameters per second) can be noninvasively assessed by M-mode echocardiography. This measurement, termed the mean velocity of circumferential fibre shortening (Vcf), is normalized for LV end-diastolic dimension and can be obtained from the following equation:

$$Vcf = \frac{[LVEDD - LVESD]}{[LVEDD \times LVET]}$$

where LVEDD represents LV end-diastolic dimension, LVESD represents LV end-systolic dimension, and LVET represents LV ejection time. It can be simplified to:

$$Vcf = \frac{SF}{LVET}$$

Reported normal values for mean Vcf are 1.5±0.04 circumferences/s for neonates and 1.3±0.03 circumferences/s for children aged 2–10 years (SAHN et al. 1974; RUBAY et al. 1997).

To normalize Vcf for variation in heart rate, LVET is divided by the square root of the R–R interval to derive a rate-corrected mean velocity of circumferential fibre shortening (Vcf$_c$). Normal Vcf$_c$ has been reported to be 1.28±0.22 and 1.08±0.14 circumferences/s in neonates and children, respectively (COLAN et al. 1984). Because Vcf$_c$ values are corrected for heart rate, a significant decrease in Vcf$_c$ between neonates and children has been attributed to increased systemic afterload with advancing age. Thus, shortening fraction alone may underestimate ventricular function in newborns. In patients with congenital heart lesions resulting in LV volume overload, mean Vcf$_c$ has been shown to increase, most likely secondary to increased LVEDD as well as augmented LV contractility with increased LV preload. In contrast, patients with dilated cardiomyopathy with decreased LV systolic function have been reported to have significantly decreased Vcf$_c$.

The majority of ejection phase indices, including shortening fraction, ejection fraction and Vcf$_c$, are dependent upon the underlying loading state of the LV. Colan and colleagues (1984) have previously described a stress–velocity index which is an inverse linear relationship between Vcf$_c$ and end-systolic wall stress (which most accurately measures left ventricular afterload) (LIPSHULTZ et al. 1991). The stress-velocity index, unlike shortening/ejection fractions or Doppler-derived blood flow velocities, is independent of preload, is normalized for heart rate, and incorporates afterload resulting in a noninvasive measure of LV contractility which is independent of ventricular loading conditions. Since contractility is the intrinsic ability of the myofibres to generate force, this stress-velocity index can therefore differentiate states of increased ventricular afterload from decreased myocardial contractility. The stress-velocity index has demonstrated significant increases in LV afterload with concomitant decreases in myocardial contractility in patients receiving doxorubicin for treatment of childhood leukaemia (Thomas and Weyman 1991). More recently, this index has demonstrated improved LV contractility and decreased end-systolic wall stress with amrinone infusion in neonates with postoperative congestive heart failure (CALABRO et al. 1999).

Although this methodology is theoretically sound and scientifically valid, it is somewhat more tedious to perform compared to other methodologies since the ejection time needs to be obtained from an indirect carotid or brachial artery pulse tracing (CREPAZ et al. 1998; MYRENG and SMISETH 1990; GARCIA et al. 1996a, 1996b; SABBAH et al. 1987; WATANABE et al. 2003). In addition, its interpretation needs to take age into account (as the neonatal myocardium exhibits a higher basal contractile state and a greater sensitivity to changes in afterload) (ZOGHBI and QUINONES 1986; SABBAH et al. 1987; MYRENG and SMISETH 1990; GARCIA et al. 1996a, 1996b; WATANABE et al. 2003).

13.8.3
Doppler Tissue Imaging (DTI) and Strain Rate Imaging

Quantitative assessment of regional LV function has centred upon evaluation of segmental endocardial excursion and LV wall thickening (GARCIA et al. 1996b). These semi-quantitative methods often fail to discriminate between active and passive myocardial motion. Newer echocardiographic modalities such as Doppler tissue imaging (DTI) and strain rate imaging offer a potentially more quantitative and accurate approach to the assessment of regional myocardial contraction and relaxation and can correlate with myocardial performance (ZOGHBI and QUINONES 1986; SABBAH et al. 1987; PINAMONTI et al. 1993; GARCIA et al. 1996; WATANABE et al. 2003;).

Doppler tissue imaging (DTI) is a relatively novel method of assessing quantitative longitudinal ventricular function by measuring pulsed wave Doppler velocities directly from underlying myocardium. It is load independent and has systolic and diastolic components. The systolic velocity (S) is always positive and starts with the first heart sound but ends before the second heart sound. The velocities are heterogeneous depending on ventricular wall and position. The diastolic filling waves, therefore, consist of the early filling wave (Ea) and the late filling wave (Aa) of mitral inflow. Finally, there are also isovolumic Doppler signals that are low-velocity biphasic waves during isovolumic contraction and relaxation. These velocities are influenced by sample location as velocities tend to be higher in lateral left ventricular wall and at the base (compared to the apex).

In assessing systolic function, an increase in inotropic state increases DTI velocities while impaired systolic function is manifested by decreased DTI velocities. The rate of annular descent of the atrioventricular valve and the degree of long-axis ventricular shortening have been shown to be sensitive echocardiographic indices of ventricular function (SNIDER et al. 1985; ALAM et al. 1992; O'LEARY et al. 1998; NII et al. 2002). Recent studies have demonstrated significant changes in mitral annular DTI velocities in adult patients with LV dysfunction and elevated LV filling pressures (QUINONES et al. 1981; MORI et al. 2000). There are changes in these LV wall motion velocities with heart rate and age in the paediatric population. Marked differences in velocities in children with dilated and hypertrophic cardiomyopathy have allowed discrimination between patients with poorer clinical outcomes (MCMAHON et al. 2004a, 2004b).

The deformation or strain of a myocardial tissue segment occurs over the cardiac cycle and the rate of this deformation is termed the strain rate. Strain rate imaging is also a new echocardiographic technique used to measure regional elongation and shortening of myocardial tissue segments (HEIMDAL et al. 1998). Preliminary studies have demonstrated regional differences in strain rate in adult patients after myocardial infarction and measurements of radial and longitudinal strain rate have also recently been reported in normal children (WEIDEMANN et al. 2002). In addition, quantification of regional right and left ventricular function by ultrasonic strain rate and strain indexes after surgical repair of tetralogy of Fallot in children demonstrated that RV deforma-

tion abnormalities are associated with electrical depolarization abnormalities (XIE et al. 1994). Further studies are needed to identify potential applications of strain rate imaging in the regional assessment of myocardial function of both right and left ventricles in children with heart failure.

13.9
Left Ventricular Diastolic Dysfunction

Because diastolic dysfunction often precedes systolic dysfunction, careful quantitative assessment of LV diastolic function is mandatory in the noninvasive diagnosis and serial evaluation of patients with heart failure. LV diastolic dysfunction is associated with abnormalities of ventricular compliance and relaxation and can be demonstrated by characteristic changes in both mitral inflow and pulmonary venous Doppler flow patterns as well as newer modalities including Doppler tissue imaging and colour Doppler flow propagation velocity (NISHIMURA et al. 1989; VIGNON et al. 1996; NAGUEH et al. 1997; RUBAY et al. 1997; VASAN et al. 1999). There are inherent limitations with these methodologies that continue to be refined and studied to yield the most accurate evaluation of diastolic function.

13.9.1
Doppler-Derived Indices

Mitral inflow Doppler, obtained from the apical four-chamber view by positioning a pulse-wave Doppler sample at the leaflet tips of the mitral valve (in order to obtain signals for maximal transvalvar velocity), represents the diastolic pressure gradient between the left atrium (LA) and left ventricle. Among indices studied are peak filling velocities, acceleration and deceleration rates and times, velocity ratios, and areas under the diastolic filling curve.

The early phase of diastole is based on active relaxation. The early diastolic filling wave, or E-wave, is the dominant diastolic wave and represents the peak pressure gradient between the LA and LV at the onset of diastole. This E-wave portion of the diastolic curve is usually 65±4% of the total area of the diastolic curve but is less in disease states that lead to LV noncompliance (SAHN et al. 1997). The deceleration time of the mitral E-wave reflects the time period needed for equalization of LA and LV pressure. The late phase of diastole is the passive filling phase. The late diastolic filling wave, or A-wave, represents the peak pressure gradient between the LA and LV in late diastole at the onset of atrial contraction.

Normal mitral inflow Doppler is characterized by a dominant E-wave, a smaller A-wave, and a ratio of E and A waves (E:A ratio) between 1.0 and 3.0. The normal duration of mitral deceleration as well as isovolumic relaxation time vary with age and have been reported in both paediatric and adult populations (Byrg et al. 1987; Bessen and Gardin 1990; Ota et al. 1999). For assessment of diastolic function, mitral inflow Doppler velocities are not only impacted by changes in relaxation and compliance components of diastolic function but also by a variety of additional anatomic and physiologic factors including loading conditions, contractility, heart rate, interventricular interaction, valve mobility, respiratory phase and age (Stugaard et al. 1994). Interpretation of characteristic patterns of mitral inflow must be carefully evaluated with particular attention given to the potential impact of each of these factors on mitral inflow Doppler velocities.

Diastolic dysfunction is manifested by characteristic mitral inflow Doppler patterns. The earliest stage of LV diastolic dysfunction demonstrated by mitral inflow Doppler is termed abnormal relaxation. Factors that affect relaxation include loading conditions, contractile state and elastic recoil properties of the ventricle as well as age, hypertrophied ventricles, myocardial ischaemia, or infiltrative cardiomyopathy with normal atrial pressure. Abnormal relaxation, therefore, is characterized by a reduced E-wave velocity, increased A-wave velocity, reversed E:A ratio (<1.0), and a prolonged mitral deceleration time and isovolumic relaxation time (IVRT).

As diastolic dysfunction progresses, further changes in both ventricular relaxation and compliance occur, leading to an increase in LA pressure. Factors that affect compliance include myocardial properties, interventricular interaction and ventricular geometry. Increased LA pressure normalizes the initial transmitral gradient between the LA and LV producing a transitional "pseudo-normalized" mitral inflow Doppler pattern with increased E-wave velocity and E:A ratio and normalized mitral deceleration and isovolumic relaxation time intervals. The pathophysiology is abrupt cessation of early filling as the left ventricular diastolic pressure is increased. This pseudo-normal Doppler pattern may be difficult to distinguish from normal mitral inflow Doppler;

additional evaluation of pulmonary venous inflow Doppler, however, can be complementary in helping to unmask this advanced degree of LV diastolic dysfunction since the pulmonary venous pattern will be abnormal (i.e. forward flow in systole is decreased, forward flow in diastole is increased, and atrial diastolic reversal is also more significant).

Further deterioration of LV diastolic function results in restrictive ventricular filling with an additional increase in LA pressure and a concomitant decrease in ventricular compliance. The Doppler pattern of restrictive LV filling is characterized by additional increases in E-wave velocity, reduction in A-wave velocity, an increased E:A ratio >2.0, and significant shortening of both mitral deceleration time and IVRT.

Adult studies have demonstrated that heart failure patients with altered mitral inflow Doppler, and most importantly a restrictive filling pattern, have significantly increased morbidity and mortality (Yamamoto et al. 1997). Reversal of this restrictive filling pattern with medical therapy to a pattern characteristic of either abnormal relaxation or pseudo-normalization has correlated with improved long-term survival in adult heart failure patients Teshima et al. 2002).

Pulmonary venous Doppler, combined with mitral inflow Doppler, provides a more comprehensive assessment of LA and LV filling pressures (Klein and Tajik 1991; Oki et al. 1997). Pulmonary venous inflow consists of three distinct Doppler waves: a systolic wave (S-wave), a diastolic wave (D-wave) and a reversal wave with atrial contraction (Ar-wave). In normal adolescents and adults, the characteristic pattern of pulmonary venous inflow consists of a dominant S-wave, a smaller D-wave and a small Ar-wave of low velocity and brief duration. In neonates and younger children, a dominant D-wave is often present with a similar brief low-velocity, or even absent, Ar-wave.

With worsening LV diastolic dysfunction, LA pressure rises, leading to diminished systolic forward flow into the LA from the pulmonary veins with relatively increased diastolic forward flow resulting in a diastolic dominance of pulmonary venous inflow. More importantly, both the velocity and duration of the pulmonary venous atrial reversal wave are increased. Paediatric and adult studies have demonstrated that an Ar-wave duration >30 ms longer than the corresponding mitral A-wave duration or a ratio of pulmonary venous Ar-wave to mitral A-wave duration >1.2 is predictive of elevated LV filling pressure.

Early diastolic DTI velocities (Ea) at the lateral mitral annulus have demonstrated clinical utility in patients with LV dysfunction. With increasing diastolic dysfunction, LA and LV filling pressures rise, leading to an increased mitral E-wave velocity; however, these same changes have been shown to have little impact on DTI E-wave velocity at the mitral annulus. DTI velocities have also been demonstrated to be less significantly impacted by changes in ventricular filling pressure and loading conditions compared to mitral inflow Doppler velocities (CHOONG et al. 1988; SPENCER et al. 1999). While mitral E-wave velocity alone is less reliable as an index of abnormal diastolic function, a ratio of mitral E-wave to DTI E-wave velocity (E/Ea) >15 has been shown to be more predictive of elevated pulmonary capillary wedge pressure in adult patients. In addition, early diastolic myocardial velocity was found to be the single best discriminator between control subjects and patients with diastolic dysfunction (FARIAS et al. 1999). Lastly, this methodology to assess diastolic dysfunction needs to consider that there is substantial heterogeneity in measured velocities within individual myocardial segments consistent with known spatial distribution of myocardial fibres (GALIUTO et al. 1998). In addition to DTI, a continuous-wave Doppler velocity profile of mitral regurgitation can yield negative LV dP/dt and thus the time constant of relaxation (τ) (CHEN et al. 1994). Lastly, pulsed Doppler detection of abnormal LV posterior wall diastolic motion dynamics (by placing the sample volume apical to the mitral valve sulcus and within the LV endocardium) can also gain insight into global LV diastolic performance (ISAAZ et al. 1989b).

13.9.2
Color M-Mode Flow Propagation Velocity (Vp)

Recently, colour M-mode Doppler echocardiography has been demonstrated to provide information about diastolic function by measurement of sequential mitral inflow filling waves during propagation from base to apex (BORDER et al. 2003). Specifically, the flow propagation velocity of early transmitral flow from colour M-mode recordings inversely correlated with the time constant of relaxation τ (MOLLER et al. 2000). As opposed to mitral inflow Doppler, this propagation velocity has been shown to be less dependent on changes in heart rate, LA pressure and loading conditions and may therefore more

accurately reflect changes in myocardial relaxation. Numerous studies have demonstrated a significant decrease in flow propagation velocity in patients with diastolic dysfunction of varying aetiology. The ratio of the mitral annular Doppler tissue E-wave velocity to flow propagation velocity is a significant predictor of outcome in patients after myocardial infarction (MOLLER et al. 2001). This ratio of flow propagation and DTI velocity may also be helpful in distinguishing a normal mitral inflow pattern from one of pseudo-normalized mitral inflow.

13.10
Global Left Ventricular Dysfunction

Systolic and diastolic dysfunction may coexist, so a combined measure of LV performance may be more reflective of overall ventricular dysfunction. The myocardial performance or Tei index (MPI) is a Doppler-derived quantitative measure that incorporates both systolic and diastolic time intervals. This index measures the ratio of total time spent in isovolumic activity divided by the time spent in ventricular ejection. The MPI is defined as the sum of isovolumic contraction time (ICT) and isovolumic relaxation time (IRT) divided by ejection time (ET):

$$MPI = \frac{(ICT + IRT)}{ET}$$

The components of this index are measured from routine pulse-wave Doppler signals at the atrioventricular valve and ventricular outflow tract of either left or right ventricle. To derive the sum of ICT and IRT, the Doppler-derived ejection time for either ventricle is subtracted from the Doppler interval between the cessation and onset of the respective atrioventricular valve inflow signal (from the end of the Doppler A-wave to the beginning of the Doppler E-wave of the next cardiac cycle). The Doppler time intervals should be obtained as close to simultaneously as possible and consecutive Doppler intervals should not vary by more than 5–15 ms. This measure is invalid in the setting of arrhythmias.

A validation study demonstrated that the MPI (and especially the ratio of shortening fraction/MPI) closely correlate with dP/dt over a range of haemodynamic conditions in animal models (BROBERG et al. 2003). The higher the MPI (or Tei) value the greater the global ventricular dysfunction. In adults, normal LV and RV MPI values are 0.39±0.05 and 0.28±0.04 respectively, while in children similar values for the LV and RV are reported to be 0.35±0.03 and 0.32±0.03 respectively (TEI et al. 1996b). This index is relatively load independent making it particularly appealing in this patient population.

13.11
Right Ventricular Dysfunction

Echocardiographic assessment of ventricular function in the morphological right ventricle is important for several paediatric patient populations, including patients with transposition of the great arteries who had an atrial switch (Senning or Mustard), those with tetralogy of Fallot who have pulmonary insufficiency, and patients with single ventricle anatomy of right ventricular morphology.

The asymmetric and crescentic geometric shape of the right ventricle complicates echocardiographic assessment of ventricular function. Doppler echocardiography has historically been useful in the noninvasive prediction of RV systolic and pulmonary artery pressures. Quantification of RV systolic function by M-mode or 2-D echocardiography has relied on a qualitative assessment of relative RV wall motion or semiquantitative measurements of fractional area change in RV dimension or volume (KAUL et al. 1984). Newer echocardiographic modalities, which show promise in quantifying RV function, include additional Doppler measures of RV performance (myocardial performance index, RV dP/dt, and DTI) as well as acoustic quantification and 3-D echocardiography.

As described previously, the MPI is a Doppler-derived measure of global ventricular function that can be applied to any ventricular geometry. The MPI has demonstrated prognostic power in discriminating outcome in patients with either RV or LV failure (YU and SANDERSON 1997). In patients with congenital heart disease with altered RV preload or afterload, the RV MPI has been shown to be relatively independent of changes in loading conditions making it particularly appealing in this subset of patients.

Similar to the MR and calculation for LV dP/dt, the RV dP/dt or the rate of RV pressure change over time can also be used as a measure of RV systolic function in patients with tricuspid regurgitation. The change in RV pressure can then be divided by the change in time between the two Doppler velocities (1 and 2 m/s) to derive the RV dP/dt [so that RV dP/dt=$(4\times2^2-4\times1^2)$/time in seconds or 12 mmHg/time in seconds]. (Note that 2 m/s is used as the second Doppler velocity rather than 3 m/s as with the LV.) RV dP/dt has been shown to have correlation with invasive measures of RV performance and is helpful in the serial assessment of RV function in children with hypoplastic left heart syndrome.

A relatively new addition to the quantitative evaluation of RV function is Doppler tissue imaging (DTI). Tricuspid annular motion has been shown to correlate with RV function in several studies (FROMMELT et al. 2002). DTI has been shown to be a reproducible noninvasive method of assessing systolic and diastolic annular motion and RV function. Unlike conventional Doppler inflow velocities, preliminary studies with DTI in adults and children have demonstrated these velocities to be relatively independent of loading conditions (MORI et al. 2002). Comparative measurements of annular and inflow velocities reveal that the ratio of late-to-early diastolic tricuspid annular velocity showed a higher correlation with RV end-diastolic pressure.

Acoustic quantification utilizes automated border detection techniques to measure the absolute change and rate of change in RV volume. This modality has been shown to correlate with other invasive methods of RV functional assessment in adults with abnormalities of global RV function. Automated border methods have shown good correlation with MRI in assessing changes in RV volume and systolic function. Feasibility of acoustic quantification in the noninvasive evaluation of RV function in normal children has also been reported. This technique needs to be studied further in the identification and serial evaluation of RV dysfunction in heart failure.

The recent advent of 3-D echocardiography has enabled noninvasive evaluation of RV volume and function. Because 3-D echocardiography can evaluate RV geometry in multiple spatial planes, accurate assessment of changes in RV volume during the cardiac cycle is possible. Such data collection needs to be rapid, efficient and automated with minimal motion effects. Application of this new modality to the evaluation of RV systolic failure in adults and children has not yet been reported but appears to be promising.

13.12
Univentricular Hearts and Assessment of Ventricular Function

Quantitative echocardiographic assessment is limited by complex ventricular geometry often with associated abnormalities of wall motion. Similar to novel techniques used to assess RV function, Doppler echocardiography holds promise in the potential evaluation of global single ventricle function. However, only limited studies to date have addressed either dP/dt or the MPI in patients with functional single ventricles. One study showed improved function after cavopulmonary anastomosis in single-ventricle patients when the operation is performed at less than 1 year of age when using MPI as a measurement of ventricular function. Although there are limited data on these new Doppler indices to predict outcome in patients with complex single-ventricle anatomy, early studies demonstrate the feasibility of Doppler-derived indices for assessment of single-ventricle function.

13.13
Tissue Harmonic Imaging

This technique enhances image clarity by focusing transducer frequencies on higher harmonic frequencies rather than lower frequencies (McMAHON et al. 2001). This results in a significant improvement in image resolution.

13.14
Fetal Echocardiography

This is more challenging than conventional echo cardiography as the fetus is often in motion and fetal positioning with the spine upwards may make image acquisition difficult. The segmental cardiac approach should be applied as in the child (GARLAND et al. 1991; LANG et al. 1991; ALLAN 1993). The determination of cardiac situs, an apical four-chamber view, imaging of the systemic and pulmonary venous drainage, the atrioventricular valves, interventicular and atrial septa, outflow tracts, the aortic arch and ductus arteriosus are then sequentially scanned. Fetal ventricular function is assessed using M-mode to determine LV shortening fraction. The presence of tachyarrhythmias or AV block is recorded using M-mode (TWORETSKY et al. 2001).

13.15
Transoesophageal Echocardiography

Transoesophageal echocardiography (TOE) allows imaging clarity rarely offered by transthoracic views (YANG et al. 2000). The basal long-axis, mid-oesophagus long-axis and transgastric long-axis views are initially obtained. Rotation of the probe in each of these views allows complete intra-cardiac evaluation. Imaging of the aortic arch may be limited using TOE. TOE is primarily used in the postoperative setting but also has a clinical role in the intensive care setting and in patients with poor echocardiographic windows.

13.16
Conclusions

Ultrasound of the heart has progressed to be the primary imaging modality for assessing cardiac anatomy in children with congenital and acquired heart disease. A sequential logical approach is mandatory in all patients to avoid errors in diagnosis and consequently patient management. Increasingly new noninvasive imaging tools are becoming available to provide further data regarding ventricular function.

References

Alam M, Hoglund C, Thorstrand D (1992) Longitudinal systolic shortening of the left ventricle: an echocardiographic study in subjects with and without preserved global function. Clin Physiol 12:443–453

Allen HD, Gutgesell HP, Clark EB, Driscoll DJ (2000) Echocardiography. In: Moss and Adams' heart disease in infants, children, and adolescents: including the fetus and young adult, 6th edn. Lipincott, Williams and Wilkins, Baltimore, Md., pp 204–233

Allan LD (1993) Fetal diagnosis of fetal congenital heart disease. J Heart Lung Transplant 12:S159–S160

Anderson RH, Freedom RM (2005) Normal and abnormal structure of the ventriculo-arterial junctions. Cardiol Young 1:3–16

Anderson RH, McCarthy K, Cook AC (2001) Continuing medical education. Double outlet right ventricle. Cardiol Young 11:329–344

Anjos RT, Ho SY, Anderson RH (1990) Surgical implications of juxtaposition of the atrial appendages. A review of forty-nine autopsied hearts. J Thorac Cardiovasc Surg 99:897–904

Bargiggia GS, Bertucci C, Recusani F, Raisaro A, de Servi S, Valdes-Cruz LM, Sahn DJ, Tronconi L (1989) A new method for estimating left ventricular dp/dt by continuous wave Doppler-echocardiography. Circulation 80:1287–1292

Bessen M, Gardin JM (1990) Evaluation of left ventricular diastolic function. Cardiol Clin 8:15–32

Bevilacqua M, Sanders SP, Van Praagh S, Colan SD, Parness I (1991) Double-inlet left ventricle: echocardiographic anatomy with emphasis on the morphology of the atrioventricular valves and ventricular septal defect. J Am Coll Cardiol 18:559–68

Border WL, Michelfelder EC, Glascock BJ, Witt SA, Spicer RL. Beekman RH, Kimball TR (2003) Color M-mode and Doppler tissue evaluation of diastolic function in children: Simultaneous correlation with invasive indices. J Am Soc Echocardiogr 16:988–94

Boxt LM (1996) MR imaging of congenital heart disease. Magn Reson Imaging Clin N Am 4:327–359

Broberg CS, Pantely GA, Barber BJ, Mack GK, Lee K, Thigpen T, Davis LE, Sahn D, Hohimer AR (2003) Validation of the myocardial performance index in mice: a noninvasive measure of left ventricular function. J Am Soc Echocardiogr 16:814–823

Byrg RJ, Williams GA, Labvitz AJ (1987) Effect of aging on left ventricular diastolic filling in normal subjects. Am J Cardiol 59:971–974

Calabro R, Piscane C, Pacileo G, Russo MG (1999) Left ventricular midwall mechanics in healthy children and adolescents. J Am Soc Echocardiogr 12:932–940

Chen C, Rodriguez L, Guerrero JL, Marshall S, Levine RA, Weyman AE, Thomas JD (1991) Noninvasive estimation of the instantaneous derivative of left ventricular pressure using continuous wave Doppler echocardiography. Circulation 83:2102–2110

Chen C, Rodriguez l, Lethor JP, Levine RA, Semigran MS, Fifer MA, Weyman AE, Thomas JD (1994) Continuous wave Doppler echocardiography for noninvasive assessment of left ventricular left ventricular dP/Dt and relaxation time constant from mitral regurgitant spectra in patients. J Am Coll Cardiol 23:970–976

Choong CY, Abascal VM, Thomas JD, Guerrero JL, McGlens S, Weyman AE (1988) Combined influence of ventricular loading and relaxation on the transmitral flow velocity profile in dogs measured by Doppler echocardiography. Circulation 78:672–683

Cintron G, Johnson G, Francis G, Cobb F, Cohn JN (1993) Prognostic significance of serial changes in left ventricular ejection fraction in patients with congestive heart failure. Circulation 87:17–23

Cohn JN, Johnson GR, Shabetai R, Loeb H, Tristani F, Rector T, Smith R, Fletcher R (1993) Ejection fraction, peak exercise oxygen consumption, cardiothoracic ratio, ventricular arrhythmias, and plasma norepinephrine as determinants of prognosis in heart failure. Circulation 87:V5–V16

Colan SD, Borow KM, Newmann A (1984) Left ventricular end-systolic wall stress-velocity of fibert shortening relation: a load independent index of myocardial contractility. J Am Coll Cardiol 4:715–724

Corti R, Binggeli C, Turina M, Jenni R, Luscher TF, Turina J (2001) Predictors of longterm survival after valve replacement for chronic aortic regurgitation: is M-mode echocardiography sufficient? Eur Heart J 22:866–873

Crepaz R, Pitscheider W, Radetti G, Gentili L (1998) Age-related variation in left ventricular myocardial contractile state expressed by the stress-velocity relation. Pediatr Cardiol 19:463–467

Danielson GK, Tabry IF, Ritter DG, Fulton RE (1979) Surgical repair of criss-cross heart with straddling atrioventricular valve. J Thorac Cardiovasc Surg 77:847–851

Eidem BW, O'Leary P, Tei C, Seward JB (1998) Nongeometric quantitative assessment of right and left ventricular function: myocardial performance index in normal children and patients with Ebsteins anomaly. J Am Soc Echocardiogr 11:849–856

Farias CA, Rodriguez L, Garcia MJ, Sun JP, Klein AL, Thomas JD (1999) Assessment of diastolic function by tissue Doppler echocardiography: comparison with standard transmitral and pulmonary venous flow. J Am Soc Echocardiogr 12:609–617

Frommelt PC, Ballweg JA, Whitestone BN, Frommelt MA (2002) Usefulness of Doppler tissue imaging analysis of tricuspid annular motion for determination of right ventricular function in normal infants and children. Am J Cardiol 89:610–613

Galiuto L, Ignone G, DeMaria AN (1998) Contraction and relaxation velocities of the normal left ventricle using pulsed-wave tissue Doppler echocardiography. Am J Cardiol 81:609–614

Garcia MJ, Rodriguez L, Ares M, Griffin BP, Thomas JD, Klein AL (1996a) Differentiation of constrictive pericarditis from restrictive cardiomyopathy: assessment of left ventricular diastolic velocities in longitudinal axis by Doppler tissue imaging. J Am Coll Cardiol 27:108–114

Garcia MJ, Rodriguez L, Ares M, Griffin BP, Klein AL, Stewart WJ, Thomas JD (1996b) Myocardial wall velocity assessment by pulsed Doppler tissue imaging: characteristic findings in normal subjects. Am Heart J 136:648–656

Gardin JM, Iseri LT, Elkayam U, Tobis J, Childs W, Burn CS, Henry WL (1983) Evaluation of dilated cardiomyopathy by pulsed Doppler echocardiography. Am Heart J 106:1057–1065

Geva T (1975) Segmental approach to the diagnosis of congenital heart disease. In: Freedom RM, Braunwald E (eds) Atlas of heart disease, Vol XII (Congenital heart disease). Mosby, Philadelphia, Pa., pp 5.1–5.15

Goldberg BB, Kimmelman BA (eds) (1988) Medical diagnostic ultrasound: a retrospective on its 40th anniversary. Eastman Kodak, Rochester, N.Y., pp 2–19

Gonzalez-Vilchez F, Ares M, Ayuela J, Alonso L (1999) Combined use of pulsed and color M-mode Doppler echocardiography for the estimation of pulmonary capillary wedge pressure: an empirical approach based on an analytical relation. J Am Coll Cardiol 34:515–523

Haendchen RV, Wyatt HL, Maurer G, Zwehl W, Bear M, Meerbaum S, Corday E (1983) Quantitation of regional cardiac function by two-dimensional echocardiography. I. Patterns of contraction in the normal left ventricle. Circulation 67:1234–1245

Harrison MR, Clifton GD, Sublett KL, DeMaria AN (1989a) Effect of heart rate on Doppler indices of systolic function in humans. J Am Coll Cardiol 14:929–935

Harrison MR, Clifton GD, Berk MR, DeMaria AN (1989b) Effect of blood pressure and afterload on Doppler echocardiographic measurements of left ventricular systolic function in normal subjects. Am J Cardiol 64:905–908

Hatle L, Angelsen B (1995) Doppler ultrasound in cardiology: physical principles and clinical applications, 2nd edn. Lea and Febiger, Philadelphia, Pa., pp 1–96

Heimdal A, Stoylen A, Torp H, Skjaerpe T (1998) Real-time strain rate imaging of the left ventricle by ultrasound. J Am Soc Echocardiogr 11:1013–1019

Henry WL, Gardin JM, Ware JH (1980) Echocardiographic measurements in normal subjects with from infancy to old age. Circulation 62:1054–1061

Icardo JM, Sanchez de Vega MJ (1991) Spectrum of heart malformations in mice with situs solitus, situs inversus and associated visceral heterotaxy. Circulation 84:2547–2558

Isaaz K, Ethevenot G, Admanti P, Brembilla B, Pernot C (1989a) A new Doppler method for assessing left ventricular ejection force in congestive heart failure. Am J Cardiol 64:81–87

Isaaz K, Thompson A, Ethevenot G, Choez JL, Brembilla B, Pernot C (1989b) Doppler echocardiographic measurement of low velocity motion of the left ventricular posterior wall. Am J Cardiol 64:66–75

Jiang I, Siu C, Handschmacher S, Luis Guergerro J, Vasquez de Prada JA, King ME, Picard MH, Weyman AE, Levine RA (1994) Three-dimensional echocardiography: in vitro validation for right ventricular volume and function. Circulation 89:2342–50

Jindal RC, Saxena A, Kothari SS, Juneja R, Shrivastava S (2000) Congenital severe aortic stenosis with congestive heart failure in late childhood and adolescence: effect on left ventricular function after balloon valvuloplasty. Catheter Cardiovasc Interv 51:168–72

Kaul S, Tei C, Hopkins JM, Shah PM (1984) Assessment of right ventricular function using two-dimensional echocardiography. Am Heart J 107:526–31

Klein AL, Tajik AJ (1991) Doppler assessment of pulmonary venous flow in healthy subjects and in patients with heart disease. J Am Soc Echocardiogr 4:379–92

Lang D, Oberhoffer R, Cook A, Sharland G, Allan L, Fagg N, Anderson RH (1991) Pathologic spectrum of malformation s of the tricuspid valve in prenatal and postnatal life. J Am Coll Cardiol 17:1161–7

Lipshultz SE, Colan SD, Belber RD, Gelber RD, Perez-Atayde AR, Sallan SE, Sanders SP.(1991) Late cardiac effects of doxorubicin therapy for acute lymphoblastic leukemia in childhood. N Engl J Med 324;843–5

McMahon CJ, Fraley K, Kovalchin JP (2001) Use of tissue harmonic imaging in pediatric echocardiography. Cardiol Young 11:562–4

McMahon CJ, Nagueh SF, Eapen RS, Dreyer WJ, Finkelshtyn I, Cao X, Eidem BW, Bezold LI, Denfield SW, Towbin JA, Pignatelli RH (2004a) Echocardiographic predictors of adverse clinical events in children with dilated cardiomyopathy: a prospective clinical study. Heart 90:908–915

McMahon CJ, Nagueh SF, Pignatelli RH, Denfield SW, Dreyer WJ, Price JF, Clunie S, Bezold LI, Hays AL, Towbin JA, Eidem BW (2004b) Characterization of left ventricular diastolic function by tissue Doppler imaging and clinical status in children with hypertrophic cardiomyopathy. Circulation 109:1756–62

Moller JE, Sondergaard E, Seward JB Appleton CP, Egstrup K (2000) Ratio of left ventricular peak E wave velocity to flow propagation assessed by color Doppler echocardiography in first myocardial infarction. J Am Coll Cardiol 35:363–70

Moller JE, Sondergaard E, Poulsen SH Seward JB, Appleton CP, Egstrup K (2001) Color M-mode and pulsed wave tissue Doppler echocardiography: powerful predictors of cardiac events after first myocardial infarction. J Am Soc Echocardiogr 14:757–63

Mori K, Hayabuchi Y, Kuroda Y, Nii M, Manabe T (2000) Left ventricular wall motion velocities in healthy children measured by pulsed wave Doppler tissue echocardiography: norml values and relation to age and heart rate. J Am Soc Echocardiogr 13:1002–1011

Myreng V, Smiseth OA (1990) Assessment of left ventricular relaxation by Doppler echocardiography. Circulation 81:1260–1266

Nagueh SF, Middleton KJ, Kopelen HA, Zoghbi WA, Quinones MA (1997) Doppler tissue imaging: a noninvasive technique for evaluation of left ventricular relaxation and estimation of filling pressures. J Am Coll Cardiol 30:1527–1533

Nii M, Mori K, Kuroda Y (2002) Quantification of the myocardial velocity gradient and myocardial wall thickening velocity in healthy children: a new indicator of regional myocardial wall motion. J Am Soc Echocardiogr 15:624–632

Nishimura RA, Abel MB, Hatle LK, Tajik AJ (1989) Assessment of diastolic function of the heart: background and current applications of Doppler echocardiography. Part II. Clinical studies. Mayo Clin Proc 64:181–204

Oki T, Tabata T, Yamada H, Wakatsuki T, Shinohara H, Nishikado A, Luchi A, Fukuda N, Ito S (1997) Clinical application of pulsed Doppler tissue imaging for assessing abnormal left ventricular relaxation. Am J Cardiol 79:921–928

O'Leary PW, Durongpisitkul K, Cordes TM, Bailey KR, Hagler DJ, Tajik J, Seward JB (1998) Diastolic ventricular function in children: a Doppler echocardiographic study establishing normal values and predictors of increased ventricular end-diastolic pressure. Mayo Clin Proc 73:616–628

Ota T, Fleishman CE, Strub M, Stretten G, Ohazama CJ, von Ramm OT, Kisslo J (1999) Real-time, three-dimensional echocardiography: feasibility of dynamic right ventricular volume measurement with saline contrast. Am Heart J 137:958–966

Pinamonti B, DiLenarda A, Sinagra G, Camerini F (1993) Restrictive left ventricular filling pattern in dilated cardiomyopathy assessed by Doppler echocardiography: clinical, echocardiographic and hemodynamic correlations and prognostic indications. Heart Muscle Disease Study Group. J Am Coll Cardiol 22:808–815

Quinones MA, Waggoner AD, Reduto LA, Nelson JG, Young JB, Winters WL, Ribeiro LG, Miller RR (1981) A new simplified and accurate method for determining ejection fraction with two-dimensional echocardiography. Circulation 64:744–753

Raines RA, LeWinter MM, Covell JW (1976) Regional shortening patterns in canine right ventricle. Am J Physiol 231:1395–1400

Rice MJ, Seward JB, Edwards WD, Hagler DJ, Danielson GK, Puga FJ. Tajik AJ (1985) Straddling atrioventricular valve: two-dimensional echocardiographic diagnosis, classification and surgical implications. Am J Cardiol 55:505–513

Rowland DG, Gutgesell HP (1995) Noninvasive segmental assessment of myocardial contractility, preload and afterload in healthy newborn infants. Am J Cardiol 75:18–21

Rubay JE, Shango P, Clement S, Ovaert C, Matta A, Vliers A, Sluysfians T (1997) Ross procedure in congenital results and left ventricular function. Eur J Cardiothorac Surg 11:92–99

Ruscazio M, Van Praagh S, Marrass AR, Catani G, Iliceto S, Van Praagh R (1998) Interrupted inferior vena cava in asplenia syndrome and a review of the hereditary patterns of visceral situs abnormalities. Am J Cardiol 81:111–116

Sabbah HN, Gheorghiade M, Smith ST, Frank DM, Stein PD (1987) Rate and extent of recovery of left ventricular function in patients following acute myocardial infarction. Am Heart J 114:516–524

Sahn DJ, Deely WJ, Hagan AD, Friedman DM (1974) Echocardiographic assessment of left ventricular performance in normal newborns. Circulation 49:232–236

Sahn DJ, Vaucher Y, Williams DE, Allen HD, Goldberg SJ, Friedman WF (1976) Echocardiographic detection of large left to right shunts and cardiomyopathy in infants and children. Am J Cardiol 38:73–79

Sahn DW, Chai IH, Lee DJ, Kim HC, Kim HS, Oh BH, Lee MM, Park YB, Choi YS, Seo JD, Lee YW (1997) Assessment of mitral annulus velocity by tissue Doppler imaging in evaluation of left ventricular diastolic function. J Am Coll Cardiol 30:474–480

Schiller NB, Shah PM, Crawford M, DeMaria A, Devereux R, Feigenbaum H, Gutgesell H, Reichek N, Sahn D, Schnittger I (1989) Recommendation for quantitation of the left ventricle by two-dimensional echocardiography. J Am Soc Echocardiogr 2:358–367

Sebbag I, Rudski LG, Therrien J, Hirsch A, Langleben D (2001) Effect of chronic infusion of epoprostenol on echocardiographic right ventricular myocardial performance index and its relation to clinical outcome in patients with primary pulmonary hypertension. Am J Cardiol 88:1060–1063

Sharland GK, Chita SK, Fagg NL, Anderson RH, Tynan M, Cook AC, Allan LD (1991) Left ventricular dysfunction in the fetus: relation to aortic valve anomalies and endocardial fibroelastosis. Br Heart J 66:419–424

Silverman NH (1983) An ultrasonic approach to the diagnosis of cardiac situs, connections, and malpositions. Cardiol Clin 1:473–486

Snider AR, Ritter S (2000) Doppler echocardiography. In Allen HD, Gutgesell HP, Clark EB, Driscoll DJ (eds) Moss and Adams' heart disease in infants, children, and adolescents: including the fetus and young adult, 6th edn. Lipincott, Williams and Wilkins, Baltimore, Md., pp 234–263

Snider AR, Gidding SS, Rocchini AP, Rosenthal A, Dick M, Crowley DC, Peters J (1985) Doppler evaluation of left ventricular diastolic filling in children with systemic hypertension. Am J Cardiol 56:921–926

Snider AR, Serwer GA, Ritter SB (eds) (1997) Echocardiography in pediatric heart disease, 2nd edn. Mosby-Year Book, St. Louis, Mo., pp 27–52

Soto B, Becker AE, Moulaert AJ, Lie JT, Anderson RH (1980) Classification of ventricular septal defects. Br Heart J 43:332–343

Spencer KT, Garcia MJ, Weinart L, Vignon P, Lang R (1999) Assessment of right ventricular and right atrial systolic and diastolic performance using an automated border detection. Echocardiography 16:643–652

Stoddard MF, Pearson AC, Kearn MJ, Ratcliff J, Mrosek DG, Labovitz AJ (1989) Influence of alteration in preload on the pattern of left ventricular diastolic filling assessed by Doppler echocardiography in humans. Circulation 79:1226–1236

Stugaard M, Brodahl U, Torp H, Ihlen H (1994) Abnormalities of left ventricular filling in patients with coronary artery disease: assessment by colour Doppler technique. Eur Heart J 15:318–327

Tei C, Dujardin KS, Hodge DO, Bailey KR, McGoon MD, Tajik AJ, Seward SB (1996a) Doppler echocardiographic index for assessment of global right ventricular function. J Am Soc Echocardiogr 9:838–847

Tei C, Dujardin KS, Hodge DO, Kyle RA, Tajik AJ, Seward JB (1996b) Doppler index combining systolic and diastolic myocardial performance: clinical value in cardiac amyloidosis. J Am Coll Cardiol 28:658–664

Teshima H, Tobita K, Yamamura H, Takeda A, Motomura H, Nakazawa M (2002) Cardiovascular effects of a phosphodiesterase III inhibitor, amrinone, in infants: non-invasive echocardiographic evaluation. Pediatr Int 44:259–263

Thomas JD, Weyman AE (1991) Echo Doppler evaluation of left ventricular diastolic function: physics and physiology. Circulation 84:977–990

Tworetsky W, McElhinney DB, Reddy VM, Brook MM, Hanley FL, Silverman NH (2001) Improved outcomes after fetal diagnosis of hypoplastic left heart syndrome. Circulation 103:1269–1273

Vasan RS, Larson MG, Benjamin EJ, Evans JC, Reiss CK, Levy D (1999) Congestive heart failure in subjects with normal versus reduced left ventricular ejection fraction. Prevalence and mortality in a population based cohort. J Am Coll Cardiol 33:1948–1955

Vignon P, Spencer K, Mor-avi V et al (1996) Quantification of regional systolic and diastolic right ventricular function using color kinesis. Circulation 94 [Suppl I]:1–668

Watanabe M, Ono S, Tomomasa T, Okada Y, Kobayashi T, Suzuki T, Morikawa A (2003) Measurement of tricuspid annular diastolic velocities by Doppler tissue imaging to assess right ventricular function in patients with congenital heart disease. Pediatr Cardiol 24: 463–467

Weidemann F, Eyskens B, Mertens L, Dommke Cm Kowalski M, Simmons L, Claus P, Bijnens B, Gewillig M, Hatle L, Sutherland GR (2002) Quantification of regional right and left ventricular function by ultrasonic strain rate and strain indexes after surgical repair of tetralogy of Fallot. Am J Cardiol 90:133–138

Xie GY, Berk MR, Smith MD, Gurley JC, DeMaria AN (1994) Prognostic value of Doppler transmitral flow patterns in patients with congestive heart failure. J Am Coll Cardiol 24:132–139

Yamamoto K, Nishimura RA, Chaliki HP, Appleton CP, Holmes DR, Redfield MM (1997) Determination of left ventricular filling pressures by Doppler echocardiography in patients with coronary artery disease: critical role of left ventricular systolic function. J Am Coll Cardiol 30:1819–1826

Yang SG, Novello R, Nicolson S, Steven J, Gaynor JW, Spray TL, Rychik J (2000) Evaluation of ventricular septal defect repair using intraoperative transesophageal echocardiography: frequency and significance of residual defects in infants and children. Echocardiography 17:681–684

Yu CM, Sanderson JE (1997) Right and left ventricular diastolic function in patients with and without heart failure: effect of age, sex, heart rate, and respiration on Doppler-derived measurements. Am Heart J 34:426–434

Zoghbi W, Quinones MA (1986) Determination of cardiac output by Doppler echocardiography: a critical appraisal. Herz 11:258–268

Magnetic Resonance Imaging in Congenital Heart Disease

CHRISTIAN J. KELLENBERGER

CONTENTS

14.1
Introduction

Congenital heart disease (CHD) occurs in 7–9 per 1000 live births (PRADAT et al. 2003) with the more complex anomalies often presenting during the newborn period. Initial investigation of neonates with CHD requires imaging for defining the cardiovascular anomalies and planning further clinical management. Echocardiography provides a full morphologic and functional evaluation in most neonates, but sometimes the acoustic windows may be insufficient for definite delineation of all vascular abnormalities. Further investigation has traditionally been performed by angiocardiography, which is invasive due to radiation exposure and catheterization with a considerable complication rate in neonates (VITIELLO et al. 1998). Although computed tomography angiography (CTA) with current mul-

C. J. KELLENBERGER, MD
Department of Diagnostic Imaging, University Children's Hospital, Steinwiesstrasse 75, 8032 Zurich, Switzerland

tirow-detector technology allows excellent assessment of the extracardiac thoracic vasculature, it still poses a substantial radiation exposure that should be avoided in neonates.

In current practice, cardiovascular magnetic resonance (MR) is an established noninvasive imaging modality for assessing the morphology and physiology of specific heart defects and vascular anomalies in older children and adults (PENNELL et al. 2004). With the necessary adjustments of the technique to the small size and fast heart rates of babies, MR can also provide valuable complementary morphologic and functional information in neonates and represents a veritable alternative to angiocardiography and CTA (KASTLER et al. 1990; KELLENBERGER et al. 2007; TSAI-GOODMAN et al. 2004). In this chapter the current techniques and common indications of cardiovascular MR in neonates with CHD will be discussed.

14.2
Techniques

14.2.1
General Setting

The MR scanner can be considered a hostile environment for a sick neonate and therefore the MR study should be as short as possible, tailored to the specific questions that need to be answered. The vital functions of the baby must be ensured by monitoring the heart rate, blood pressure, blood oxygen saturation, respiration and body temperature. As neonates are at risk of becoming hypothermic during an MR study, we place commercially available hotpacks, preheated to body temperature, around the head, pelvis and legs, and cover the baby with a blanket. A constant body temperature can be ensured by monitoring the skin temperature with a sensor or by measuring the ear temperature before and after the imaging. In order to avoid motion artefacts, neonates have to be immobilized for an MR study. Our and other paediatric anaesthesiologists and intensive care physicians prefer general anaesthesia with intubation to sedation in sick neonates with complex CHD, because the vital functions can be better controlled within the scanner (Tsai-Goodman et al. 2004). In addition, the combination of intubation and relaxation allows the induction of short periods of apnoea which are important for achieving the best image quality without degradation by respiratory motion.

Adequate spatial resolution of the MR imaging sequences is another essential factor for obtaining diagnostic image quality in neonates. The small size of the heart and vessels in a baby requires a high spatial resolution (in-plane resolution ~1 mm²), which is achieved by using a relatively small field of view (FOV = 18–20 cm), a sufficiently large matrix, and thin slices. In order to receive enough signal from the resulting small voxels, appropriate coil selection is crucial. The best coil for imaging the neonatal chest is the smallest coil that covers the entire chest and provides the highest signal-to-noise ratio (SNR). A small phased-array coil with a maximum FOV of approximately 20–25 cm and multi-element design allowing parallel imaging would be optimal for improving spatial resolution or shortening imaging time. Unfortunately, such coils are not yet

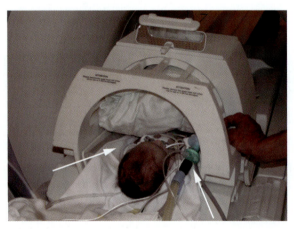

Fig. 14.1. Adult quadrature head coil used for cardiovascular MR imaging of a neonate. The intubated baby is positioned in the middle of the coil. The baby is covered with a blanket and preheated hot packs wrapped in a sheet (*arrows*) are placed around its body to prevent hypothermia

widely available. Depending on the MR system, an adult phased-array shoulder coil, a multi-channel knee coil, or a head coil into which the neonate fits, can be alternatives. On our system, we achieve the best results with a transmit/receive quadrature head coil (Fig. 14.1).

14.2.2
Pulse Sequences

With the advent of strong and fast gradient systems, various pulse sequences that allow detailed anatomic and functional assessment of CHD have become routinely available on most MR systems (Chung 2000; Fogel 2000; Powell and Geva 2000). The following discussion reflects the author's clinical experience using a 1.5 T Signa MR/i Twinspeed scanner (General Electric Medical Systems, Milwaukee, Wis., USA) at the University Children's Hospital in Zurich, Switzerland. Table 14.1 shows typical selected technical parameters for a cardiovascular MR study in neonates at our institution.

Every cardiovascular MR study is started with the acquisition of non-gated steady-state free precession (SSFP) sequences in the coronal, axial and sagittal planes covering the entire chest. These bright-blood SSFP images are acquired in less than 2 min and serve as localizers for the subsequent imaging. They also provide a basic overview of the situs, the cardiac and vascular anatomy. Since the cardiac anatomy has usually already been well defined by echocardiography before the MR study, we seldom perform further more detailed morphologic imaging of the heart.

In earlier days of cardiovascular MR imaging, both intracardiac and vascular anatomy used to be assessed with black-blood imaging using conventional spin-echo T_1-weighted sequences with electrocardiographic (ECG) gating and multislice acquisition (Chung 2000; Kastler et al. 1990). Shorter scan times can today be achieved with hybrid T_1-weighted spin-echo sequences and echoplanar read-out. Higher spatial resolution can be obtained with the more recently available ECG-gated double inversion recovery fast spin-echo sequences with single slice acquisition. Fast spin-echo sequences also allow different image contrasts (T_1-weighted, proton density, T_2-weighted) by using one or two RR intervals as repetition time (TR) and varying the echo time (TE). Fat saturation is possible by adding a third inversion pulse (triple inversion recovery) or a spec-tral saturation pulse. T_1-weighted, T_2-weighted and T1-weighted images following intravenous administration of gadolinium are valuable for evaluation of the extent and tissue characteristics of a tumour. Black-blood images are also useful for delineating the anatomy of the central airways. Slice thickness should not exceed 3 mm and black-blood imaging can be performed during free breathing with multiple signal averages.

In our experience, contrast-enhanced MR angiography (MRA) and cine imaging have replaced static black-blood imaging for morphologic evaluation in all patients with CHD except for those with tumours. Contrast-enhanced MRA is the most efficient sequence for a detailed study of the entire thoracic vasculature. Three-dimensional (3D) image data is acquired in continuous partitions with a 3D

fast spoiled gradient echo sequence (FSPGR) after intravenous administration of gadolinium. From the 3D data set, it is possible to display a specific vessel in any oblique plane with sub-volume maximum intensity projection (MIP) reconstructions and to accurately measure the vessel dimensions (VALSANGIACOMO BUCHEL et al. 2005). For illustration purposes, 3D volume-rendered MRA images can excellently demonstrate the often complex vascular anatomy in patients with CHD.

For MRA in neonates, we use a double or triple dose of gadolinium (0.2–0.3 mmol/kg bodyweight). Because of the small contrast volumes, we usually dilute the contrast with saline up to a total volume of 2 ml and inject manually through any available peripheral intravenous line. The diluted contrast bolus is injected over 6–8 s and is followed by the

Table 14.1. Selected technical parameters for cardiovascular MR in neonates. (2D Two-dimensional, 3D three-dimensional, ECG electrocardiogram, FIESTA fast imaging employing steady-state acquisition, FSPGR fast spoiled gradient echo, FSE fast spin-echo, SSFP steady-state free precession, T_1w T_1 weighting, T_2w T_2 weighting)

	Localizers	Black-blood imaging	Cine imaging		Flow measurement	MR angiography
Pulse sequence	SSFP (2D FIESTA)	Double inversion recovery FSE	SSFP (2D FIESTA)	Fast gradient echo (Fast cine)	Phase contrast (Fast cine PC)	3D FSPGR
Gating	None	ECG	ECG	ECG	ECG	None
Repetition time	3.5 ms	1–2 RR intervals	4 ms	8.3 ms	8 ms	3.3 ms
Echo time	1.4 ms	5 ms (for T_1w) 85 ms (for T_2w)	1.6 ms	3.7 ms	3.6 ms	1.0 ms
Bandwidth	±100 kHz	±62.5 kHz	±100 kHz	±31.25 kHz	±31.25 kHz	±62.5 kHz
Flip angle	45°	90°	45°	20°	15°	30°
Field-of-view	25 cm	18–20 cm	22 cm	18–20 cm	18–20 cm	18–20 cm
Phase field-of-view	0.75	0.8	0.75	0.75	0.75	0.8
Matrix	160×192	320×224	192×224	256×160	256×160	256×160
Slice thickness	5 mm	3 mm	5 mm	3 mm	4 mm	1.2–2.0 mm
Other parameters	–	Echotrain length 32 ± fat saturation	–	–	–	40 partitions Zero interpolation
Number of signal averages	0.75	3–4	1	2–3	2	1
Views per segment adjusted to heart rate	–	–	12 (<100 bpm) 10 (100–120 bpm) 8 (>120 bpm)	6 (<80 bpm) 4 (80–120 bpm) 2 (>120 bpm)	2 (<120 bpm) 1 (>120 bpm)	–
Scan time (s)	~60 s (three planes)	~15–20 s/slice	~10 s/slice	~30–60 s/slice	~80–160 s/slice	~15 s/ dynamic

same volume of saline. In order to achieve a sufficient injection rate, the contrast and saline bolus cannot be administered through an air filter. Hence, great care has to be taken to not inject any air. Exact timing of the MRA image acquisition is crucial for obtaining angiographic images with a high SNR. In our experience, the best results are achieved with an automated bolus detection method such as Smartprep (Foo et al. 1997) or MR fluoroscopic triggering (RIEDERER et al. 2000) combined with elliptic-centric k-space filling. Because the neonatal aorta and pulmonary trunk are too small, we place the region of interest for detecting the contrast bolus arrival in the right ventricle and initiate the MRA image acquisition after a delay of 5 s. If no real-time triggering method is available, image acquisition can be performed with sequential k-space filling and started together with the contrast injection. To ensure that all vessels including the systemic veins are opacified, the image acquisition is repeated twice. The need for bolus timing can be eliminated by using "time-resolved" MRA, which consists of a series of consecutive short 3D volume acquisitions (dynamics) (CHUNG 2005). With parallel imaging or advanced k-space filling schemes, it has become possible to obtain one dynamic in less than 3–5 s. However, with current "time-resolved" MRA techniques, the improved temporal resolution is traded for a lower true spatial resolution ($\sim 1.5 \times 1.5 \times 2$–$3 \text{ mm}^3$) than is possible by means of conventional MRA techniques with an imaging time of 10–20 s. With a conventional 3D FSPGR sequence, we achieve a sub-millimetre spatial resolution by using a section thickness of 1.2–2 mm, a FOV of 180–200 mm, a matrix of 256×160, and zero interpolation resulting in a reconstructed voxel size of $0.45 \times 0.55 \times 0.3$–$0.5 \text{ mm}^3$ (true spatial resolution $0.9 \times 1.1 \times 1.2$–$2 \text{ mm}^3$). The larger thoracic vessels such as the aorta and normal-sized pulmonary arteries are shown sufficiently during free breathing, but accurate delineation of hypoplastic pulmonary arteries, pulmonary veins and aortopulmonary collateral arteries requires image acquisition during breath-holding. An apnoea of 30–45 s is sufficient for running two to three dynamics and is usually well tolerated after a short period of hyperoxygenation before the image acquisition.

Cine imaging with ECG-gated SSFP or fast gradient echo sequences provides bright-blood multiphase images that show cardiac contraction and valvular motion in multiple frames throughout the cardiac cycle. We occasionally use cine SSFP sequences in the axial plane for a better assessment of the cardiac anatomy than is achieved with the non-gated SSFP localizers. In neonates with tumours, cine SSFP sequences in various planes aligned to the heart (short-axis plane, vertical or horizontal long-axis planes, and ventricular outflow tract planes) are used to assess impairment of the cardiac function. For assessing ventricular function, cine imaging is performed in the short-axis plane covering the heart from the base to the apex. Ventricular function can be quantified by measuring the ventricular volumes and ejection fractions with commercially available post-processing software. For accurate volume measurements of the small neonatal ventricles, we prefer the cine fast gradient echo sequence as it allows acquisition of thinner slices (3 mm) than the cine SSFP sequence (5 mm). Cine imaging is usually performed during free breathing with multiple signal averages (two to four) for cancellation of respiratory motion artefacts and achieving adequate SNR.

Velocity encoded cine phase-contrast (PC) sequences allow quantitative measurements of blood flow volumes. Differential blood flow to the lungs can be assessed by measuring the flow volume in the right and left pulmonary arteries (POWELL and GEVA 2000; ROMAN et al. 2005). Intracardiac or extracardiac shunts can be quantified by the systemic-to-pulmonary flow ratio (Q_P/Q_S), which is calculated from flow measurements in the pulmonary trunk and the ascending aorta. If the anatomy is complex with vascular or valvular atresia, a patent ductus arteriosus, systemic pulmonary blood supply, or anomalous pulmonary venous connections, additional flow measurements in systemic or pulmonary veins, in the ductus arteriosus, or in collateral arteries may be necessary to determine the Q_P/Q_S and the blood supply to each lung.

The fast heart rates in neonates (100–150 bpm) require a high temporal resolution (20–40 ms) to obtain a sufficient number of frames per heart beat. For accurate ventricular volume measurements and flow measurements we want to acquire more than 15 frames per heart beat. If a segmented k-space technique is used for cine imaging or cine PC, it is necessary to adjust the number of lines or views per segment (LPS/VPS) to the heart rate and TR to obtain the desired temporal resolution. The temporal resolution is calculated as TR × VPS for cine imaging, and 2 × TR × VPS for a PC sequence with one flow encoding direction. Table 14.1 shows how we adjust the VPS to the heart rate for the cine imaging and PC sequences with different repetition times.

14.3
Clinical Indications

14.3.1
Thoracic Vasculature

Patients with CHD frequently have complex abnormalities of the thoracic vasculature. Accurate delineation of the vascular anatomy is essential for diagnosis and surgical planning. Although the mediastinal vessels in neonates are usually well visualized by echocardiography, vessels surrounded by aerated lung cannot be assessed and sometimes the acoustic windows may be insufficient for definite delineation of all vessels in complex congenital anomalies. Investigation of the thoracic vasculature is now a major indication for MR imaging in neonates with CHD, due to the ability of contrast-enhanced MRA to noninvasively visualize all thoracic vessels with a single intravenous injection of Gadolinium (Masui et al. 2000; Tsai-Goodman et al. 2004).

In patients with anomalies of the aorta, including vascular rings, coarctation (Fig. 14.2) and interrupted aortic arch (Fig. 14.3), the anatomy and size of the aortic arch, the branching pattern of the head and neck arteries, and the patency of the ductus arteriosus can be clearly shown by MRA (Eichhorn et al. 2004; Roche et al. 1999). Identification of the anatomic details is important for selecting the proper operative approach and, in our experience, 3D illustration of the aortic arch morphology with volume-rendered images is of great help to the surgeon for planning the reconstruction of the aortic arch.

In tetralogy of Fallot and in pulmonary atresia with ventricular septal defect, the size of the pulmonary arteries results from the amount of pulmonary blood flow during the prenatal period. If there is severe obstruction of the right ventricular outflow tract, such as in pulmonary infundibular stenosis or pulmonary valve atresia, the pulmonary arteries may be hypoplastic or atretic and blood flow to the lungs can be maintained through persistent embryonic vessels arising from the thoracic aorta, so-called major aortopulmonary collateral arteries (MAPCAs). The anatomy of the pulmonary arteries, of a patent ductus arteriosus and of the MAPCAs determines if repair with a right ventricle-pulmonary artery shunt or unifocalization of the MAPCAs is feasible. Precise knowledge of the anatomy of all blood supply to the lungs is crucial for the choice of the appropriate surgical technique, and accurate preoperative mapping of the MAPCAs can reduce cardiopulmonary bypass time. When the pulmonary arteries are severely hypoplastic and not well visualized on echocardiography, MRA is useful to delineate the presence, size and continuity of the mediastinal pulmonary artery segments, the presence of a patent ductus arteriosus and the exact anatomy of MAPCAs (Fig. 14.4) (Geva et al. 2002; Holmqvist et al. 2001).

In truncus arteriosus a single arterial vessel arises from the heart and supplies the systemic, coronary and pulmonary circulations. Based on the origins of the pulmonary arteries and anatomy the aortic arch, truncus arteriosus is grouped into three categories that affect the approach of surgical repair (Jacobs 2000). In the first category, the pulmonary arteries arise together or separately from the truncus. In the second category, one pulmonary artery arises from the descending aorta or a patent ductus arteriosus. In the third category, the aortic arch is interrupted or there is severe coarctation. When both pulmonary arteries are visualized, evaluation with echocardiography is usually sufficient. If one pulmonary artery is not visualized at echocardiography or there is interruption of the aortic arch, MRA may be necessary to delineate the origins of the pulmonary arteries and morphology of the aortic arch (Fig. 14.5).

Accurate visualization of abnormal pulmonary veins is challenging and delineation of all pulmonary veins may be incomplete by using both echocardiography and angiocardiography. MRA has been shown to be the most accurate imaging modality for visualizing the entire course of all pulmonary veins in the mediastinum as well as in the lungs (Greil et al. 2002; Valsangiacomo et al. 2003). Anomalous connections of a single, multiple or all pulmonary veins to a supracardiac or infracardiac systemic vein or the portal venous system are well shown by the large FOV provided by MRA (Figs. 14.2, 14.6). The presence of pulmonary venous obstruction can be assessed and intrinsic congenital stenosis can be differentiated from extrinsic compression by another vascular structure or the diaphragm.

Patients with visceral heterotaxy syndrome (polysplenia and asplenia) may have an associated complicated heart anomaly with unusual veno-atrial connections that need to be accurately delineated before surgery or catheter-guided intervention. With MRA identification of the hepatic, systemic and pulmonary veins, their relationship to both atria is usually better shown than with echocardiography or angiocardiography (Fig. 14.6).

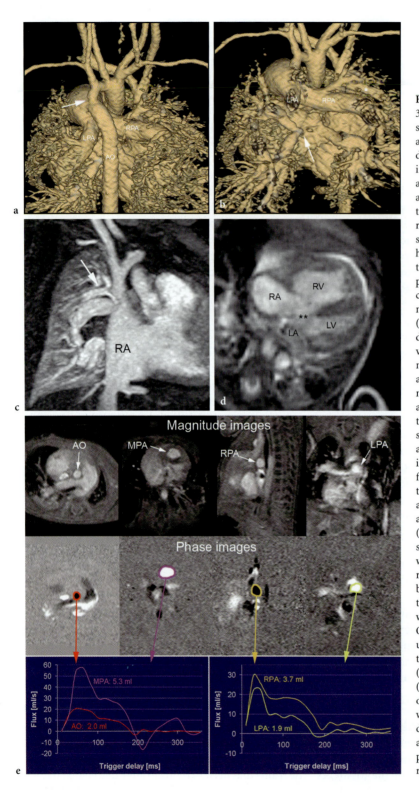

Fig. 14.2a–e. Aortic coarctation in a 3-week-old girl with atrioventricular septum defect (AVSD). Pulmonary vein anomalies were suspected at echocardiography. **a** Horizontal long-axis cine image shows the AVSD (******). (LA=Left atrium, LV=left ventricle, RA=right atrium, RV=right ventricle.) **b,c** Posterior volume-rendered magnetic resoance angiography (MRA) images show a patent ductus arteriosus, a hypoplastic aortic arch and the coarctation (*arrow* in **b**). The anatomy of the pulmonary veins is clearly defined as a common orifice of the left-sided pulmonary veins, which is also stenotic (*arrow* in **c**), and partial anomalous drainage of the right upper pulmonary vein (***). (AO=Aorta, LPA=left pulmonary artery, RPA=right pulmonary artery.) **d** Coronal oblique sub-volume maximum intensity (MIP) MRA image demonstrates the connection of the right upper pulmonary vein to the superior vena cava (*arrow*). (*RA*=Right atrium.) **e** Magnitude images, phase images and graphs demonstrate how flow volume measurements are obtained perpendicular to the ascending aorta (*AO*), pulmonary trunk (MPA), and right and left pulmonary arteries (*RPA, LPA*). The flow measurements show a significant left-to-right shunt with a pulmonary-to-systemic flow ratio (Q_P/Q_S) of 3.3 and asymmetric blood flow to the lungs with a right-to-left ratio of 66%:34%. In this case with a patent ductus arteriosus the Q_P/Q_S is calculated from the flow volumes in the aorta (Q_{AO}), pulmonary trunk (Q_{MPA}) and pulmonary arteries (Q_{RPA}, Q_{LPA}). Q_P is $Q_{RPA}+Q_{LPA}$ and Q_S is $(Q_{AO}+Q_{MPA})-(Q_{RPA}+Q_{LPA})$. On the basis of the MR findings the coarctation was repaired first with closure of the ductus arteriosus, and 3 weeks later, at the time of the AVSD repair, the pulmonary veins were augmented or reimplanted into the left atrium

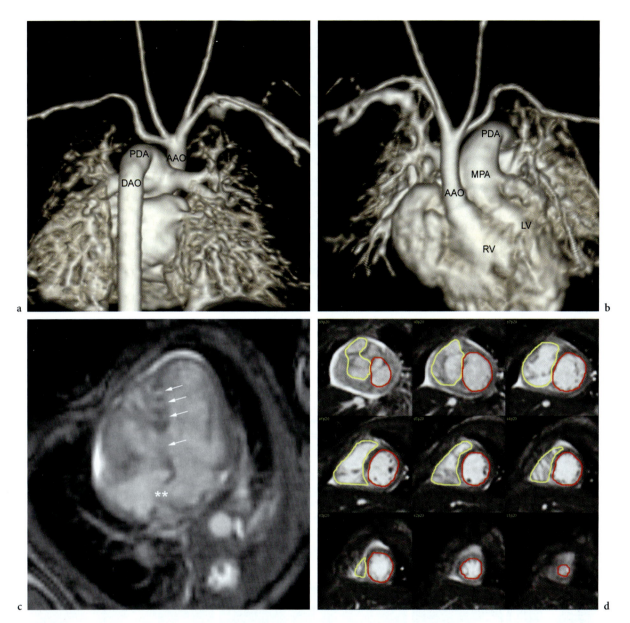

Fig. 14.3a–d. Interrupted arch in a 3-day-old girl with transposition of the great arteries, ventricular septum defects (VSDs) and an atrial septum defect (ASD). Severe aortic coarctation and hypoplasia of the right ventricle were suspected at echocardiography. **a,b** Posterior (**a**) and anterior (**b**) volume-rendered MRA images show interruption of the aortic arch distal to the left subclavian artery (type A). The descending aorta is supplied by the patent ductus arteriosus (*PDA*). The gap that needs to be reconstructed between the ascending aorta (*AAO*) and the descending aorta (*DAO*) is well illustrated. Transposition of the great arteries, with the aorta arising from the right ventricle (*RV*) and the pulmonary trunk (*MPA*) from the left ventricle (*LV*), is clearly shown. **c** Horizontal long-axis cine image shows multiple VSDs (*arrows*) and the ASD (******). **d** Short-axis cine images with measurement of the end-diastolic ventricular volumes demonstrate equally sized ventricles. On the basis of the MR findings reconstruction of the aortic arch and pulmonary banding were performed on day 4. Biventricular repair including arterial switch operation and closure of the ASD and VSDs was performed 3 weeks later

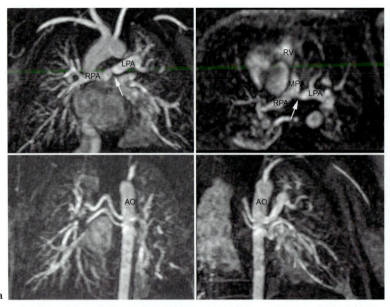

a

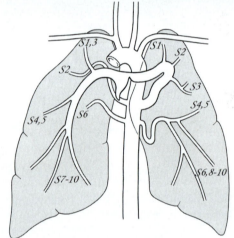

b

Fig. 14.4a,b. Multicentric pulmonary blood supply in a 3-week-old girl with pulmonary atresia and ventricle septum defect. **a** Sub-volume maximum intensity (*MIP*) MR angiographic images in different oblique planes demonstrate multiple major aortopulmonary collateral arteries (*MAPCAs*) arising from the descending aorta (*AO*) and supplying both lungs. The native pulmonary arteries (*RPA, LPA*) are confluent and there is a stenosis at the origin of the left pulmonary artery (*arrows*). (*MPA*=Patent distal portion of the pulmonary trunk, *RV*=infundibulum of the right ventricle.). **b** A composite drawing of the MAPCAs and native pulmonary arteries, derived from viewing the 3D MRA dataset with sub-volume MIP images on the workstation, can be helpful to the surgeon for planning the unifocalization procedure. (*S1–10*=Pulmonary segments)

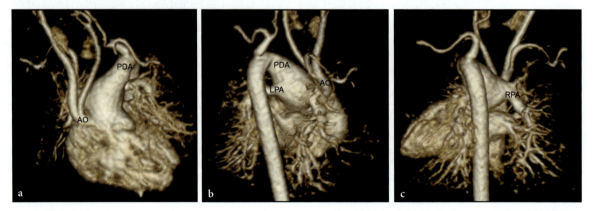

Fig. 14.5a-c. Truncus arteriosus in a 1-day-old boy. **a** Anterior, **b** right posterior oblique and **c** posterior volume-rendered MRA images show a single arterial vessel arising from the heart. The ascending aorta (*AO*) originates from the base of the truncus. The right and left pulmonary arteries (*RPA, LPA*) arise separately and widely spaced from the posterior wall of the truncus. The aortic arch is interrupted beyond the left carotid artery (type B) and the descending aorta is supplied by a patent ductus arteriosus (*PDA*)

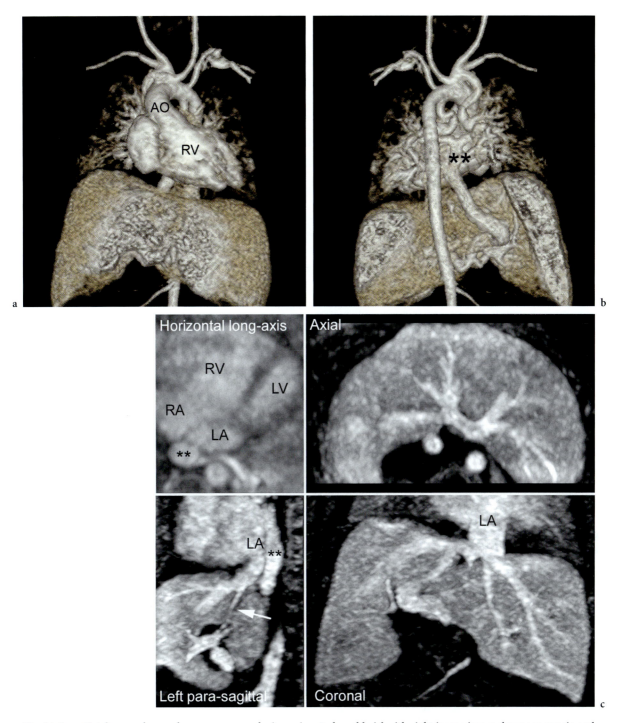

Fig. 14.6a–c. Total anomalous pulmonary venous drainage in a 3-day-old girl with right isomerism, pulmonary atresia and atrioventricular septum defect. **a** Anterior and **b** posterior volume-rendered MRA images show a transverse liver and asplenia. The aorta (*AO*) is in a right anterior position arising from the right ventricle (*RV*). The pulmonary arteries are supplied by bilateral patent arterial ducts with the left arterial duct arising from the aortic isthmus and the right arterial duct arising from the right brachiocephalic artery. The individual pulmonary veins connect to a retrocardiac venous confluence (****) that drains unobstructed into the portal venous system. **c** Sub-volume maximum intensity projection (*MIP*) images in different planes demonstrate that all hepatic veins drain into the left atrium (*LA*). The venous confluence (****) is separated from the left atrium. Note the patent ductus venosus Arantii (*arrow*). (*LV*=Left ventricle, *RA*=right atrium, *RV*=right ventricle)

14.3.2
Ventricular Size

In patients with a small right or left ventricle, the size of the smaller ventricle determines prognosis and is an important parameter for deciding on biventricular repair or single ventricle palliation (DE OLIVEIRA et al. 2005; SCHWARTZ et al. 2001). MR cine imaging in short-axis view is considered more accurate than echocardiography for assessing the ventricular size, as it provides a 3D measurement of the ventricular volumes and does not rely on geometrical assumptions. Exact measurement of the ventricular volumes by MR cine imaging has been recommended in patients with a borderline small ventricle, such as in hypoplastic left heart complex or unbalanced atrioventricular septal defect, because the results are so crucial for further management. In our experience, volumetry of the ventricles by MR cine imaging has modified decisions that were based on echocardiography (Fig. 14.3).

14.3.3
Tumours

Primary cardiac tumours are uncommon in neonates and mostly of benign histology (BEGHETTI et al. 1997; FREEDOM et al. 2000). However, cardiac tumours may cause significant morbidity due to blood flow obstruction, ventricular dysfunction or arrhythmia. The most common tumour is rhabdomyoma, which is often associated with tuberous sclerosis. Other tumours include fibroma, haemangioma and pericardial teratoma. A rhabdomyoma is usually well characterized as a hyperechoic mass on echocardiography, which is superior to MR if the tumour is small and intramural (Fig. 14.7). If the tumour is larger, MR is useful in defining the anatomy, involvement and functional impairment (Fig. 14.8). Black-blood imaging with different weightings and following intravenous application of gadolinium demonstrates tumour extension and may help identify the likely tissue type of the tumour (KIAFFAS et al. 2002). Further, gadolinium-enhanced sequences can differentiate enhancing tumour from non-enhancing thrombus. Cine imaging is used for assessing the presence of inflow or outflow obstruction, compression of adjacent vascular structures and ventricular function.

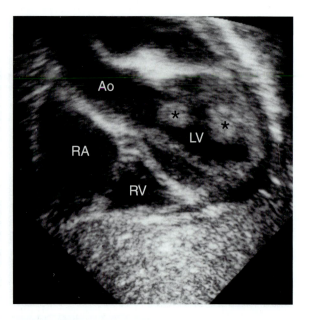

Fig. 14.7. Rhabdomyoma. Subcostal echocardiographic image shows two hyperechoic tumours (*) in the left ventricle (*LV*). (*Ao*=Aorta, *RA*=right atrium, *RV*=right ventricle)

14.4
Conclusion

Cardiovascular MR is a powerful imaging tool providing morphologic, functional and haemodynamic information which can be decisive for the management of neonates with CHD. Excellent quality images can be obtained when the MR techniques are adjusted to the small size and fast heart rates of the neonates. In our experience, MR is the noninvasive imaging modality of choice for neonates with CHD in whom echocardiography fails to fully depict the necessary clinically relevant information. The ability of MR to accurately demonstrate complex abnormalities of the entire thoracic vasculature can obviate potentially harmful cardiac catheterization in many cases.

References

Beghetti M, Gow RM, Haney I et al (1997) Pediatric primary benign cardiac tumors: a 15-year review. Am Heart J 134:1107–1114

Chung T (2000) Assessment of cardiovascular anatomy in patients with congenital heart disease by magnetic resonance imaging. Pediatr Cardiol 21:18–26

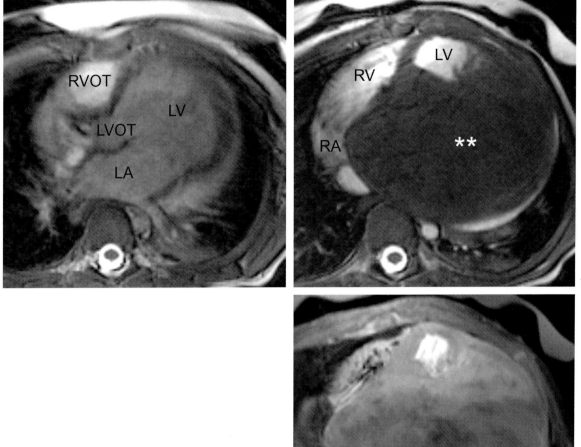

Fig. 14.8a–c. Fibroma. **a,b** Axial cine images show a large mass *(**)* involving the posterior and inferior wall of the left ventricle *(LV)* and the ventricular septum. The ventricular inflow and outflow tracts are not obstructed. *(LA=*Left atrium, *LVOT=*left ventricular outflow tract, *RA=*right atrium, *RV=*right ventricle, *RVOT=*right ventricular outflow tract.) **c** Axial T1-weighted image with fat suppression and following administration of gadolinium shows inhomogeneous enhancement of the tumour with relative sparing of its core, which is considered characteristic of a fibroma

Chung T (2005) Magnetic resonance angiography of the body in pediatric patients: experience with a contrast-enhanced time-resolved technique. Pediatr Radiol 35:3–10

De Oliveira NC, Sittiwangkul R, McCrindle BW et al (2005) Biventricular repair in children with atrioventricular septal defects and a small right ventricle: anatomic and surgical considerations. J Thorac Cardiovasc Surg 130:250–257

Eichhorn J, Fink C, Delorme S et al (2004) Rings, slings and other vascular abnormalities. Ultrafast computed tomography and magnetic resonance angiography in pediatric cardiology. Z Kardiol 93:201–208

Fogel MA (2000) Assessment of cardiac function by magnetic resonance imaging. Pediatr Cardiol 21:59–69

Foo TK, Saranathan M, Prince MR et al (1997) Automated detection of bolus arrival and initiation of data acquisition in fast, three-dimensional, gadolinium-enhanced MR angiography. Radiology 203:275–280

Freedom RM, Lee KJ, MacDonald C et al (2000) Selected aspects of cardiac tumors in infancy and childhood. Pediatr Cardiol 21:299–316

Geva T, Greil GF, Marshall AC et al (2002) Gadolinium-enhanced 3-dimensional magnetic resonance angiography of pulmonary blood supply in patients with complex pulmonary stenosis or atresia: comparison with X-ray angiography. Circulation 106:473–478

Greil GF, Powell AJ, Gildein HP et al (2002) Gadolinium-enhanced three-dimensional magnetic resonance angiography of pulmonary and systemic venous anomalies. J Am Coll Cardiol 39:335–341

Holmqvist C, Hochbergs P, Bjorkhem G et al (2001) Preoperative evaluation with MR in tetralogy of fallot and pulmonary atresia with ventricular septal defect. Acta Radiol 42:63–69

Jacobs ML (2000) Congenital Heart Surgery Nomenclature and Database Project: truncus arteriosus. Ann Thorac Surg 69:S50–S55

Kastler B, Livolsi A, Germain P et al (1990) Magnetic resonance imaging in congenital heart disease of newborns: preliminary results in 23 patients. Eur J Radiol 10:109–117

Kellenberger CJ, Yoo SJ, Buchel ER (2007) Cardiovascular MR imaging in neonates and infants with congenital heart disease. Radiographics 27:5–18

Kiaffas MG, Powell AJ, Geva T (2002) Magnetic resonance imaging evaluation of cardiac tumor characteristics in infants and children. Am J Cardiol 89:1229–1233

Masui T, Katayama M, Kobayashi S et al (2000) Gadolinium-enhanced MR angiography in the evaluation of congenital cardiovascular disease pre- and postoperative states in infants and children. J Magn Reson Imaging 12:1034–1042

Pennell DJ, Sechtem UP, Higgins CB et al (2004) Clinical indications for cardiovascular magnetic resonance (CMR): Consensus Panel report. Eur Heart J 25:1940–1965

Powell AJ, Geva T (2000) Blood flow measurement by magnetic resonance imaging in congenital heart disease. Pediatr Cardiol 21:47–58

Pradat P, Francannet C, Harris JA et al (2003) The epidemiology of cardiovascular defects, part I: a study based on data from three large registries of congenital malformations. Pediatr Cardiol 24:195–221

Riederer SJ, Bernstein MA, Breen JF et al (2000) Three-dimensional contrast-enhanced MR angiography with real-time fluoroscopic triggering: design specifications and technical reliability in 330 patient studies. Radiology 215:584–593

Roche KJ, Krinsky G, Lee VS et al (1999) Interrupted aortic arch: diagnosis with gadolinium-enhanced 3D MRA. J Comput Assist Tomogr 23:197–202

Roman KS, Kellenberger CJ, Farooq S et al (2005) Comparative imaging of differential pulmonary blood flow in patients with congenital heart disease: magnetic resonance imaging versus lung perfusion scintigraphy. Pediatr Radiol 35:295–301

Schwartz ML, Gauvreau K, Geva T (2001) Predictors of outcome of biventricular repair in infants with multiple left heart obstructive lesions. Circulation 104:682–687

Tsai-Goodman B, Geva T, Odegard KC et al (2004) Clinical role, accuracy, and technical aspects of cardiovascular magnetic resonance imaging in infants. Am J Cardiol 94:69–74

Valsangiacomo ER, Levasseur S, McCrindle BW et al (2003) Contrast-enhanced MR angiography of pulmonary venous abnormalities in children. Pediatr Radiol 33:92–98

Valsangiacomo Buchel ER, DiBernardo S, Bauersfeld U et al (2005) Contrast-enhanced magnetic resonance angiography of the great arteries in patients with congenital heart disease: an accurate tool for planning catheter-guided interventions. Int J Cardiovasc Imaging 21:313–322

Vitiello R, McCrindle BW, Nykanen D et al (1998) Complications associated with pediatric cardiac catheterization. J Am Coll Cardiol 32:1433–1440

Chest Radiography in Congenital Heart Disease

15

Bjarne Smevik

CONTENTS

15.1
Introduction

Modern radiological imaging has opened up new areas for precise diagnosis of congenital heart disease. The most important and most frequently performed radiological examination is still chest radiography, but magnetic resonance imaging and multislice spiral computed tomography have gained much ground over the more invasive angiocardiography. Invasive studies are still needed in the more complex conditions or as postoperative controls, and also as part of the increasingly performed interventional procedures. In this chapter, the approach to interpreting the chest radiograph of patients with congenital heart and great vessel disease will be presented.

The incidence of congenital heart disease (CHD) is reported to be between 3 and 12 per 1000 live births (HOFFMAN 1995; SAMANEK and VORISKOVA 1999). Most investigators report a higher incidence after echocardiography with colour Doppler making it feasible to detect and characterize asymptomatic lesions. This has been paralleled by the access to trained paediatric cardiologists for a larger percentage of the population in many regions of the world. The more recent reports are therefore more accurate than old estimates based on severe symptoms and invasive studies used selectively in the more obvious cases. This is also reflected in the fact that no significant change in the incidence of the severe forms of CHD has been found. A number of factors greatly influence the reported incidence in the different studies, and two will be mentioned here. If asymptomatic and mild forms of ventricular septal defects (VSD) are detected and included, this will significantly influence the whole picture. The same is true for patent arterial duct (PDA) which will be reported very differently depending on inclusion or not of the increasing number of premature low-birth-weight infants with PDA and minute ducts as a surprise finding in children with physiological murmurs examined with colour Doppler.

In a study including more than 800,000 live born children in BOHEMIA, SAMANEK and VORISKOVA (1999) found that the most frequent conditions were VSDS (41.6%), atrial septal defect (8.7%), aortic (7.8%) and pulmonary (5.8%) stenoses. Transposition of the great arteries was found in 5.4%, coarctation of the aorta in 5.3% and persistent arterial duct in 5.1%.

Many syndromes are associated with congenital heart or great vessel disease, and a few of the best

B. SMEVIK, MD
Section of Paediatric Radiology, Department of Radiology, Rikshospitalet Radiumhospitalet hf, The National Hospital, Sognsvannsveien 20, 0373 Oslo, Norway

known will be briefly mentioned. Patients with Down's syndrome may have 11 pairs of ribs and a double manubrial centre, and close to 50% are reported to have cardiac lesions such as atrioventricular septal defect, VSD or tetralogy of Fallot. Goldenhar syndrome is also seen in patients with tetralogy of Fallot. Turner's syndrome is associated with coarctation of the aorta or aortic or pulmonic stenosis. Fewer than half the patients with Williams-Beuren syndrome with the characteristic "elfin face" have supravalvular aortic stenosis and/or peripheral pulmonary stenosis; Alagille's syndrome patients also may have peripheral pulmonary stenosis and vertebral anomalies. In DiGeorge syndrome abnormalities of the large vessels such as conotruncal malformation or interrupted aortic arch may be found. Hurler syndrome is associated with cardiomyopathy. In Holt-Oram syndrome septal defects may be found between the atria or the ventricles. The CATCH-22 syndrome consists of cardiac defects, abnormal facies, thymic hypoplasia, cleft palate and hypocalcemia from deletions in chromosome 22 (O'BRIAN 1985). Only 8% of the congenital heart defects are believed to be caused by chromosome or single-gene defects, 2% are caused by environmental teratogens, and 90% are unknown or multifactorial (NORA 1993).

Many of the important congenital heart defects are better understood by studying the embryology behind the malformation.

15.2
Clinical Information

Every referral for a chest radiograph of a patient suspected of congenital heart and/or great vessel disease to the radiological department should include adequate clinical information. Are there signs of poor weight gain and failure to thrive? Is the child cyanotic? Are there respiratory problems such as tachypnoea? Is the liver enlarged? Is there a blood pressure difference between arms and legs? Does the child lie in opisthotonus, stretching and thereby stiffening the trachea?

One very common reason for suspicion of congenital heart defect is a heart murmur. The location and character may give important clues as to whether the murmur is physiological or caused by heart disease. It is also well known that the complex changes that take place in the circulation of the newborn may give rise to loud/pronounced murmurs without clinical importance, while on the other hand serious congenital heart defects may be completely "silent". If there is a clinical suspicion of CHD in a newborn, the patient is frequently seen by a paediatric cardiologist who will add a diagnosis or important information based upon echocardiography including Doppler recordings of the heart and great vessels.

The age of the child when the clinical symptoms become obvious may give some clue to the underlying lesion. The most frequently encountered lesions manifest within the first few days of extrauterine life include coarctation of the aorta or critical aortic valvular stenosis, complete transposition of the great arteries and hypoplastic left heart syndrome, in addition to some very complex conditions. In a patient aged 1–4 weeks, heart failure as the presenting problem is most likely caused by complete transposition of the great arteries, a large left-to-right shunt, cardiomyopathy or coronary artery anomalies.

15.3
Chest Radiography

The first radiological study performed in a newborn is usually chest radiography. It is readily available, and still serves as one of the basic screening tests. The digital era has replaced the nicely tuned traditional film/screen combinations, which were excellently suited for their purpose. Phosphor plates are being used on an increasing scale as picture archiving and communication systems (PACS) take over more and more in modern hospitals. Direct digital radiography has the advantage over phosphor plates in that cassette handling is eliminated. However, even in the most modern environment, phosphor plates are still very important for chest radiography of infants in incubators and for bedside studies.

15.3.1
Technical Considerations

Special precautions for obtaining high-quality radiographs from premature babies in incubators include special wrapping for the cassette and the infant in commercially available covering known not to interfere with diagnostic quality. It is essential that the quality of the chest radiograph allows differentiation of very fine details, and the resolution needed in premature babies could easily be compared to the resolution needed for mammography. A direct digital radiography system should perform better than 3.5 line pairs per mm. The radiation dose must be kept as low as possible, and if possible it should be recorded and documented. Under- and overexposed films have become a much smaller problem since the introduction of digital radiography. Still a few basic principles must be adhered to: the exposure must be made during sufficient inspiration, indicated by the projection of the right hemidiaphragm below the posterior eighth rib; the child must not be rotated; in the anterio-posterior (AP) projection, which is routinely used in neonates and small children, the bony ends of the ribs must be as symmetrical as possible, and in the lateral view the distance between the posterior margins of the right and left ribs must be small. Another good indicator is to look for symmetry in the medial ends of the clavicles. A good example of a chest radiograph well suitable for interpretation is shown in Figure 15.1. Excessive lordosis as shown in Figure 15.2. or kyphosis will also influence the appearance of the heart contours and must be avoided. Again, it is important to look at the clavicles. If they are projected high above the first ribs, the radiograph is made in lordosis, and a projection well below the thoracic aperture means kyphosis. Some controversy still exists about the number of exposures, but there are reasons to advocate the "old" cardiac series in some cases, with frontal, lateral and two oblique films, all with barium in the oesophagus. In older children, a posterio-anterior film should be preferred in accordance with the European guidelines on quality criteria for diagnostic radiographic images in paediatrics (KOHN et al. 1996).

15.3.2
Evaluation

The evaluation of the heart and lungs is much more difficult in a neonate or premature baby than in an older child. There is no co-operation, and the frequency of respiration is much higher. Respiratory assistance such as respirators or high-frequency oscillators and central arterial and venous lines and feeding tubes may interfere with adequate projection and positioning of the patient.

Careful interpretation of the chest radiograph in a neonate suspected of having cardiovascular disease includes the following well-known points of interest: lung vessels, aeration, the heart, lung parenchyma, large airways, oesophagus, aorta and pulmonary trunk, the skeleton and arrangement of the organs.

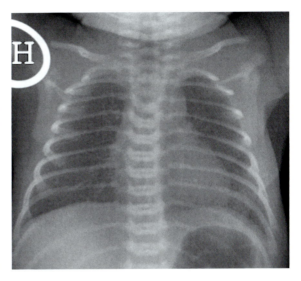

Fig. 15.1. A 1-day-old girl. Correct chest radiograph. The clavicles and ribs are symmetrical, and the diaphragm is at the level of the ninth posterior costae. Gastric air is seen in normal position

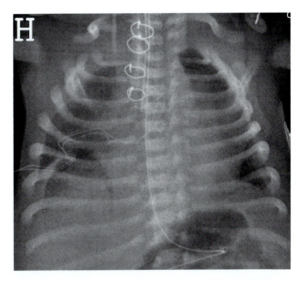

Fig. 15.2. A 10-day-old boy. Postoperative chest radiograph exposed with the patient in lordosis. The anterior rib ends curve cranially instead of caudally. The heart contours are different from a normal projection, with the apex lifted. Note the clavicles projected high above the first ribs

15.3.2.1
Lung Vessels

Are the lung vessels large, small, normal or uneven? There is no exact objective way of assessing the size of the lung vessels, so experience and caution are very important to make this part of the interpretation useful. Nevertheless, it is important that radiologists make their opinion on these difficult issues outspoken should they wish to be of help to the clinician. Especially in the neonate, the evaluation of lung vessels is extremely difficult before the pressure in the lung vessels is normalized after a few days. In persistent fetal circulation, the shunt is from right to left through the open arterial duct until the resistance in the pulmonary vascular bed drops.

If the chest radiograph indicates a left-to-right shunt with enlarged lung vessels, the relation between pulmonary and systemic blood flow is usually larger than 2:1 (Fig. 15.3). Increased blood volume in the lungs is caused either by difficulties of getting blood out of the lungs (as in mitral stenosis or congestive heart failure) or because there is an excessive volume of blood passing through the lungs (left-to-right shunt). The first situation will affect mainly the pulmonary veins (congestion), the latter more the arteries (plethora).

Heart failure in the neonate may be caused by such different conditions as volume overload of the left ventricle from a large right-to-left shunt, incompetent aortic or mitral valves, coarctation of the aorta, peripheral arteriovenous malformations and iatrogenic fluid overload. Abnormal myocardium with ischaemia or myocarditis or myocardial failure caused by an anomalous coronary artery, Kawasaki's disease or glycogen storage disease may also give rise to the signs of distended pulmonary vessels and interstitial and alveolar oedema (MARKOWITZ and FELLOWS 1998).

Is there congestion or pleural or pericardial effusion? If the problem is pulmonary venous obstruction, the picture may be more blurred, with increased interstitial markings, perivascular and alveolar oedema and pleural effusion. The underlying cause may be total anomalous pulmonary venous drainage, especially the infradiaphragmatic type, stenosis of pulmonary veins (Fig. 15.4) or cor triatriatum (Fig. 15.5) and different forms of restriction in the mitral valves.

Hypoperfusion of the lungs may occur in pulmonary atresia or the more severe forms of tetralogy of Fallot. Tricuspid atresia and other heart malformations with restrictive access to the pulmonary artery will also result in reduced flow through the lungs. As was the case with increased lung perfusion, there is

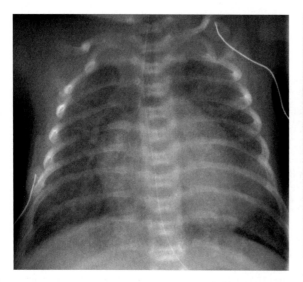

Fig. 15.3. A 3-week-old girl with atrial and ventricular septal defects and an open arterial duct. The heart is enlarged, and the lung vessels markedly increased

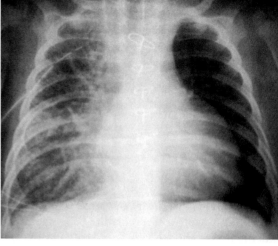

Fig. 15.4. A 5-month-old boy with stenosis of the lung veins from the right side. The patient had a single right ventricle with double outlet and a hypoplastic aortic arch. At re-operation the marked stenosis of the veins from the right lung at the entrance to the left atrium were described

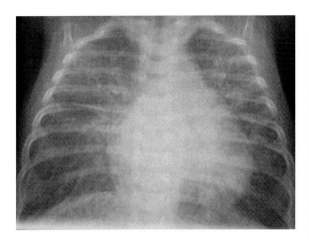

Fig. 15.5. A 4-month-old girl with cor triatriatum. Chest radiograph shows marked bilateral pulmonary venous congestion

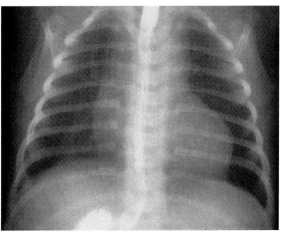

Fig. 15.6. A 3-month-old girl with tetralogy of Fallot, and levocardia in situs inversus. There is obvious pulmonary hypoperfusion with very small lung vessels

no objective way of making the diagnosis of oligaemia, and again experience is important for a reliable assessment. Pronounced hypoperfusion is usually quite evident, as shown in Figure 15.6.

Patients with atresia of the pulmonary artery may sometimes have very uneven vascular patterns in the lungs, with marked asymmetry, reflecting asymmetric artery distribution, e.g. caused by collaterals from systemic to pulmonary arteries (Fig. 15.7). They are frequently stenotic either at their origin from the aorta, or at the connection to the pulmonary artery. This may result in a mixture of hypoperfusion and plethora.

15.3.2.2
Aeration

Another feature that must be taken into account is aeration of the lungs. Reduced lung size may be the result of ipsilateral atresia or severe hypoplasia of the pulmonary artery (Fig. 15.8). In some patients with enlarged heart or with large vessels compressing airways, atelectasis of segments or lobes may occur, and in the postoperative period, nerve injury may result in paralysis of the hemidiaphragm and subsequent atelectasis (Fig. 15.9).

It is important to differentiate true oligaemia from hyperlucency caused by hyperinflation. Hyperinflation may be general or local affecting a lobe or even the whole lung. This may be caused by a valve mechanism resulting from vessels compressing the airway. Hyperinflated lungs may also be seen associated with a significant left-to-right shunt

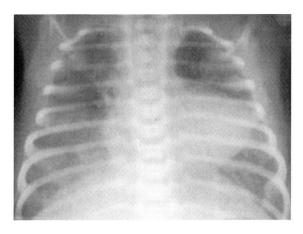

Fig. 15.7. A 1-day-old boy with pulmonary atresia and a large ventricular septal defect (VSD). Chest radiograph shows elevated apex and concave contour at the level of the pulmonary artery. The pulmonary arteries turned out to be missing completely, and three MAPCAs were going from the descending aorta to the right lung and one to the left. The patient was operated with unifocalization of the MAPCAs. These arteries were fed from the aorta through a 4-mm central Gore-Tex shunt

causing enlargement of the pulmonary arteries and perivascular oedema compressing the smaller airways (Fig. 15.10). This will result in retention of air and a compensatory increase in respiratory work which manifests itself by an increase in respiration rate and shallow fast breathing with greater effort and sometimes wheezing: cardiac asthma.

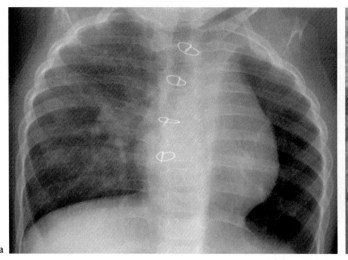
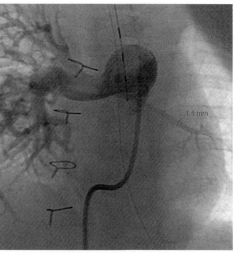

Fig. 15.8a,b. A 14-month-old boy with hypoplasia of the left lung. Chest radiograph shows small left hemi-thorax and very small lung vessels. Angiography with injection of contrast medium into the main pulmonary artery shows large vessels in the right lung, and only one very small branch to the left lung

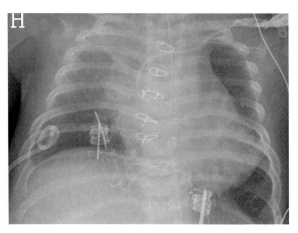

Fig. 15.9. A 5-month-old girl with Down's syndrome, atrioventricular septal defect (AVSD), anomalous pulmonary venous drainage, tracheal stenosis and Mb. Hirschsprung. A pigtail catheter drains pleural effusion on the right side, and there is atelectasis of the right upper lobe

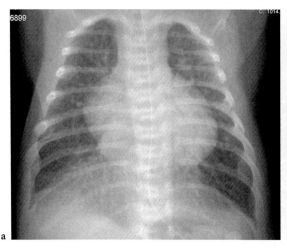
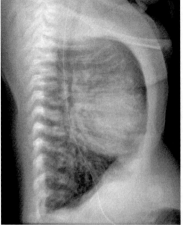

Fig. 15.10a,b. A 1-month-old girl with Down's syndrome and AVSD. The heart is enlarged and the lung vessels increased, indicating a large left-to-right shunt. The lungs are hyperinflated

15.3.2.3
The Heart

What are the size, shape and position of the heart? The appearance of all these variables depends heavily on projection criteria. Assessment of the heart size may be difficult, and it is even more difficult in neonates than in older children. Some institutions use the cardiothoracic ratio as a guide: if the transverse cardiac diameter to maximum internal diameter of the thorax ratio exceeds 60% in an infant, the heart is considered enlarged. Cardiomegaly is a useful sign in detecting CHD, but highly unspecific (Fig. 15.11).

All of the following criteria depend upon the normal presence and orientation of the large vessels and the heart chambers. An increase in the size of the left atrium is often detectable on plain chest radiographs with barium in the oesophagus. In the lateral view, the oesophagus is displaced posteriorly at the level of the left atrium. The left main bronchus may be displaced superiorly and posteriorly. Left ventricular enlargement displaces the oesophagus dorsally on the lateral film, and the cardiac apex downward and to the left in the frontal projection. However, oesophageal displacement can also result from a normal left ventricle being pushed by a big right ventricle, thus mimicking left ventricular enlarge-

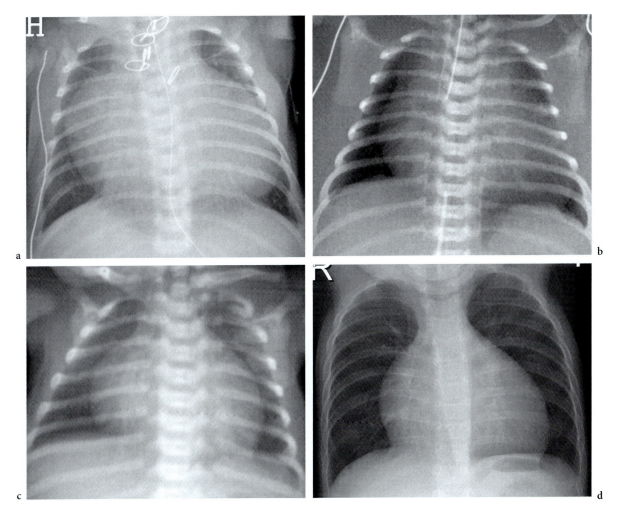

Fig. 15.11a–d. A large heart is suggestive of congenital heart disease, but unspecific. **a** A 14-day-old boy with pulmonary atresia, and dysplastic tricuspid valve. At surgery, a central shunt from the aorta to the pulmonary arteries was established. Note the oblique sternal sutures due to osteomyelitis of the sternum. **b** A 1-day-old boy with enlarged but otherwise normal heart. There was a large arteriovenous malformation in the left leg. **c** An 18-day-old girl with pericardial effusion. Enlarged heart with prominent right contour and straightening of the normal angle between the diaphragm and the heart. **d** An 11-month-old boy with enlarged heart due to Ebstein's anomaly

ment. Right atrial enlargement may cause a prominent right heart contour. A large right ventricle will lift the cardiac apex because the left ventricle is displaced, and in the lateral film, the heart is in greater than usual contact with the sternum.

The shape of the heart contours is frequently not a very useful sign, especially in the more complex lesions, like the patient shown in Figure 15.12. The main task of the radiologist first encountering such a patient is to report haemodynamic information and to initiate further studies such as echocardiography and possibly heart catheterization. In tetralogy of Fallot, the "classical" boot shape of the heart may be seen, but the heart may just as well look perfectly normal. This is illustrated in Figure 15.13. The appearance of a heart with an atrial septal defect (ASD) depends of course on the size of the shunt. In some patients the heart has a broad base, like a sand-bag placed on the diaphragm (Fig. 15.14). This is mainly due to dilatation, and not a sign of hypertrophy. Cardiomegaly is not very apparent unless there is coexistent mitral regurgitation, sometimes in conjunction with mitral valve prolapse. In atrioventricular septal defect (AVSD) most patients have enlargement of the heart with dominance on the right side. The right atrium is enlarged, resulting in an angular contour of the right atrium in a frontal projection (Fig. 15.15). The right ventricle is also enlarged, giving rise to a large area of contact between the heart and the sternum in the lateral projection. Vascular markings in the lungs are usually markedly increased, and the lungs may be hyper-inflated. The "typical" shape of different congenital anomalies of the heart listed in the literature is not seen very often, especially not in the neonate. In chest radiographs of patients with complete transposition of the great arteries the classical appearance of "egg on side" with a narrow superior mediastinum (Fig. 15.16) is not so frequently seen anymore, probably because the narrow pedicle depends on involution of the thymus caused by severe stress, and this is counteracted by early palliation. Still, some knowledge about the different shapes associated with the heart defects may be helpful.

15.3.2.4
Lung Parenchyma

In the premature, changes caused by respiratory distress syndrome (RDS) will frequently dominate the appearance of the lungs with micro-atelectases

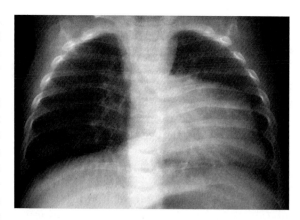

Fig. 15.12. A 6-month-old boy with prominent left heart contour and small pulmonary arteries. The final diagnosis was double-outlet right ventricle, hypoplastic left ventricle, valvular pulmonic stenosis, and anomalous pulmonary artery with the right pulmonary artery branching off the main pulmonary artery immediately above the stenotic valves

and more or less white lungs. Changes brought on by cardiac failure or an open arterial duct may be very difficult to detect. One sign may be that lungs that had started to clear as the production of surfactant increases opacify again as the left-to-right shunt through the open duct increases.

A sequester will be seen as a density close to the spine (Fig. 15.17).

15.3.2.5
Large Airways

Does the trachea look normal, or is there dislocation or compression? Are the main bronchi visible, and is there a short right and long left main stem bronchus? Is the calibre of the trachea and of the bronchi normal? Tracheobronchomalacia may of course be the reason for breathing difficulties in the neonate, and high-quality pulsed fluoroscopy will usually confirm the diagnosis. On rare occasions, bronchoscopy in combination with bronchography may be necessary to reveal a vascular compression or short stenosis, but in most cases the less invasive modalities of computed tomography or magnetic resonance imaging will provide the necessary information. On the other hand, if a patient with a history of respiratory symptoms is undergoing heart catheterization under general anaesthesia anyway, a small amount of nonionic contrast medium in the airways may be a simple and quick way to clarify the situation, as shown in Figure 15.18.

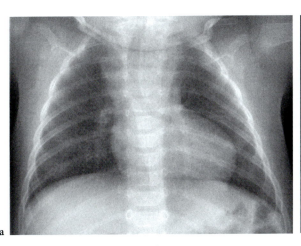
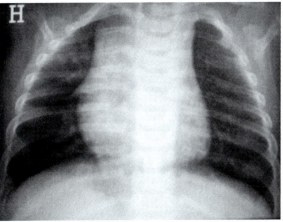

Fig. 15.13a,b. Two patients with tetralogy of Fallot illustrating the different presentations on plain chest radiography. **a** "Classical" boot shape of the heart in a 3-month-old boy. **b** Normal heart contour and prominent right lobe of the thymus in a 4-month-old boy

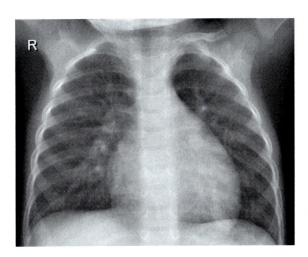

Fig. 15.14. An 18-month-old boy with atrial septal defect in the oval fossa. The enlarged heart "sits" broad-based on the diaphragm

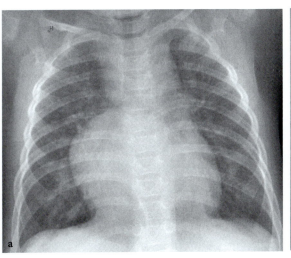
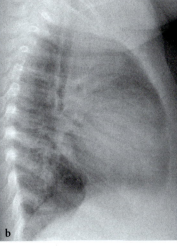

Fig. 15.15a,b. A 10-month-old girl with atrioventricular septal defect. The enlarged right atrium gives a shelf-like upper right contour (*arrows*)

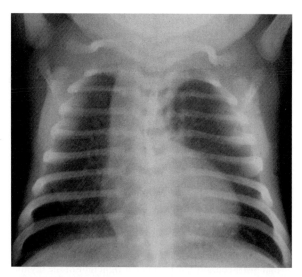

Fig. 15.16. A 2-month-old boy with transposition of the great arteries. Chest radiograph shows narrow superior mediastinum and the egg-like appearance of the heart

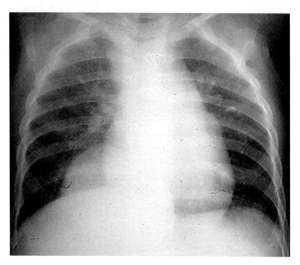

Fig. 15.17. A 2-year-old boy with a sequester. Chest radiograph shows a large mass close to the spine in the lower right lung

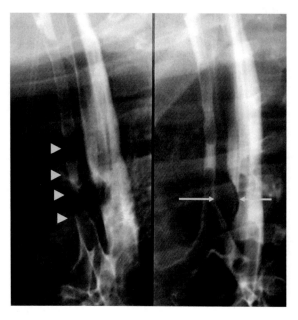

Fig. 15.18. A 6-month-old boy with pulmonary sling and tracheomalacia (*arrowheads*). The left pulmonary artery passes between the trachea and the oesophagus at the level of the arrows

15.3.2.6
Oesophagus

The oesophagus should preferably be visualized in at least two projections at the first study. This can give important clues to the diagnosis of vascular anomalies in the mediastinum, and the costs and the discomfort to the patient are negligible. Whenever suspicion of heart or great vessel disease is accompanied by respiratory distress, it should be obligatory to perform an oesophagogram. Pathologic conditions in need of surgical relief, such as a double aortic arch (Fig. 15.19) or Kommerell's diverticulum, could easily be picked up on the basis of such a study. The impression from arteria lusoria (Fig. 15.20) is usually much smaller than the double aortic arch, and this anomaly does usually not require surgery.

15.3.2.7
Aorta and Pulmonary Trunk

Is the aortic arch on the right or on the left side? Is the normal contour of the pulmonary artery present? In newborn babies, the thymus frequently obscures the view of the great arteries, and this is illustrated in Figure 15.21. The most important clue to determine the position of the aorta may sometimes be the distance from the lateral border of the trachea to the mediastinal contour. It is largest at the side where the aorta is located. A right-sided aortic arch is frequently associated with tetralogy of Fallot with severe stenosis of the pulmonary artery (Fig. 15.22). Uneven distribution of lung vessels in combination with a concave left heart contour raises the suspicion of pulmonary atresia with collateral circulation from the aorta to the pulmonary arteries. Both absent and prominent pulmonary trunk must be related to the clinical information of cyanosis and the appearance of the pulmonary vasculature before the true meaning of this sign can be evaluated. In postoperative patients, asymmetric lung vessels may be caused by iatrogenic occlusion of parts of the pulmonary artery tree (Fig. 15.23).

15.3.2.8
Skeleton

Are vertebral anomalies or bony abnormalities of the chest wall visible? In Alagille's syndrome butterfly vertebrae and peripheral pulmonary stenosis frequently coexist (Fig. 15.24). Scoliosis is reported

in 6% of children with cyanotic congenital heart defects as opposed to 0.4% in the general population (LUKE and McDONNELL 1968). The well-known rib notching in coarctation of the aorta is a relatively late sign, rarely encountered in children below 8 years of age. Widened, tortuous subcostal arteries eroding the ribs (Fig. 15.25) is the causing factor. Two manubrial centres and 11 pairs of ribs are associated with Down's syndrome, which is one of many syndromes associated with CHD.

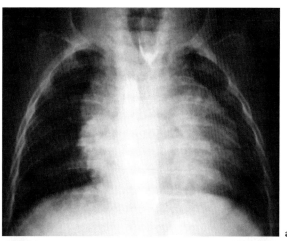
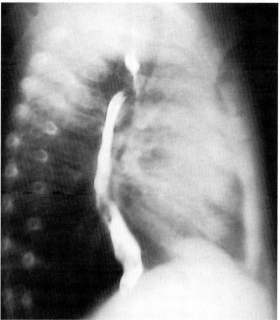

Fig. 15.19a,b. A 6-month-old boy with marked impression in the oesophagus and trachea from a double aortic arch

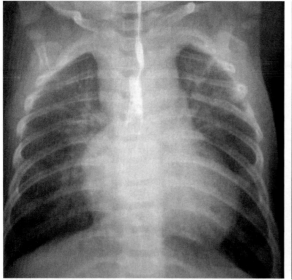 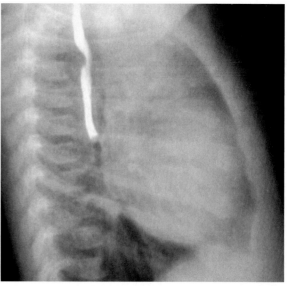

a   b

Fig. 15.20a,b. A 3-month-old boy with typical impression in the oesophagus caused by an aberrant subclavian artery. **a** Frontal chest radiograph shows compression of the oesophagus from the vessel coming from the left side and crossing the oesophagus as it courses upwards to reach the right arm as the right subclavian artery. **b** Lateral chest radiograph shows an impression in the posterior aspect of the oesophagus

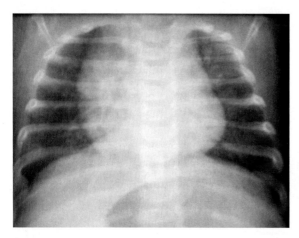 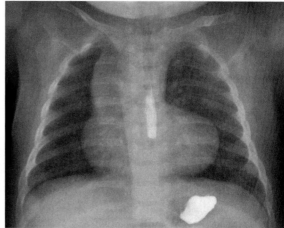

Fig. 15.21. A 3-month-old boy with valvular pulmonic stenosis. The large thymus makes assessment of the aorta and central pulmonary arteries virtually impossible

Fig. 15.22. A 3-month-old girl with right-sided aortic arch (*arrowheads*) in tetralogy of Fallot

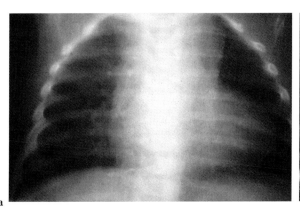
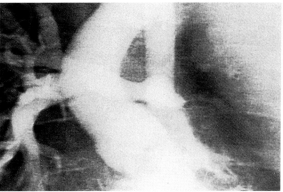

a

b

Fig. 15.23a,b. A 14-month-old girl after shunt operation for tetralogy of Fallot. **a** Asymmetrical lung vasculature with small lung vessels on the left side. **b** Angiography after injection into the right ventricle shows occlusion of the left pulmonary artery. There were no visible collaterals from the systemic circulation to the pulmonary arteries in the left lung

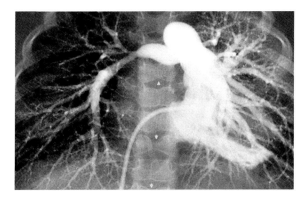
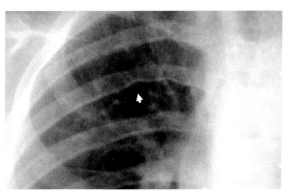

Fig. 15.24. Alagille's syndrome (arteriohepatic dysplasia). Peripheral pulmonary artery stenosis and butterfly vertebrae (*arrowheads*)

Fig. 15.25. A 9-year-old boy with coarctation of the aorta and rib notching (*arrowhead*)

15.3.2.9
Arrangement of the Organs

Where are the liver, spleen and the stomach located? What is the position of the heart and the descending aorta, and are the bronchi visible? The atria may be considered the key cardiac structures, and must fit with the situs determined for a particular patient. In situs solitus (usual position), the heart as well as the viscera have normal morphology as well as normal position. This also means that the right atrium is on the right side with its characteristic broad-based triangular appendage. In situs inversus, the arrangement of all viscera is completely mirror-imaged both in the thorax and the abdomen. In situs inversus the risk for cardiac anomalies is doubled compared to the normal arrangement. When the patient does not contain both a left and right half, the term situs ambiguus

(indeterminate) has been used. In such a case that patient is either double-left or double-right. This has implications for unilateral organs: sinus node (right) and spleen (left). Since the former has two sinus nodes and the latter none, both are prone to rhythm disturbances. It has been advocated to replace the "ambiguous" term by naming the condition in accordance with the atrial morphology: left atrial isomerism is also known as the polysplenia syndrome, and right atrial isomerism is termed asplenia syndrome (ANDERSON and Ho 1990).

The position of the apex of the heart can also vary. In the usual arrangement the apex is on the left side (levocardia), and in the mirror-image arrangement it is on the right (dextrocardia) (Fig. 15.26). Sometimes the apex is in the midline (mesocardia). It is good advice to look for the position of the apex as well as the position of the gastric air (Fig. 15.27).

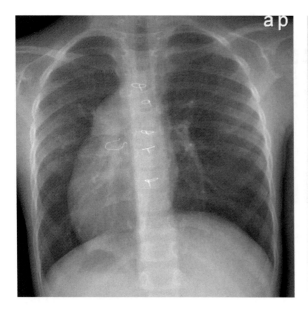

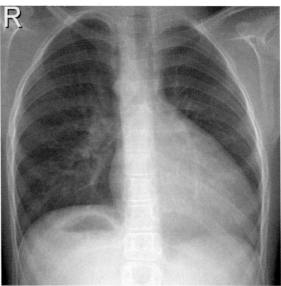

Fig. 15.26. A 6-year-old girl with situs inversus – mirror-image arrangement of all organs

Fig. 15.27. A 9-year-old girl with levocardia. Note gastric air on the right side. The patient also had atrial septal defect, double-outlet right ventricle, pulmonic stenosis and anomalous pulmonary venous drainage

15.4
Conclusion

As a rule a definite diagnosis of a specific heart malformation should not be based upon the chest radiograph alone. However, this does not mean that the different signs should be ignored. The main task of the radiologist interpreting the chest radiograph is to raise suspicion of a possible CHD based upon the criteria mentioned in this chapter. Most experienced paediatric radiologists will use heart size and the appearance of lung vessels as the strongest indicators of pathology, but, as LAYA et al. (2006) reported, the chest radiograph alone is not diagnostic of specific congenital cardiac lesions, and has a low accuracy of 71%. Our approach to patients with CHD has changed profoundly over the last 20 years, with a much stronger impact from echocardiography and magnetic resonance imaging (HIGGINS 2006). Multislice computed tomography with angiography and 3D reconstruction is increasingly important. Still, chest radiography is frequently performed, and may give essential haemodynamic information. Further, it is necessary both in the differentiation between heart and lung disease and in the postoperative period.

References

Anderson RH, Ho SY (1990) Cardiac situs and malpositions: echocardiographic evaluation. In: Higgins CB, Silverman NH, Kersting-Sommerhoff BA, Schmidt K (eds) Congenital heart disease. Echocardiography and magnetic resonance imaging. Raven, New York, pp 73–88

Higgins CB (2000) Cardiac imaging. Radiology 217:4–10

Hoffman JIE (1995) Incidence of congenital heart disease: I. Postnatal incidence. Pediatr Cardiol 16:103–113

Kohn MM, Moores BM, Schibilla H et al (1996) European guidelines on quality criteria for diagnostic radiographic images in paediatrics. EUR 16261 EN

Laya BF, Goske MJ, Morrison S et al (2006) The accuracy of chest radiographs in the detection of congenital heart disease and in the diagnosis of specific congenital cardiac lesions. Pediatr Radiol 36:677–681

Luke MJ, McDonnel EJ (1968) Congenital heart disease and scoliosis. J Pediatr 73:725–733

Marin-Garcia J, Tandon R, Lucas RV Jr et al (1975) Cor triatriatum. Study of 20 cases. Am J Cardiol 35:59–66

Markowitz RI, Fellows KE (1998) The effect on congenital heart disease on the lungs. Semin Roentgenol 23:126–135

Nora JJ (1993) Causes of CHD. Old and new modes, mechanisms, and models. Am Heart J 125:1409–1418

O'Brian KM (1985) Congenital syndromes with congenital heart disease. Semin Roentgenol 20:104–105

Samanek M, Voriskova M (1999) Congenital heart disease among 815569 children born between 1980 and 1990 and their 15-year survival: a prospective Bohemia survival study. Pediatr Cardiol 20:411–417

Angiocardiography and Intervention in Congenital Heart and Great Vessel Disease

16

Bjarne Smevik and Per G. Bjørnstad

16

CONTENTS

16

B. Smevik, MD
Section of Paediatric Radiology, Department of Radiology, Rikshospitalet Radiumhospitalet HF, The National Hospital, Sognsvannsvn 20, 0373 Oslo, Norway
P. G. Bjørnstad, MD, PhD
Section of Paediatric Cardiology, Department of Paediatrics, Rikshospitalet Radiumhospitalet HF, The National Hospital, Sognsvannsvn 20, 0373 Oslo, Norway

16.1 Introduction

There are different ways to visualize the heart before and during interventions. Traditionally, the first methods were fluoroscopy and angiocardiography, but other possible methods will also be mentioned in this context. One of the major issues in modern imaging is to choose the right tool for the question to be answered. To be able to do this, one must be aware of the advantages and disadvantages of every single method. During one type of intervention echocardiography may be indispensable; for another, echocardiography would not be of any importance at all. Thus, knowledge of the advantages and disadvantages of every method is of vital importance.

The heart is a complex three-dimensional organ with walls, valves and vessels, all in different shapes of curved surfaces positioned at some angle to each one of the other parts of the heart. In the end, visualization with whatever method should result in a virtual three-dimensional picture displayed in the examiner's brain, be it M-mode or two-dimensional echocardiography, chest radiography, angiocardiography or two- or three-dimensional reconstruction from computerized methods. This requires a deep understanding of the cardiac anatomy in the normal and malformed heart and the capability to direct the planes of the investigating tool to optimize the visualization of the part of the heart in question. The days have passed when it was possible to perform every single angiocardiographic recording in two planes: the anterior-posterior and the lateral ones. Today the X-ray tubes in a catheterization laboratory may be rotated and angled in a multitude of ways to best outline the structure of interest. This feature gives us the possibility of making pictures that enable us to understand the nature of the malformation and to demonstrate it to others. But the many possibilities of projection also require an understanding of the cardiac structures, their spatial orientation and interrelationship. Only with such an understanding may the tubes be steered into the optimal position for angiocardiography and fluoroscopy. This means that workers in the field need a high degree of three-dimensional thinking and imagination as well as detailed anatomical knowledge and familiarity with all the different imaging modalities and their advantages and disadvantages.

16.2
Different Modes of Visualization

16.2.1
Ultrasonography

Ultrasonographic imaging has evolved over the latest three to four decades and now echocardiography is an indispensable tool in diagnostics and interventions in cardiac disease. The heart can be viewed from all available "windows", i.e. from all positions where air in the lungs or the thickness of bone do not prevent visualization of cardiac structures. The possible positions may be on the chest, in the jugular or supraclavicular fossae or even within the oesophagus. Such examinations are in most cases performed by paediatric cardiologists or their technicians. The transducer emits and receives ultrasound waves either in a single beam or with multiple beams in a waveform, the former producing a time/distance curve, the latter a moving two-dimensional picture. The recordings display cardiac motion and distances between the different structures. Thus one may measure cavity dimensions and wall thickness and even their rates of change. Echocardiography has become increasingly important, and the dynamic presentation of studies from easily available digital storage has made a big difference in the assessment of congenital heart disease. Application of the Doppler principle yields information about velocity and direction of blood flow that may be recorded. Colour-flow Doppler imaging enables us to visualize flow related to structures in a two- or one-dimensional display. Flow away from the transducer is normally coded in shades of blue, flow towards the transducer in shades of red. Abnormal flow will easily be demonstrated in such a system. Blood flow velocity measured by Doppler ultrasound has a constant relation to systolic pressure gradients across short stenoses. The flow velocity through a stenosis is mirroring the drop in pressure. The systolic pressure gradient is calculated from the simplified Bernoulli equation which says that the gradient (in mmHg) is $4 \times v^2$, where v is the trans-stenotic velocity in metres per second. It may be given as peak gradient (peak instantaneous gradient) or mean gradient. Such gradients are different to the invasive measurement of peak-to-peak gradients: the peak gradient shows the gradient at peak flow, which is early in systole, and the mean gradient incorporates each gradient throughout the whole ejection.

Ultrasonography is routinely performed in the radiological department to study the preoperative intracranial status prior to heart surgery in neonates. In the first postoperative days the study may be repeated whenever clinical suspicion of intracranial pathology arises. Also ultrasonographic abdominal screening is frequently performed in such patients. Many well-known syndromes include significant abdominal pathology, and this ranges from mirror-image orientation of organs with asplenia or polysplenia to changes in the appearance of the abdominal aorta (e.g. Kawasaki disease) and the absence of a normal right-sided inferior vena cava. Patients with congenital cardiac malformations also have a higher incidence of abnormalities in the renal system. Enlargement of the liver and distension of liver veins and the inferior vena cava may indicate right-sided heart failure. Screening of the internal jugular vein and other large peripheral veins before placement of central venous catheters is recommendable, especially if the patient has had a previous central venous line. Ultrasonography is also used in patients with congenital heart disease for the evaluation and, if needed, drainage of pleural and pericardial effusions, which may occur in the postoperative period after heart surgery. Some patients may have significant production of ascites that may be monitored and sometimes drained under ultrasonographic guidance. Ultrasonography may also be used to evaluate the movement of both hemidiaphragms, particularly in the postoperative patient.

Finally, ultrasonography is used as an imaging guide to puncture veins and arteries not easily accessible in obese patients and in patients after multiple previous procedures, or where the pulse is very weak. The vessel is imaged in colour Doppler mode and, after finding the exact course longitudinally, the puncture is performed with the vessel in transverse section. This enables evaluation of where the needle is entering the circumference of the vessel, but the drawback is that the needle is not visible before it is close to the vessel wall. By using this technique to enter the internal jugular vein, puncture of the main carotid artery may be avoided. Such an error is reported to happen in approximately 10% of cases, even with trained operators, if the "landmark" method is used.

16.2.2
Fluoroscopy

During catheter intervention fluoroscopy plays an important role. Catheters are moved around and manipulated into proper positions under fluoroscopic guidance. In most cases it will be recommendable, if not mandatory, to have a biplane catheter laboratory to create the virtual three-dimensional display in the operator's mind. There have been reports on interventions having taken place without any X-ray being involved; for example, atrial septal defects (ASDs) being closed solely on the basis of echocardiography. This shows it is possible but in our opinion it is not recommendable as additional information and thus increased safety are derived from concomitant fluoroscopy. The introduction of pulsed fluoroscopy with as few as three frames per second has led to a significant reduction in radiation dose to the patient. Experience shows that for the bigger part of the invasive study this rate is sufficient. This dose

reduction is of course important in all invasive studies, but particularly for the sometimes very long and complicated interventional procedures.

16.2.3
Angiocardiography

Most patients with congenital heart disease will be adequately handled on the basis of the knowledge derived from clinical and biochemical studies, electrocardiography (ECG), echocardiography including Doppler and chest radiography. This will suffice to determine whether to treat conservatively, to perform an intervention or to operate and, if so, when that operation should be performed. Conditions usually managed along these lines include both simple and complex malformations, such as persistent arterial duct, atrial and ventricular septal defects (VSDs), transposition of the great arteries, tetralogy of Fallot, and hypoplastic left heart syndrome.

Heart catheterization with angiocardiography is still frequently needed in more complex lesions. It is important to record pressure and oxygen saturation in different locations in the heart and great vessels and to compare the physiologic values with the anatomic information from the recorded injections of contrast medium.

Although it is fashionable to state that angiocardiography is being replaced by echocardiography, magnetic resonance imaging (MRI) with cine- and angio-sequences with and without gadolinium contrast media, as well as multislice computed tomography (MCT), it is still a fact that some of the more complex situations need all available modalities. Even after all modalities have been used unsolved questions may remain.

Furthermore, the number of catheter-based interventions is increasing, even within a few days or weeks after birth (KRETSCHMAR et al. 2000). In fact, the intervention first introduced was just in neonates. The growing population of adults with late effects and complications after surgery also makes it necessary to maintain skills in angiocardiography. The reasons for performing heart catheterization in patients with congenital heart disease have changed. Because the number of catheter-based interventions has increased at the same rate as purely diagnostic catheterizations have decreased, the total number of procedures in our institution has remained remarkably stable at about 300 per year. This covers the needs of a population of about 4.5 million people.

16.2.3.1
Technique

Modern digital equipment allows up to 50 frames per second in biplane to be recorded, and this competes favourably with the old cine-angiography systems that performed at 75 frames per second. Post-processing possibilities are especially important in extracting as much information as possible from the study, and in addition to measurements of sizes and ejection fraction of the ventricles, change of window/level, brightness and contrast, inversion and edge enhancement should be used actively. The use of modern low-osmolar contrast media ensures high-quality angiocardiograms and minimal discomfort to, and complications for, the patient. As a rule of thumb, the total amount of contrast medium injected for each series is 1.5 ml per kilogram body weight in the large cavities on the left side of the heart, and this is increased to 2 ml per kilogram body weight on the right side. In vessels such as the aorta, pulmonary arteries or smaller branches, the amount must be adapted to the calibre of the vessel and the neighbouring vascular bed. The volume may even be increased beyond this when the contrast medium is diluted into the volume of two circuits, as in the common arterial trunk. Opacification depends on how much contrast medium is injected per second as well as the concentration of the contrast medium. The concentration is usually 300 mg I/ml, and the flow rate is set to inject the volume indicated above in about 1.5 s. It is obviously important to use the least toxic contrast media available (STAKE et al. 1991). The projection is adjusted according to the suspected lesion, and the size of the patient. The information obtained from echocardiography is used to individualize the projection.

A VSD in the membranous portion of the septum may be best visualized in the "four-chamber view", which is a left anterior oblique view with a 75° left and 25° cranial angulation. If it is located in the outlet portion of the septum, a true lateral view may localize it best. Inlet portion defects are best shown in a modest left anterior oblique projection with 25° left and at least 45° cranial angulation. In the newborn, the aortic arch frequently runs in the sagittal plane, and consequently it may be best seen in a lateral projection. In older children, the best projection for the aortic arch is as a rule a left anterior oblique view. As can readily be seen from a lateral view of the main pulmonary artery, it runs at an angle of approximately 45° to the sternum, and hence the frontal projection should be angled accordingly in the cranial direction.

16.2.3.2
Complications

The complications that may occur in an invasive study such as angiocardiography include injury to the vessel of entry. These include compression from haematomas after removal of vascular sheaths, spasm and occlusion of the femoral artery or vein. Guide wires and catheters may perforate the heart or great vessels (Fig. 16.1). Vessels may be occluded through damage of the vessel wall or by emboli, resulting in ischaemic injury to organs such as the brain or the heart. A combination of ischaemia and the toxic effect of contrast media may cause substantial damage to the kidneys. Extrasystoles occur in most procedures, but real problems with arrhythmia through manipulation of catheters or the influence of contrast medium injections are rarely seen. Allergic reactions to the contrast medium used have been reported, as well as complications caused by sedation, general anaesthesia or the different drugs used for various tests.

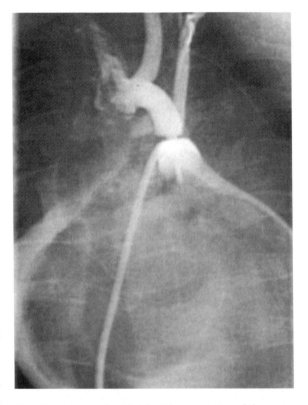

Fig. 16.1. A 2-month-old girl with coarctation of the aorta. After perforation contrast medium has collected in the pericardial cavity. The patient did not have clinical symptoms, and the study could be completed with visualization of the coarctation and the hypoplastic posterior aortic arch after inflation of a balloon in the descending aorta

16.2.4
Other Imaging Modalities

MRI and MR angiography (MRA) as well as MCT and CT angiography (CTA) are not included in this chapter, but clearly these modalities are very helpful in the planning of interventional procedures. MRI with flow measurements will be able to estimate the gradient in stenotic lesions not very well seen by echocardiography and thus help to decide if intervention is appropriate. Both MRA and CTA are very useful in planning balloon size and stent size in vascular stenosis before the interventional procedure (e.g. peripheral pulmonary stenosis, recoarctation of the aorta). Both modalities may also provide a useful map of collaterals that may need embolization.

16.3
Intervention in Congenital Heart Disease

The introduction of transcatheter interventional procedures has saved an increasing number of patients the burden of thoracotomy, sternotomy and heart operation. But also the catheter-based and much less invasive procedures do require manual training and skills as well as angiographic training and optimal radiological equipment. An intervention is monitored with fluoroscopy, angiocardiography and in many cases also echocardiography, most often with the transoesophageal, but sometimes with transthoracic or even intracardiac approach.

Practice differs from one institution to another, depending on the personal views and skills amongst the different members of the team taking care of children with congenital heart disease. There is no uniform approach and much is decided on personal preferences. The goal is to propose the best solution for each individual patient based on the experience in each single centre. The catheter-based treatment is normally performed instead of a surgical operation. In premature and low-body-weight infants, however, the goal of transcatheter intervention is frequently to postpone rather than replace surgery or to stabilize the haemodynamic situation prior to surgery, as illustrated in Figure 16.2.

From analysis of material consisting of 27 transcatheter interventions performed in 24 patients with a body weight under 2.5 kg, KRETSCHMAR et al. (2000) reported that surgery was effectively postponed in nine patients with pulmonary stenosis, valvular aortic stenosis and aortic coarctation. Only three patients had no benefit from the intervention. Femoral arterial complications occurred in 30% of arterial catheterizations. There has been a steady increase in the number of catheter-based options for definite treatment of congenital heart defects. This development has been paralleled by a significant improvement in the safety and efficacy of the methods. In practice, the closure of the open duct, excluding premature babies, has been completely taken over by the catheter methods, thus saving thoracotomy in all these children. Balloon treatment of valvular pulmonic stenosis is the method of choice. A few valves, however, are resistant to such treatment and heart surgery must be performed. Atrial septal defects in the oval fossa can be closed with catheter-based techniques in 75% of cases. Closure of VSDs is increasingly being performed with catheters. Extracardiac applications of catheter-based methods include closure of surgical shunts and aorticopulmonary or venous collaterals. The introduction of different types of retrievable coils has made such procedures much safer and accessible to new groups of patients. For widening of narrow passages in veins, arteries or surgical channels balloons may be used, but more often it is recommendable to use some kind of a stent to maintain the opened area even after the balloon has been deflated.

Every interventional procedure carries some risk of injury to the patient. Balloon dilatations may cause rupture, avulsion of valves and injury to surrounding tissue (e.g. lung parenchyma) if the balloon bursts. Sometimes a balloon will rupture transversely and may have to be removed surgically. Embolization may cause the post-embolization syndrome consisting of leucocytosis, hyperpyrexia, and pain or discomfort. Implants may be misplaced, dislodge or embolize. In many cases, though, such material can be retrieved with different types of snares or forceps.

The following sections deal with situations within congenital heart disease where intervention may be considered, is used occasionally, or even represents the preferred treatment.

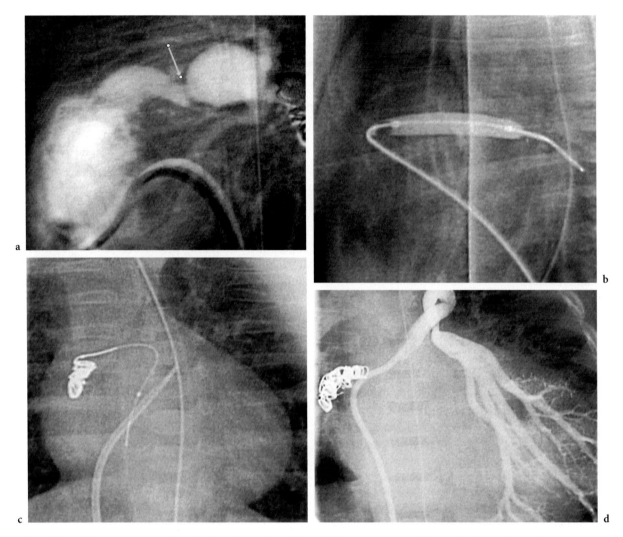

Fig. 16.2a–d. Premature 1-month-old girl with a body weight of 2400 g at the time of the study. The patient had severe pulmonic stenosis with a gradient of 50 mmHg. Intervention was considered necessary to stabilize the clinical condition before operative measures could be undertaken. **a** Lateral view shows stenosis of the pulmonary artery (*arrow*). **b** Balloon dilatation with a balloon of 6 mm diameter. **c** Coil occlusion of large collateral from the aorta to the pulmonary artery. **d** Another collateral was the only feeding artery to the left lower lobe

16.4
Transposition of the Great Arteries

In complete transposition of the great arteries (TGA) the aorta arises from the anterior right ventricle, and the pulmonary artery from the posterior left ventricle. Because the superior and inferior vena cava, the pulmonary veins, the atria and the ventricles are normally connected, blood returning from the lungs to the left atrium re-enters the pulmonary artery from the left ventricle. Blood returning from the body through the inferior and superior caval veins returns to the body via the right ventricle and the aorta. Thus two independent circuits exist. Survival is only possible if mixing between the two parallel circulations occurs, most commonly through a patent oval foramen and/or an open arterial duct. Desoxygenation is always present, but may be less visible if a VSD is present.

Echocardiography establishes the diagnosis and demonstrates associated lesions. The patient will be referred for a switch procedure: the great arteries are transected, switched and sutured to the stump of the artery leaving the ventricle from which they were supposed to originate. Also the origin of the coronary arteries is moved and reimplanted into the aorta to be. If the coronary artery anatomy is unclear from echocardiographic studies, it should be studied by angiocardiography. A balloon septostomy (Rashkind's procedure) may be performed at the same time, but this procedure is now mostly performed with echocardiographic support alone. Abnormalities of the coronary arteries may occasionally make a switch operation difficult or impossible. Angiography may also be appropriate to rule out stenosis of the coronary arteries after a switch procedure (Fig. 16.3). The earlier operations for complete TGA, the Mustard or Senning procedure, both essentially switched the circulation at the atrial level leading red blood from the pulmonary veins into the right ventricle giving rise to the aorta and leading desoxygenated blood into the left ventricle from which the pulmonary artery would lead it to the lungs for reoxygenation. The Mustard operation used Dacron® patches; the Senning operation used the atrial walls for this re-routing. These operations are still occasionally used in special patients.

16.4.1
Transcatheter Intervention

In addition to the Rashkind procedure already described, the postoperative patient may need intervention for stenosis in the venous channels following an atrial switch operation. In such cases, balloon dilatation followed by stenting is the preferred procedure. After an arterial switch operation the suture site may become stenotic, especially in the new, low-pressure pulmonary artery. Such stenoses may be effectively treated with balloon dilatation.

16.5
Tetralogy of Fallot

The tetralogy of Fallot consists of a subaortic VSD and obstruction of the right ventricular outflow tract. The infundibular septum is displaced anteriorly and causes the subpulmonic obstruction and an "overriding" of the aorta. The degree of over-

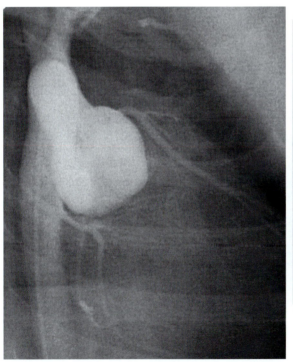
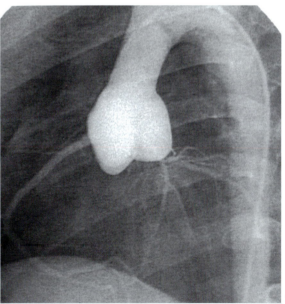

Fig. 16.3a,b. A 20-month-old boy operated for transposition of the great arteries (TGA) with a switch procedure of the great arteries. Angiography of the ascending aorta. The anastomosis between the pulmonic root and the ascending aorta as well as the appearance of the implanted coronary arteries is inconspicuous

riding has no influence on haemodynamics. The degree of cyanosis depends solely on the degree of obstruction. The thickened right ventricular wall is a normal reaction to the systemic pressure in the right ventricle. The aortic arch is right-sided in one-quarter of cases. The narrow outflow tract from the right ventricle may involve the whole infundibulum, and in addition the pulmonary valve may be stenotic with a small annulus. Supravalvular and branch stenoses are also often found. General hypoplasia of the pulmonary tree or unilateral agenesis of the pulmonary artery may be encountered. Pulmonary atresia with VSD can be considered the ultimate form of tetralogy. The classical Fallot is rarely diagnosed before 3 months of age, the ones with earlier diagnosis often present with the more complex lesions and multi-level stenoses.

In the regular case echocardiography makes the diagnosis, measures the size of the defect and is able to visualize the outflow tract obstruction and the proximal pulmonary arteries. For detailed imaging of the pulmonary tree and possible collateral arteries angiocardiography or CTA is needed. Also angiocardiography shows the right ventricle and the degree and level of stenoses. Special attention is paid to the angiocardiographic presentation of the coronary arteries. Coronary artery anomalies occur in

4%–5% of patients. The most important one is the right coronary artery giving rise to the left anterior descending branch, which crosses the infundibulum of the right ventricle. This is the region where correction of the outflow tract obstruction may occur, and such a course of the artery may prohibit complete repair. The cardiac surgeon at least should be forewarned. It is important to visualize the infundibulum of the right ventricle and the pulmonary arteries (Fig. 16.4). The pulmonary valve annulus as well as any stenosis in the pulmonary tree is measured. If the pulmonary arteries are small, the Nakata index should be reported (NAKATA et al. 1984). This is the sum of the area of the right and left pulmonary arteries divided by body surface area. The Nakata index is an indication of whether the patient will tolerate repair or first must be treated with a shunt from a systemic artery to the pulmonary tree to allow the pulmonary arteries to grow. The palliative treatment mostly used today is the central prosthetic shunt between the ascending aorta and the main stem of the pulmonary artery or a modified Blalock-Taussig anastomosis. This involves placing a tube of synthetic material between the subclavian artery and the right or left pulmonary artery (Fig. 16.5). Potts' and Waterston's anastomoses are obsolete.

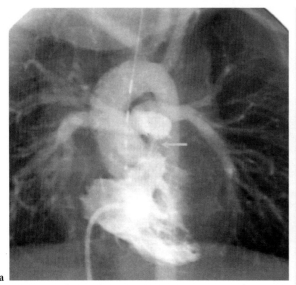
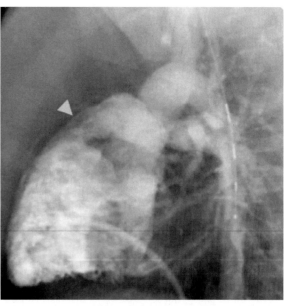

Fig. 16.4a,b. A 3-year-old girl with tetralogy of Fallot. The main pulmonary artery is hypoplastic and the right and left pulmonary arteries are small. **a** Angiocardiography of the right ventricle shows hypertrophy with a dynamic infundibulum contracting markedly in systole (*arrow*). **b** Infundibulum relaxing in diastole (*arrowhead*)

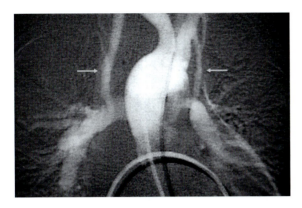

Fig. 16.5. A 4-year-old boy. Angiography shows open bilateral modified Blalock–Taussig shunt (*arrows*)

Repair involves patch closure of the VSD and relief of the obstruction(s). The outflow stenoses may be resected, the valve opened and often left with a slight stenosis. The outflow tract and/or pulmonary artery may be enlarged with a patch, sometimes transannular, and left with or without a valvular structure in the passage. Last, the outflow tract and proximal pulmonary artery may be exchanged with a conduit with a valve or a homograft.

There have been attempts to repair the Fallot with interventional techniques (SIDERIS et al. 2005). As yet this is not an established treatment. But operative treatment may sometimes be successfully postponed by balloon dilatation of the infundibulum and the pulmonary valve. Some patients with severe pulmonic stenosis develop collaterals that may need transcatheter closure after surgical repair of the pulmonary artery.

16.6
Pulmonary Atresia with Ventricular Septal Defect

The difference between pulmonary atresia with VSD and tetralogy of Fallot is the lack of continuity between the right ventricle and the pulmonary artery. The blood supply to the lungs is through a patent arterial duct, major aorticopulmonary collateral arteries (MAPCAs), or a surgically created anastomosis in isolation or combination. The internal mammary artery on both sides and the bronchial arteries may also contribute. The central pulmonary

arteries have variable presentations, and the main pulmonary artery, the confluence and the right or left pulmonary artery may be absent, hypoplastic and/or stenotic.

Angiocardiography is frequently the only modality allowing complete visualization of all the different large and small branches supplying the pulmonary artery circulation, although preoperative MCT may also be a valuable tool. Figure 16.6. illustrates a case where a multitude of small vessels supplies the pulmonary circulation. When the various collaterals are considered disadvantageous to the patient, they may be embolized.

16.7
Pulmonary Atresia with Intact Ventricular Septum

The heart is nearly always in a normal left position with a left-sided aortic arch. The right ventricle is usually hypoplastic, but may, at least initially, be quite sizeable. The tricuspid valve may be both abnormal and obstructive. Persistent right ventricular myocardial sinusoidal-coronary artery connections are frequently reported in association with this condition (CORNELL 1966; FREEDOM and MOES 1985). The flow is usually from the ventricle to the coronary artery through these sinusoids as shown in Figure 16.7. The blood returning from the body enters the right atrium and must be able to shunt over to the left side of the heart if the patient is to survive. This is most frequently through an ASD but also in part through existing sinusoids. The lungs must be perfused through an open arterial duct. The diagnosis can often be reliably established with echocardiography, but angiocardiography will be better able to exclude or depict in detail fistulous connections from the right ventricular cavity through the sinusoids to the coronary arteries. The pulmonary arteries may be visualized through an injection in the aortic arch or – entering from the left ventricle and through the aortic arch – into the descending aorta with an inflated balloon blocking its lumen and forcing the contrast medium up the aorta, through the arterial duct and into the pulmonary arteries. Efforts must be made to ensure pulmonary blood flow either through a surgical shunt or by placing a stent to keep the duct open.

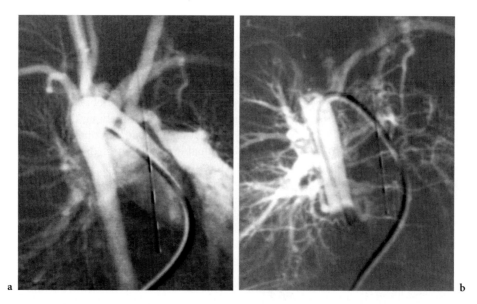

Fig. 16.6a,b. A 3-day-old girl with pulmonary atresia and ventricular septal defect (VSD). **a** Angiocardiography shows right-sided aorta and collaterals to the lungs. **b** Numerous small collaterals from the descending aorta and the left subclavian artery become evident after the run-off of contrast medium is blocked by inflating a balloon in the descending aorta

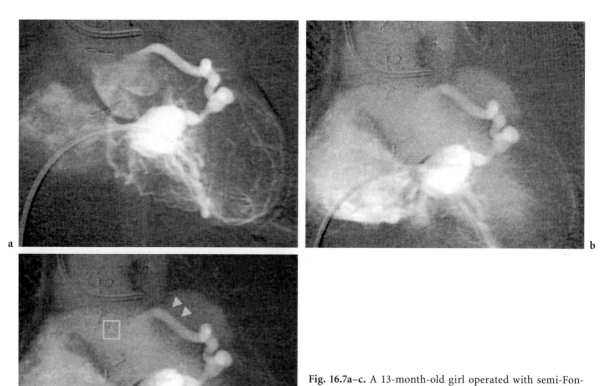

Fig. 16.7a–c. A 13-month-old girl operated with semi-Fontan procedure. Sinusoids are shown to communicate with the left coronary artery. **a** Injection of contrast medium into the right ventricle fills multiple small channels (sinusoids). **b** Retrograde filling of the left coronary artery (*arrowheads*) and the ascending aorta (A) via the sinusoids. **c** Injection in the ascending aorta verifies the appearance of the left coronary artery

Another approach is to try to open the pulmonary valve provided it is a valvular atresia and the pulmonary artery is intact all the way from the atretic valve. Such valves may be opened by means of radiofrequency energy applied through special catheters (ROSENTHAL et al. 1993). After having established an opening of the valve a guide wire is introduced through it into the pulmonary artery. This wire is used as a guide for the following balloon-tipped catheter that will be inflated in the usual way to dilate the now severely stenotic valve. Often it is possible to achieve quite good results from such therapy without surgical intervention and the use of the heart lung machine.

16.8
Tricuspid Atresia

One important point in the classification of tricuspid atresia is to decide if the tricuspid valve is atretic or absent. If the valve is present, albeit imperforate, it is theoretically possible to create a connection from the right atrium to the right ventricle. Almost exclusively, though, the right ventricle is far too small to accept a sufficient volume and create a relevant output. The most common form involves absent tricuspid valve with a separation of the right atrium from the right ventricle by a wedge of fatty tissue, frequently also containing the right coronary artery. The right ventricle is hypoplastic but contains the three parts of a ventricle: inflow, sinus and outflow parts. The VSD necessary for survival of the patient – if there is no open arterial duct – may be restrictive. In addition, infundibular hypoplasia and/or pulmonary valve stenosis may reduce the pulmonary blood flow. The great arteries may be in normal position (70%) or transposed (30%).

In a patient with tricuspid atresia the blood returning from the body to the right atrium must pass through the atrial septum to the left atrium and into the left ventricle. A VSD or an open arterial duct is necessary for the blood to enter the pulmonary arteries. The right ventricle has no function other than being a transit chamber for the blood flow through the VSD. The more restrictive the VSD, infundibulum and pulmonary valves, the more dependent the patient is on blood flow through an open arterial duct.

Angiocardiography with injection of contrast medium into the right atrium will define the lack of flow through the tricuspid valve and mostly show enlargement of the right atrium with back-flow into the inferior vena cava, the hepatic veins and sometimes also into the often widened coronary sinus. The left ventricle is enlarged, compensating for the hypoplastic right ventricle. Both the size of the VSD and the total size of the right ventricle as well as its connection to the pulmonary artery must be evaluated, and this is best achieved in the left anterior oblique view with left ventricular injection. Most important is to accurately define the size of the pulmonary arteries before surgery. Sometimes stenting of the arterial duct may be considered.

16.9
Single Ventricle

The original "pure" single ventricle is a lesion in which the inflow part of one of the ventricles is missing. It may have one or two inlets and one or two outlets, and has accordingly been called single/double-inlet and single/double-outlet single ventricle. The main ventricle is a complete ventricle, mostly of left (75%) but sometimes of right ventricular type (20%). Occasionally, the type of ventricle cannot be defined (FREEDOM et al. 1984a,b). The malformed, diminutive ventricle contains just the sinus and outlet portion. It is deprived of the vicinity to the atrium and is situated under one of the large arteries as a "rudimentary outflow chamber". If there is an artery originating from this outlet chamber, it needs a communication with the main ventricle. Such a communication is called the "bulboventricular foramen" and is in function a VSD. This term of "single ventricle" has been contaminated with other entities and now often includes all situations with only one functional ventricle. Thus it has increasingly become an expression without a solid definition and often only a convenient term for all types of lesions that cannot be repaired to become a four-chambered heart. Such a malformation may be combined with valvular stenoses or regurgitation. Other co-existent malformations are abnormal systemic venous connections, and anomalies of the atrial septum and appendages and the atrioventricular junction.

Echocardiography should define both the anatomy and the haemodynamic characteristics of the single ventricle. Connections are seen, the number of valves counted and their size measured. Their position is being visualized and the degree of stenosis or regurgitation is measured. If possible, the different veins and their draining site should be documented. Even trained echocardiographers will sometimes be unable to visualize all the details in such a complex structure, and will ask for complementary support from angiocardiography or MCT and MRI.

Angiocardiography should at least demonstrate the ventricular anatomy, the position of the outlet chamber, and the type of ventriculoarterial connection. The pulmonary artery and the aortic arch as well as the coronary arteries must be visualized, and the venous drainage must also be included in the study. CT and MRI may be superior to other techniques in defining the systemic and pulmonary venous drainage.

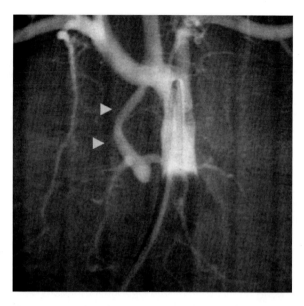

Fig. 16.8. A 3-day-old girl with hypoplastic left heart syndrome. Angiography through the patent ductus arteriosus (PDA) shows retrograde filling of a thin ascending aorta acting as a connection to the two coronary arteries

16.10
Hypoplastic Left Heart Syndrome (HLHS)

This syndrome is a complicated entity with the main functional feature of a left heart of insufficient size to allow adequate systemic circulation. This was originally termed the hypoplastic left ventricle syndrome by SINHA et al. (1968). The central anatomical features are atresia or severe stenosis of the aortic and/or mitral valve and a very small or absent left ventricle. Right-sided heart structures will be correspondingly enlarged. The blood from the left atrium will escape the left atrium by a communication through the atrial septum. The systemic circulation is supplied from the right side of the heart through the arterial duct and distributed both to the descending aorta and through the arch into the ascending aorta which is very small, functioning as "common coronary artery" (Fig. 16.8).

The patients typically present with mild cyanosis, tachypnoea and tachycardia. Peripheral pulses may be normal, diminished, or absent. The liver is enlarged. With closure of the arterial duct, the patient dies. If the duct does not close, the patients die from severe pulmonary hyperflow and reduced coronary blood flow paralleling the fall in pulmonary vascular resistance. Patency of the duct is achieved with continuous infusion of prostaglandin E1.

Echocardiography is the diagnostic tool of choice for hypoplastic left heart syndrome, and both intra-cardiac anatomy and the anatomy of the ascending aorta and aortic arch are usually well depicted. Colour Doppler imaging will give important information regarding regurgitation through the tricuspid valve, which is reported in more than 50%. Initial treatment is surgical with the so-called Norwood procedure (NORWOOD and JAKOBS 1994). The ultimate goal is the Fontan procedure because there is only one functioning ventricle. The initial Norwood palliation must ensure that: (1) the aorta has a direct and unobstructed connection from the right ventricle through the proximal pulmonary artery, (2) pulmonary blood flow is adequate with a sufficient aorticopulmonary shunt, and (3) free flow out of the pulmonary circuit is provided by creating a large interatrial connection. A few centres performed this first step with either purely catheter-based techniques or with hybrid procedures. Such treatment will include stenting of the open duct and implantation of flow-reducing devices in the side branches of the pulmonary artery or bands applied around the side branches by the thoracic surgeon.

Angiocardiography is not routinely used for the initial diagnosis in hypoplastic left heart syndrome, but is very important during follow-up. Not infrequently, stenosis at the anastomosis between the neo-aorta and the posterior native aorta develops, and this may be treated with balloon dilatation.

16.11
Balloon Dilatation of Valvar Stenoses

16.11.1
Pulmonary Valve Stenosis

The pulmonary valve may be stenotic as an isolated lesion or as part of more complex anomalies. The valve is as a rule tricuspid, but both bicuspid valves and four leaflets have been described. When the cusps are fused, they form a dome with a central opening that varies in size. Sometimes the leaflets may be dysplastic and thicker than normal. This is frequently seen in patients with Noonan's syndrome. Because of the extra workload against the stenotic valves, the right ventricle will develop hypertrophy, and this may be very pronounced in the infundibulum, sometimes resulting in an additional, secondary stenosis. The jet of blood coming through the narrow opening tends to dilate the main pulmonary artery, frequently also involving the left pulmonary artery, a direct continuation of the main trunk. The initial diagnosis is made by echocardiography but the visualization of the stenosis and detailed anatomy of the stenosis and the adjacent structures is made by angiocardiography with injection of contrast medium into the right ventricle. For optimizing the information through precise angulation of the X-ray tubes one has to recall the orientation of the right ventricular outflow tract and the pulmonary artery indicated above. The branching of the pulmonary artery originates from the same region at the same level, but the left branch courses more dorsally and a little higher than the right branch. This has to be reflected in the angulation in two planes: the lateral view should be almost perpendicular to the outflow tract of the right ventricle and align well with the pulmonary valve ring. If the visualization also must separate the side branches, the lateral projection should be oblique with its axis closer to the right shoulder on the right side, more caudal on the left. For the inspection of the dilatation itself, the lateral projection is the one most often preferred.

The first report of a successful balloon dilatation of pulmonic stenosis was from SEMB et al. (1979). The modern technique for treating congenital pulmonary-valve stenosis was presented by KAN et al. (1982). Balloons were constructed to create defined radial forces within defined diameters. The first results were promising and after some years balloon treatment of stenosed pulmonary valves became the method of choice. The catheter must have a balloon of appropriately selected width, and the length is usually 2 cm in the neonate and small infant, 3 cm in the bigger child and up to 4 cm in an adult. Such a catheter is placed over a guide wire so that the middle of the balloon is at the site of the stenosed valve. The width of the balloon should exceed the diameter of the valve ring by 25%–40%. In a successful case one would appreciate on fluoroscopy or on recorded film how the stenosed valve produces a waist in the balloon filled with diluted contrast medium. This waist suddenly disappears as the balloon forces the stenosed valve open (Fig. 16.9). As soon as the valve has been seen to open, the balloon is deflated as rapidly as possible. The interruption of the pulmonary circulation during the time of dilatation results in reduced filling of the left ventricle and a drop in the systemic blood pressure. For this limited period of time such an alteration is normally very well tolerated.

The results are typically good. As early as 1986 RADTKE et al. reported a 74% reduction in gradient. But even after a successful dilatation, the immediate gradient reduction may be disappointing, because a dynamic subpulmonary stenosis is triggered by the relief of the stenosis. The complication rate has been low, and STANGER et al. (1990) reported a mortality rate of 0.2% and only three other major complications (0.4%) among 822 procedures. In infants with critical pulmonary valve stenosis such a balloon procedure can be life saving. In some of these cases it may be difficult to access the pulmonary artery with a wire and a catheter. In such cases the balloon treatment may be performed as a hybrid solution with surgeons in the operating theatre gaining access to the pulmonary artery through the right ventricular outflow tract without using the heart-lung machine (Fig. 16.10).

16.11.2
Aortic Valve Stenosis

In children, this is a congenital lesion. The aortic valve is stenotic, but the narrowing is caused by a malformed valve. If the stenosis is relieved, be it by surgery or by catheter intervention, the valve is still malformed. Clinical symptoms vary with the severity of the lesion, but in the newborn a critical aortic stenosis may present with dramatic, sometimes life-threatening, symptoms. If the left ventricle is not able to deliver sufficient systemic cardiac output through the aortic valve the newborn is dependent on additional blood from the pulmonary artery through the arterial duct. If the duct then reacts normally and closes shortly after birth, symptoms will be severe. Occasionally, such neonates may have enormously enlarged heart contours and cardiac failure (Fig. 16.11). The diagnosis is made with echocardiography, and the severity estimated with Doppler ultrasonography velocity measurements. Echocardiography does not always give the detailed anatomy of the aortic valve. The number of cusps and the degree of dysplasia may be difficult to depict. The accompanying hypertrophy of the left ventricle and sometimes fibroelastosis of the endocardium are usually well appreciated with ultrasound imaging.

Today angiocardiography of the left ventricle and the aorta is only performed as part of necessary balloon dilatation. The angiocardiograms are also able to visualize the hypertrophy of the left ventricle and a valve with reduced movement (Fig. 16.12). A jet of contrast medium is often seen through the narrow opening. Some of these patients, especially neonates, are definitely high-risk candidates for surgery and dilatation with a balloon catheter may be a good alternative. Exposing a very sick neonate to an open heart operation with the use of the heart-lung machine carries a significant risk, and an opening of a stenosis in a malformed valve is in any case palliative treatment. The indication for treatment should not be linked to a certain level of pressure gradient over the valve. A pressure gradient depends on the capacity of the ventricle to eject blood out through the stenosis. A failing ventricle will result in falling gradients, thus sometimes the sickest patient will be the one with the smallest gradient. The indication should be based on a sum of all available parameters from the clinical status and the different examinations. Producing aortic insufficiency will be a risk factor for any treatment.

The aortic valve can be accessed in two different ways: either retrogradely from an artery in the groin or on the neck, or with access from the femoral vein through the right atrium, foramen ovale, left atrium, mitral valve, left ventricle and the aortic valve into the ascending aorta. The stenotic opening is easier to pass from the ventricle,

but to make the turn in the ventricular apex may be a problem in a small ventricle. With the arterial approach it is often difficult to pass the small or minute opening on the top of the cone formed by the stenotic valves. The femoral artery is small in the newborn and sometimes premature babies, but in the regular case the modern balloon catheters will create no access problem. Such an access may, though, lead to occlusion of the used artery. Using the larger right common carotid artery to insert a balloon of proper size is an alternative. Borghi et al. (2001) have found that the right common carotid artery was well preserved after neonatal surgical cutdown in 17 patients, with only occasional asymptomatic obstruction present. One problem with the balloon is the tendency of ventricular systole to eject the balloon before it is fully inflated. The diameter of the balloon should not exceed the diameter of the aortic annulus, and the length of the balloon must be appropriate to the size of the patient.

The results following dilatation will mainly depend on the valvular anatomy (Pedra et al. 2004). One complication feared more than in angioplasty of valvular pulmonic stenosis is the creation of severe regurgitation. It may happen if a tear or avulsion of a cusp occurs and in the neonate the only solution will be to perform a Ross operation.

16.11.3
Mitral Valve Stenosis

Congenital mitral stenosis is most frequently associated with anomalies of the subvalvular apparatus of chordae and papillary muscles. It may be very well described with echocardiography. Such a stenotic valve is not accessible to dilatation techniques. In rheumatic mitral stenosis, though, there is a normally constructed but diseased valve with fusions of the leaflets. Such a valve, also diagnosed with ultrasound, may be treated very well with the Inoue balloon technique (Flores et al. 2006). The Inoue balloon catheter is entered by the venous route into the left ventricle over a guide wire. The left atrium is accessed either by transseptal puncture or through the atrial septum's open foramen.

The most distal balloon is inflated and pulled back until it stops in the mitral opening. Then the proximal balloon is inflated quickly and both balloons deflated.

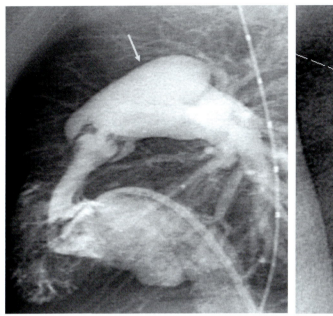
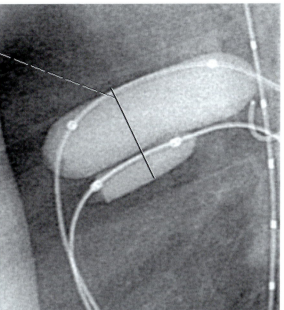

a   b

Fig. 16.9a,b. A 6-month-old boy with valvular pulmonary stenosis. **a** The thickened valves open incompletely, and the jet through the narrow opening has contributed to the widening of the main pulmonary artery (*arrows*). **b** Balloon dilatation with two balloons to avoid introducing sheaths and catheters that are too large for the femoral vein

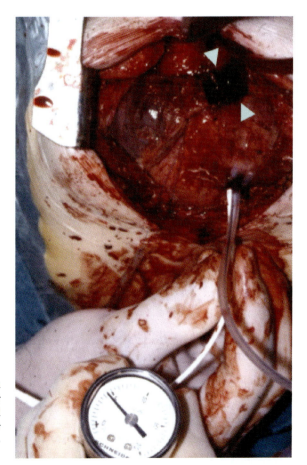

Fig. 16.10. Intra-operative balloon dilatation in a newborn with extremely narrow pulmonary stenosis. The catheter was inserted with the Seldinger technique through the wall of the right ventricle, and the balloon inflated while proper positioning was ascertained by palpation. A small haematoma is visible just beneath the valves (*arrowheads*)

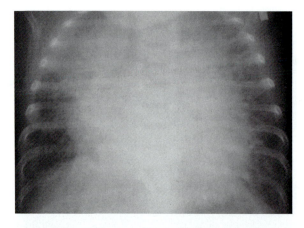

Fig. 16.11. A 1-day-old triplet with valvular aortic stenosis. Note enlarged heart and severe congestion. Echocardiography revealed poor function of the left ventricle

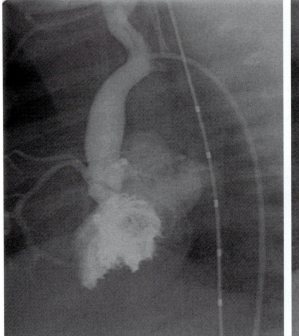

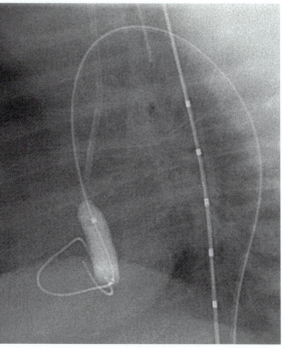

a   b

Fig. 16.12a,b. Severe valvular aortic stenosis in a 7-day-old girl. **a** Angiography depicted the stenotic valve and allowed precise measurements. The left ventricle had very poor contractions. **b** Balloon inflated within the stenotic area

16.12
Treatment of Stenoses in Arteries or Veins – Balloons and Stents

16.12.1
Pulmonary Artery Banding

In patients with a large VSD the treatment is mainly surgical with closure of the defect itself, but there are alternatives in certain cases. If the patient is too sick to tolerate repair, at least the pulmonary arteries should be protected from the high pressure and the left ventricle from an intolerable volume load by performing a banding procedure on the pulmonary artery. As the patient grows a stepwise debanding may be performed by balloon dilatation (Fig. 16.13) if the initial procedure prepared for this possibility (BJØRNSTAD et al. 1993).

16.12.2
Peripheral Pulmonary Artery Stenosis

The pulmonary arteries may be stenotic as a result of congenital heart disease, or following surgery. Sometimes neighbouring structures compress the artery and create a localized stenosis. Many groups have been reluctant to treat peripheral pulmonary artery stenosis with balloon dilatation alone, because the recommended balloon diameter is so much larger than the diameter of the stenosis and adjacent vessel. Stents may be of advantage in this situation, and preferably a type of stent that allows re-dilatation if needed (Fig. 16.14). Modern stents have sizes that may fit the biggest vessels in adult patients.

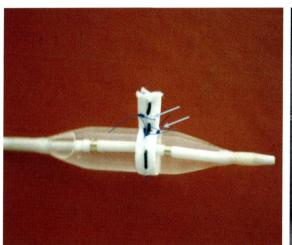
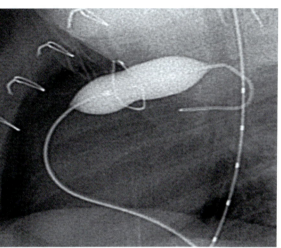

a
b

Fig. 16.13a,b. Stepwise balloon debanding of the pulmonary artery. **a** The principle of staged debanding is based upon the double 5.0 prolene sutures (*arrows*) that keep the band together. **b** In time, the inner suture may be burst by a balloon with the proper size, without bursting the outer suture, as shown in this 3-month-old boy

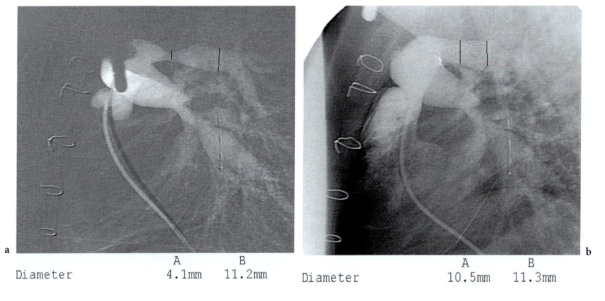

a
b

	A	B
Diameter	4.1mm	11.2mm

	A	B
Diameter	10.5mm	11.3mm

Fig. 16.14a,b. Peripheral pulmonary artery stenosis. **a** Marked narrowing in the central part of the left pulmonary artery. **a** Stent that may be re-dilated if needed is placed in the stenotic area

16.12.3
Supravalvular Aortic Stenosis

The most common association with supravalvular aortic stenosis is the Williams-Beuren syndrome, but it may also be seen in other patients. The location of the stenosis is at, or distal to, the origin of the coronary arteries. Three different types have been described: the hourglass, the membranous and the hypoplastic type (the whole of the aorta and its branches are hypoplastic). Dysplastic changes in the aortic leaflets are seen in about one-third of patients (FREEDOM et al. 1984a,b). In some patients, particularly those with Williams-Beuren syndrome, accompanying stenoses of the pulmonary artery branches and other major arteries may be seen. Also the ostium of the coronary arteries may be affected.

Angiocardiography with an injection into the aortic base should also depict the aortic arch. In addition, the abdominal aorta should be studied to rule out abdominal coarctation or stenosis in major conducting arteries, provided MCT or MRA did not rule out this possibility. At present there is no indication for catheter-based treatment.

16.12.4
Coarctation of the Aorta

The narrowing in coarctation of the aorta is regularly located at the aortic isthmus between the left subclavian artery and the level of the arterial duct. A ridge-like, eccentric infolding of aortic tissue causes the stenosis. Distal to the coarctation the aorta may be dilated. In infants, the posterior arch is frequently hypoplastic, and the arterial duct is open (Fig. 16.15). The length of the hypoplastic segment varies, but it may cover the whole distance back to the innominate artery. The aetiology is still debatable. One theory suggests that a sling of ductal tissue extends into the aortic wall and contracts after birth (HO and ANDERSON 1979). Others suggest that a vessel injury before birth results in smooth muscle and fibrous tissue proliferation (BALIS et al. 1967). Collaterals may develop even in utero if the coarctation lies distal to the arterial duct. In infancy, large collaterals may sometimes be encountered if the coarctation is severe and is the only lesion (MATHEW et al. 1972).

The coarctation may become evident as the duct closes in the neonate with a collapse as the first

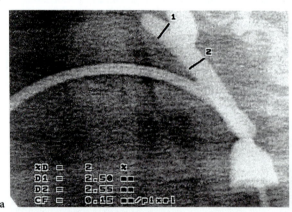
a

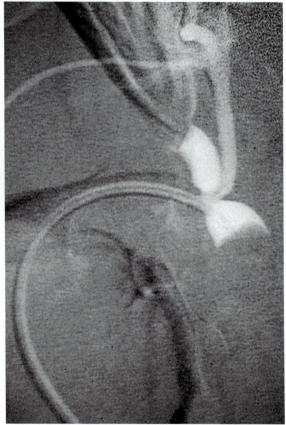
b

Fig. 16.15. a A 3-month-old girl with post-ductal coarctation of the aorta and marked hypoplasia of the posterior aortic arch. In addition, the patient had a double-outlet right ventricle. b A 2-month-old girl with coarctation of the aorta located at the orifice of the left subclavian artery. The posterior arch is slightly hypoplastic, and the catheter has been passed from the right atrium and right ventricle through the main pulmonary artery and the open ductus arteriosus into the descending aorta

symptom. There may be severe congestive heart failure, and the patient may be critically ill and rescued with prostaglandin infusion opening the duct. Typically, the radial pulses will be prominent and the femoral pulses weak or absent. Blood pressure differences are present and measurements in all extremities indicate the localization of the stenosis.

The diagnosis is made on clinical suspicion and echocardiographic findings. In several instances, however, echocardiographic images are insufficient for detailing the anatomy, especially in the complicated case. Doppler studies for calculation of the gradient across the stenosis are inaccurate, since the type of stenosis does not conform to the theoretical base for gradient calculations. Nevertheless, echocardiographic examinations may be sufficient to prepare the patient for treatment.

Either angiocardiography or three-dimensional reconstructions from CTA or MRA may present detailed images of the lesion. Frequently the coarctation occurs as part of very complex intracardiac malformations and angiocardiography needs to be performed. On properly angulated angiocardiography varying from a lateral view to a left anterior oblique projection the coarctation is usually very well seen (Fig. 16.16). Frequently the coarctation occurs as part of very complex intracardiac malformations and angiocardiography needs to be performed. On properly angulated angiocardiography varying from a lateral view to a left anterior oblique projection the

coarctation is usually very well seen. In infants, we recommend performing the study by the venous approach. The open arterial duct will in most cases allow a balloon-tipped catheter with side holes proximal to the balloon to pass into the descending aorta. Inflating the balloon will force the injected contrast volume to flow in a retrograde fashion both into the aortic arch and the pulmonary arteries. Also the left ventricle should be visualized in the same study. This may typically be achieved by passing the catheter through the open oval foramen into the left atrium and proceed through the mitral valve into the left ventricle. If one – second best – has to rely on imaging of the left ventricle after recirculation through the lungs, modern digital angiographic equipment with subtraction will frequently allow sufficient detail of the left ventricle and its outflow tract to be seen.

It is rare to encounter coarctation of the aorta in other locations. However, it has been described proximal to the innominate artery, in the descending thoracic and in the abdominal aorta. In the abdomen, gas may sometimes make ultrasound difficult or impossible, but CTA or MRA with three-dimensional reconstruction will give the diagnosis.

Treatment of coarctation of the aorta is still controversial. Surgical techniques include resection and end-to-end anastomosis, the obsolete subclavian flap techniques, extended anastomosis of the distal aorta to the under-surface of the aortic arch if the aortic arch is hypoplastic, and patch graft aortoplasty. The

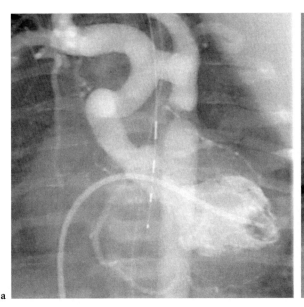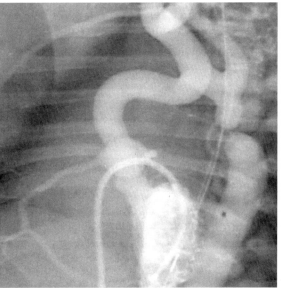

a   b

Fig. 16.16a,b. A 5-day-old boy with marked coarctation and elongated, tortuous aortic arch. **a** Angiocardiography in frontal projection. **b** Angiocardiography in left anterior oblique projection

results after surgery depend on the method used and the surgeon's skill. Aneurysm formation has been seen after patch graft aortoplasty. Generally, the mortality and morbidity of surgical repair of native coarctation is very low, and the main complication is re-coarctation. This may be seen after all surgical techniques, and is more common in patients who were operated on in infancy. Its incidence has been reported to be between 11% and 42% (STARK 1994). Intervention is considered necessary if the gradient is 30 mmHg or more. Balloon dilatation of native coarctation is controversial, as reported by PATEL et al. (2001). Some centres will reserve balloon dilatation for patients at high risk for surgical repair or even implant a stent as a palliative measure. TYNAN et al. (1990) reported results after dilatation of native coarctation remarkably similar to those who had angioplasty for re-coarctation.

As surgery of re-coarctation may be technically difficult, and as balloon dilatation generally is considered a safer procedure in re-coarctation than in native coarctation, transcatheter techniques are usually preferred.

After prior diagnostic measurements and imaging through the femoral artery, the technique is to cross the coarctation with a soft guide wire followed by a suitable catheter with a balloon as short as possible to avoid unnecessary stretching and straightening of the posterior aortic arch. The diameter should be 3–4 times the diameter of the coarctation, but not much more than the diameter of the normal adjacent aorta. The balloon is inflated until the waist disappears or maximum inflation pressure is reached. The diameter of the dilated stenosis is measured before and after the procedure (Fig. 16.17). Residual peak-to-peak gradients demonstrate a significant reduction, as reported by HELLENBRAND et al. (1990). Growth of the dilated segment with the patient has been observed. After this intra-arterial procedure, about one-third of the patients lose the pulse in the lower extremity. Anticoagulants and thrombolysis will restore the blood flow in most patients. Another feared complication is the development of aneurysms, and the reported incidence varies between 0% and 40%. TYNAN et al. (1990) reported 8 aneurysms in 93 patients. Neurological complications have also been reported.

Sometimes it may be necessary to place a stent after balloon dilatation if the re-coarctation is recoiling (Fig. 16.18). If no significant additional growth is expected, the method of choice probably should be to use a covered stent.

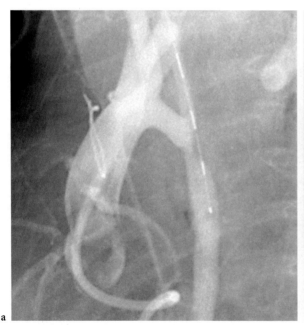
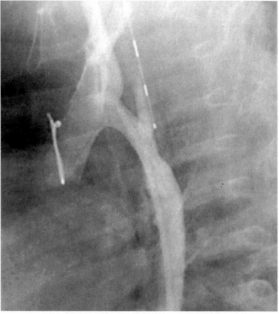

a   b

Fig. 16.17a,b. A 3-month-old boy with re-coarctation of the aorta. **a** The smallest diameter was 2 mm before dilatation. **b** The balloon was inflated to 6 mm diameter, and the diameter increased to 4 mm after dilatation

16.12.5
Stenosis in Veins

16.12.5.1
Vena Cava

Stenosis in the superior or inferior vena cava is mostly encountered after surgery in children. Both the Fontan repair in single ventricle situations and the Mustard and Senning procedure in patients with TGA may occasionally give rise to stenoses. These are now preferably treated with stents (Fig. 16.19).

16.12.5.2
Pulmonary Vein Stenosis

In this rare congenital anomaly, the stenosis may be localized at the venoatrial junction, or more proxi-

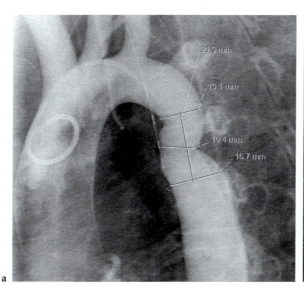
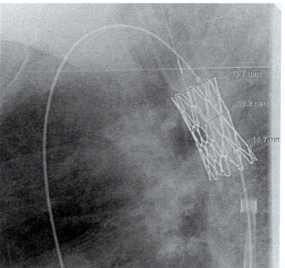

a   b

Fig. 16.18a,b. A 12-year old girl with re-coarctation of the aorta. **a** Angiography of the aortic arch shows kinking and narrowing of the aorta. **b** Stent distended within the re-coarctation

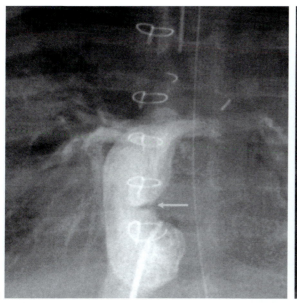
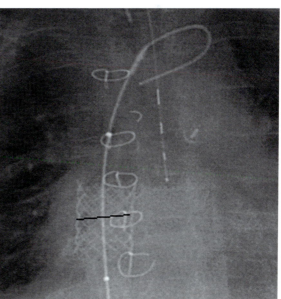

a   b

Fig. 16.19a,b. Narrowing of the inferior vena cava after a Fontan operation. **a** Stenosis within the atrial tunnel (*arrow*). **b** Stent properly placed to relieve the narrowing

mal into the lung vein(s). The narrowing may be long or short, a true stenosis or a diaphragm. Sometimes the pulmonary vein(s) may be hypoplastic and even atresia may occur. In atresia, large lymphatic channels persist from fetal life and helps to clear interstitial fluid. Such a stenosis will not create a pressure gradient or increase the pressure in the pulmonary arteries, but will redistribute flow to the non-stenosed area. The patients may have pulmonary symptoms.

Echocardiography may not be able to visualize the stenoses, especially the longer ones or the generally hypoplastic veins. Angiocardiography may be used to outline the full extent of the stenosis. Injection into the pulmonary artery with the subtraction technique will show delayed venous return from the affected segments and may show the unequal distribution of flow. Injection into the pulmonary vein itself may depict the detailed anatomy. Poor visualization or no opacification of the affected veins strengthens the suspicion of severe stenosis or atresia. In mild to moderate stenosis the subtraction angiography will be able to demonstrate the lesion directly. The best visualization of the length of the stenosis is usually achieved after entering the vein in question from the left atrium and injecting contrast material directly. If the pulmonary veins are extremely hypoplastic, the ipsilateral pulmonary artery is usually small as well. Pulmonary artery wedge injection may demonstrate the veins in such a situation (KINGSTON et al. 1983).

Also CT with three-dimensional reconstruction may give valuable anatomical information

(Fig. 16.20). In the postoperative patient, venous stenosis may be dilated and stented as shown in Figure 16.21. The vein is entered from the left atrium and a stent of appropriate size is implanted over a guide wire under fluoroscopic and angiocardiographic control.

16.12.6
Stent in Ductus Arteriosus

Some patients have a circulation depending on the presence of an open arterial duct. The duct is important for pulmonary blood flow in pulmonary atresia or severe stenosis, but on the other hand also for the systemic circulation in cases with severe left ventricular outflow obstructions. Under such duct-dependent circumstances stenting of the arterial duct prevents it from closing (SCHNEIDER et al. 1991). This will in the former group allow the lung vessels to be perfused and to grow; in the latter, a duct kept open by a stent will improve systemic cardiac output. This forms an alternative to a surgical shunt. The stent alternative will allow more definite surgery to be undertaken at a later stage without the difficulties created by a previous operation.

If the pulmonary artery is not open the easiest access to the duct in most cases will be through the left subclavian artery originating close to the duct. Sometimes the access is easier from the femoral artery. After angiocardiographic imaging and measurements a coronary stent of appropriate length is

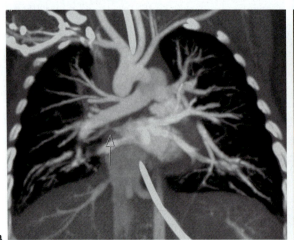 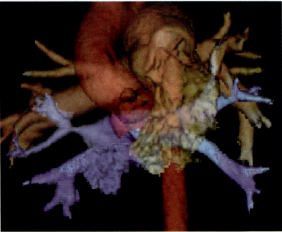

a   b

Fig. 16.20a,b. CTA shows a hypoplastic and stenotic upper right lung vein in a 3-month-old girl. **a** Coronal reconstruction shows the stenosis very well (*arrow*). **b** Three-dimensional reconstruction gives a very precise impression of the anatomy. This model may be rotated to better show the interrelationship with important neighbouring structures

precrimped on a balloon catheter of chosen width and introduced over a guide wire into the right pulmonary artery. Its position is documented with hand injections. When in proper position the balloon is inflated and the stent placed. Care must be taken not to displace the stent during retraction of the balloon. After initial problems (GIBBS et al. 1999) it seems that the results now are acceptable for offering this method to selected patients (GEWILLIG et al. 2004).

16.13
Closure of Atrial Septal Defects

Atrial septal defects are divided into three subgroups. The most common defect is the one in the region of the oval fossa. It is not an excessively open foramen allowing a left-to-right shunt, but a malformation with deficient creation of the interatrial wall. The second most common is the so-called primum ASD, a defect with no distance to the atrioventricular valves. In fact, it is an atrioventricular malformation with involvement of the atrioventricular valves themselves. The third group of ASD is the sinus venosus defects either close to the inferior vena cava and tricuspid valve or high up towards the superior vena cava and right pulmonary artery, always involving drainage of at least one pulmonary vein to the wrong side of the circulation. A patient with ASD is frequently asymptomatic, and the diagnosis may be delayed for months or years, even sometimes first recognized in old-aged patients. On the other hand it may in certain cases create respiratory problems and lead to failure to thrive even in the first year of life.

In childhood transthoracic echocardiography will suffice for a complete understanding of the defect's anatomy, and together with chest radiography it will reflect the haemodynamic load. Catheterization and angiocardiography for the diagnosis of ASD is no longer performed. Treatment of ASDs has for half a century been surgical. It still is for the sinus venosus defects and the incomplete atrioventricular septal defect. For the defects in the oval fossa, however, percutaneous closure has become the method of choice.

Catheterization is now exclusively performed with the aim of therapeutic closure. Such a procedure is offered if, by transthoracic or transoesophageal echocardiographic criteria, the size, shape and location of the ASD are considered suitable for transcatheter treatment. This is the case for approximately three-quarters or more of all such patients. Several devices are currently on the market. By far most chosen device for such closures

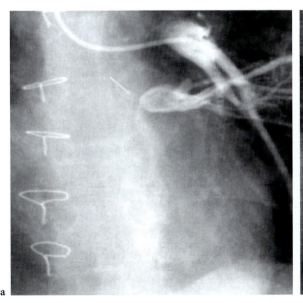
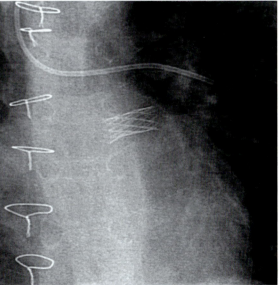

a   b

Fig. 16.21a,b. A 22-month-old boy has a severe stenosis at the common opening into the left atrium of both lung veins on the left side. **a** Contrast medium injected into the left lung artery shows the very stenotic entrance of the vein to the left atrium (*arrow*). **b** Stent placed within the stenosis effectively relieved the stenosis

is the Amplatzer Device® (BJØRNSTAD et al. 1997; MASURA et al. 1997; FISCHER et al. 2003) but the StarFLEX® (CARMINATI et al. 2001) and Helex® (LATSON et al. 2000, 2005) devices are alternatives. Some implant without using angiography at all, some inject into the upper right pulmonary vein in four-chamber view to get an overview of the atrial septum and the shunt localization, and some perform an angiocardiogram of the pulmonary artery to exclude anomalous pulmonary venous return which may be missed on echocardiography alone. The closure procedure is monitored with fluoroscopy and transoesophageal echocardiography. The two methods supplement each other; echocardiography with distinct imaging of walls and devices in the two-dimensional plane, fluoroscopy with its overall view. It has been possible to perform the sizing and closure procedure based on echo alone, but the combination of the two imaging methods enhances the control over the procedure and improves safety.

The sizing of the defect is more critical with the Amplatzer Device® than with the two others. The Amplatzer Device® may close defects up to 40 mm across. One-third of ASDs in paediatric patients exceed 20 mm. The dimension of the defect is either measured directly on echocardiography or by inflating a soft balloon within the defect and measuring it on echocardiography or fluoroscopy. Some stop the inflation when no more flow is seen on echocardiography; some prefer an indentation in the contours of the balloon (Fig. 16.22). The measurements are compared. A third possibility is to note the volume within the balloon, and inject the exact same volume into the balloon after its removal from the patient. By matching the diameter with the holes in a plastic board, yet another indication for the proper diameter of the device is found. In the umbrella-type devices the measurement is doubled to select their size. Using the Amplatzer Device® the connecting waist is selected with the measured diameter. Thus its cylindrical core will fill the defect for complete closure and provide a self-centring function during placement. There are really no practical size or age limits for the use of such methods, but most patients will be treated after their first year of life. In many places closure is recommended only in patients above 4 or 5 years of age.

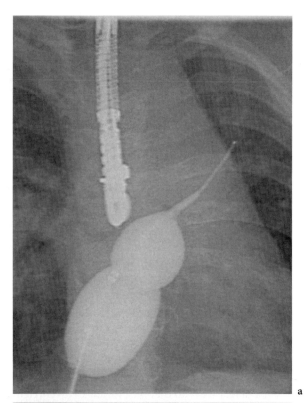

a

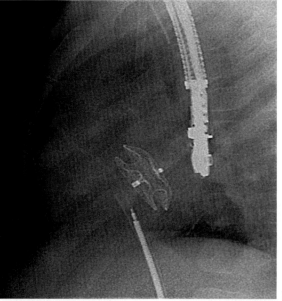

b

Fig. 16.22a,b. Procedure for measuring ASD before selecting the proper size of the Amplatzer® ASD occluder. **a** Balloon sizing of ASD by measuring the waist in the balloon. **b** Amplatzer® device in proper position after release

16.13.1
Fenestrations in Fontan's Operation

When the surgeons perform total cavopulmonary connections – the so-called Fontan operation – they often, for the safety of the patient, leave an opening between the venous channel leading to the lungs and the right atrium. This leaves the possibility for the patient to have some blood to bypass the lung circuit if the volume should become critical in the period of adaptation to the new flow situation. But such a communication is also a source of desoxygenation. Some of these so-called fenestrations close spontaneously. Others stay open and may counteract a good operative result, leaving the patient cyanotic. After some time it may be decided to close such communications with catheter-based techniques. Depending on the size and localization of the defect several devices may be used, but usually a device designed for ASD closure is selected. The size of the communication is decided from an angiocardiographic frame, often by measuring the jet of contrast medium passing from one side to the other. The role of echocardiography in such a case is limited. The procedure will differ depending on the device selected, but in principle the device is left with parts on either side of the surgical wall and thus obstructs and closes the communication (Fig. 16.23).

16.14
Closure of Ventricular Septal Defects

The interventricular septum consists of two main parts: the membranous and the muscular component. The membranous septum is located immediately beneath the aortic valve at a distance of 2–3 mm and just above the tricuspid valve. The area of the membranous septum is relatively small with a diameter of 5 mm in an adult (Soto et al. 1985). The muscular part of the ventricular septum is divided into the inlet septum, the trabecular portion and the outlet septum. Based on the anatomy of the septum, a VSD may be perimembranous, muscular or in the outlet septum. The latter is committed to both arteries and therefore sometimes called "doubly committed" but also called a "subpulmonic" or "supracristal" defect. It is characterized by the separation from the membranous septum of the muscular supraventricular crest. The muscular defect may be situated in different parts of the muscular septum, sometimes in the middle, sometimes more to its margins. The perimembranous (or membranous) VSD used to be called "subaortic" because it sits below the aortic valves, but in fact the outlet septum defect is closer to the aorta than the perimembranous "subaortic" one. An important trait with the

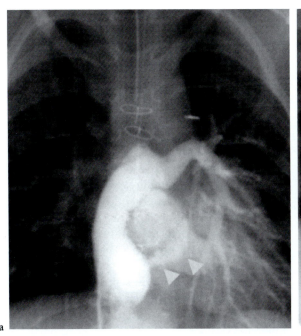
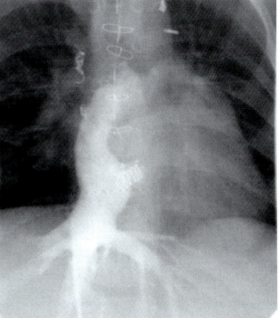

a

b

Fig. 16.23a,b. Open fenestration after Fontan operation. **a** Angiocardiography in inferior vena cava shows jet of contrast medium through the fenestration (*arrowheads*). **b** A coil intended for closure of the arterial duct effectively closes the connection

perimembranous defects is its close vicinity with the conduction system. This runs in the caudal part of the defect on the left side of the septum. Surgeons know this and try to avoid injury during repair, but this anatomical feature may be a limiting factor for the use of present devices to close such defects.

Symptoms of a VSD may be severe or absent, depending on the size of the left-to-right shunt. In utero, the circulation in a fetus with VSD is not affected. After birth the left-to-right shunt in a non-restrictive VSD will increase as the pulmonary artery resistance decreases. The degree of volume load to the left heart and pulmonary circuit decides the severity of the malformation.

Echocardiography and chest radiography assess the shunt volume and thus the load to the heart. The "flow ratio" is a term dating back to catheterization measures with relatively inaccurate oximetry calculations. Now better ways should be found to assess the severity of a VSD. For the diagnosis of the VSD both heart catheterization and angiocardiography at present play a very limited role. Still angiocardiography may sometimes be performed if the situation is complicated by other defects and therefore less well shown by echocardiography. Depending on where the defect is located, a left anterior oblique projection may depict the perimembranous defects and most of the muscular defects (Fig. 16.24). A pure lateral view or sometimes a right anterior oblique view may show the doubly committed/supracristal/subpulmonic/outlet septum VSD (Fig. 16.25).

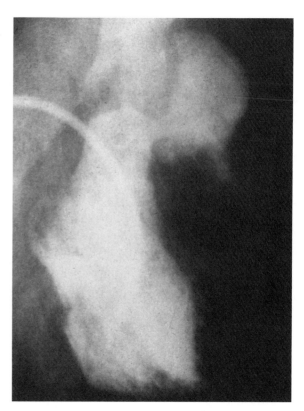

Fig. 16.25. A 5-year-old girl. Right anterior oblique projection showing subpulmonic VSD. This defect is located above the crista supraventricularis, and the flow is directed upwards into the pulmonary artery. Note that almost no contrast medium flows down into the right ventricle

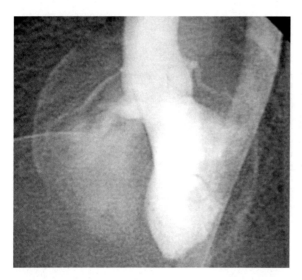

Fig. 16.24. A 14-year-old girl with VSD. Left anterior oblique projection showing subaortic diverticulum measuring 11 mm at the base and a VSD of approximately 2 mm at the top

If the defect is to be closed by intervention, one has to bear in mind that not every hole is circular. Only one of the diameters – top/bottom – is measured on angiocardiography, whereas the echocardiographic picture may be rotated in several projections, thus giving a series of different diameters.

The majority of VSDs are still closed surgically. Late effects of untreated VSD include aortic regurgitation caused by prolapse of a valve, endocarditis and congestive heart failure. Some 8% of patients with a large VSD are reported to develop stenosis of the right ventricular outflow tract (Soto et al. 1985) caused by hypertrophy of the infundibulum.

Transcatheter closure for VSD has been a challenge to interventionists, both in the muscular and the membranous portions of the septum. A series of different devices have been used since Rashkind's first attempts: Lock's Clamshell®/CardioSEAL®/STARflex® umbrellas (Lock et al. 1988; Knauth et al. 2004), the buttoned device (Sideris et al. 1997), the Rashkind Ductal Umbrella® (Vogel et al. 1996) and Gianturco

Coils® (LATIFF et al. 1999) have been used for closure of VSDs of different kinds. The common denominator for all these devices is that they have not been designed for the specific anatomy of a VSD. A breakthrough came with the specially designed Amplatzer® devices created for both muscular and perimembranous VSDs. The muscular defect devices are symmetrical with a central core of 7 mm length and different diameters according to the defect's width. The discs on both the right and left sides have a diameter of 6 mm more than the waist. The device for the membranous VSD is asymmetrically made with the left-sided disc almost in flush with the core of the device in the part facing the aortic valve, and the "shirt" facing the apex is 6 mm long. The length of the core of the device also pays respect to the much thinner membranous septum and is only 1.5 mm long.

The implantation procedure is technically more demanding than the closure of ASDs and is even more dependent on imaging support. Both angiocardiography and transoesophageal echocardiography are necessary for localizing and sizing the defect as well as for defining correct position of the device during implantation and before release. The procedure is normally carried out with access from both the artery and the vein in the inguinal region. For some muscular defects the implantation is easier if the venous access is from the right jugular vein. The retrograde catheter from the femoral artery is brought into the left ventricle, through the defect and into the right ventricle. A long exchange wire is passed through the catheter either into the pulmonary artery or one of the caval veins. The guide wire is snared after transvenous access and pulled out of the femoral vein. Thus a guide loop is created where both ends of the guide are outside the patient: one end out of the vein, the other out of the artery. This wire passes through two valves and is always covered by a catheter to avoid injury. Then, the delivery sheath is passed from the femoral vein, through the defect and manipulated into the apex of the left ventricle. The retention shirt is unfolded, and pulled back towards the septum under echocardiographic and fluoroscopic control. When the left-sided disc has reached the septum, the central core and the right-sided disc are exposed. At this point another angiocardiography with injection into the left ventricle is performed. The angle of the projections is often adjusted according to the projection of the device still fixed to the delivery cable. Only after having confirmed the right position both with angiography and echocardiography will the device be released (Fig. 16.26).

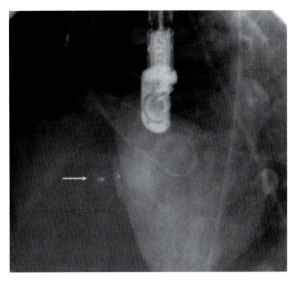

Fig. 16.26. Angiography of a 12-year-old boy with a muscular VSD. The injection in the left ventricle shows that the defect is completely closed and that the VSD plug is in the proper position (*arrow*)

The method is used in many centres (BASS et al. 2003), but not yet generally accepted, especially not for the membranous VSD because of concerns that the procedure may cause heart blocks (BUTERA et al. 2006).

16.15
Closure of Arteries and Arteriovenous Connections

16.15.1
Persistent Arterial Duct

The open arterial duct is a necessary prerequisite for a normal circulation and heart development prior to birth. It normally closes during the first weeks of life through muscular contraction and obliteration with tissue. Small premature babies lack such muscles and thus the duct will remain open as a part of their prematurity. Some newborns with duct-dependent circulation because of congenital heart disease may be helped by infusions of prostaglandin. In some children the duct remains open and causes pulmonary overflow. Then it represents a malformation with effect on the central circulation and is considered a heart disease. Surgeons have been closing such defects with continuous murmur since 1938 (GROSS and HUB-BARD 1939). Through the years all diagnosed ducts have been closed, but only ducts having a continuous murmur were diagnosed. The problem of indication for closure did arise the moment a lot of small ducts were diagnosed because colour-flow Doppler became available. These were "silent" and were not diagnosed before the mid 1980s. There is no common policy on whether such ducts should be closed or not. The argument for increased risk of endocarditis in such ducts is questioned (VAN DER MEER 2002).

The patent duct is usually a short connection between the distal aortic arch and the pulmonary tree. It typically starts with a cone from the aorta and drains with a much narrower part into the roof of the pulmonary artery near the origin of the left branch. There are, however, lots of variations in sizes, shapes and lengths. It may even be bilateral, reflecting its origin from the sixth brachiocephalic arch. Its course is sometimes in the sagittal plane but often it may point to the left or, less often, to the right from its origin in the aorta.

Through this communication part of the saturated blood from the aorta flows back to the pulmonary artery. The amount of flow is determined by the size of the duct and the resistance in the pulmonary circuit. Depending on these factors the overflow and symptoms related to the increased volume load are very different from patient to patient. The size of the pulmonary arteries and the left-sided heart chambers reflect the volume load. The bigger the duct, the bigger the shunt and the more pronounced the findings. The shunt pattern differs from the situation in ASD and VSD since the shunt though a duct is both systolic and diastolic, and the duct is the only shunt lesion affecting the aorta.

Angiocardiography is no longer performed to establish the primary diagnosis, but interventional closure of the open arterial duct with coils or other devices needs fluoroscopy and angiocardiography. Echocardiography is important for the primary diagnosis, but has no place during intervention. When the main direction of the duct is in the sagittal plane, a pure lateral projection will give good visualization of the shape of the duct and the size of the different portions. The more the main direction is deviating from the sagittal plane, the less reliable the information. Usually a straight lateral projection and the frontal plane rotated 20° to the right will be a good choice. In most cases this will give a good view in one of the two planes. The "easiest" ducts are the ones with a well developed cone towards the aorta and a distinct opening into the pulmonary artery.

The first commercial available device for ductal closure was the Rashkind Ductal Umbrella® (RASHKIND et al. 1987). It had a significant number of residual shunts, especially in the bigger ducts. When the "un-controlled" Gianturco Coils® and the Cook Detachable Coils® – screwed on to the delivery wire – were introduced (GALAL et al. 1996; TOMETZKI et al. 1996) the use of the Rashkind Umbrella® declined. The smaller ducts are effectively closed by coils (Fig. 16.27). The main problem was initially the bigger ducts above 2.5–3 mm minimal width. Several solutions were launched, mostly based on the use of multiple coils (GRIFKA et al. 1995). Other types of coils were also suggested (GRABITZ et al. 1998). The problem with the bigger ducts was solved with the Amplatzer Duct Occluder®, where one plug effectively closes even the largest ducts (Fig. 16.28) (MASURA et al. 1998). The shallower the ampulla, the more critical the size of the part of the device left there. In such a case devices not made for ductal closure may be considered (Fig. 16.29). Another problem is the tubular, long duct, sometimes with sequential narrowings along its course. In such a case a coil may be put into the middle of the tubular part.

By the end of the millennium the closure of ducts had been completely transferred from the operation theatre to the catheterization laboratory except in premature babies. In small premature babies, extrapleural surgical closure with clips on the duct is still the preferred method.

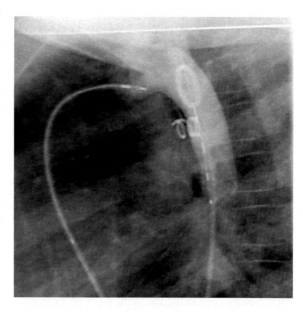

Fig. 16.27. Closure of PDA with detachable coil. After release of the coil the duct is occluded

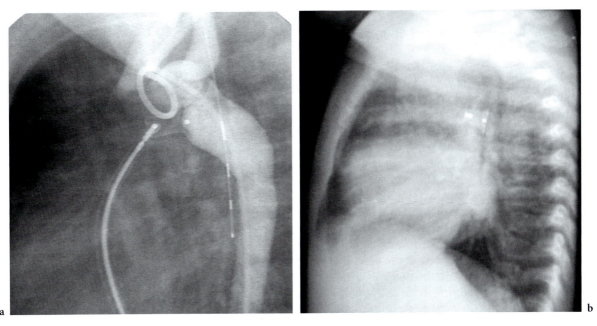

Fig. 16.28a,b. Closure of PDA with Amplatzer® plug in a 5-month-old boy. **a** Correct position is verified before release of the plug. **b** Follow-up the day after closure shows plug in good position

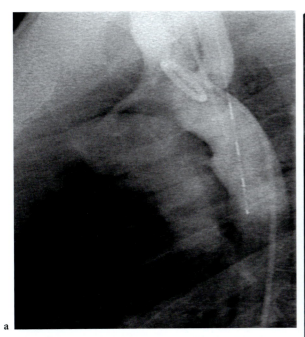

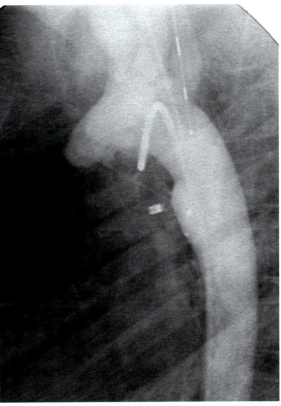

Fig. 16.29a,b. A 5-year-old boy referred for closure of an arterial duct. **a** Open arterial duct with shallow aortic ampulla will make the plug or coil normally used protrude too much into the lumen of the aorta. **b** Closure with device intended for VSD closure

16.15.2
Systemic to Pulmonary Artery Shunts and Collaterals

The lungs receive all their blood from systemic arteries in pulmonary atresia. As a rule, the largest feeding arteries originate directly from the aorta, and this is also the case in truncus arteriosus and hemitruncus. In lung hypoplasia, dual lung arterial supply often occurs. A systemic artery may feed a segment, lobe or entire lung, and the supply of blood may come entirely from the systemic side or from both the pulmonary artery and the systemic collateral. This is frequently seen in patients with tetralogy of Fallot and severe pulmonary artery stenosis, and other complex lesions with seriously impaired filling of the pulmonary artery. Many of these patients are operated with a conduit from the right ventricle to the native pulmonary artery bifurcation. Instead of extending the operation in order to find and ligate all systemic feeding arteries the patient is referred for trans-catheter embolization. After Fontan operation or Norwood operation, collaterals to the lung and pleura may develop, causing pleural and pericardial effusion as well as ascites caused by protein-losing enteropathy.

16.15.2.1
Surgical Shunts

The modified Blalock-Taussig anastomosis may be embolized by coils or vascular plugs when surgical correction has been performed (Fig. 16.30). Also direct surgical anastomoses between the ascending aorta and the main stem of the pulmonary artery may be closed with devices.

16.15.2.2
Systemic MAPCAs

MAPCAs are persistent segmental arteries that develop by the 40th day of fetal life and normally disappear 10 days later. They may persist and enlarge when the normal blood supply to the lungs is absent or too small. After creating a connection from the right ventricle to the pulmonary artery, MAPCAs may be closed either surgically or by embolization. Because the origin may be from the aorta both above and below the diaphragm, they may be difficult or impossible to reach for the surgeon performing the correction, and the logical approach will be embolization after ascertaining that the vessel has a communication with the pulmonary artery (Fig. 16.31).

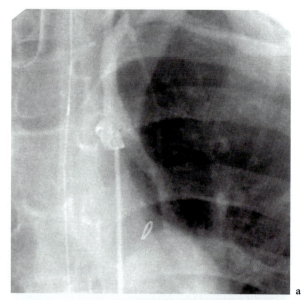

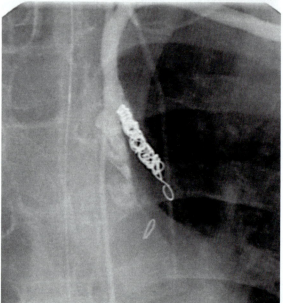

Fig. 16.30a,b. Closure of surgical shunt by embolization. **a** Selective angiography demonstrates open modified Blalock–Taussig shunt. **b** Complete occlusion after coil embolization

16.15.2.3
Arteria Mammaria Interna

When the arteria mammaria interna develop significant collaterals to the pulmonary artery before surgical correction, the surgeon may treat by placing a clip on the artery during the same operation because they are easily reached from the same inci-

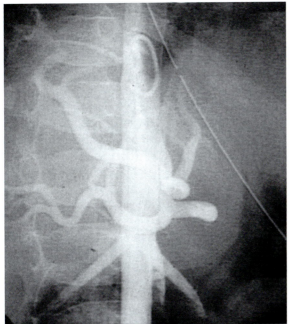

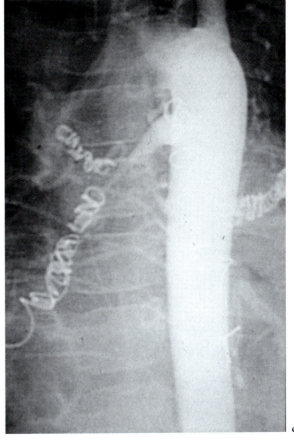

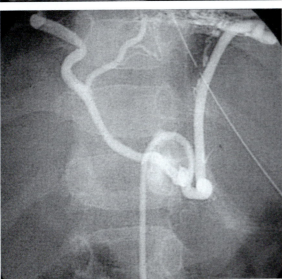

Fig. 16.31a–c. Major aorticopulmonary arteries (MAPCAs) present in a wide variety of shapes and sizes. **a** A complete map is made covering the aortic arch, the descending thoracic and the upper abdominal aorta. **b** Selective injection shows the sometimes long and tortuous course of the MAPCAs. **c** Embolization, in this case by coils

sion. Occasionally, the arteries are embolized during diagnostic angiography or at a later stage postoperatively if they become significant contributors to the left-to-right shunt (Fig. 16.32).

16.15.2.4
Bronchial Arteries

Bronchial collateral circulation develops mainly after birth in cyanotic patients. There may be indication for embolization on rare occasions (Fig. 16.33).

16.15.3
Anomalies of the Coronary Arteries with a Shunt

Coronary artery fistulas are defined as abnormal coronary-cameral communications that may involve any chamber and one or all coronary arteries. Abnormal connections from the coronary arteries have been described not only to the four heart chambers, but also to the pulmonary artery and the superior vena cava. The right coronary artery is involved more than the left, and more than 90% of the fistulae drain into the right side of the heart. Such

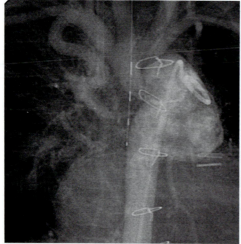

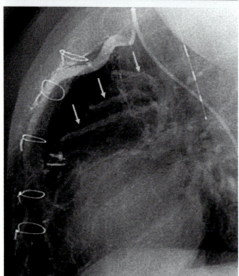

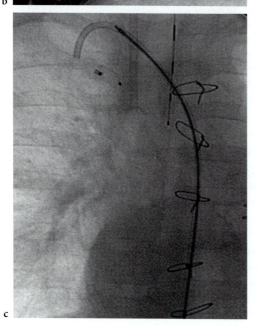

communications are often asymptomatic, but may cause ischemia and ST changes during a stress test. Echocardiography may be able to define the communication, its localization and its draining site, but is in most cases insufficient for detailed planning and performance of its closure. In many cases the treatment may be catheter based, by placing a type of detachable coil (Fig. 16.34) or sometimes other devices to close the communication. If catheter access is technically difficult to achieve because of tortuousity of vessels, if the device may occlude an important coronary artery branch or may have a non-obstructive opening into the right heart giving no support to a device making device embolization an imminent risk, surgery may be a better solution.

16.15.4
Lung Sequester

A lung sequester is a congenital anomaly with nonfunctioning lung tissue. The arterial supply is through one or more arteries originating from the aorta or its branches. In most cases, the venous drainage is into a systemic vein, but drainage into the pulmonary veins is also seen (CORBETT and HUMPHREY 2004; CURROS et al. 2000). Treatment may be surgical or interventional by embolization of the feeding arteries (Fig. 16.35).

16.15.5
Intrapulmonary Arteriovenous Fistula

This is a fistula from the pulmonary artery to the pulmonary veins, draining into the left atrium without appropriate oxygenation of the blood. It is frequently called pulmonary arteriovenous malformation. The lesion may be isolated or multiple fistulae may be found. It is associated with syndromes such as hereditary haemorrhagic telangiectasia (Rendu-Weber-Osler syndrome). These patients frequently also have other lesions located mainly in the gastrointestinal canal and in the skin. Depending on the

Fig. 16.32a–c. A significant shunt to the pulmonary circulation from a very large arteria mammaria interna on the right side in a 14-month-old girl after semi-Fontan operation. **a** Selective injection into right arteria mammaria interna shows communication to the pulmonary circulation in the frontal projection. **b** Lateral view shows even better the arterial branches (*arrows*) connecting to the pulmonary artery. **c** Closure by a vascular plug

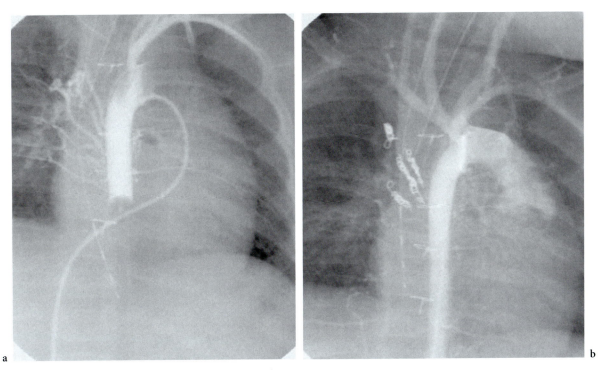

Fig. 16.33a,b. A 13-month-old girl with shunt from the systemic to the pulmonary circulation after a surgical connection of the superior vena cava to both pulmonary arteries. **a** Angiography of the descending aorta with balloon occlusion technique shows bronchial arteries connecting to the pulmonary arteries. **b** Control angiography shows occlusion after coil embolization of three bronchial arteries and the arteria mammaria interna on the right side

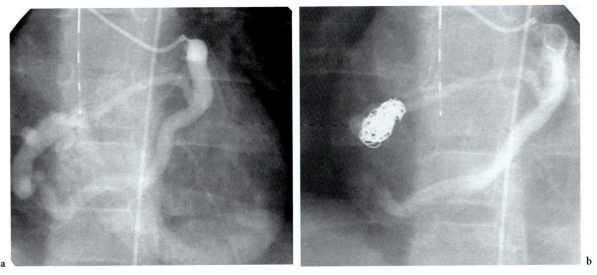

Fig. 16.34a,b. A 4-year-old girl with coronary artery fistula. **a** A large fistula from the left coronary artery connects to the right ventricle. **b** Complete closure after embolization

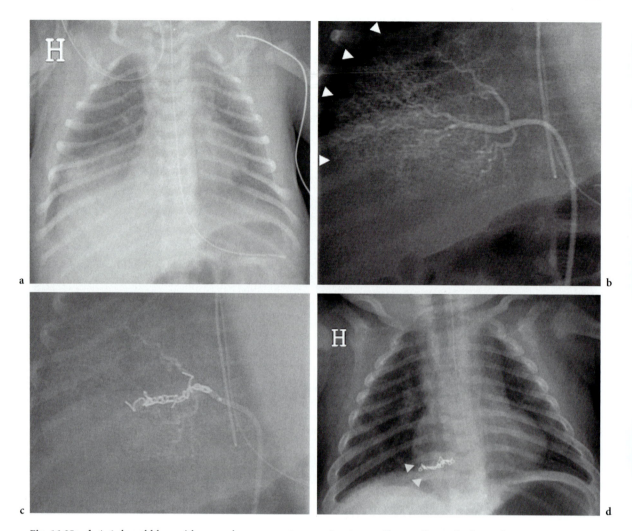

Fig. 16.35a–d. A 6-day-old boy with a very large sequester seen in utero. **a** Chest radiograph shows the sequester occupying much of the base of the right lung. **b** One week later selective injection into the feeding artery shows the extent of the sequester (*arrowheads*). **c** Control angiography during embolization. **d** Chest radiograph at 4 months of age shows marked shrinkage of the sequester (*arrowheads*)

size of the right-to-left shunt, the patient will have varying degrees of hypoxia or even heart failure. Well-known complications are cerebral symptoms such as infarcts or abscesses. The lesion is suspected from changes in the lung parenchyma on the chest radiograph in combination with the clinical symptoms. MCT with contrast enhancement may prove the vascular nature of the lesion and depict cerebral lesions, and angiography with selective injection in the pulmonary artery will also give a definitive diagnosis. Because new lesions frequently develop with time, surgery with lobectomy is not an attractive alternative, and embolization is now the treatment of choice (De Cillis et al. 2006). Since the pulmonary artery often has a wide connection to the pulmonary

vein as shown in Figure 16.36, it is extremely important to ascertain that no embolization device passes to the left atrium and the systemic circulation. This may be achieved by using an occlusion device that can be safely placed, checked for stable position, and if needed repositioned before release, e.g. Interlocking Detachable Coils® or Jackson® coils.

16.15.6
Large Arteriovenous Malformations in Other Locations

Occasionally, a newborn may develop cardiac failure immediately after birth because of a massive

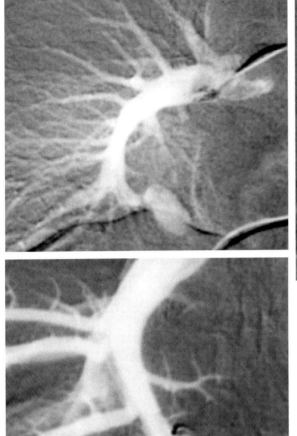

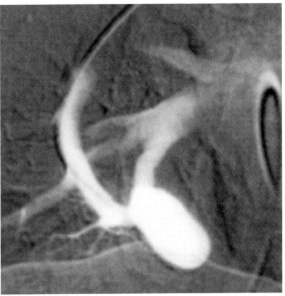

Fig. 16.36a–c. Patient with pulmonary arteriovenous malformation. **a** Injection into the right pulmonary artery shows aneurysmatic lesion in lower right lung. **b** Selective injection into the feeding artery shows the aneurysm draining into the lower right lung vein and left atrium. **c** Complete occlusion after placement of detachable coils

left-to-right shunt through a large arteriovenous malformation (Fig. 16.37).The lesion may be located in the liver, or associated with the gastrointestinal tract. Multiple imaging modalities are frequently needed because of the complexity of the lesions (BURROWS et al. 2001). Sometimes, a large number of small feeding arteries may be visualized, making complete resection impossible. When the lesion is located in the liver, MCT with contrast enhancement demonstrates which liver segments are involved and the relationship to the liver veins and portal vein branches. Embolization may sometimes treat the liver lesion completely; sometimes its purpose is to facilitate the surgical resection and reduce blood loss during the operation.

Another location of arteriovenous fistula is the choroid plexus within the roof of the third ventricle. These fistulae lead to the massive dilation of the vein of Galen (Fig. 16.38). The diagnosis is sometimes made by fetal ultrasonography, sometimes by ultrasonography with colour Doppler imaging shortly after birth when clinical symptoms become manifest. The lesion is difficult to treat, but successful embolization has been reported from some centres. BORTHNE et al. (1997), in a series of 14 vein-of-Galen vascular malformations, reported 90% successful embolization in 10 patients older than 1 year. Of the four patients embolized on vital indication during the first week of life, only one survived with marked improvement of cardiac symptoms.

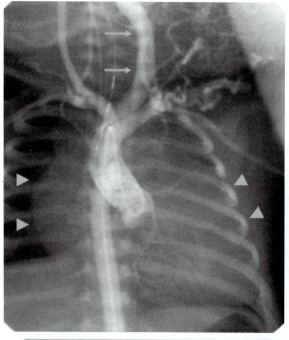

a

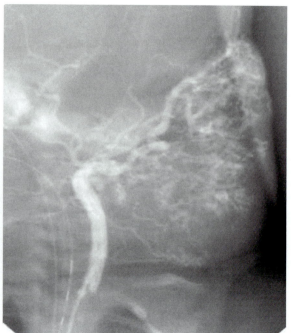

b

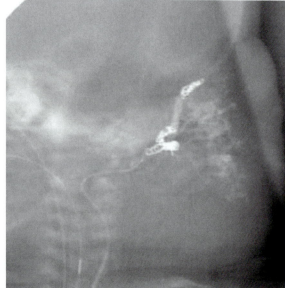

c

Fig. 16.37a–c. A 4-day-old girl with heart failure and huge arteriovenous malformation (AVM) on the left side of the neck. **a** Cardiomegaly (*arrowheads*) and enlarged left common carotid artery (*arrows*) with the same diameter as the descending aorta. **b** Selective angiography shows the extent of the AVM before embolization. **c** After embolization the cardiac failure improved quickly, and the patient was doing well with no cardiac symptoms on follow-up 15 months after the procedure

16.16
Closure of Veins

The embryology of the cardinal venous system is beyond the scope of this presentation, but this is clearly an area where the embryology helps in understanding the different variants. These abnormalities do not usually give any signs on the chest radiograph, and are found either at echocardiography or during heart catheterization.

The right superior vena cava may be absent in combination with persistence of the left superior vena cava. It may connect to the left instead of the right atrium, and it may enter the right atrium lower than normal. The upper left caval vein persists quite commonly and drains into the right atrium through the coronary sinus. It may also drain partly or totally into the left atrium. The coronary sinus may be partially unroofed and thus drain also into the left atrium (left atrial-coronary sinus window). The

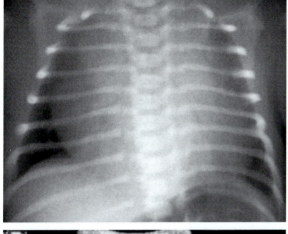

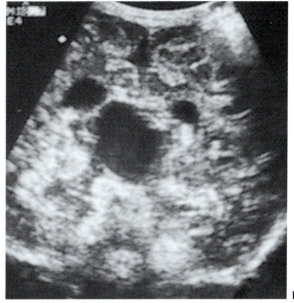

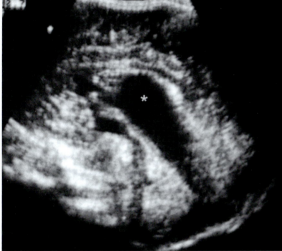

Fig. 16.38a–c. Newborn boy with serious cardiac failure. **a** Chest radiograph on the first day of life shows enlarged heart and congestion. **b** Coronal cerebral ultrasonography shows large midline vascular structure compatible with vein of Galen aneurysm. **c** Mid-sagittal ultrasonography image shows aneurysmatic vein of Galen (*asterisk*)

opening of the coronary sinus into the right atrium may be stenotic or atretic.

The inferior caval vein may also show a number of anomalies. Infrahepatic interruption with either azygos or hemi-azygos continuation is among the well-known and not uncommon anomalies. Parallel to what is seen in the superior vena cava, the inferior vena cava may insert abnormally high in the right atrium, or there may be an anomalous connection to the left atrium or to the coronary sinus.

The hepatic veins may also connect abnormally to the heart in four different ways: the common hepatic vein may connect to the right or left atrium, and the left hepatic vein may enter the left atrium or coronary sinus. Drainage into the right atrium or coronary sinus is of no haemodynamic significance.

Veins draining into the wrong side of the heart, as mentioned above, leave the patient cyanotic. Such communications may be diagnosed with echocar-

diography, but more often cardiac catheterization is necessary. That gives the possibility of occluding the communication following its exact diagnosis. Often a vascular plug is chosen and implanted through a guiding catheter.

16.16.1
Postoperative Abnormal Venous Connections

Following the Fontan operation with increased venous filling pressure the venous blood sometimes tries to find an escape route to a lower pressure system. Such a system can be found in the pulmonary venous atrium. Therefore veno-venous collaterals may be created connecting mostly the upper caval vein to the pulmonary veins. This will result in desoxygenation or even cyanosis in such patients. For the benefit of the patients such significant communications should be closed if possible (Fig. 16.39). Mostly they can be closed with either occlusion coils or with vascular plugs. The results are good, but may be limited with time as new collaterals may arise.

From time to time, bizarre veno-venous connections are found in the postoperative patient, and if a substantial part of the venous blood drains away from a Fontan connection of systemic venous return to the pulmonary artery, closure may be indicated (Fig. 16.40).

After the Fontan operation some patients develop protein-losing enteropathy and ascites. Norwood thought that such effusions might be caused by increased liver capsule pressure, and started to let a part of the liver drain into the functional left atrium when completing the Fontan operation. This led to a significant intrahepatic right-to-left shunt and the patients became cyanotic. Instead of performing repeat surgery, such drainage could be closed with catheter-based approaches: access from the right jugular vein, puncturing the venous channel with a trans-septal needle and introducing a delivery sheath into the venous drainage into the anatomical right, functional left atrium and implanting an occlusion device.

16.17
Removal of Intracardiac or Intravascular Foreign Body

From time to time, foreign bodies have to be removed from the cardiovascular system. Fragments from both diagnostic and therapeutic catheters may be found in various parts of the circulation. Guide wires and electrodes may break, and of course coils used for embolization, vascular plugs and other closure devices and stents may dislodge or be misplaced. When removal is possible, usually a snare is used (Fig. 16.41). Sometimes a dislodged stent may be redilated and fixed to the vessel wall in a position that will not cause any harm. It may also sometimes be snared and brought to a position where surgical removal is easier. Even large devices, such as the Amplatzer® ASD occluder, may be retrieved with double venous access (Fig. 16.42).

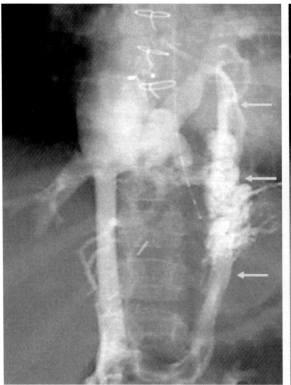 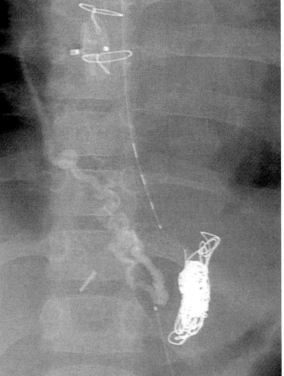

a   b

Fig. 16.39a,b. A 6-year-old girl with uni-ventricular heart. A Fontan procedure and closure of a fenestration has been performed. **a** Injection of contrast medium in the inferior vena cava reveals that collaterals have developed between the left renal vein and the left atrium (*arrows*). **b** After embolization the main shunt is closed, but small collaterals still remain open

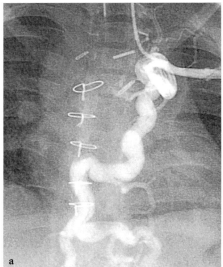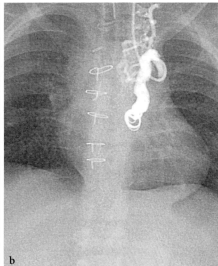

Fig. 16.40a,b. A 4-year-old girl with significant vein bypassing the Fontan circulation. **a** Selective injection into the vein shows diffuse drainage into venous structures below the diaphragm. **b** Closure with coil embolization

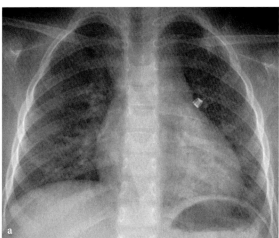

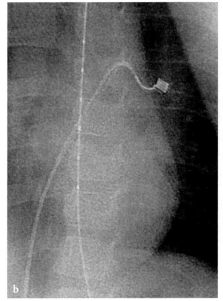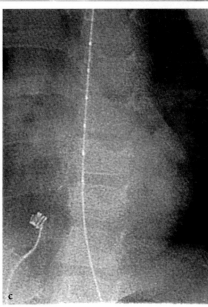

Fig. 16.41a–c. A 5-year-old girl treated for open arterial duct with coil embolization. **a** Chest radiograph 1 day after the procedure showed that the coil had embolized into a branch of the left pulmonary artery. **b** Using a snare through a selective catheter the coil is caught. **c** The coil is removed, and the open arterial duct was closed with a plug in the same setting

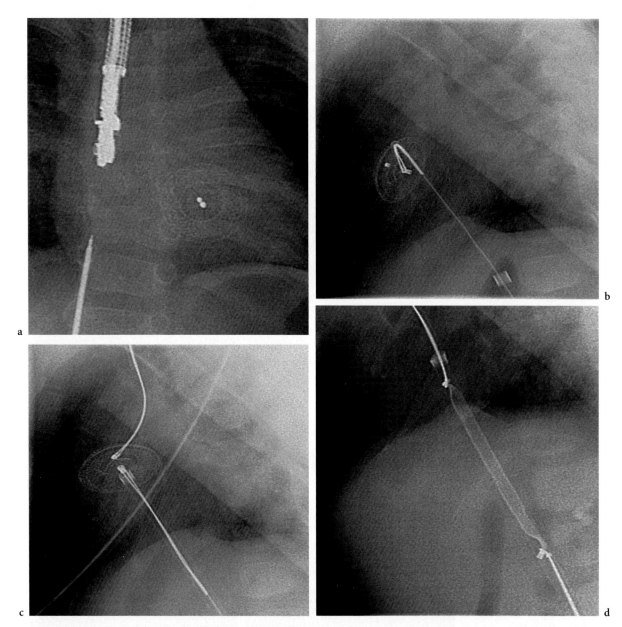

Fig. 16.42a–d. A 14-month old girl with ASD. **a** The Amplatzer® ASD closure device was misplaced in the right atrium and quickly moved with the blood stream into the infundibulum of the right ventricle. **b** A large long sheath and a catheter with a snare were brought in via the inferior vena cava, and one end of the device was caught. **c** Another catheter and snare were introduced through the right internal jugular vein and superior vena cava, and the other end was snared. **d** The device was stretched, brought into the long sheath, and removed. After careful inspection, the device was re-introduced and closed the ASD

Table 16.1. Cardiovascular catheter-based therapeutic procedures. (MAPCAs Major aorticopulmonary collateral arteries)

Balloon dilatation	Pulmonary stenosis	Valvular
		Banding of the pulmonary artery
		Peripheral (primary or after surgery)
	Intraoperative balloon dilatation	
	Mitral valve stenosis	
	Aortic stenosis	Valvular
	Coarctation of the aorta	Native
		Re-coarctation
	Surgical shunts	All types
	Venous stenosis	After surgery
		Native
Occlusions	Atrial septal defect	Defects in the oval fossa
		Fontan fenestrations
	Ventricular septal defect	Perimembranous and muscular
	Persistent patency of the arterial duct	Native
		After previous treatment
Embolization	Coronary artery fistula	
	Surgical systemic to pulmonary artery shunts	
	Systemic to pulmonary artery collaterals	MAPCA
		Bronchial arteries
		A.mammaria interna
	Feeding artery to sequester	
	Pulmonary arteriovenous malformations	
	Arteriovenous malformation of the liver	
Stents	Pulmonary artery branches	
	Stenosis of superior and inferior vena cava	
	Stenosis after Senning and Fontan procedures	
	Re-coarctation of the aorta	
Balloon rupturing	Atrial septostomy (Rashkind procedure)	In transposition of the great arteries and other malformations demanding interatrial communication.
Removal of intracardiac or intravascular foreign body	Catheter fragments	
	Guide wires	
	Electrodes	
	Coils	
	Plugs	

16.18
Conclusion

The possibilities in cardiovascular diagnosis and intervention have increased considerably over the last decade. Transcatheter cardiovascular interventions are currently used in a wide variety of lesions summarized in Table 16.1. It is of importance to every radiologist reading paediatric chest radiographs to be familiar with the possibilities that exist today. The appearance of the various devices on the chest radiograph should be recognized (WILLIAMS et al. 2006). Safe practice in this field requires an experienced team and sufficient volume of procedures to maintain skills.

References

Balis JU, Chan AS, Conen PE (1967) Morphogenesis of human aortic coarctation. Exp Mol Pathol 6:25–28

Bass JL, Kalra GS, Arora R et al (2003) Initial human experience with the Amplatzer perimembranous ventricular septal occluder device. Catheter Cardiovasc Interv 58:238–245

Bjørnstad PG, Lindberg HL, Smevik B (1993) Staged expanding pulmonary artery band. Ann Thorac Surg 55:566–567

Bjørnstad PG, Smevik B, Fiane AE et al (1997) Catheter-based closure of atrial septal defects with a newly developed nitinol double disc: an experimental study. Cardiol Young 7:220–224

Borghi A, Agnoletti G, Poggiani C (2001) Surgical cutdown of the right carotid artery for aortic balloon valvuloplasty in infancy: midterm follow-up. Pediatr Cardiol 22:194–197

Borthne A, Carteret M, Baraton J et al (1997) Vein of Galen vascular malformations in infants: clinical, radiological and therapeutic aspect. Eur Radiol 7:1252–1258

Burrows PE, Dubois J, Kassarjian A (2001) Pediatric hepatic vascular anomalies. Pediatr Radiol 31:533–545

Butera G, Massimo C, Mario C (2006) Late complete atrio-venous block after percutaneous closure of a perimembranous ventricular septal defect. Catheter Cardiovasc Interv 67:938–941

Carminati M, Chessa M, Butera G et al (2001) Transcatheter closure of atrial septal defects with the STARFlex device: early results and follow-up. J Interv Cardiol 14:319–324

Corbett HJ, Humphrey GM (2004) Pulmonary sequestration [Review]. Paediatr Respir Rev 5:59–68

Cornell SM (1966) Myocardial sinusoids in pulmonary valvular atresia. Radiology 86:421–424

Curros F, Chigot V, Emond S et al (2000) Role of embolisation in the treatment of bronchopulmonary sequestration. Pediatr Radiol 30:769–773

De Cillis E, Burdi N, Bortone AS et al (2006) Endovascular treatment of pulmonary and cerebral arteriovenous mal-

formations in patients affected by hereditary haemorrhagic telangiectasia [Review]. Curr Pharmaceut Design 12:1243–1248

Fischer G, Stieh J, Uebing A et al (2003) Experience with transcatheter closure of secundum atrial septal defects using the Amplatzer septal occluder: a single centre study in 236 consecutive patients. Heart (Br Cardiac Soc) 89:199–204

Flores FJ, Ledesma VM, Palomo Villada JA et al (2006) Long-term results of mitral percutaneous valvuloplasty with Inoue technique. Seven-years experience at the Cardiology Hospital of the National Medical Center "Siglo XXI", IMSS [Spanish]. Arch Cardiol Mexico 76(1):28–36

Freedom RM, Moes CAF (1985) The hypoplastic right heart complex. Semin Roentgenol 20:169–183

Freedom RM, Culham JAG, Moes CAF (1984a) Left ventricular outflow tract obstruction (valve, subvalve, or supravalve). In: Freedom RM, Culham JAG, Moes CAF (eds) Angiocardiography of congenital heart disease. Macmillian, New York, pp 369–388

Freedom RM, Culham JAG, Moes CAF (1984b) Single ventricle. In: Freedom RM, Culham JAG, Moes CAF (eds) Angiocardiography of congenital heart disease. Macmillian, New York, pp 593–628

Galal O, de Moor M, Al Fadley F et al (1996) Transcatheter closure of the patent ductus arteriosus: comparison between the Rashkind occluder device and the anterograde Gianturco coils technique. Am Heart J 131:368–373

Gewillig M, Boshoff DE, Dens J et al (2004) Stenting the neonatal arterial duct in duct-dependent pulmonary circulation: new techniques, better results. J Am Coll Cardiol 43:107–112

Gibbs JL, Uzun O, Blackburn ME et al (1999) Fate of the stented arterial duct. Circulation 99:2621–2625

Grabitz RG, Freudenthal F, Sigler M et al (1998) Double-helix coil for occlusion of large patent ductus arteriosus: evaluation in a chronic lamb model. J Am Coll Cardiol 31:677–683

Grifka RG, Mullins CE, Gianturco C et al (1995) New Gianturco-Grifka vascular occlusion device. Initial studies in a canine model. Circulation 91:1840–1846

Gross RE, Hubbard JH (1939) Surgical ligation of a patent ductus arteriosus: report of first successful case. J Am Med Assoc 112:729

Hellenbrand WE, Allen HD, Golinko RJ et al (1990) Balloon angioplasty for aortic recoarctation: results of valvuloplasty and angioplasty of congenital anomalies registry. Am J Cardiol 65:793–797

Ho SY, Anderson RH (1979) Coarctation, tubular hypoplasia and the ductus arteriosus. Histological study of 45 specimens. Br Heart J 41:268–274

Kan JS, White RJ, Mitchell SE et al (1982) Percutaneous balloon valvuloplasty: a new method for treating congenital pulmonary-valve stenosis. New Engl J Med 307:540–542

Kingston HM, Patel RG, Watson GH (1983) Unilateral absence or extreme hypoplasia of pulmonary veins. Br Heart J 49:148–153

Knauth AL, Lock JE, Perry SB et al (2004) Transcatheter device closure of congenital and postoperative residual ventricular septal defects. Circulation 110:501–507

Kretschmar O, Dähnert I, Berger F et al (2000) Percutaneous transcatheter interventions in the treatment of congenital heart disease in infants with a body weight below 2.5 kilograms. Z Kardiol 89:1126–1132

Latiff HA, Alwi M, Kandhavel G et al (1999) Transcatheter closure of multiple muscular ventricular septal defects using Gianturco coils. Ann Thorac Surg 68:1400–1401

Latson LA, Zahn EM, Wilson N (2000) Helex septal occluder for closure of atrial septal defects. Curr Interv Cardiol Reports 2:268–273

Latson LA, Jones TK, Jacobson J et al (2005) Analysis of factors related to successful transcatheter closure of secundum atrial septal defects using the HELEX septal occluder. Am Heart J 151:1129e 7–11

Lock JE, Block PC, McKay RG et al (1988) Transcatheter closure of ventricular septal defects. Circulation 78:361–368

Masura J, Gavora P, Formanek A et al (1997) Transcatheter closure of secundum atrial septal defects using the new self-centering Amplatzer septal occluder: initial human experience. Catheter Cardiovasc Diagnosis 42:388–393

Masura J, Walsh KP, Thanopoulous B et al (1998) Catheter closure of moderate- to large-sized patent ductus arteriosus using the new Amplatzer duct occluder: immediate and short-term results. J Am Coll Cardiol 31:878–882

Mathew R, Simon G, Joseph M (1972) Collateral circulation in coarctation of aorta in infancy and childhood. Arch Dis Child 47:950–953

Nakata S, Imai Y, Takanashi Y et al (1984) A new method for the quantitative standardization of cross-sectional areas of the pulmonary arteries in congenital heart diseases with decreased pulmonary blood flow. J Thorac Cardiovasc Surg 88:610–619

Norwood WI, Jakobs ML (1994) Hypoplastic left heart syndrome. In: Stark J, de Laval M (eds) Surgery for congenital heart defects. Saunders, Philadelphia, Pa., pp 587–598

Patel HT, Madani A, Paris YM et al (2001) Balloon angioplasty of native coarctation of the aorta in infants and neonates: is it worth the hassle? Pediatr Cardiol 22:53–57

Pedra CAC, Sidhu R, McCrindle BW et al (2004) Outcomes after balloon dilation of congenital aortic stenosis in children and adolescents. Cardiol Young 14:315–321

Radtke W, Keane JF, Fellows KE et al (1986) Percutaneous balloon valvotomy of congenital pulmonary stenosis using oversized balloon. J Am Coll Cardiol 8:909–915

Rashkind WJ, Mullins CE, Hellenbrand WE et al (1987) Nonsurgical closure of patent ductus arteriosus: clinical application of the Rashkind PDA Occluder System. Circulation 75:583–592

Rosenthal, E.Qureshi SA, Chan KC et al (1993) Radiofrequency-assisted balloon dilatation in patients with pulmonary valve atresia and an intact ventricular septum. Br Heart J 69:347–351

Schneider M, Zartner P, Sidiropoulos A et al (1991) Stent implantation of the arterial duct in newborns with duct-dependent circulation. Eur Heart J 12:1401–1409

Semb BKH, Tjønneland S, Stake G et al (1979) "Balloon valvulotomy" of congenital pulmonary valve stenosis with tricuspid valve insufficiency. Cardiovasc Radiol 2:239–241

Sideris EB, Walsh KP, Haddad JL et al (1997) Occlusion of congenital ventricular septal defects by the buttoned device. "Buttoned device" Clinical Trials International Register. Heart 77:276–279

Sideris EB, Macuil B, Justiniano S et al (2005) Total percutaneous correction of a tetralogy of Fallot variant with dominant pulmonary valve stenosis. Heart 91:345–347

Sinha SN, Rusnak SL, Sommers HM et al (1968) Hypoplastic left ventricle syndrome. Am J Cardiol 21:166–173

Soto B, Bargeron LM Jr, Diethelm E (1985) Ventricular septal defect. Semin Roentgenol 20:200–213

Stake G, Smevik B, Westvik J (1991) The role of X-rays in children with congenital heart disease. In: Nitter Hauge S, Allison D (eds) Cardiac imaging X-ray, MR and ultrasound. Elsevier, Amsterdam, pp 21–31

Stanger P, Cassidy SC, Girod DA et al (1990) Balloon pulmonary valvuloplasty: results of Valvuloplasty and Angioplasty of Congenital Anomalies Registry. Am J Cardiol 65:775–783

Stark J (1994) Coarctation of the aorta. In : Stark J, de Laval M (eds) Surgery for congenital heart defects. Saunders, Philadelphia, Pa., pp 285–298

Tometzki A, Chan K, De Giovanni J et al (1996) Total UK multi-centre experience with a novel arterial occlusion device (Duct Occlud pfm). Heart 76:520–524

Tynan M, Finley JP, Fontes V et al (1990) Balloon angioplasty for the treatment of native coarctation: results of Valvuloplasty and Angioplasty of Congenital Anomalies Registry. Am J Cardiol 65:790–792

Van der Meer JTM (2002) Prophylaxis of endocarditis. Netherl J Med 60:423–427

Vogel M, Rigby ML, Shore D (1996) Perforation of the right aortic valve cusp: complication of ventricular septal defect closure with a modified Rashkind umbrella. Pediatr Cardiol 17:416–418

Williams RJ, Levi DS, Moore JW et al (2006) Radiographic appearance of pediatric cardiovascular transcatheter devices. Pediatr Radiol 36:1231–1241

Computed Tomography in Congenital Heart Disease

Laureen Sena and Hyun Woo Goo

CONTENTS

L. Sena, MD
Department of Radiology, Children's Hospital, Boston, 300
Longwood Avenue, Boston MA 02115, USA
H. W. Goo, MD
Department of Radiology, Asan Medical Center,
University of Ulsan College of Medicine, 388–1 Songpa-gu
Poongnap-2dong, Seoul, Korea

17.1
Introduction

Over the past two decades, technological improvements have significantly advanced the role of multidetector computed tomography (MDCT) in noninvasive imaging of children with congenital heart disease (CHD). From the early use of helical CT for imaging congenital anomalies of the extracardiac thoracic vasculature (Hopkins et al. 1996; Westra et al. 1999), MDCT has become an important complementary modality to echocardiography and magnetic resonance imaging (MRI) for the morphologic evaluation of CHD (Goo et al. 2003). In addition, MDCT can now be used to assess coronary artery anatomy, measure regional and global cardiac function (Juergens et al. 2004), and provide morphologic and functional evaluation following operative and catheter intervention for many forms of congenital heart disease (Kawano et al. 2000). MDCT has rapidly evolved to systems which generate isotropic volume data and there are now much improved and faster post-processing techniques for visualizing the vasculature as compared with previously used methods. Current MDCT scanners have gantries that can spin faster than two revolutions per second, which further increases the speed of data acquisition. The increased speed of scanning can be used for increased volume coverage and improved longitudinal (z-axis) spatial resolution. The need for sedation or anaesthesia when imaging younger children who cannot lie still or voluntarily suspend respiration has been significantly reduced. In addition, the increased speed of scanning can now be used to scan faster than the heart rate in order to produce motion-free images of the heart and vasculature.

The driving force behind the rapid development of MDCT for cardiac imaging has been the noninvasive detection of adult coronary artery disease using coronary MDCT angiography with electrocardiography

(ECG) gating (Schoepf et al. 2004; Schoenhagen et al. 2004). Dedicated cardiac reconstruction algorithms have been developed that have broadened the clinical applications for MDCT beyond evaluation of extracardiac vascular morphology to the assessment of intracardiac morphology and ventricular function. In addition, dose modulation techniques (Jakobs et al. 2002; Goo and Suh 2006) have been developed that have significantly reduced radiation exposure during scanning. This chapter will focus on the technical aspects of cardiovascular imaging with MDCT for morphological assessment of CHD. The relative merits of cardiovascular imaging with MRI versus MDCT will be discussed with regards to specific issues pertaining to imaging patients with CHD.

17.2
Technical Considerations

17.2.1
Spatial and Temporal Resolution

The spatial resolution of a CT image is equivalent to the thinnest axial slice that can be reconstructed based on the CT detector configuration. Current MDCT scanners have improved spatial resolution and many systems have an in-plane spatial resolution that is sub-millimetre depending on the reconstruction algorithm. As compared with prior MDCT systems, the introduction of 16 MDCT with faster rotation speeds resulted in routine imaging with higher, sub-millimetre spatial resolution in the longitudinal plane as well (Mahesh 2002). For the first time, CT imaging data are being acquired with equal resolution in all three imaging planes. Images are therefore comprised of isotropic voxels so that there is significantly less misrecording of the anatomy when the imaging data are reconstructed with arbitrary obliquities. Isotropic cardiovascular imaging with MDCT has led to a vast improvement in the quality of processing techniques for visualizing the vasculature with multiplanar reformatting, maximum intensity projection as well as 3-D reconstruction with volume rendering.

Producing motion-free images of the heart and coronary arteries with high spatial resolution is one of the major challenges to be overcome for successful cardiac imaging, and requires the imaging modality to produce images faster than the heart rate, or with an increased temporal resolution or frame rate. In MDCT,

the temporal resolution is equivalent to half the gantry rotation time, because each reconstructed image requires CT data from half of a complete gantry rotation. To generate a smooth cine image of cardiac motion throughout systole and diastole, the temporal resolution has to be improved so that more images can be reconstructed per RR interval with a shorter time between them. This is accomplished with multisegment image reconstruction (Horiguchi et al. 2002). Imaging data acquired over several heartbeats is added to generate a single image during every half revolution of the gantry. Multiple images can then be reconstructed during systole and diastole and can be displayed as a cine loop to assess ventricular function.

There are a few drawbacks of multisegment reconstruction which are of particular concern when imaging children who have faster heart rates and are inherently more susceptible to the effects of ionizing radiation. Multisegment reconstruction requires a much lower CT pitch, which results in greater data oversampling and a higher radiation dose. Also, since multiple heartbeats are used to fill the 180° gantry rotation necessary for image reconstruction, fluctuation of the heart rate during the scan can cause significant motion artefact in the reconstructed images.

Prospective ECG triggering and retrospective ECG gating are two different processing methods for synchronizing the patient's ECG tracing and imaging data that are simultaneously acquired with MDCT. With prospective triggering, the gantry rotation is initiated during a predefined moment in the cardiac cycle from the QRS complex when there is less motion, typically during diastole. This technique delivers a very low radiation dose because the x-ray tube is only turned on when data needed for image reconstruction are acquired. The technique can be used successfully when static images of moving structures are desired, as in confirming anomalous coronary arteries in infants with rapid heart rates.

Retrospective ECG gating is more commonly used with current MDCT scanners because it allows multiple phases to be acquired throughout the cardiac cycle for more accurate depiction of the coronary arteries and for cine imaging of ventricular function, wall motion and motion of valves (Achenbach et al. 2000; Flohr et al. 2005). In order to freeze cardiac motion, images are reconstructed retrospectively using a short temporal segment that is located in the same position of the RR interval over multiple cardiac cycles. The duration of the temporal segment or phase is equal to the highest temporal resolution of the scanner. Reconstructing multiple phases requires oversampling of image data and reducing the pitch to 0.2–0.35, resulting in longer scan times and increased radiation exposure to the patient.

17.2.2
Radiation Dose Considerations

It is well known that children are more sensitive to the effects of ionizing radiation than adults, and have a longer life-span with a correspondingly greater potential for the development of radiation-induced malignancies. It is important to limit the indications for cardiac-related MDCT examinations to those in which the useful diagnostic information cannot be obtained from an alternative imaging modality such as echocardiography or MRI. MDCT examinations should be performed with techniques that provide acceptable and diagnostic image quality with the lowest possible radiation exposure. The use of MDCT for paediatric cardiac applications should therefore be approached in terms of what needs to be seen, rather than what can be seen. Important scanning parameters affecting image quality and radiation dose include tube current, pitch, beam collimation, tube voltage, table speed and gantry rotation time (DONNELLY and FRUSH 2003; KALRA et al. 2004). The most important factor for reducing radiation exposure is to use techniques that adjust the tube current according to the weight of the child (DONNELLY et al. 2001). In addition, recently manufactured MDCT scanners are now equipped with a dose modulation application that is able to modulate the dose based on the size of the patient. Automatic tube current modulation is a dose-reduction technique that automatically adjusts the tube current depending on the size, shape and density of the scanning region (KALRA et al. 2004) (Fig. 17.1). When scanning the thorax for cardiac applications, excluding the arms from the scan range in children, and scanning from caudal to cranial will allow an even greater tube current reduction when using combined tube current modulation (Goo and SUH 2006; GREESS et al. 2002)

A reduction in the x-ray tube voltage in contrast-enhanced MDCT studies in smaller children will allow a further dose saving while maintaining image contrast (SIEGEL et al. 2004). Other important measures to decrease radiation dose when scanning children include confining the study to the anatomical area of interest, avoiding multiphase examinations, using faster gantry cycle times and higher pitch (FRUSH 2002), and restricting the use of ECG-gated acquisitions to only a few select indications.

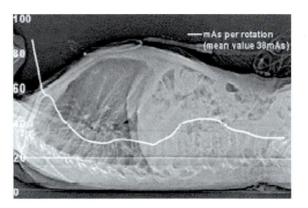

Fig. 17.1. Automatic exposure control with multidetector computed tomography (*MDCT*). Lateral topogram (scout view) for thoraco-abdominal CT in a 6-year-old child. The curve represents the automatically adapted milliampere-seconds value as a function of z-axis position during scanning with spiral CT. Although the standard adult protocol was used, the average milliampere-seconds value throughout the scan was adjusted to 38 mAs with automatic exposure control (FLOHR et al. 2005, used with permission)

Knowing that the use of ECG gating increases radiation dose as much as four- to fivefold over that of routine nongated MDCTA using appropriate weight-based protocols and tube current modulation, there are only a few specific indications for cardiovascular imaging in young children in which a gated acquisition should be considered. Based on these authors' experience as well as others (SIEGEL 2003), MDCT angiography can be performed without ECG gating for general evaluation of the extracardiac vasculature, including the thoracic aorta, systemic and pulmonary veins and arteries. MDCT with prospective ECG triggering can be used for more precise evaluation of the morphology of the heart chambers, including assessment of ventricular aneurysms, cardiac thrombi and tumours, for motionless imaging of the aortic root and ascending aorta if there is a suspicion of dissection, or evaluation of small aortopulmonary collaterals. MDCT for detection of anomalous coronary origin can be performed with either prospective ECG triggering or retrospective ECG gating (Fig. 17.2). However, fairly reliable visibility of the coronary artery origins was shown in a study using nongated MDCT angiography with a 16 detector scanner (Goo et al. 2005), and it is conceivable that 64 MDCT with fast gantry rotation times synchronized to the heart rate will prove even more useful in evaluating intracardiac morphology and diagnosing anomalous coronary artery origins in the future (Fig. 17.3). Therefore, coronary artery im-

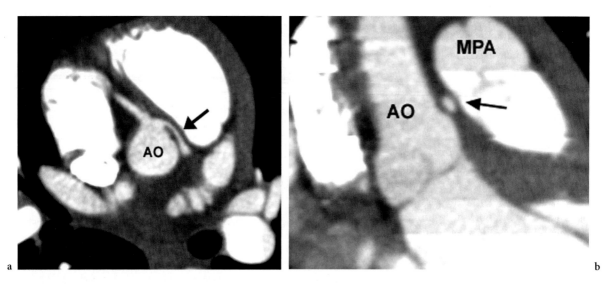

Fig. 17.2a,b. Anomalous left coronary artery. **a** Axial and **b** coronal maximum intensity projection (*MIP*) images obtained from a retrospectively gated coronary CT angiography (*CTA*) demonstrate an anomalous left coronary artery (*large arrow*) arising from the right coronary sinus and passing between the aorta (*AO*) and main pulmonary artery (*MPA*)

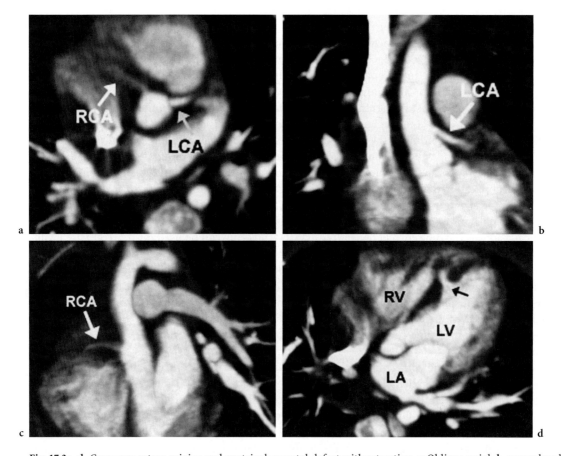

Fig. 17.3a–d. Coronary artery origins and ventricular septal defect without gating. **a** Oblique axial, **b** coronal and **c** sagittal MIP images demonstrate a high origin of the left coronary artery (*LCA*) above the sinotubular junction and a normal origin of the right coronary artery (*RCA*) from the right sinus without ECG gating. The origin of the RCA can be defined despite some blurring due to motion artefact. A mid-muscular ventricular septal defect (*VSD*) closed by right ventricular trabeculations is also present (*arrow* in **d**). Images were acquired with a 64 MDCT system at a heart rate of 150 bpm

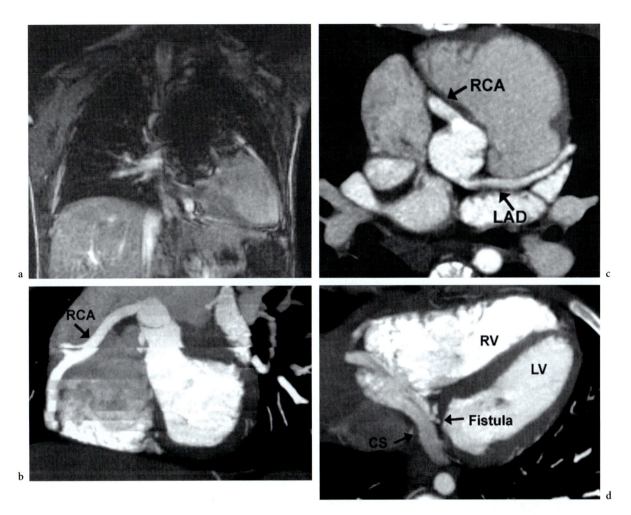

Fig. 17.4a–d. Coronary artery fistula in a 9-year-old girl with Noonan syndrome. **a** Coronal SSFP MR image demonstrates a large imaging artefact due to a stainless steel coil used to occlude a patent ductus arteriosus (*PDA*). **b** Oblique coronal and **c, d** oblique axial images from a retrospectively gated coronary CTA demonstrate diffuse enlargement of the right coronary artery (*RCA*) with a tortuous distal branch that enters a dilated coronary sinus (*CS*). Flow through the fistulous connection was coil-occluded to prevent coronary steal. (*LAD* Left anterior descending coronary artery)

aging with MDCT angiography with retrospective ECG gating and multi sector reconstruction (radiation-intensive approach) can be reserved for indications which require motionless images with high spatial resolution, such as for detection of coronary artery fistula (Fig. 17.4) and stenosis (Fig. 17.5) or aneurysms in patients with Kawasaki disease.

17.2.3
Scanning Technique for MDCT Angiography for Infants and Small Children

With the development of faster MDCT scanners, it is now vital for the radiologist performing and interpreting the CT examination to review any information pertaining to the child's form of CHD and surgical repair or palliation prior to scanning. Patients can have extremely variable sources of pulmonary blood flow, from pulmonary atresia with aortopulmonary collaterals arising from the descending aorta, to Glenn shunts or a cavopulmonary anastomosis between the SVC and the pulmonary arteries in patients with single-ventricle physiology. The knowledge of the patient's intracardiac anatomy and relevant surgeries will make planning of the timing of scanning after contrast administration much more accurate in order to effectively opacify the extracardiac vasculature, and avoid the mistake of scanning partially opacified vessels and confus-

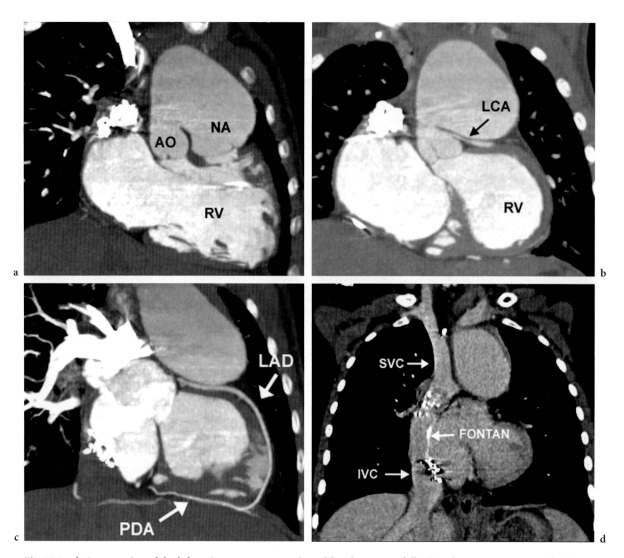

Fig. 17.5a–d. Compression of the left main coronary artery by a dilated neoaorta following the Fontan operation for hypoplastic left heart syndrome. **a** Coronal oblique MIP images show a markedly dilated reconstructed neoaorta (*NA*) arising from the right ventricle (*RV*) that is connected by a patent Stansel anastomosis to the native aorta (*Ao*). **b** A moderately compressed proximal left main coronary artery (*LCA*) passes inferior to the dilated neoaorta. The left main coronary could not be accessed at cardiac catheterization. **c** This is a left dominant coronary system with the left anterior descending coronary artery (*LAD*) giving rise to the posterior descending coronary artery (*PDA*). **d** Delayed venous phase coronal oblique image demonstrates patent Fontan pathway between the inferior vena cava (*IVC*) and superior vena cava (*SVC*) and RPA (not shown) with streak artefacts from closure devices placed for prior baffle leaks

ing them with thrombus. Knowledge of the patient's anatomy will help the choice of the best level in the chest to image for tracking the bolus prior to scanning the entire chest for the angiogram. For example, in patients with pulmonary atresia and major aortopulmonary collateral arteries (MAPCAs), timing off the ascending aorta should be adequate to opacify the collateral vessels, and there is often back filling of the branch pulmonary arteries (if they are present) from the collaterals (Fig. 17.6).

Another important consideration for the timing of contrast injection and scanning is in the patient who is status post Fontan operation. These patients have a single functioning ventricle which supports the aorta and receives the pulmonary venous return. The systemic venous return is directly routed into the pulmonary arteries without an intervening ventricular chamber. When performing MDCT angiography of Fontan patients, potential aortopulmonary collateral vessels from the aorta need to be imaged, as well as the systemic venous pathway from the IVC and SVC to the pulmonary arteries. One may decide to acquire only one set of images at 50–60 s after initial contrast administration, which will be in the venous phase with homogeneous but relatively less opacification of the entire vasculature (Fig. 17.7). Alternatively, one may acquire two sets of images, the first earlier in the arterial phase at about 20 s to more adequately enhance potential

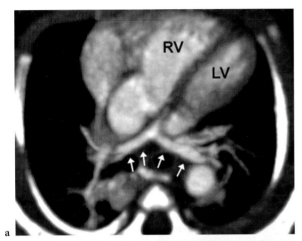

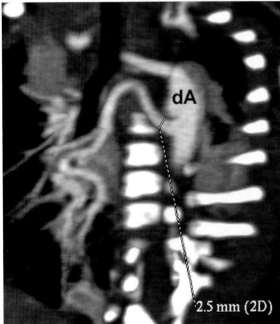

Fig. 17.6a, b. Pulmonary atresia with major aortopulmonary collateral vessels. **a** Oblique axial image demonstrates hypoplastic confluent central pulmonary arteries (*arrows*). **b** Oblique coronal image demonstrates an aortopulmonary collateral artery arising from the descending aorta (*dA*) and supplying the right lung

aortopulmonary collaterals, as well as for better visualization of the pulmonary venous system if pulmonary vein stenosis is suspected. In order to decrease radiation exposure and acquire images with more dense and homogeneous opacification of both the pulmonary and systemic vasculature, it is best to perform the examination with simultaneous injections through catheters placed in both the upper and lower extremities. This provides a better evaluation of the branch pulmonary arteries out to the subsegmental level for possible pulmonary embolism, since patients with CHD are at increased risk for pulmonary embolism (PE), particularly those with the Fontan circulation (BABYN et al. 2005) (Fig. 17.8).

Nongated MDCT angiography and gated acquisitions for imaging the coronaries or cardiac function are usually performed with dual injection of nonionic contrast followed by a saline or dilute contrast flush. Scanning of the heart at peak contrast enhancement during the saline flush reduces the streak artefact of dense contrast material passing through the SVC into the right heart. Injection rates in children will necessarily be different depending on the size of the catheter able to be placed and the amount of contrast to be injected (usually a maximum of 2 ml/kg). Table 17.1 provides a guideline for contrast injection rates by size of catheter. A 24 gauge catheter is satisfactory for infants and young children who will receive smaller volumes of contrast according to their body weight. The injection rate can be adjusted so that the total volume of contrast is administered in 20 s or less.

In the majority of patients with CHD, all of the vascular anatomy needs to be evaluated, including pulmonary and systemic arteries and veins, so that scanning later into the injection rather than earlier is generally better for more uniform opacification of the vasculature. Since current MDCT systems can acquire images through the chest in small children quite rapidly, the need for general anaesthesia with breath-holding capability is becoming less of a necessity and excellent imaging can be performed during quiet breathing. However, if there is any chance that there could be body movement during the acquisition time for MDCT angiography, sedation will be necessary. A child who is asleep without sedation may often move during or after the contrast injection, and any motion will significantly degrade oblique reconstructions of the 3D data that were acquired.

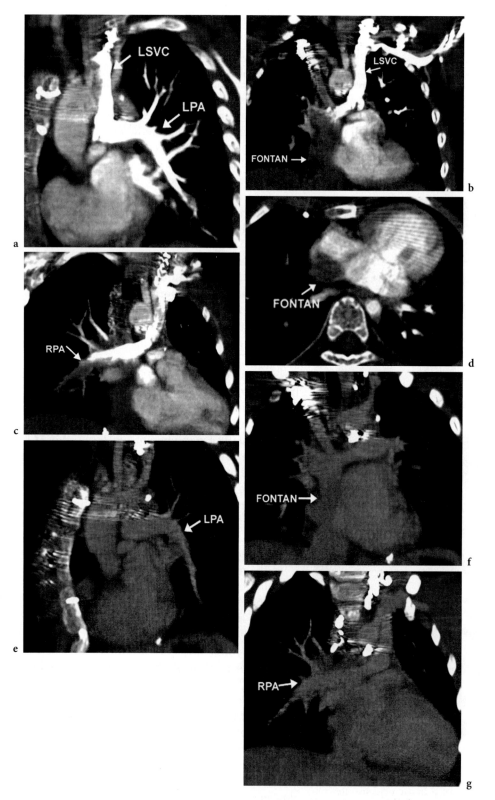

Fig. 17.7a–g. Lack of opacification of the Fontan pathway during arterial phase of scanning. **a** Coronal and axial oblique MIP images demonstrate dense contrast in the LPA via a left-sided SVC after a left arm injection. **b, d** The Fontan pathway from the IVC and the **c** distal RPA are incompletely opacified. Coronal oblique images reconstructed from the venous phase demonstrate homogeneous opacification of the LPA (**e**) Fontan pathway (**f**) and RPA (**g**)

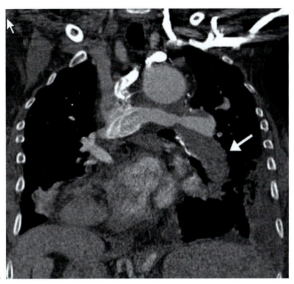
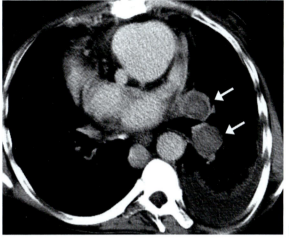

Fig. 17.8a, b. Coronal reformatted (**a**) and axial (**b**) images of a Fontan patient demonstrate extensive thrombus (*arrows*) extending from the Fontan pathway into the main and segmental branches of the LPA (courtesy of Rajesh Krishnamurthy)

Table 17.1. Intravenous contrast injection rates

Catheter size (g)	Flow rate (ml/s)
18	5–6
20	4–5
22	3–4
24	1–2

17.3
Complementary Role of MDCT and MRI for Cardiac Imaging

It is generally preferable to use echocardiography and/or MRI as a first approach to obtain adequate morphologic and functional information when imaging patients with known or suspected CHD. MRI is currently superior to MDCT for the evaluation of intracardiac anatomy, flow and function. However, there continues to be limited access to MRI scanners for paediatric cardiovascular exams in many hospitals and institutions, and the imaging is time consuming and requires technical expertise to perform routine quality examinations. In addition, infants and young children generally require sedation or anaesthesia more often for MRI (ODEGARD et al. 2004) than for MDCT, and assistance by anaesthesia

personnel may not be as readily available at a given clinical institution. For the initial evaluation of CHD in infants and young children, echocardiography often provides a complete assessment of intracardiac morphology, flow and ventricular function. The remaining clinical questions may only pertain to the morphology of the extracardiac vasculature, including the pulmonary arteries, thoracic aorta and branches, and pulmonary and systemic veins. MDCT angiography currently provides accurate imaging of the extracardiac vasculature that is clearly comparable to MRI with shorter procedure times and less need for sedation and general anaesthesia (LAMBERT et al. 2005). MDCT angiography is especially helpful with regards to imaging of airway compromise in patients who have suspected vascular rings or patients who have persistent respiratory symptoms or prolonged requirement for mechanical ventilation following cardiac surgery (KIM et al. 2002).

MRI becomes increasingly utilized in the non-invasive evaluation of CHD when echocardiography becomes more difficult to perform in older and larger children who have had multiple chest surgeries. The information provided by MRI can be used for serial follow-up of post-operative children who may need further catheter-based or surgical intervention, and can limit or completely obviate the radiation exposure required for diagnostic catheterization. Unfortunately, MR evaluation of patients with CHD can become severely compromised by susceptibility artefact if prior treatment has required placement of embolization coils, stents and occlusion devices (Fig. 17.4). In addition, indwelling pacemakers and automatic implantable cardio-defibrillator (AICD) devices remain contraindications for MRI.

MDCT is considered to be the best noninvasive imaging alternative for follow-up of cardiac morphology and function in those patients who have poor echocardiographic windows and indwelling devices that are contraindications to or would severely limit MRI. MDCT angiography also permits reliable visualization of the vascular lumen inside stents, and provides a noninvasive assessment of stent patency (EICHHORN et al. 2006). In the past, motion and streak artefacts related to the high-density material of the stent limited this application. The faster tube rotation time of current systems reduces the frequency of motion artefacts so that gat-

ing is usually not required. These features allow assessment of stent patency in larger stents with high confidence (Fig. 17.9).

17.4
Clinical Applications

17.4.1
Aortic Arch Anomalies

17.4.1.1
Coarctation

Coarctation is a congenital maldevelopment of the aorta presenting with variable degrees of hypoplasia of the distal transverse arch and focal or long segment narrowing of the aortic isthmus. Similar to

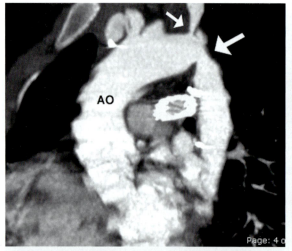

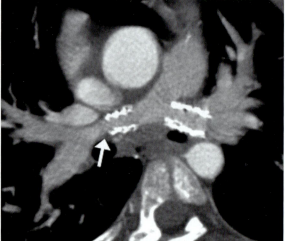

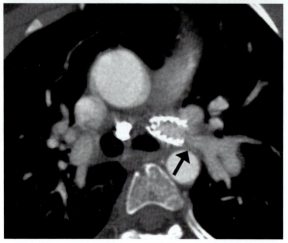

Fig. 17.9a–c. Tetralogy of Fallot and coarctation status post repair. a Sagittal oblique MIP image shows recurrent stenosis at the aortic isthmus (*large arrow*) and proximal left subclavian artery (*small arrow*) following an end-to-end anastomosis for coarctation repair. Oblique axial MIP images show patent bilateral proximal branch PA stents with narrowing of the RPA (*arrow* in **b**) and LPA (*arrow* in **c**) distal to the stents

MRI, MDCTA demonstrates the location and length of the coarctation segment, the degree of hypoplasia of the transverse arch and post-stenotic dilatation and co-lateralization to the descending aorta. Accurate delineation of the relationship of the origins of the left and right subclavian arteries to the coarctation segment is also defined on MDCT. A focal coarctation at the isthmus and tubular hypoplasia of the transverse arch can occur together or independently (Figs. 17.9, 17.10). Tubular hypoplasia or diffuse, long segment narrowing of the aortic arch is more often seen in neonates. A diffuse coarctation is also referred to as complex, due to an increased association with intracardiac defects such as VSD, ASD, valvar and subvalvar aortic stenosis (bicuspid aortic valve) and congenital mitral stenosis. In the hypoplastic left heart syndrome, the entire left side of the heart and aorta are underdeveloped, and the mitral and aortic valves are severely stenotic or atretic (Fig. 17.11).

17.4.1.2
Interrupted Aortic Arch

Interrupted aortic arch is defined as a complete separation of the ascending and descending aorta that results from an abnormal involutional pattern of the paired dorsal aorta during embryonic development. Type A is an interruption that occurs distal to the second subclavian artery that arises from the transverse arch; type B occurs between the second carotid and ipsilateral subclavian artery; and type C occurs between the two carotid arteries. Each of these three types is further subdivided: subtype 1 has a normal subclavian artery; subtype 2 has an aberrant subclavian artery; and subtype 3 has an isolated subclavian artery that arises from the ductus arteriosus. To determine

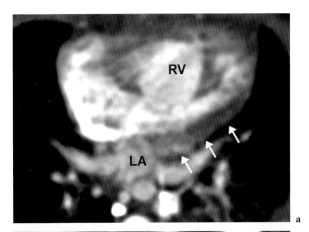

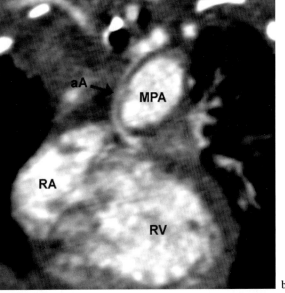

Fig. 17.11a, b. Hypoplastic left heart syndrome. An oblique axial image (a) demonstrates an enlarged apex forming right ventricle (*RV*), and marked hypoplasia of the left atrium (*LA*) and left ventricle (*LV*). Oblique coronal image (b) demonstrates severe hypoplasia of the ascending aorta (*aA*) and an enlarged MPA which is supporting the systemic and pulmonary circulation via an enlarged ductus arteriosus (not shown)

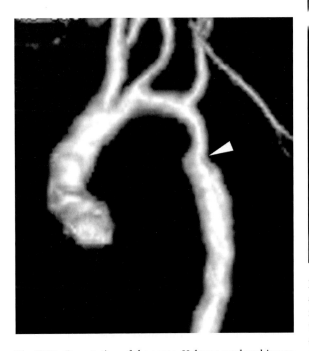

Fig. 17.10. Coarctation of the aorta. Volume rendered image demonstrates diffuse narrowing or tubular hypoplasia of the aortic arch and isthmus (*arrowhead*)

arch sidedness, the usual convention of noninterrupted arches is followed with the order of the branching brachiocephalic vessels: the first branch of the aorta proximal to the interruption contains the carotid artery opposite the side of the presumptive arch, and an aberrant or isolated subclavian artery is always opposite the side of the presumptive arch. The importance of arch sidedness in the setting of an interrupted aortic arch is the association of DiGeorge syndrome in all cases of an interrupted right arch. Type A interruptions tend to occur with aortopulmonary window or transposition of the great arteries (Fig. 17.12). Type B interruptions are

much more common than type A and are often associated with a VSD and subaortic obstruction. Type C interruptions are very rare. In addition to characterizing the type of interrupted aortic arch and the distance between the interrupted segments, left ventricular outflow tract patency and other intracardiac abnormalities need to be detected for appropriate surgical planning.

Following surgical repair of coarctation or interrupted aortic arch, MDCTA can be used to evaluate for possible complications such as anastomotic stenosis, re-coarctation (Fig. 17.8) or aneurysm formation at the repair site.

17.4.1.3
Truncus Arteriosus and Aortopulmonary Window

Truncus arteriosus is characterized by a single arterial trunk that arises from the base of the heart and gives origin to the systemic, pulmonary and coronary arteries. Truncus arteriosus has a single arterial valve, and this is the feature that differentiates truncus arteriosus from pulmonary or aortic valve atresia, which are both conditions in which a single arterial vessel receives the entire output of both ventricles, but a second atretic semilunar valve is present (Fig. 17.14). Aortopulmonary window is a defect in the septum that separates the aorta and pulmonary artery during embryologic development and the defect most often occurs midway between the semilunar valves and the pulmonary bifurcation (Fig. 17.15). Both truncus arteriosus and aortopulmonary window result in large, usually continuous left-to-right shunts when the pulmonary vascular resistance decreases in the newborn period. In hemitruncus, one of the branch pulmonary arteries (usually the right) originates from the ascending aorta and one arises from the main pulmonary artery (Fig. 17.16).

17.4.2
Coronary Artery Anomalies

17.4.2.1
Anomalous Coronary Artery

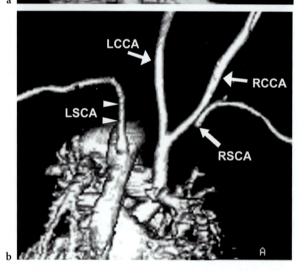

Fig. 17.12a,b. Interrupted aortic arch. Posterior volume rendered images demonstrate a type A1 arch interruption (**a**) just distal to the left subclavian artery (*LSCA*) and a second patient with a type B3 arch interruption between the left common carotid (*LCCA*) and left subclavian artery. An isolated right subclavian artery (*RSCA*) is also seen (**b**)

Congenital anomalous coronary arteries, although rare, are a well-recognized cause of myocardial ischaemia and sudden death in children and young adults, with an increased prevalence in patients with CHD, especially tetralogy of Fallot (TOF), transposition of the great arteries (TGA) and congenitally corrected TGA. Coronary artery anomalies include anomalous left or right coronary artery from the pulmonary artery, anomalous origin from the contralateral facing sinus (Fig. 17.2) and coronary artery fistula (Fig. 17.4). When one of the coronary arteries arises from the contralateral sinus, defining the exact proximal course of the coronary arteries with respect to the aorta and pulmonary artery is essential because this is the most important indicator of risk of ischaemia and determines treatment. The increased risk of ischemia/infarction in patients

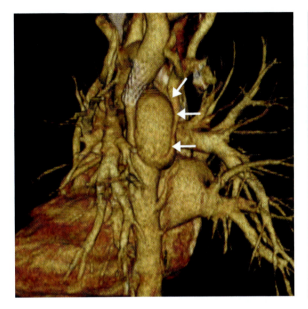

Fig. 17.13. Dissection and pseudoaneurysm of the thoracic aorta following balloon dilatation and stenting of coarctation. Oblique volume rendered image demonstrates a stent at the aortic isthmus with a dissection and large pseudoaneurysm (*arrows*) protruding from the aorta. The patient required an additional covered stent to be placed which closed the entrance of the pseudoaneurysm into the thoracic aorta. The pseudoaneurysm was shown to be thrombosed on subsequent imaging

Fig. 17.14. Truncus arteriosus. Combined oblique coronal and volume rendered image demonstrates a truncus arteriosus (*TA*) giving rise to the ascending aorta (*aA*) and the pulmonary trunk (*PT*)

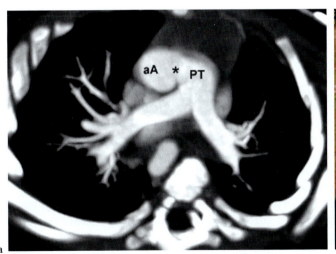
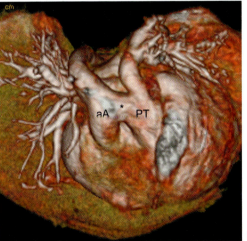

Fig. 17.15a,b. Aortopulmonary window. Oblique axial MIP (**a**) and VR (**b**) images demonstrate the abnormal connection (*) between the ascending aorta (*aA*) and pulmonary trunk (*PT*)

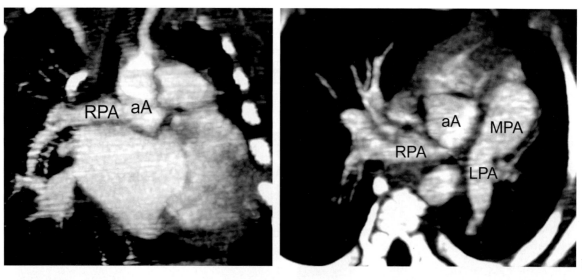

Fig. 17.16a,b. Hemitruncus or anomalous origin of one pulmonary artery from the ascending aorta. Oblique coronal (**a**) and axial (**b**) reformatted images demonstrate an anomalous RPA arising from the ascending aorta (*aA*) and LPA arising from the MPA

with anomalous coronary arteries is thought to be due to the intra-arterial course of the coronary artery between the aorta and the pulmonary artery and/or a tangential origin of the coronary artery from the aortic sinus that passes within the aortic wall and results in narrowing of the ostium (KIM et al. 2006). Defining the course and distribution of the coronary arteries is also important prior to repair of CHD, because the surgical approach to the repair may have to be altered if a coronary artery has an aberrant course that traverses a potential ventriculostomy site.

Echocardiography with colour Doppler has replaced cardiac catheterization as the standard method of visualizing the proximal coronary arteries in infants and children (SATOMI et al. 1984), but visualization can become more limited in adolescents and adults.

MDCT is now widely available and coronary CTA is being increasingly performed in many medical centres (GERBER et al. 2002), due to its relative ease of use and rapid image acquisition times compared with MRI. MDCT coronary angiography can be used to confirm anomalous coronary origins detected at echocardiography in young children. MDCT is advantageous for rapid diagnosis in patients presenting with acute symptoms including palpitations, dizziness, atypical or typical exertional chest pain, and dyspnoea on exertion, especially young athletes (DEIBLER et al. 2004). The

anomalous origin of the coronary artery arising from the contralateral aortic sinus and an interarterial course between the aorta and the pulmonary artery can be reliably detected on gated coronary MDCTA (Fig. 17.2).

17.4.2.2
Kawasaki Disease

Kawasaki disease is an acute vasculitis of unknown origin that occurs most often in young children. It begins as a pancarditis with vasculitis of small vessels (stage 1), progresses to vasculitis of the epicardial coronary arteries (stage 2), followed by resolution of vascular inflammation with a decrease in size of the aneurysms (stage 3), and scarring of the coronary arteries with stenoses (stage 4) (FUJIWARA and HAMASHIMA 1978). Coronary artery aneurysms can develop in up to 15%–25% of untreated cases and can be associated with thrombotic events leading to myocardial ischaemia and infarction in adulthood (KATO et al. 1996). Although current therapy with intravenous gamma-globulin and high-dose aspirin has reduced the mortality rate and incidence of coronary artery abnormalities, there continue to be cardiac sequelae in about 13% of patients with Kawasaki disease (YANAGAWA et al. 1999). An autopsy study has shown an association between post coronary arteritis lesions, especially focal aneurysms, and development of premature atherosclerosis (TAKAHASHI et al. 2001).

Serial follow-up of patients with Kawasaki disease is essential because the size of aneurysms and severity of coronary artery stenosis can change over time. Transthoracic echocardiography is now used frequently to follow small children for the development of aneurysms, but adequate visualization of the proximal coronaries tends to diminish with increasing age and size of the patients. Good correlation of the presence of stenosis and size of aneurysms of the proximal coronary arteries between MRI and cardiac catheterization has been reported (GREIL et al. 2002) but current MRI techniques have limited spatial resolution for reliable detection of coronary wall thickening, plaque formation, and abnormalities of the distal portions of the coronary arteries compared with ECG- gated MDCT. This has clinical relevance, as there is evidence of persistent intimal thickening at sites of prior aneurysms that have regressed (IEMURA et al. 2000), a higher rate of coronary abnormalities and significant cardiovascular complications with recurrent disease (MOMENAH et al. 1998), and in older children there have been documented fatalities due to myocardial infarction related to diffuse arteritis in the absence of aneurysms (BURKE et al. 1998).

In a study of adolescents with Kawasaki disease (SATO et al. 2003), ECG-gated MDCT coronary angiography accurately demonstrated all aneurysms, complete occlusions and stenosis that were present on invasive angiography (Fig. 17.17). In addition, MDCT can demonstrate abnormalities of the coronary wall, including diffuse intimal irregularity with a "braid-like" or artery-within-artery appearance, calcification and soft plaque, consistent with the sequelae of vasculitis that could lead to premature atherosclerosis (GOO et al. 2006; TAKAHASHI et al. 2001).

17.4.3
Pulmonary Vasculature

17.4.3.1
Pulmonary Artery Anomalies

In patients with right ventricular outflow tract obstructive lesions, such as tetralogy of Fallot and pulmonary atresia, precise preoperative delineation of the presence, size and confluency of the pulmonary arteries, and aortopulmonary collateral vessels from the aorta is necessary for surgical planning. In recent years, diagnostic cardiac catheterization has been almost completely replaced by Doppler echocardiography and cardiac MRI. Slow acquisition times and increased motion artefacts, especially in rapidly breathing infants and young children, compromised early acceptance of nonhelical CT in the evaluation of pulmonary arteries. With the development of helical CT, early studies showed high specificity, sensitivity and accuracy in the assessment of stenotic and nonconfluent central pulmonary arteries, and revealing the extent of aortopulmonary artery collaterals compared with echocardiography and angiography (HOPKINS et al. 1996; WESTRA et al. 1999). Current MDCT scanners now allow higher spatial resolution imaging compared with MRA, and two- and three-dimensional reconstruction techniques permit very accurate assessment of the vasculature (GOO et al. 2005; GREIL et al. 2006) (Fig. 17.18). Other abnormalities of the branch pulmonary arteries that are well depicted on MDCT include an abnormal origin or course such as in truncus arteriosus or pulmonary artery sling (Fig. 17.19). The branch pulmonary arteries can be atretic (Fig. 17.19), stenotic or hypoplastic related to decreased blood flow during growth (Fig. 17.20), due to extrinsic compression or the result of a surgically altered course or anastomosis such as a palliative shunt between the systemic and pulmonary artery circulation. Intrinsic stenosis of the pulmonary arteries can also be associated with genetic syndromes, such as Williams and Alagille (Fig. 17.21).

17.4.3.2
Pulmonary Vein Anomalies

Pulmonary venous anomalies include anomalous connections, normal connections with abnormal drainage and stenotic connections. Anomalous connections of all or some of the pulmonary veins to a systemic vein, the right atrium or the portal vein can occur due to an abnormal persistence of primitive connections between the pulmonary veins of the developing lung buds and the cardinal and umbilicovitelline venous systems. Total anomalous pulmonary venous connection (TAPVC) results when all of the pulmonary veins connect to a common confluence that then connects to a systemic vein. TAPVC is described as supracardiac, intracardiac or infracardiac depending on the level of connection to the systemic veins, and the abnormal venous connection can most often be fully characterized on echo-

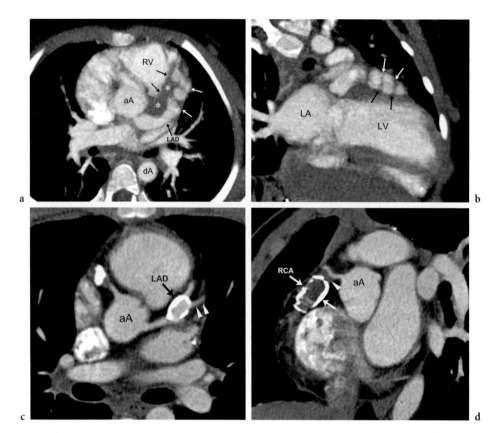

Fig. 17.17a–d. Kawasaki disease. Two patients with coronary artery aneurysms and stenosis. Oblique axial (**a**) and sagittal (**b**) MIP images from a gated MDCT angiogram of a 4-year-old girl demonstrate a string of aneurysms (*arrows*) with intervening areas of stenosis involving the left anterior descending coronary artery (*LAD*). A hypodense thrombus is present in the medial aspect of the aneurysm (*arrows* and *asterisks* in **a**). Oblique axial (**c**) and sagittal (**d**) images of a 13-year-old boy demonstrate large calcified coronary artery aneurysms of the proximal LAD and right coronary artery (*RCA*). The LAD and first diagonal (*arrowheads* in **c**) are unobstructed. The RCA proximal to the aneurysm is totally occluded by hypodense thrombus (*arrowhead* in **d**)

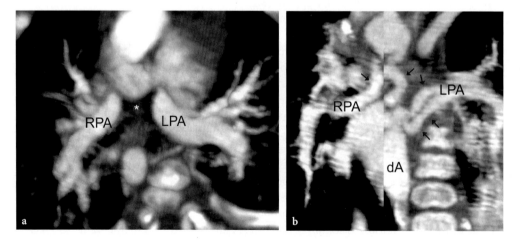

Fig. 17.18a,b. Pulmonary atresia with nonconfluent pulmonary arteries. **a** Axial MIP image demonstrates the absence of the confluent portion of the central pulmonary artery (*asterisk* in **a**) between the branch pulmonary arteries. **b** Combined coronal MIP images demonstrate major aortopulmonary collateral vessels (*arrows*) arising from the descending aorta (*dA*) and supplying the branch pulmonary arteries

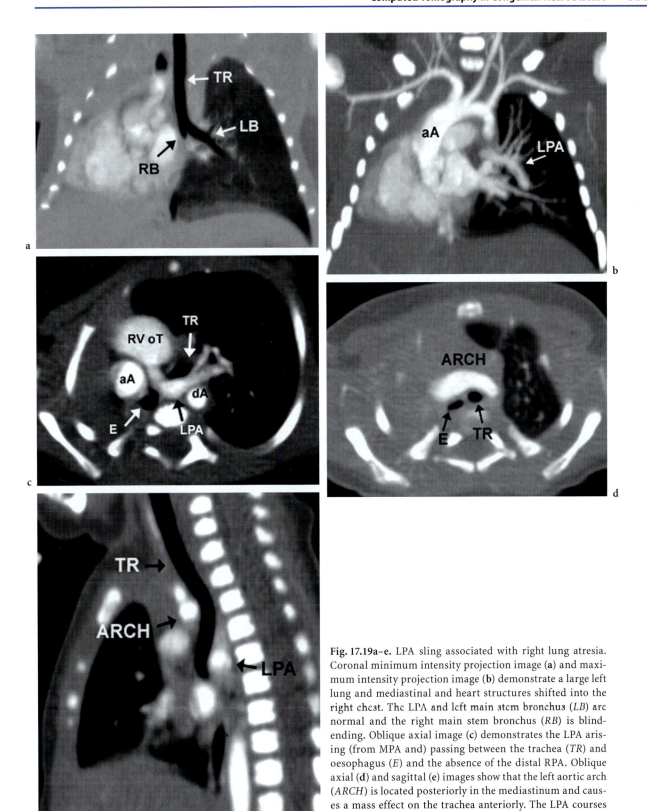

Fig. 17.19a–e. LPA sling associated with right lung atresia. Coronal minimum intensity projection image (**a**) and maximum intensity projection image (**b**) demonstrate a large left lung and mediastinal and heart structures shifted into the right chest. The LPA and left main stem bronchus (*LB*) are normal and the right main stem bronchus (*RB*) is blind-ending. Oblique axial image (**c**) demonstrates the LPA arising (from MPA and) passing between the trachea (*TR*) and oesophagus (*E*) and the absence of the distal RPA. Oblique axial (**d**) and sagittal (**e**) images show that the left aortic arch (*ARCH*) is located posteriorly in the mediastinum and causes a mass effect on the trachea anteriorly. The LPA courses posterior to the trachea (**e**)

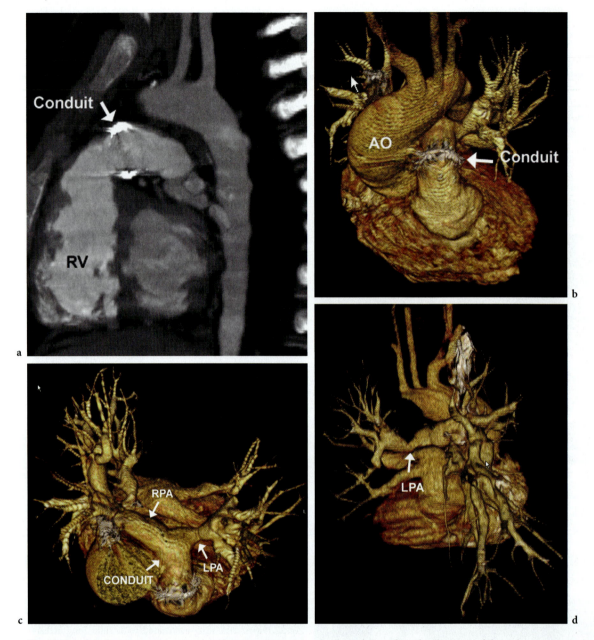

Fig. 17.20a–d. Pulmonary artery atresia status post RV to PA valved conduit and unifocalization of the pulmonary arteries. Reconstructed sagittal oblique MIP (**a**) and 3D volume rendered image (**b**) demonstrate a valved conduit arising from the RV causing only a mild discrete artefact. Additional 3D volume rendered anterior (**c**) and posterior (**d**) images demonstrate focal stenosis of the LPA

cardiography. In the mixed form of TAPVC, there may be more than one abnormal pulmonary venous connection to the systemic veins, or the abnormal pulmonary venous channel may course through the lung (Fig. 17.22). These latter forms of TAPVC may not be able to be fully depicted on echocardiography, and either MDCT or MR angiography can be used as an adjunct for imaging when echocardiog-

raphy is limited in order to identify the number and course of anomalously connecting or draining veins (Kim et al. 2000). In partial anomalous pulmonary venous connection, one or more pulmonary veins from some of the lobes have an anomalous connection to the systemic veins, most often to the innominate vein on the left and the SVC on the right (Fig. 17.23).

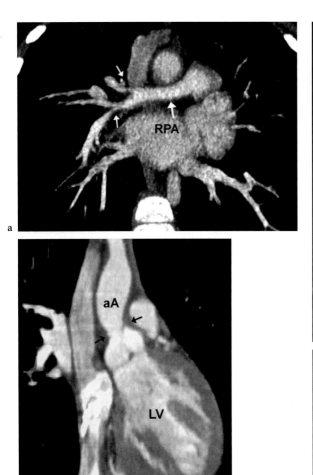

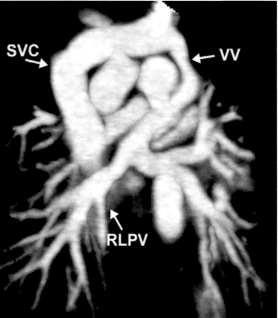

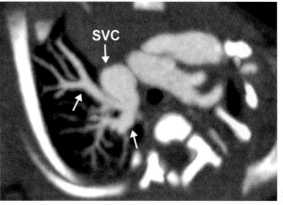

Fig. 17.21a,b. Williams Syndrome. Peripheral pulmonary stenosis and supravalvular aortic stenosis. Coronal reformatted image (a) shows diffuse hypoplasia of the RPA and multiple stenoses of distal branches (*arrows*). Coronal oblique image (b) shows an hourglass deformity of supravalvular stenosis of the ascending aorta (*aA*) characteristic of William syndrome

Fig. 17.22a,b. Mixed total anomalous pulmonary venous connection. Oblique coronal MIP image (a) demonstrates the right lower pulmonary vein (*RLPV*) and the left upper and lower pulmonary veins (*arrows*) joining to an ascending vertical vein (*VV*) which connects to a dilated left innominate vein to right superior vena cava (*SVC*). Oblique axial image (b) demonstrates branches of the right upper pulmonary vein (*arrows*) connecting directly into the right SVC

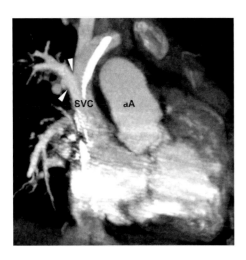

Fig. 17.23. Partial anomalous pulmonary venous connection (*PAPVC*): coronal oblique image demonstrates the right upper lobe pulmonary vein (*arrowheads*) connecting to a right SVC. All other pulmonary veins connected normally to the left atrium (not shown)

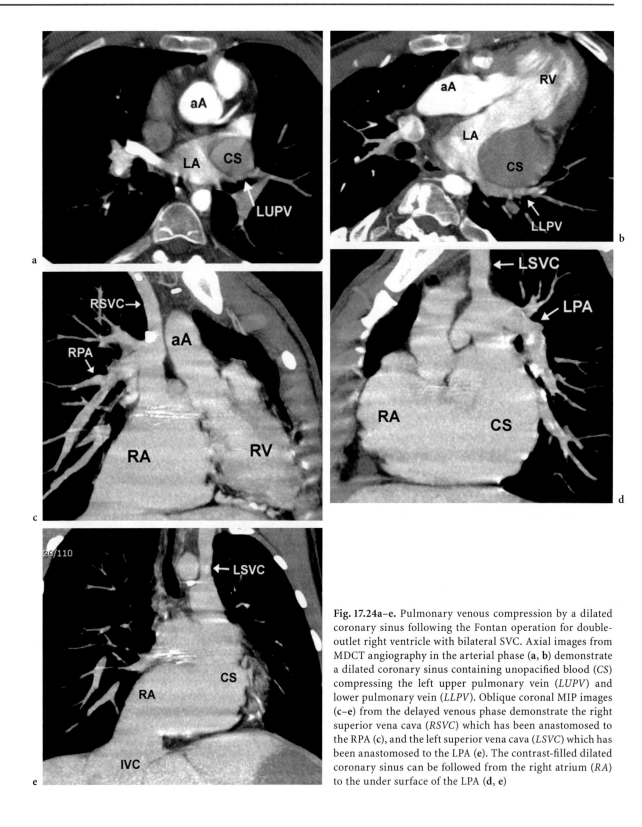

Fig. 17.24a–e. Pulmonary venous compression by a dilated coronary sinus following the Fontan operation for double-outlet right ventricle with bilateral SVC. Axial images from MDCT angiography in the arterial phase (**a, b**) demonstrate a dilated coronary sinus containing unopacified blood (*CS*) compressing the left upper pulmonary vein (*LUPV*) and lower pulmonary vein (*LLPV*). Oblique coronal MIP images (**c–e**) from the delayed venous phase demonstrate the right superior vena cava (*RSVC*) which has been anastomosed to the RPA (**c**), and the left superior vena cava (*LSVC*) which has been anastomosed to the LPA (**e**). The contrast-filled dilated coronary sinus can be followed from the right atrium (*RA*) to the under surface of the LPA (**d, e**)

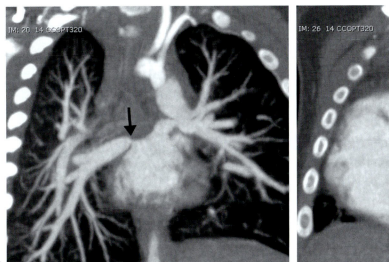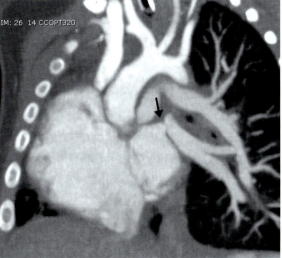

Fig. 17.25a,b. Total anomalous pulmonary venous return status post repair with pulmonary venous stenosis. Coronal oblique MIP images demonstrate focal stenosis (*arrows*) of the right (**a**) and left (**b**) pulmonary veins. (Courtesy of Sjirk Westra)

When associated with CHD, pulmonary vein stenosis (PVS) is most often extrinsic due to compression by other vascular structures (Fig. 17.24) or associated with the site of a prior surgical anastomosis. PVS can rarely be intrinsic and rapidly progressive and refractory to all forms of surgical (Caldarone et al. 1998) and/or a catheter-based intervention (Driscoll et al. 1982). Progressive PVS can occur as a complicating feature of CHD (Breinholt et al. 1999) (Fig. 17.25) or can occur in isolation in infants and children with otherwise normal hearts. PVS is a diagnostic consideration in any patient presenting with recurrent infection, haemoptysis, unexplained pulmonary hypertension, and/or interstitial lung disease. MDCT can detect the presence of PVS and the extent of associated involvement of the lung parenchyma and can be used as a noninvasive method to follow-up these patients for disease progression.

17.4.4
Airway Compromise in Patients with CHD

The most common types of vascular anomalies to cause symptomatic tracheal and oesophageal compression are the right aortic arch with aberrant left subclavian artery and the double aortic arch. In infants and children with these anomalies, symptoms can vary from wheezing to frank respiratory failure, related in part to the direct effect of vascular compression as well as secondary tracheobronchomalacia that can result from prolonged compression. If the vascular ring exhibits less compression, it may be diagnosed in the older child with symptoms primarily of oesophageal compression.

MDCT provides imaging in multiple planes to completely characterize the anomalous vasculature and the extent of airway compression. The current trend of performing minimally invasive surgery for repair of the vascular ring using video-assisted thorascopic or robotic endoscopic techniques has advantages over lateral thoracotomy including a smaller incision, improved visualization inside the chest cavity, reduced postoperative pain and risk of chest wall deformity. These less invasive techniques require more precise delineation of the size, patency and location of the vascular structures preoperatively (Lambert et al. 2005), and therefore there is now increased utilization of CT or MRI prior to surgical repair.

In addition to the above-described vascular anomalies, there are more rare conditions that can result in symptomatic airway and/or oesophageal compression, including pulmonary artery sling (Fig. 17.19), innominate artery compression (Fig. 17.26), circumflex aorta and cervical aortic arch. Patients with tetralogy of Fallot and absent pulmonary valve syndrome can have severe pulmonary regurgitation, which can lead to markedly enlarged pulsatile pulmonary arteries that can cause severe bronchial compression associated with bronchomalacia (Ditchfield and Culham 1995) (Fig. 17.27).

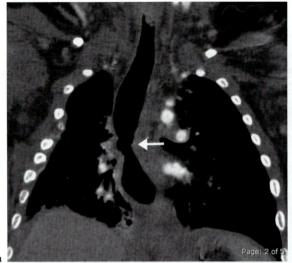

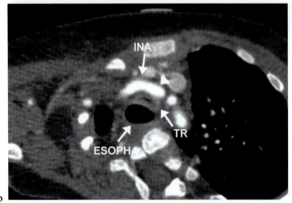

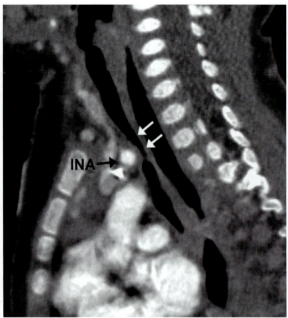

Fig. 17.26a–c. Innominate artery compression of the trachea following tracheoesphageal fistula repair. Coronal (**a**), oblique axial (**b**) and sagittal (**c**) MIP images demonstrate diffuse distension of the oesophagus (*ESOPH*) with a mild narrowing at the site of surgical anastomosis (*arrow* in **a**) and severe anterior tracheal compression (*arrows* in **b, c**) by the innominate artery (*INA*) as it courses from left to right across the mediastinum

MDCT provides a rapid assessment of the intensive care unit patient for potential causes of failed extubation in the early postoperative period following surgery for CHD (Lambert et al. 2005). The airway compression may be related to the patient's intrinsic anatomy, such as in TOF with a right aortic arch and markedly dilated ascending aorta (McElhinney et al. 1999) (Fig. 17.28), or due to surgically reconstructed vessels, such as with the arterial switch operation for TGA (Robotin et al. 1996) and aortic arch reconstruction following the Norwood operation. Other complications that can be rapidly diagnosed by MDCT in the early postoperative period include mediastinitis with abscess, mediastinal haematoma (Fig. 17.29) or a seroma, which is commonly associated with a Blalock-Taussig shunt and can also cause airway compression.

MDCT is also helpful to evaluate for airway or pulmonary parenchymal abnormalities in postoperative patients with chronic respiratory symptoms. Surgically altered position of the vasculature, conduits and vascular stents can cause compression of the trachea, main stem and lobar bronchi that may lead to chronic symptoms of airway compression that can worsen over time (Fig. 17.30). Dynamic airway studies can differentiate between stenosis related to vascular compression and intrinsic stenosis due to tracheal and/or bronchomalacia.

17.4.5
Postoperative Congenital Heart Disease

The evaluation of surgical results and possible complications involving palliative shunts, conduits and intracardiac baffles and the patency of the pulmonary arteries has become a major application of noninvasive imaging of postoperative CHD. CT is most often utilized if a full evaluation of the postoperative vascular morphology is limited on MRI due to artefacts from indwelling ferromagnetic materials such as stents, coils and occlusion devices or when there

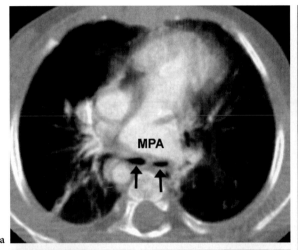

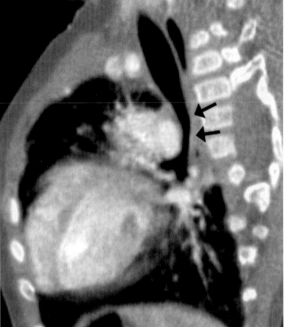

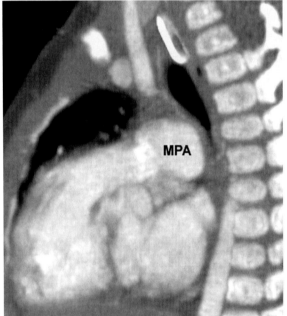

Fig. 17.27a–c. Tetralogy of Fallot with absent pulmonary valve syndrome status post repair. Axial (**a**) and sagittal oblique (**b, c**) MIP images from a MDCTA demonstrate severe dilatation of the main pulmonary artery (*MPA*) and proximal branch PAs causing severe compression of the distal trachea and proximal main stem bronchi (*arrows*)

is patient claustrophobia, which tends to be more of an issue with older patients.

Extracardiac conduits are prosthetic or homograft tubes used to create venoarterial, ventriculoarterial and arterioarterial connections when the structures to be connected are too far away from each other to allow a direct anastomosis. There are three different mechanisms of conduit obstruction: formation of a thick endothelial peal, scarring at sites of anastomosis and relative narrowing of the conduit associated with growth of structures at either end. Both MDCT and MR angiography allow a more complete visualization of conduits in their entirety than echocardiography or angiography due to a wide field of view and 3D imaging capability. Right ventricle to pulmonary artery conduits are used for repair of tetralogy of Fallot in patients who have severe pulmonary stenosis or atresia (Fig. 17.20) or anomalies of the coronary arteries limiting safe access to the right ventricular outflow tract, in the Rastelli operation for TGA with pulmonary valve stenosis, and in repair of truncus arteriosus. MDCTA is especially helpful for detection of in-stent stenosis when narrowing of the conduit has required stenting (Fig. 17.30) (EICHHORN et al. 2006).

There are two main types of intracardiac baffles used to redirect venous blood flow through the heart – the atrial inversion procedure (Mustard or Senning operations) for transposition of the great

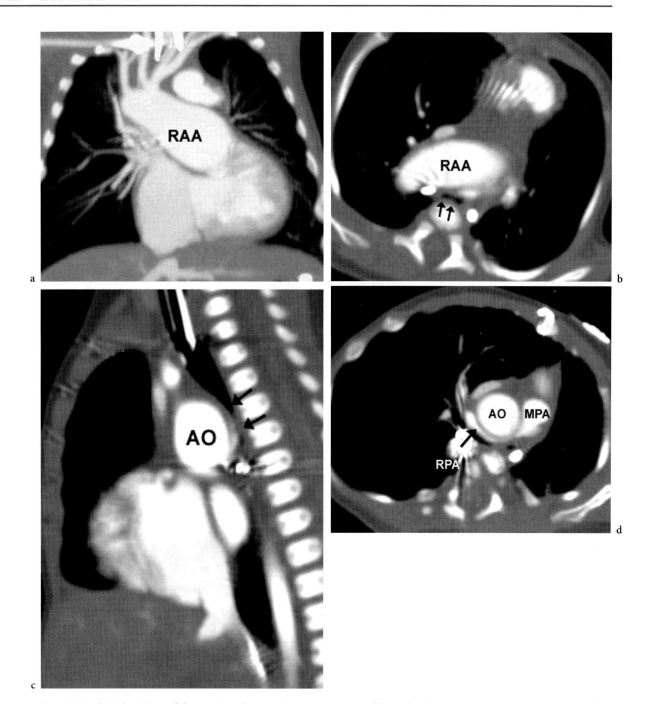

Fig. 17.28a–d. Malposition of the aortic arch causing severe airway and branch pulmonary artery narrowing in an infant with severe respiratory compromise following repair of tetralogy of Fallot and pulmonary atresia. Coronal (**a**), axial (**b, d**) and sagittal (**c**) oblique MIP images demonstrate a markedly dilated right aortic arch (*RAA*) positioned posteriorly within the chest, resulting in severe compression of the distal trachea and carina (*small arrows*), as well as the right pulmonary artery (*arrow* in **d**)

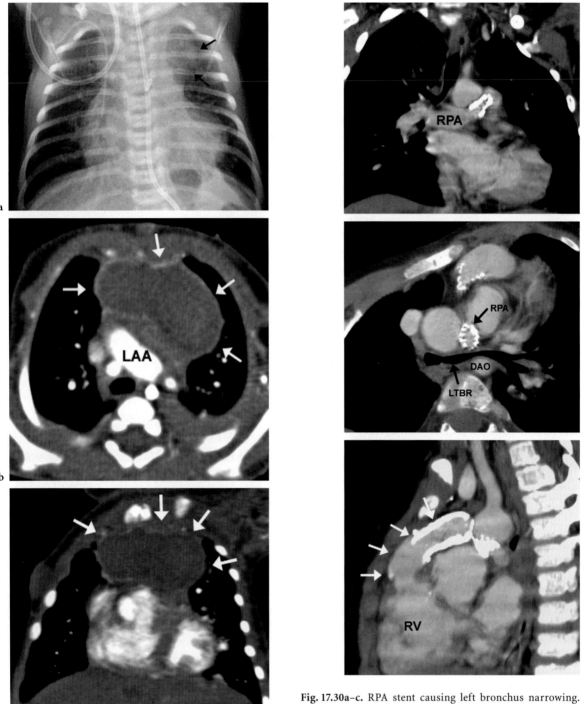

Fig. 17.29a–c. Mediastinal haematoma. Infant with TGA and subpulmonary stenosis status post right modified Blalock–Taussig shunt with large hypoechoic fluid collection noted on echocardiography and mediastinal widening on chest X-ray (*arrows* in **a**). Axial (**b**) and coronal reformatted (**c**) CT images demonstrate a large hypodense collection (*arrows*) with an enhancing wall filling the anterior mediastinum. A post-operative haematoma was evacuated at surgery. LAA (left aortic arch)

Fig. 17.30a–c. RPA stent causing left bronchus narrowing. Truncus arteriosus with interrupted aortic arch status post repair with an RV to PA conduit. Postoperative RPA stenosis treated with balloon dilation and stenting followed by development of recurrent left lower lobe pneumonia. Coronal (**a**) and axial oblique (**b**) MIP images demonstrate a patent stent in the proximal RPA and moderate narrowing of the left main stem bronchus (*LTBR*) as it courses between the stented portion of the RPA and the descending aorta (*DAO*). Sagittal oblique MIP image (**c**) demonstrates the RV to PA conduit with indwelling stent (*arrows*)

arteries and the Fontan procedure for functionally univentricular hearts. In the Mustard or Senning operation, the native intra-atrial septum is excised and a baffle is inserted to direct superior and inferior vena cava blood flow to the mitral valve. The pulmonary venous blood passes around the baffle and is directed towards the tricuspid valve. Both systemic and pulmonary venous pathways have the potential for obstruction, which can be assessed by CT (Fig. 17.31).

In the Fontan operation, a surgically created pathway reroutes the systemic venous return from the IVC and SVC directly to the pulmonary arteries. Possible complications include pulmonary arteriovenous malformations and pulmonary venous obstruction due to extrinsic compression by an intra- or extracardiac baffle or an enlarged cardiac structure such as the coronary sinus (Fig. 17.16) used for the Fontan pathway. Narrowing of the pulmonary artery can occur at the level of the cavopulmonary anastomosis or due to distortion from a prior shunt or surgical pulmonary artery reconstruction. Imaging evaluation is directed to establish the overall patency of the Fontan pathway. In the early versions of the Fontan operation, the right atrium is incorporated into the systemic venous to pulmonary artery connection, and not infrequently patients can develop thrombus in the pathway due to relative stasis of slow flowing blood (Fig. 17.8).

Many patients with CHD can develop conduction abnormalities or arrhythmias related to the surgical repair (especially following the Mustard or Senning or Fontan operations) or inherent to abnormal intracardiac connections, such as in congenitally corrected TGA. An indwelling pacemaker or retained pacing leads are contraindications for MR imaging, and CT can be used as an alternative method for both morphologic and functional imaging in these patients.

17.5
Conclusion

In summary, MDCT provides a number of important advantages for morphological and functional assessment of the cardiovascular system, including isotropic high-resolution volume imaging, high volume coverage, and improved temporal resolution with dose reduction methods. MDCT is now a major

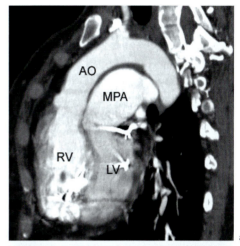

a

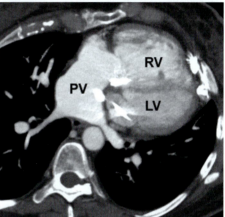

b

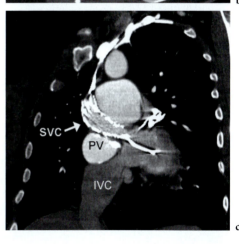

c

Fig. 17.31a–c. D-TGA status post Senning. Sagittal oblique (**a**) MIP image demonstrates the characteristic morphology of D-TGA with the anterior aorta arising from the RV and posterior main pulmonary artery arising from the LV. Axial MIP image (**b**) demonstrates the pulmonary venous (*PV*) pathway that directs oxygenated blood to the systemic RV positioned anteriorly. Coronal reformatted image (**c**) demonstrates the typical "pant leg" configuration of the IVC and SVC (with stent) pathway directed to the left ventricle separated by an intra-atrial baffle from the PV pathway

diagnostic tool in children with CHD, and, when performed for appropriate indications with proper technical parameters, the benefits can far exceed the very small individual risk.

References

Achenbach S, Ulzheimer S, Baum U, Kachelriess M, Ropers D, Giesler T, Bautz W, Daniel WG, Kalender WA, Moshage W (2000) Noninvasive coronary angiography by retrospectively ECG-gated multislice spiral CT. Circulation 102:2823–2828

Babyn PS, Gahunia HK, Massicotte P (2005) Pulmonary thromboembolism in children. Pediatr Radiol 35:258–274

Breinholt JP, Hawkins JA, Minich LA, Tani LY, Orsmond GS, Ritter S, Shaddy RE (1999) Pulmonary vein stenosis with normal connection: associated cardiac abnormalities and variable outcome. Ann Thorac Surg 68:164–168

Burke AP, Virmani R, Perry LW, Li L, King TM, Smialek J (1998) Fatal Kawasaki disease with coronary arteritis and no coronary aneurysms. Pediatrics 101:108–112

Caldarone CA, Najm HK, Kadletz M, Smallhorn JF, Freedom RM, Williams WG, Coles JG (1998) Relentless pulmonary vein stenosis after repair of total anomalous pulmonary venous drainage. Ann Thorac Surg 66:1514–1520

Deibler et al. (2004)

Ditchfield MR, Culham JA (1995) Assessment of airways compression by MR imaging in children with aneurysmal pulmonary arteries. Pediatr Radiol 25:190–191

Donnelly LF, Frush DP (2003) Pediatric multidetector body CT. Radiol Clin North Am 41:637–655

Donnelly LF, Emery KH, Brody AS, Laor T, Gylys-Morin VM, Anton CG, Thomas SR, Frush DP (2001) Minimizing radiation dose for pediatric body applications of single-detector helical CT: strategies at a large Children's Hospital. AJR Am J Roentgenol 176:303–306

Driscoll DJ, Hesslein PS, Mullins CE (1982) Congenital stenosis of individual pulmonary veins: clinical spectrum and unsuccessful treatment by transvenous balloon dilation. Am J Cardiol 49:1767–1772

Eichhorn JG, Long FR, Hill SL, O'Donovan J, Chisolm JL, Fernandez SA, Cheatham JP (2006) Assessment of in-stent stenosis in small children with congenital heart disease using multi-detector computed tomography: a validation study. Catheter Cardiovasc Interv 68:11–20

Flohr TG, Schaller S, Stierstorfer K, Bruder H, Ohnesorge BM, Schoepf UJ (2005) Multi-detector row CT systems and image-reconstruction techniques. Radiology 235:756–773

Frush DP (2002) Strategies of dose reduction. Pediatr Radiol 32:293–297

Fujiwara H, Hamashima Y (1978) Pathology of the heart in Kawasaki disease. Pediatrics 61:100–107

Gerber TC, Kuzo RS, Karstaedt N, Lane GE, Morin RL, Sheedy PF, Safford RE, Blackshear JL, Pietan JH (2002) Current results and new developments of coronary angiography with use of contrast-enhanced computed tomography of the heart. Mayo Clin Proc 77:55–71

Goo HW, Suh DS (2006) Tube current reduction in pediatric non-ECG-gated heart CT by combined tube current modulation. Pediatr Radiol 36:344–351

Goo HW, Park IS, Ko JK, Kim YH, Seo DM, Yun TJ, Park JJ, Yoon CH (2003) CT of congenital heart disease: normal anatomy and typical pathologic conditions. Radiographics 23 [Spec No]:S147–S165

Goo HW, Park IS, Ko JK, Kim YH, Seo DM, Yun TJ, Park JJ (2005) Visibility of the origin and proximal course of coronary arteries on non-ECG-gated heart CT in patients with congenital heart disease. Pediatr Radiol 35:792–798

Goo HW Park IS, Ko JK, Kim YH (2006) Coronary CT angiography and MR angiography of Kawasaki Disease. Pediatric Radiol 36:699–700

Greess H, Nomayr A, Wolf H, Baum U, Lell M, Bowing B, Kalender W, Bautz WA (2002) Dose reduction in CT examination of children by an attenuation-based on-line modulation of tube current (CARE Dose). Eur Radiol 12:1571–1576

Greil GF, Stuber M, Botnar RM, Kissinger KV, Geva T, Newburger JW, Manning WJ, Powell AJ (2002) Coronary magnetic resonance angiography in adolescents and young adults with kawasaki disease. Circulation 105:908–911

Greil GF, Schoebinger M, Kuettner A, Schaefer JF, Dammann F, Claussen CD, Hofbeck M, Meinzer HP, Sieverding L (2006) Imaging of aortopulmonary collateral arteries with high-resolution multidetector CT. Pediatr Radiol 36:502–509

Hopkins KL, Patrick LE, Simoneaux SF, Bank ER, Parks WJ, Smith SS (1996) Pediatric great vessel anomalies: initial clinical experience with spiral CT angiography. Radiology 200:811–815

Horiguchi J, Nakanishi T, Tamura A, Ito K, Sasaki K, Shen Y (2002) Technical innovation of cardiac multirow detector CT using multisector reconstruction. Comput Med Imaging Graph 26:217–226

Iemura M, Ishii M, Sugimura T, Akagi T, Kato H (2000) Long term consequences of regressed coronary aneurysms after Kawasaki disease: vascular wall morphology and function. Heart 83:307–311

Jakobs et al. (2002)

Juergens KU, Grude M, Maintz D, Fallenberg EM, Wichter T, Heindel W, Fischbach R (2004) Multi-detector row CT of left ventricular function with dedicated analysis software versus MR imaging: initial experience. Radiology 230:403–410

Kalra MK, Maher MM, Toth TL, Hamberg LM, Blake MA, Shepard JA, Saini S (2004) Strategies for CT radiation dose optimization. Radiology 230:619–628

Kato H, Sugimura T, Akagi T, Sato N, Hashino K, Maeno Y, Kazue T, Eto G, Yamakawa R (1996) Long-term consequences of Kawasaki disease. A 10- to 21-year follow-up study of 594 patients. Circulation 94:1379–1385

Kawano et al. (2000)

Kim SY, Seo JB, Do KH, Heo JN, Lee JS, Song JW, Choe YH, Kim TH, Yong HS, Choi SI, Song KS, Lim TH (2006) Coronary artery anomalies: classification and ECG-gated multi-detector row CT findings with angiographic correlation. Radiographics 26:317–333; discussion 333–314

Kim TH, Kim YM, Suh CH, Cho DJ, Park IS, Kim WH, Lee YT (2000) Helical CT angiography and three-dimensional reconstruction of total anomalous pulmonary venous connections in neonates and infants. AJR Am J Roentgenol 175:1381–1386

Kim YM, Yoo SJ, Kim TH, Park IS, Kim WH, Lee JY, Han MY (2002) Three-dimensional computed tomography in children with compression of the central airways complicating congenital heart disease. Cardiol Young 12:44–50

Lambert V, Sigal-Cinqualbre A, Belli E, Planche C, Roussin R, Serraf A, Brunaiux J, Angel C, Paul JF (2005) Preoperative and postoperative evaluation of airways compression in pediatric patients with 3-dimensional multislice computed tomographic scanning: effect on surgical management. J Thorac Cardiovasc Surg 129:1111–1118

Lawler LP, Corl FM, Fishman EK (2002) Multi-detector row and volume-rendered CT of the normal and accessory flow pathways of the thoracic systemic and pulmonary veins. Radiographics 22 [Spec No]:S45–S60

Lee EY, Siegel MJ, Sierra LM, Foglia RP (2004) Evaluation of angioarchitecture of pulmonary sequestration in pediatric patients using 3D MDCT angiography. AJR Am J Roentgenol 183:183–188

Mahesh (2002)

McElhinney DB, Reddy VM, Pian MS, Moore P, Hanley FL (1999) Compression of the central airways by a dilated aorta in infants and children with congenital heart disease. Ann Thorac Surg 67:1130–1136

Momenah T, Sanatani S, Potts J, Sandor GG, Human DG, Patterson MW (1998) Kawasaki disease in the older child. Pediatrics 102:108–112

Odegard KC, DiNardo JA, Tsai-Goodman B, Powell AJ, Geva T, Laussen PC (2004) Anaesthesia considerations for cardiac MRI in infants and small children. Paediatr Anaesth 14:471–476

Robotin MC, Bruniaux J, Serraf A, Uva MS, Roussin R, Lacour-Gayet F, Planche C (1996) Unusual forms of tracheobronchial compression in infants with congenital heart disease. J Thorac Cardiovasc Surg 112:415–423

Sato Y, Kato M, Inoue F, Fukui T, Imazeki T, Mitsui M, Matsumoto N, Takahashim M, Karasawa K, Ayusawa M, Kanamaru H, Harada K, Kanmatsuse K (2003) Detection of coronary artery aneurysms, stenoses and occlusions by multislice spiral computed tomography in adolescents with kawasaki disease. Circ J 67:427–430

Satomi G, Nakamura K, Narai S, Takao A (1984) Systematic visualization of coronary arteries by two-dimensional echocardiography in children and infants: evaluation in Kawasaki's disease and coronary arteriovenous fistulas. Am Heart J 107:497–505

Schoenhagen et al. (2004)

Schoepf UJ, Becker CR, Ohnesorge BM, Yucel EK (2004) CT of coronary artery disease. Radiology 232:18–37

Siegel MJ (2003) Multiplanar and three-dimensional multidetector row CT of thoracic vessels and airways in the pediatric population. Radiology 229:641–650

Siegel MJ, Schmidt B, Bradley D, Suess C, Hildebolt C (2004) Radiation dose and image quality in pediatric CT: effect of technical factors and phantom size and shape. Radiology 233:515–522

Takahashi K, Oharaseki T, Naoe S (2001) Pathological study of postcoronary arteritis in adolescents and young adults: with reference to the relationship between sequelae of Kawasaki disease and atherosclerosis. Pediatr Cardiol 22:138–142

Tomita H, Yamada O, Ohuchi H, Ono Y, Arakaki Y, Yagihara T, Echigo S (2001) Coagulation profile, hepatic function, and hemodynamics following Fontan-type operations. Cardiol Young 11:62–66

Westra SJ, Hill JA, Alejos JC, Galindo A, Boechat MI, Laks H (1999) Three-dimensional helical CT of pulmonary arteries in infants and children with congenital heart disease. AJR Am J Roentgenol 173:109–115

Woodring JH, Howard TA, Kanga JF (1994) Congenital pulmonary venolobar syndrome revisited. Radiographics 14:349–369

Yanagawa H, Tuohong Z, Oki I, Nakamura Y, Yashiro M, Ojima T, Tanihara S (1999) Effects of gamma-globulin on the cardiac sequelae of Kawasaki disease. Pediatr Cardiol 20:248–251

Chest Wall Abnormalities which Cause Neonatal Respiratory Distress

Georg F. Eich

18

18.1
Introduction

Thoracic cage abnormalities may produce respiratory problems in the neonatal period. Particularly disorders of bone growth and formation, such as in skeletal dysplasias, may restrict pulmonary development and expansion, or may distort the airways. The radiographic features of these disorders are diverse, but generally include short ribs.

Other disorders, such as neuromuscular disorders, may produce functional impairment of the chest wall with secondary respiratory distress. This latter group includes myotonia congenita, congenital myasthenia gravis, myotonic dystrophy, and Werdnig-Hoffmann disease. These disorders may show nonspecific, secondary findings such as thinning of the ribs and clavicles or diffuse pulmonary underaeration.

18.2
Anatomic, Pathophysiologic, and Nosologic Considerations

Pulmonary hypoplasia is a less common cause for respiratory distress of the neonate, but it is the commonest single abnormality found at autopsy in early neonatal deaths (WIGGLESWORTH and DESAI 1982). Pulmonary hypoplasia consists of an incomplete development of the lung. The lung is small in size and volume and shows a reduced number of bronchial branches, alveoli, and vessels. Patients with bilateral lung hypoplasia usually present immediately after birth with respiratory distress. They are difficult to resuscitate and require high inflating pressures. Pneumothorax is a common complication (GREENOUGH 1996).

G. F. EICH, MD
Division of Pediatric Radiology, Kantonsspital, 5001 Aarau, Switzerland

Pulmonary hypoplasia usually occurs in association with other malformations. Rarely it may be called primary or idiopathic. Many disorders that result in a reduction of the intrathoracic space, a reduction of fetal breathing movements, or a reduction of amniotic fluid volume produce hypoplasia of the lung (Fig. 18.1) (Thomas and Smith 1974; Greenough 1996). Reduction of the intrathoracic space may be caused by skeletal restriction of the chest or by intrathoracic space-occupying lesions as in diaphragmatic hernias.

Disorders with congenital skeletal restriction of the chest are usually classified as skeletal dysplasias (bone dysplasias or osteochondrodysplasias) (Online Mendelian Inheritance in Man; OMIM 2007; Superti-Furga et al. 2007). Skeletal dysplasias are characterized by a disturbance of cartilage and/or bone growth and development. They are grouped into different families according to their underlying gene or gene product defect, or their phenotypic

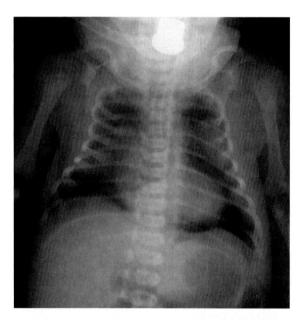

Fig. 18.1. Oligohydramnios-associated pulmonary hypoplasia (Potter). The full-term female infant was born with oligohydramnios, low birth weight, and microcephaly. Delivery was performed by caesarean section. The face and extremities were deformed. The patient was intubated because of asphyxia. She died after 3 h. The radiograph shows a small, bell-shaped chest. The tracheal tube is low in position. Bilateral pneumothorax is present. The ribs are thin. Autopsy confirmed hypoplastic lungs and cystic dysplasia of the kidneys. Decreased production of fetal amniotic fluid can be due to a renal pathology (Potter syndrome), or a uteroplacental insufficiency. The mechanism by which oligohydramnios induces pulmonary hypoplasia is not yet understood

presentation. Depending on the severity of the chest deformity and the presence or absence of additional malformations, particularly of the central nervous system, the spine, the airways, and/or the heart, some of these disorders almost invariably lead to death in utero or at birth and therefore are labeled as "lethal osteochondrodysplasias" (Spranger and Maroteaux 1990). Others are compatible with life, but respiratory distress may be a leading symptom and may eventually lead to premature death. The chest deformity of osteochondrodysplasias is predominantly due to insufficient growth of the ribs (Fig. 18.2). Alternatively it may be due to decreased rib stability, as in osteogenesis imperfecta and hypophosphatasia (Figs. 18.3, 18.4). Other parts of the skeletal system are often affected as well. Usually the patients are small, may have a narrow chest, and may show variable shortening, and/or bowing deformity of the limbs, spine, and a "dysmorphic" head (Fig. 18.5) (Lachman 2006).

The lethal osteochondrodysplasias consist of a heterogeneous group of disorders and are recognized with a frequency between 1:5000 and 1:11,000. Thanatophoric dysplasia, achondrogenesis-hypochondrogenesis, and osteogenesis imperfecta (type II) are amongst the most prevalent disorders, while others are less frequent (Orioli et al. 1986). Spranger and Maroteaux (1990) in their review of lethal osteochondrodysplasias have listed 11 groups of disorders that contain 61 individual conditions, some of which are well recognized, while others are rare or represented by isolated cases. Lethal osteochondrodysplasias belong to the "severe" end of the spectrum of abnormalities found in the different bone dysplasia families. Most lethal osteochondrodysplasias have moderate to marked shortening of the ribs in common, associated with lung hypoplasia. A lethal skeletal dysplasia condition may be suspected antenatally in fetuses that exhibit moderate or severe shortening and/or bowing of the long bones, a decreased crown-rump length, and decreased thoracic dimensions on ultrasound examination. Polyhydramnios and fetal hydrops are frequent additional features of lethal osteochondrodysplasias. Intrauterine radiographs are helpful in making a specific diagnosis and in differentiating between lethal and nonlethal disorders (Sharony et al. 1993), particularly in the third trimester. Prompt confirmation of the diagnosis of a lethal osteochondrodysplasia at birth is mandatory because of ethical implications. A multidisciplinary approach with close collaboration between the obstetrician, neonatologist, pediatrician, geneticist, and pediatric radiologist is important for preparation for the delivery, postnatal care, and for giving information to the parents. Usually a radiographic survey of the neonate will readily allow the distinction between lethal and nonlethal skeletal dysplasias and is the basis for the diagnosis of the disorder. A proper categorization is essential not only for prognostic purposes, but also for counseling of the involved family.

The following paragraphs illustrate the most common skeletal dysplasias that have restriction of the chest and hypoplastic lungs, and that are frequently associated with respiratory distress at birth and with death in utero or in early infancy. An encyclopedic coverage is not attempted. Other skeletal dysplasias that cause respiratory distress and early death due to hypoplasia and/or chondromalacia of the larynx and tracheo-bronchial tree are not included (e.g. campomelic dysplasia).

18.3
Thanatophoric Dysplasia (OMIM 187600)

Thanatophoric dysplasia is the most frequent lethal skeletal dysplasia with a reported prevalence rate of approx. 1:50,000 (ORIOLI et al. 1986). It is

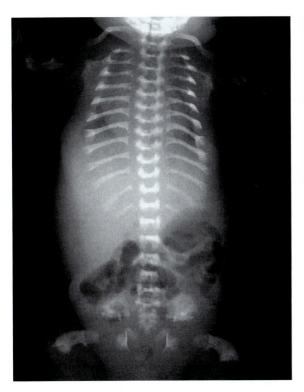

Fig. 18.2. Thanatophoric dysplasia type I. This infant boy was born in the 34th gestational week. Polyhydramnios had been diagnosed by prenatal ultrasound. In addition a large head, short limbs, and short ribs had been shown. The infant was observed in a neonatal clinic. He received oxygen by nasal administration only. Death occurred after 48 h. The postmortem radiograph shows a narrow chest with short ribs. The vertebral bodies are flat and the interpediculate distance of the lumbar spine is narrow. The pedicles and vertebral bodies resemble an "H" or "U." The ilia are small and squared with horizontal, trident-shaped acetabula, and small sacrosciatic notches. The tubular bones are short, broad, and bowed with flared metaphyses. The proximal portions of the femora are oval shaped and less dense than the shafts

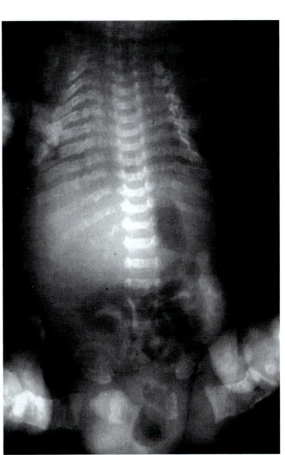

Fig. 18.3. Osteogenesis imperfecta type II A. A term born boy showed short and deformed limbs at birth. His weight, length, and head circumference were below the 3rd centile for age. Respiratory insufficiency led to his death 3 h after birth (HAWKINS 1991). The postmortem radiograph shows generalized osteopenia. The ribs are short, thick, and beaded. The vertebral bodies are flat, and the tubular bones are short, wide, and deformed simulating an accordion. Note the left inguinal hernia containing an air-filled loop of bowel

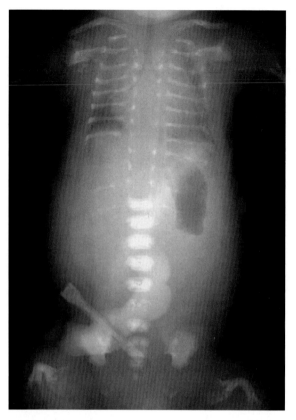

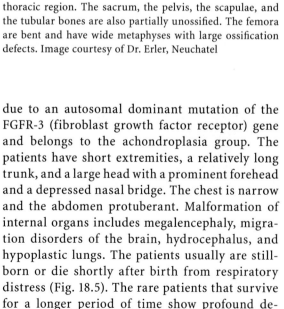

Fig. 18.4. Hypophosphatasia. This male infant was born at 35 gestational weeks. Polyhydramnios had been noted in utero. Postnatal asphyxia led to his immediate death. The postmortem radiograph shows osteopenia with deficient and irregular ossification of the skeleton. The ribs are short and thin. The vertebral bodies are unossified in the cervical and thoracic region. The sacrum, the pelvis, the scapulae, and the tubular bones are also partially unossified. The femora are bent and have wide metaphyses with large ossification defects. Image courtesy of Dr. Erler, Neuchatel

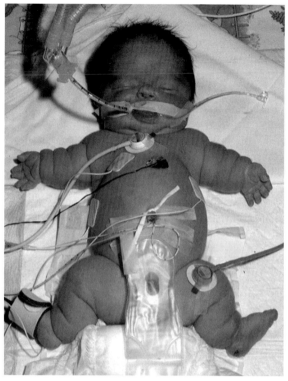

Fig. 18.5. Thanatophoric dysplasia. This infant boy was born in the 36th gestational week. Polyhydramnios, a large head, and short limbs had been shown by prenatal ultrasound. Caesarean section was performed. The boy presented with respiratory distress at birth. He was intubated and transferred to a neonatal clinic. Physical examination revealed short stature, very short limbs, a narrow chest, a relatively large head with a prominent forehead, and a depressed nasal bridge. The radiographic survey confirmed the diagnosis of thanatophoric dysplasia (not shown). The child was extubated after 12 h because of the dire prognosis and died immediately in the arms of his parents

due to an autosomal dominant mutation of the FGFR-3 (fibroblast growth factor receptor) gene and belongs to the achondroplasia group. The patients have short extremities, a relatively long trunk, and a large head with a prominent forehead and a depressed nasal bridge. The chest is narrow and the abdomen protuberant. Malformation of internal organs includes megalencephaly, migration disorders of the brain, hydrocephalus, and hypoplastic lungs. The patients usually are stillborn or die shortly after birth from respiratory distress (Fig. 18.5). The rare patients that survive for a longer period of time show profound developmental delay and growth failure (LACHMAN 2006; OMIM 2007).

The radiographic features of type I thanatophoric dysplasia consist of a narrow chest with short ribs. The vertebral bodies are flat and the interpediculate distance of the lumbar spine is narrow. The pedicles and vertebral bodies resemble an "H" or "U." The ilia are small and squared with horizontal, trident shaped acetabula, and small sacrosciatic notches. The tubular bones are short, broad, and bowed with flared metaphyses. The proximal portions of the femora are oval shaped and less dense than the shafts. The femora characteristically resemble a French telephone receiver (Fig. 18.2). Type II thanatophoric dysplasia is less common than type I. It usually is associated with a cloverleaf skull, milder skeletal changes than in type I, and milder or absent curvature of the long bones.

18.4
Osteogenesis Imperfecta (OMIM 166210)

Osteogenesis imperfecta (OI) is a disorder with a deficient synthesis of collagen type 1 mostly due to a mutation of the COL1A1 or COL1A2 gene. Autosomal dominant transmission is the rule. The spectrum of possible phenotypes is wide. OI II represents the severe end of the spectrum and belongs to the perinatally lethal osteochondrodysplasias. A further subdivision according to radiographic and prognostic features into types II A, B, and C was made, type II A bearing the worst prognosis. Patients with OI II are small, the skull is soft, the sclerae are blue, the extremities are short and bowed, and the chest is narrow. Hernias are frequent. The limbs or the head may become avulsed at birth (LACHMAN 2006; OMIM 2007).

Radiographs in OI show generalized osteopenia. The skull in OI II A is minimally ossified with multiple wormian bones, and the ribs are short, thick, and beaded. The vertebral bodies are flat, and the tubular bones are short, wide, and deformed simulating an accordion. Beading and deformity of the bones is due to countless fractures (Fig. 18.3). Type II B shows similar features to those in type II A, but usually no beading of the ribs. Type II C shows thin, fractured long bones and mildly beaded ribs. Postnatal conversion from thin to thick bones with beading can occur.

18.5
Hypophosphatasia (OMIM 241500)

Hypophosphatasia is a heritable metabolic bone disease characterized biochemically by deficient activity of the tissue-nonspecific isoenzyme of alkaline phosphatase due to a mutation in the alkaline phosphatase gene (ALPL). Hypophosphatasia results in impaired skeletal mineralization that clinically resembles rickets or osteomalacia. The spectrum of manifestation is wide. The perinatally lethal and infantile forms have an autosomal recessive trait. The length of survival is inversely related to the severity of the bone changes. At birth the patients appear short with short and deformed extremities and a soft skull. Affected newborns usually die of respiratory distress. Laboratory studies show a low serum alkaline phosphatase activity, normal calcium, and

elevated levels of phosphoethanolamine in the urine (SHOHAT et al. 1991; OMIM 2007).

Radiographs show osteopenia with deficient and irregular ossification of the skeleton. The ribs are short and thin. The calvaria, vertebrae, pelvis, and the tubular bones are partly unossified. The tubular bones have wide metaphyses with large ossification defects and may be bent (Fig. 18.4). Spur-like structures may be located symmetrically on the midshaft of the long bones and underlie skin dimples, or they may be located near the knee and elbow joints. If present, these spurs are thought to be pathognomonic for hypophosphatasia.

18.6
Short-Rib Dysplasia Group

The short rib dysplasia group is a heterogeneous group of skeletal dysplasias that are characterized by short ribs and short limbs. Polydactyly and visceral abnormalities are variable additional features. The short-rib dysplasia group comprises the following disorders: chondroectodermal dysplasia (CED, Ellis-van Creveld, OMIM 225500), short-rib-polydactyly syndrome (SRP) type 1/3 (Saldino-Noonan/Verma-Naumoff, OMIM 263510), SRP type 2 (Majewski, OMIM 263520), SRP type 4 (Beemer, OMIM 269860), oral-facial-digital syndrome type 4 (Mohr-Majewski, OMIM 258860), asphyxiating thoracic dysplasia (ATD, Jeune, OMIM 208500), and thoracolaryngopelvic dysplasia (TLPD, Barnes, OMIM 187760) (SUPERTI-FURGA et al. 2007). Autosomal recessive inheritance is recorded in all except for thoracolaryngopelvic dysplasia.

The nosology of the short-rib-polydactyly syndromes (SRP type 1–4) is still in debate, since no gene defect has yet been found. The common morphologic denominators of these disorders are variably short ribs and polydactyly; however, polydactyly is not present in all patients. Different numbering systems have been used in the past, and modifications will occur in the future. It is likely that at least part of the SRP group is caused by a single gene defect with variable expression. The perinatal lethality is related to the severity of chest constriction by the short ribs. The ribs are very short in the SRP syndromes that are invariably lethal at birth. The SRP syndromes exhibit changes in the size and shape of the tubular bones ("torpedo" and "banana peel" shape), the pelvis, and the spine (Fig. 18.6). Malformation of internal organs is frequently present, particularly pulmonary hypoplasia, congenital heart defects, malformation of the intestinal and urogenital tract, cleft lip and palate (Spranger and Maroteaux 1990; Lachman 2006; OMIM 2007).

Asphyxiating thoracic dysplasia (ATD) is usually recognized at birth in babies with a narrow chest that are in respiratory distress of variable degrees. Many patients are stillborn or die shortly after birth. Less severely affected patients survive infancy and may reach adulthood. Long-term survivors with ATD may suffer from chronic renal insufficiency related to tubulo-interstitial nephritis. Cystic changes can occur in the kidneys, liver, and pancreas. Polydactyly may be present. The limbs are short. Infants show the following variable radiographic features: short and horizontally oriented ribs, small iliac bones with horizontal and trident-shaped acetabula and small sacrosciatic notches, short limbs with mild or absent metaphyseal spurs (Fig. 18.7). The pelvic and thoracic changes regress with advancing age, but brachydactyly with cone-shaped epiphyses becomes evident in the majority of cases (Lachman 2006; OMIM 2007).

Chondroectodermal dysplasia is caused by a mutation of the EVC gene. It shares many radiographic features with asphyxiating thoracic dysplasia (Fig. 18.8). However, postaxial polydactyly is a constant feature, as is mesomelic shortening of the limbs (lower legs and forearms). Ectodermal abnormalities such as dystrophic teeth and nails, and multiple frenula are invariably present. Many patients with CED suffer from congenital heart disease, particularly atrial and ventricular septal defects. The narrow chest can lead to neonatal respiratory distress and may contribute to early death. Ossification of epiphyses, particularly of the proximal femur, may be apparent at birth in patients with CED as with ATD. CED typically is associated with accessory carpals, fusion of carpal bones, and cone-shaped phalangeal epiphyses with resultant brachydactyly. Valgus deformity of the knees and an exostosis at the medial aspect of the proximal tibial metaphysis is also characteristic for CED (Lachman 2006; OMIM 2007).

Thoracolaryngopelvic dysplasia (TLPD) is another disorder with a narrow chest, and appears similar to ATD on radiographs. TLPD, however, does not exhibit the typical iliac and acetabular features of ATD, or cone-shaped epiphyses, and is inherited with an autosomal dominant trait. Laryngeal stenosis in association with short ribs may contribute to

respiratory failure (Bankier and Danks 1983; Burn et al. 1986; OMIM 2007).

18.7
Metaphyseal Dysplasia with Pancreatic Insufficiency and Cyclic Neutropenia (Shwachman-Bodian-Diamond, OMIM 260400)

The Shwachman-Bodian-Diamond Syndrome is caused by a mutation in the SBDS gene. The salient clinical features of this syndrome with an autosomal recessive trait are failure to thrive due to exocrine

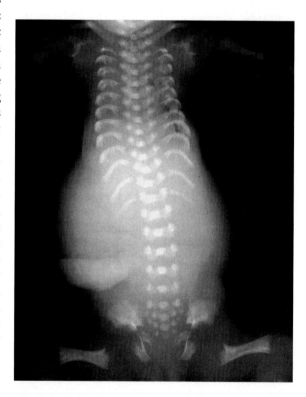

Fig. 18.6. Short-rib-polydactyly syndrome type 3 (Verma-Naumoff). This girl was born with 30 gestational weeks. Polyhydramnios was present. Macrocephaly, a cleft lip and palate, and postaxial hexadactyly were noted at birth. She suffered from perinatal asphyxia. Resuscitation was not performed. Death occurred during the first day of life. The postmortem radiograph shows very short ribs. The iliac bones are small with horizontal acetabula and small sacrosciatic notches. The tubular bones are short with spurs extending longitudinally at the metaphyses of the femora and humeri ("banana peel" appearance). Note the early ossification of the proximal epiphyses of the humeri. The spine is normal. Autopsy revealed hypoplastic lungs and duplication of the vagina and uterus. Image courtesy of Dr. Duckert, Reutlingen

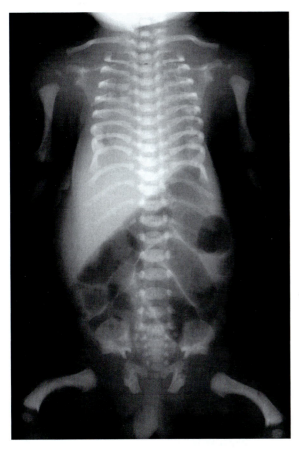 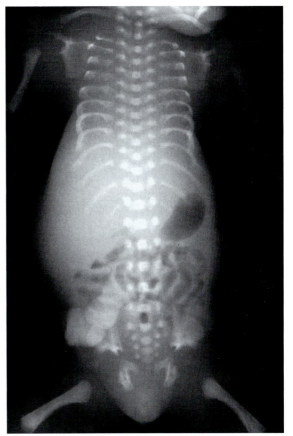

Fig. 18.7. Asphyxiating thoracic dysplasia (Jeune). This boy died of postnatal asphyxia on the first day of life. On inspection the chest was narrow, the extremities were short, the skin was normal, and polydactyly was absent. The postmortem radiograph shows a narrow chest with short ribs. The spine is normal. The ilia are small and squared with horizontal, trident-shaped acetabula and small sacrosciatic notches. Early ossification of the proximal epiphyses of the humeri and bent femora with small metaphyseal spurs are noted

Fig. 18.8. Chondroectodermal dysplasia (Ellis-van Creveld). The boy was born at 28 gestational weeks. Death occurred after 1 h. Clinical examination showed a narrow chest, short extremities, small nails, and polydactyly (pre- and postaxial). The postmortem radiograph shows short ribs, small ilia with horizontal acetabula and small sacrosciatic notches. The tubular bones are short with spurs extending longitudinally at the metaphyses of the distal femora. The metaphyses otherwise are smooth. The spine is normal. Autopsy revealed small lungs and bicuspid aortic valves. Image courtesy of Dr. Eklöf, Stockholm

pancreatic insufficiency with intestinal malabsorption, cyclic neutropenia with frequent infections, and a body height at or below the third centile. The patients may present at birth with respiratory distress. Varus deformity of the hips and mild psychomotor delay are frequent additional features (Lachman 2006; OMIM 2007).

The radiographic features at birth may include moderately short ribs with wide anterior ends (Fig. 18.9). Irregular ossification of the metaphyses usually becomes apparent by 3–4 years. Typically the proximal femoral metaphyses are most severely affected. Coxa vara and slipping of the capital femoral epiphysis may complicate the metaphyseal dysplasia.

18.8
Achondrogenesis II and Hypochondrogenesis (OMIM 200610)

Achondrogenesis II and hypochondrogenesis are part of the type II collagenopathies. These form a group of disorders with variable clinical and radiological presentation, but with a common biochemical defect of the collagen type II due to a mutation of the COL2A1 gene. Collagen type II is a glycoprotein that is a major constituent of cartilage and of the vitreous body. This may explain the association of growth failure and ocular abnormalities within this

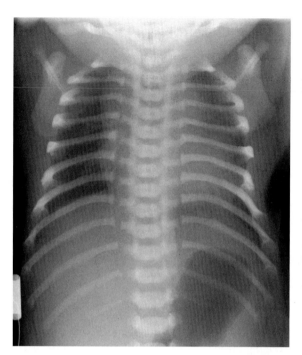

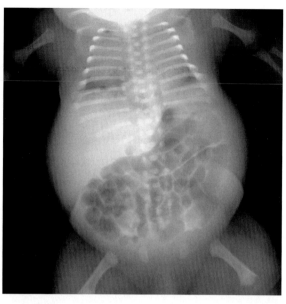

Fig. 18.9. Metaphyseal chondrodysplasia with exocrine pancreatic insufficiency and cyclic neutropenia (Shwachman-Diamond). Chest radiograph of a 3-day-old boy who presented with respiratory distress at birth. The ribs are moderately short and their anterior ends are widened. The spine is normal. Metaphyseal dysplasia became apparent at 3 years

Fig. 18.10. Hypochondrogenesis. Soon after birth at term with polyhydramnios this girl died of asphyxia. The patient was short with short extremities, a narrow chest, and a large head. The postmortem radiograph shows short and horizontal ribs (11 pairs). The vertebral bodies are small and are unossified in the lower sacral and the cervical area. The ilia are small with horizontal acetabula. The pubic bones are not ossified. The tubular bones are short with wide metaphyses. Metaphyseal spurs are present in the distal femora. Autopsy confirmed hypoplastic lungs

group. The trait is autosomal dominant. The type II collagenopathies exhibit a clinical and radiographic spectrum, the severe end of which is represented by achondrogenesis II and hypochondrogenesis that belong to the lethal osteochondrodysplasias. Kniest dysplasia and spondyloepiphyseal dysplasia congenita become apparent at birth and may also cause respiratory distress. Other disorders usually become manifest later in life. Achondrogenesis II and hypochondrogenesis are characterized by short limbs and a short trunk. The head is relatively large, the face is flat, and cleft palate is usually present (LACHMAN 2006; OMIM 2007).

The radiographic features of achondrogenesis II and hypochondrogenesis consist of absent or partial ossification of small vertebral bodies. The ribs are short and horizontally oriented. The ilia are small with horizontal acetabula. The pubic bones are not ossified. The tubular bones are moderately or severely short with wide metaphyses. Metaphyseal spurs may be present (Fig. 18.10).

18.9
Cerebro-Costo-Mandibular Syndrome (OMIM 117650)

Cerebro-costo-mandibular syndrome is a mostly sporadic disorder that is characterized by chondro-osseous defects in the posterior portion of the ribs and in extreme cases almost complete absence of rib ossification. Respiratory distress and micrognathia are also constant features. Cleft palate and glossoptosis in addition to the flail chest contribute to neonatal respiratory distress. Mental delay probably is a frequent consequence of neonatal respiratory distress with asphyxia. Spinal dysraphism may be an associated feature. Prenatal ultrasound can show micrognathia and absent or short ribs (SMITH et al. 1966; OMIM 2007).

Radiographs show mandibular hypoplasia and bilateral gaps of the posterior portion of the ribs (Fig. 18.11). Ribs 3–7 are the most commonly involved. The gaps may later become ossified in survivors.

18.10
Dyssegmental Dysplasia

Dyssegmental dysplasia is a lethal skeletal dysplasia with short limbs and trunk and a narrow chest. The disorder is inherited with an autosomal recessive trait. Cleft palate, occipital encephalocele, cardiac and urogenital malformations are recorded. There are different forms of dyssegmental dwarfism: a lethal Silverman-Handmaker type (OMIM 224410), which is caused by mutation in the perlecan gene HSPG2, and a less severe Rolland-Desbuquois type (OMIM 224400) in which survival beyond the newborn period is frequent. Perlecan is a large heparan sulfate proteoglycan that is present in all basement membranes and in other tissues such as cartilage, and is implicated in cell growth and differentiation (Fasanelli et al. 1985; OMIM 2007).

The radiographic hallmark of dyssegmental dysplasia is differences in the size and shape of the vertebral bodies (anisospondyly) that may be recognized on prenatal ultrasound examination. The ribs are short. The iliac wings are flared and the iliac bodies and sacrosciatic notches are small. The pubic and ischial bones are broad. The tubular bones are short and bowed with wide metaphyses (Fig. 18.12).

18.11
Spondylocostal Dysostosis (OMIM 277300)

Spondylocostal dysostosis belongs to a heterogeneous group of dysostoses with predominant vertebral and costal involvement. These disorders exhibit short stature with a short trunk, a nonprogressive kyphoscoliosis, segmentation defects of the spine, and rib fusions. Both autosomal dominant and autosomal recessive inheritance have been reported. Clinical examination shows a short thorax and neck with

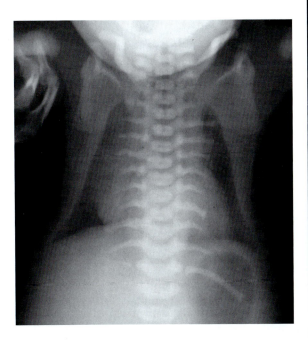

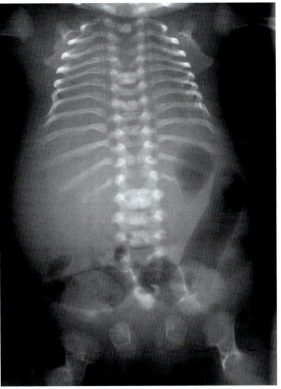

Fig. 18.11. Cerebro-costo-mandibular syndrome. The full-term male neonate required intubation for asphyxia. Death occurred after 8 h because of increasing respiratory failure. The radiograph shows a narrow chest with deficient ossification of all ribs. Ossification of the ribs is present only adjacent to the spine. Histologic examination showed gaps between the posterior, ossified portions and the anterior cartilaginous but unossified portions (Smith 1966)

Fig. 18.12. Dyssegmental dysplasia (Silverman type). Postmortem radiograph of a boy born in the 37th gestational week that had died 8 days after birth of asphyxia. The ribs are short. The ossification of the vertebral bodies is irregular and unequal with absent ossification in some (anisospondyly). The iliac wings are flared and the iliac bodies and sacrosciatic notches are small. The pubic and ischial bones are broad. The femora are short and bowed with wide metaphyses. Image courtesy of Dr. Gassner, Innsbruck

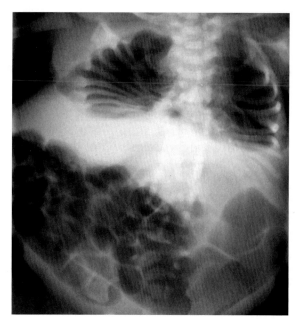

Fig. 18.13. Spondylocostal dysplasia (Jarcho-Levin type). The infant girl presented with respiratory distress at birth that required intubation. Death occurred after 44 min. The postmortem radiograph shows bilateral pneumothorax, pneumomediastinum, and distension of the abdomen. Numerous segmentation defects of the spine and ribs are present. The lower ribs are fused posteriorly and are arranged in a fan-like (crab-like) fashion. Autopsy revealed bilateral lung hypoplasia, a unilobar left lung and partial fusion of the lobes of the right lung. Additional features consisted of anal atresia with recto-vaginal fistula, cystic dysplasia of the left kidney with atresia of the ureter, and mild right hydroureteronephrosis. Image courtesy of Dr. Brühwiler, Münsterlingen

limited mobility, winged scapulae, and scoliosis or kyphoscoliosis. Affected individuals may die in infancy of respiratory failure or survive into adulthood with minimal symptoms. Associated anomalies are not common (MORTIER et al. 1996; OMIM 2007).

Radiographs show vertebral anomalies, including hemivertebrae, wedge-shaped vertebrae, butterfly vertebrae, and vertebral fusions affecting segments or the entire spine. The ribs may be partially fused and show variable thickness, size, and number. The most severe, lethal, autosomal recessive Jarcho-Levin type spondylocostal dysostosis exhibits a typical "crab-like" appearance of the thoracic skeleton (Fig. 18.13).

References

Bankier A, Danks DM (1983) Thoracic-pelvic dysostosis: a "new" autosomal dominant form. J Med Genet 20(4):276–279

Burn J, Hall C, Marsden D, Matthew DJ (1986) Autosomal dominant thoracolaryngopelvic dysplasia: Barnes syndrome. J Med Genet 23(4):345–349

Fasanelli S, Kozlowski K, Reiter S, Sillence D (1985) Dyssegmental dysplasia (report of two cases with a review of the literature). Skeletal Radiol 14(3):173–177

Greenough A (1996) Pulmonary hypoplasia. In: Greenough A, Milner AD, Roberton NRC (eds) Neonatal respiratory disorders. Arnold, London, pp 436–447

Hawkins JR, Superti-Furga A, Steinmann B, Dalgleish R (1991) A 9-base pair deletion in COL1A1 in a lethal variant of osteogenesis imperfecta. J Biol Chem 266(33):22370–22374

Lachman RS (2006) Taybi and Lachman's radiology of syndromes, metabolic disorders and skeletal dysplasias, 5th edn. Mosby, St. Louis, Mo.

Mortier GR, Lachman RS, Bocian M, Rimoin DL (1996) Multiple vertebral segmentation defects: analysis of 26 new patients and review of the literature. Am J Med Genet 61(4):310–319

Online Mendelian Inheritance in Man, OMIM (TM) McKusick-Nathans Institute for Genetic Medicine, Johns Hopkins University (Baltimore, MD) and National Center for Biotechnology Information, National Library of Medicine (Bethesda, MD), Available at http://www.ncbi.nlm.nih.gov/omim/ [accessed 25 January 2007]

Orioli IM, Castilla EE, Barbosa-Neto JG (1986) The birth prevalence rates for the skeletal dysplasias. J Med Genet 23(4):328–432

Sharony R, Browne C, Lachman RS, Rimoin DL (1993) Prenatal diagnosis of the skeletal dysplasias. Am J Obstet Gynecol 169(3):668–675

Shohat M, Rimoin DL, Gruber HE, Lachman RS (1991) Perinatal lethal hypophosphatasia; clinical, radiologic and morphologic findings. Pediatric Radiol 21(6):421–427

Smith DW, Theiler K, Schachenmann G (1966) Rib-gap defect with micrognathia, malformed tracheal cartilages, and redundant skin: a new pattern of defective development. J Pediatr 69(5):799–803

Spranger J, Maroteaux P (1990) The lethal osteochondrodysplasias. Adv Human Genet 19:1–103

Superti-Furga A, Unger S, and the Nosology Group of the International Skeletal Dysplasia Society (2007) Nosology and classification of genetic skeletal disorders: 2006 revision. Am J Med Genet A 143A:1–18

Thomas IT, Smith DW (1974) Oligohydramnios, cause of the nonrenal features of Potter's syndrome, including pulmonary hypoplasia. J Pediatr 84(6):811–815

Wigglesworth JS, Desai R (1982) Is fetal respiratory function a major determinant of perinatal survival? Lancet 1(8266):264–267

Subject Index

List of Contributors

PER G. BJØRNSTAD, MD, PhD
Section of Paediatric Cardiology
Department of Paediatrics
Rikshospitalet Radiumhospitalet HF
The National Hospital
Sognsvannsvn 20
0373 Oslo
Norway

ALISTAIR CALDER, FRCR
Department of Radiology
Great Ormond Street
Hospital for Sick Children
NHS Trust
London WCIN 3JH
UK

VERONICA DONOGHUE, MD
Consultant Paediatric Radiologist
Departments of Radiology
Children's University Hospital
Temple Street
Dublin 1
Ireland
and
The National Maternity Hospital
Holles Street
Dublin 2
Ireland

GEORG F. EICH, MD
Division of Pediatric Radiology
Kantonsspital
5001 Aarau
Switzerland

BEN EIDEM, MD, FAAC
Department of Paediatric Cardiology
Mayo Clinic
Rochester, Minnesota
USA

LAURENT GAREL, MD
Clinical Professor of Radiology
University of Montreal
Hopital Sainte-Justine
3175 Cote Sainte-Catherine
Montreal, Quebec H3T 1C5
Canada

INGMAR GASSNER, MD
Department of Paediatrics
University Hospital Innsbruck
Anichstr. 35
6020 Innsbruck
Austria

THERESA E. GELEY, MD
Department of Paediatrics
University Hospital Innsbruck
Anichstr. 35
6020 Innsbruck
Austria

HYUN WOO GOO, MD
Department of Radiology
Asan Medical Centre
University of Ulsan College of Medicine
388–1 Songpa-gu Poongnap-2dong
Seoul
Korea

CHRISTIAN J. KELLENBERGER, MD
Department of Diagnostic Imaging
University Children's Hospital
Steinwiesstrasse 75
8032 Zurich
Switzerland

DAVID MANSON, MD, FRCP
Department of Diagnostic Imaging
Hospital for Sick Children
and
Assistant Professor and Division Head
Pediatric Radiology
Department of Medical Imaging
University of Toronto
555 University Avenue
Toronto, Ontario, M5G IX8
Canada

COLIN MCMAHON, FRCPI, FAAP
Department of Paediatric Cardiology
Our Lady's Hospital for Sick Children
Crumlin
Dublin 12
Ireland

Amaka C. Offiah, BsC, MBBS, MRCP, FRCR, PhD
Consultant, Academic Paediatric Radiology
Great Ormond Street Hospital
for Children
Great Ormond Street
London WC1N 3JH
UK

Catherine M. Owens, FRCR
Department of Radiology
Great Ormond Street Hospital
for Children
NHS Trust
London WC1N 3JH
UK

Stephanie Ryan, MD
Department of Radiology
Children's University Hospital
Temple St.
Dublin 1
Ireland
and
The Rotunda Hospital
Parnell Square
Dublin 1
Ireland

Laureen Sena, MD
Department of Radiology
Children's Hospital, Boston
300 Longwood Avenue
Boston, MA 02115
USA

Bjarne Smevik, MD
Section of Paediatric Cardiology
Department of Radiology
Rikshospitalet Radiumhospitalet HF
The National Hospital
Sognsvannsvn 20
0373 Oslo
Norway

Anne Twomey, MD
Consultant Neonatologist
The National Maternity Hospital
Holles Street
Dublin 2
Ireland
and
Children's University Hospital
Temple St.
Dublin 1
Ireland

MEDICAL RADIOLOGY Diagnostic Imaging and Radiation Oncology

Titles in the series already published

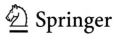

MEDICAL RADIOLOGY Diagnostic Imaging and Radiation Oncology

Titles in the series already published

RADIATION ONCOLOGY

Lung Cancer
Edited by C.W. Scarantino

Innovations in Radiation Oncology
Edited by H. R. Withers
and L. J. Peters

**Radiation Therapy
of Head and Neck Cancer**
Edited by G. E. Laramore

**Gastrointestinal Cancer –
Radiation Therapy**
Edited by R.R. Dobelbower, Jr.

**Radiation Exposure
and Occupational Risks**
Edited by E. Scherer, C. Streffer,
and K.-R. Trott

Radiation Therapy of Benign Diseases
A Clinical Guide
S. E. Order and S. S. Donaldson

**Interventional Radiation
Therapy Techniques – Brachytherapy**
Edited by R. Sauer

Radiopathology of Organs and Tissues
Edited by E. Scherer, C. Streffer,
and K.-R. Trott

**Concomitant Continuous Infusion
Chemotherapy and Radiation**
Edited by M. Rotman
and C. J. Rosenthal

**Intraoperative Radiotherapy –
Clinical Experiences and Results**
Edited by F. A. Calvo, M. Santos,
and L.W. Brady

**Radiotherapy of Intraocular
and Orbital Tumors**
Edited by W. E. Alberti and
R. H. Sagerman

**Interstitial and Intracavitary
Thermoradiotherapy**
Edited by M. H. Seegenschmiedt
and R. Sauer

Non-Disseminated Breast Cancer
Controversial Issues in Management
Edited by G. H. Fletcher and S.H. Levitt

**Current Topics in
Clinical Radiobiology of Tumors**
Edited by H.-P. Beck-Bornholdt

**Practical Approaches to
Cancer Invasion and Metastases**
**A Compendium of Radiation
Oncologists' Responses to 40 Histories**
Edited by A. R. Kagan with the
Assistance of R. J. Steckel

Radiation Therapy in Pediatric Oncology
Edited by J. R. Cassady

Radiation Therapy Physics
Edited by A. R. Smith

Late Sequelae in Oncology
Edited by J. Dunst and R. Sauer

Mediastinal Tumors. Update 1995
Edited by D. E. Wood and C. R. Thomas, Jr.

**Thermoradiotherapy
and Thermochemotherapy**
Volume 1:
Biology, Physiology, and Physics
Volume 2:
Clinical Applications
Edited by M.H. Seegenschmiedt,
P. Fessenden, and C.C. Vernon

Carcinoma of the Prostate
Innovations in Management
Edited by Z. Petrovich, L. Baert,
and L.W. Brady

**Radiation Oncology
of Gynecological Cancers**
Edited by H.W. Vahrson

Carcinoma of the Bladder
Innovations in Management
Edited by Z. Petrovich, L. Baert,
and L.W. Brady

**Blood Perfusion and
Microenvironment of Human Tumors**
Implications for Clinical Radiooncology
Edited by M. Molls and P. Vaupel

Radiation Therapy of Benign Diseases
A Clinical Guide
2nd Revised Edition
S. E. Order and S. S. Donaldson

**Carcinoma of the Kidney and Testis,
and Rare Urologic Malignancies**
Innovations in Management
Edited by Z. Petrovich, L. Baert,
and L.W. Brady

**Progress and Perspectives in the
Treatment of Lung Cancer**
Edited by P. Van Houtte,
J. Klastersky, and P. Rocmans

**Combined Modality Therapy of
Central Nervous System Tumors**
Edited by Z. Petrovich, L. W. Brady,
M. L. Apuzzo, and M. Bamberg

Age-Related Macular Degeneration
Current Treatment Concepts
Edited by W. A. Alberti, G. Richard,
and R. H. Sagerman

**Radiotherapy of Intraocular
and Orbital Tumors**
2nd Revised Edition
Edited by R. H. Sagerman,
and W. E. Alberti

Modification of Radiation Response
**Cytokines, Growth Factors,
and Other Biolgical Targets**
Edited by C. Nieder, L. Milas,
and K. K. Ang

Radiation Oncology for Cure and Palliation
R. G. Parker, N. A. Janjan,
and M. T. Selch

**Clinical Target Volumes in Conformal and
Intensity Modulated Radiation Therapy**
A Clinical Guide to Cancer Treatment
Edited by V. Grégoire, P. Scalliet,
and K. K. Ang

**Advances in Radiation Oncology
in Lung Cancer**
Edited by Branislav Jeremić

New Technologies in Radiation Oncology
Edited by W. Schlegel, T. Bortfeld,
and A.-L. Grosu

Technical Basis of Radiation Therapy
4th Revised Edition
Edited by S. H. Levitt, J. A. Purdy,
C. A. Perez, and S. Vijayakumar

**Late Effects of Cancer Treatment
on Normal Tissues**
Edited by P. Rubin, L. S. Constine,
L. B. Marks, and P. Okunieff

**Clinical Practice of Radiation Therapy for
Benign Diseases**
**Contemporary Concepts and Clical
Results**
Edited by M. H. Seegenschmiedt,
H.-B. Makoski, K.-R. Trott, and
L. W. Brady

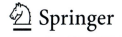